PROGRESS IN
VASCULAR SURGERY

Edited by

James S. T. Yao, MD, PhD
Magerstadt Professor of Surgery
Division of Vascular Surgery
Department of Surgery
Northwestern University Medical School
Chief, Division of Vascular Surgery
Northwestern Memorial Hospital
Chicago, Illinois

William H. Pearce, MD
Professor of Surgery
Division of Vascular Surgery
Department of Surgery
Northwestern University Medical School
Chicago, Illinois

APPLETON & LANGE
Stamford, Connecticut

Copyright © 1997 by Appleton & Lange
A Simon & Schuster Company

97 98 99 00 01   /   10 9 8 7 6 5 4 3 2 1

Prentice Hall International (UK) Limited, *London*
Prentice Hall of Australia Pty. Limited, *Sydney*
Prentice Hall Canada, Inc., *Toronto*
Prentice Hall Hispanoamericana, S.A., *Mexico*
Prentice Hall of India Private Limited, *New Delhi*
Prentice Hall of Japan, Inc., *Tokyo*
Simon & Schuster Asia Pte. Ltd., *Singapore*
Editora Prentice Hall do Brasil Ltda., *Rio de Janeiro*
Prentice Hall, *Upper Saddle River, New Jersey*

Library of Congress Cataloging-in-Publication Data

Progress in vascular surgery / edited by James S. T.
  Yao, William M. Pearce.
      p.   cm.
    Includes index.
    ISBN 0-8385-9387-9 (case : alk. paper)
    1. Blood-vessels—Surgery.   I. Yao, James S. T.   II. Pearce,
  William H.
    [DNLM: 1. Vascular Surgery.   WG 170 V331724 1997]
  RD598.5.V394   1997
  617.4'13—dc20
  DNLM/DLC
  for Library of Congress   96-36611
                                                                      CIP

ISBN 0-8385-9387-9
Acquisitions Editor: Michael Medina
Production: Spectrum Publisher Services
Designer: Janice Barsevich Bielawa

PRINTED IN THE UNITED STATES OF AMERICA

ISBN 0-8385-9387-9

90000

9 780838 593875

Contents

Contributors

William H. Baker, MD
Professor
Stritch School of Medicine
Loyola University Chicago
Chief, Department of Surgery
Division of Peripheral Vascular Surgery
Loyola University Medical Center
Maywood, Illinois

Aires A. B. Barros D'Sa, MD, FRCS, FRCSEd
Honorary Lecturer in Surgery
The Queen's University in Belfast
Consultant Vascular Surgeon, Vascular
  Surgery Unit
Royal Victoria Hospital
Belfast, United Kingdom

Jerome F. Breen, MD
Assistant Professor of Radiology
Mayo Medical School
Consultant, Division of Vascular Surgery
Mayo Clinic and Foundation
Rochester, Minnesota

Allen P. Burke, MD
Adjunct Professor
Georgetown University
Associate Chair, Division of
  Cardiovascular Pathology
Armed Forces Institute of Pathology
Washington, DC

Linda Canton, RN, BSN
Physician Extender, Division of Vascular
  Surgery
Mayo Clinic and Foundation
Rochester, Minnesota

Benjamin B. Chang, MD
Assistant Professor of Surgery
Albany Medical College
Albany Medical Center Hospital
Albany, New York

Kenneth J. Cherry, Jr., MD
Professor of Surgery
Mayo Medical School
Consultant and Chair, Division of
  Vascular Surgery
Mayo Clinic and Foundation
Rochester, Minnesota

Alexander W. Clowes, MD
Professor and Chief, Division of
  Vascular Surgery
University of Washington School of
  Medicine
Seattle, Washington

Douglas A. Coe, MD
Fellow, Vascular Surgery
Medical College of Wisconsin
Milwaukee, Wisconsin

Anthony J. Comerota, MD, FACS
Professor of Surgery
Temple University Hospital School of
  Medicine
Chief, Section of Vascular Surgery
Director, Center for Vascular Diseases
Temple University Hospital
Philadelphia, Pennsylvania

Jack L. Cronenwett, MD
Professor of Surgery
Dartmouth Medical School
Chief, Section of Vascular Surgery
Dartmouth-Hitchcock Medical Center
Lebanon, New Hampshire

Michael D. Dake, MD
Assistant Professor
Department of Radiology
Stanford University School of Medicine
Chief, Interventional Radiology
Stanford University Medical Center
Stanford, California

R. Clement Darling III, MD
Assistant Professor of Surgery
Albany Medical College
Albany Medical Center Hospital
Albany, New York

Richard H. Dean, MD
Professor and Chairman of General
  Surgery
Bowman Gray School of Medicine
Chief of Surgery
North Carolina Baptist Hospital
Winston-Salem, North Carolina

Quentin Desiron, MD
Staff Surgeon
Petié-Salpêtrière University Hospital
Paris, France

Bo Eklof, MD, PhD
Clinical Professor of Surgery
John A. Burns School of Medicine
University of Hawaii
Vascular Surgeon
Straub Clinic and Hospital
Honolulu, Hawaii

James I. Fann, MD
Clinical Assistant Professor
Department of Cardiothoracic Surgery
Stanford University School of Medicine
Staff Physician
Palo Alto Veterans Affairs Medical
  Center
Stanford, California

Andrew Farb, MD
Assistant Professor
Georgetown University
Chief, Division of Cardiovascular
  Pathology
Armed Forces Institute of Pathology
Washington, DC

Joseph Feinglass, PhD
Research Associate Professor
Division of General Internal Medicine
Northwestern University Medical School
  and Institute for Health Services
  Research and Policy Studies
Northwestern University
Chicago, Illinois

Cindy L. Felty, MSN, RN, C-ANP
Adult Nurse Practicioner
Director, Vascular Ulcer/Wound
  Healing Center
Mayo Clinic and Foundation
Rochester, Minnesota

Peter Gloviczki, MD
Professor of Surgery
Mayo Medical School
Vice-Chair, Division of Vascular Surgery
Mayo Clinic and Foundation
Rochester, Minnesota

Jerry Goldstone, MD
Professor of Surgery
Division of Vascular Surgery
University of California, San Francisco
San Francisco, California

David Green, MD, PhD
Artherosclerosis Program
Department of Medicine
Rehabilitation Institute of Chicago and
  Northwestern University Medical
  School
Chicago, Illinois

Richard M. Green, MD
Professor of Surgery
University of Rochester School of
  Medicine
Attending Surgeon
Strong Memorial Hospital
Rochester, New York

Kimberley J. Hansen, MD
Associate Professor of Surgery
Bowman Gray School of Medicine
North Carolina Baptist Hospital
Winston-Salem, North Carolina

John P. Harris, MS, FRACS, FACS
Associate Professor of Surgery
University of Sydney
Head, Division of Surgery
Head, Department of Vascular Surgery
Royal Prince Albert Hospital
Sydney, Australia

Ulf Hedin, MD, PhD
Associate Professor
Department of Surgery
University of Washington School of
  Medicine
Seattle, Washington
  and
Karolinski Institute
Stockholm, Sweden

William R. Hiatt, MD
Professor of Medicine
Section of Vascular Medicine
University of Colorado School of
  Medicine
University of Colorado Health Sciences
  Center
Denver, Colorado

K. Wayne Johnston, MD, FRCS(C)
Professor of Surgery and Biomedical
  Engineering
University of Toronto
Head, Division of Vascular Surgery
The Toronto Hospital
Toronto, Ontario, Canada

Edouard Kieffer, MD
Professor of Surgery
Petié-Salpêtrière University Medical
  School
Chief, Department of Vascular Surgery
Petié-Salpêtrière University Hospital
Paris, France

Robert L. Kistner, MD
Clinical Professor of Surgery
John A. Burns School of Medicine
University of Hawaii
Vascular Surgeon
Straub Clinic and Hospital
Honolulu, Hawaii

Dainis K. Krievins, MD
Department of Surgery
Stanford University School of Medicine
Stanford, California

Robert P. Leather, MD
Professor of Surgery
Head of Vascular Surgery
Albany Medical College
Albany Medical Center Hospital
Albany, New York

Thomas F. Lindsay, MD, FRCS(C)
Assistant Professor
University of Toronto
Vascular Surgeon, General Division
The Toronto Hospital
Toronto, Ontario, Canada

M. Ashraf Mansour, MD
Assistant Professor
Stritch School of Medicine
Loyola University Chicago
Division of Peripheral Vascular Surgery
Loyola University Medical Center
Maywood, Illinois

Michael L. Marin, MD
Associate Professor of Surgery
Albert Einstein College of Medicine
Attending in Surgery
Montefiore Medical Center
New York, New York

Elna M. Masuda, MD
Vascular Surgeon
Straub Clinic and Hospital
Honolulu, Hawaii

Jon S. Matsumura, MD
Assistant Professor of Surgery
Northwestern University Medical School
Attending Surgeon
Northwestern Memorial Hospital
Chicago, Illinois

James May, MS, FRACS, FACS
Bosch Professor of Surgery
University of Sydney
Vascular Surgeon
Royal Prince Albert Hospital
Sydney, Australia

Walter J. McCarthy, MD
Associate Professor
Northwestern University Medical School
Attending Surgeon
Northwestern Memorial Hospital
Chicago, Illinois

David D. McPherson, MD
Associate Professor—Medicine and
  Cardiology
Northwestern University Medical School
Director, Research Cardiology and
  Image Processing Laboratory
Co-Director, Echocardiography
Northwestern Memorial Hospital
Chicago, Illinois

Mark H. Meissner, MD
Assistant Professor of Surgery
Division of Vascular Surgery
University of Washington, School of
  Medicine
Harborview Medical Center
Seattle, Washington

Sunil S. Menawat, MD
Fellow in Vascular Surgery
Mayo Medical School
Mayo Clinic and Foundation
Rochester, Minnesota

D. Craig Miller, MD
Professor
Department of Cardiothoracic Surgery
Stanford University School of Medicine
Stanford University Medical Center
Stanford, California

R. Scott Mitchell, MD
Associate Professor
Department of Cardiothoracic Surgery
Stanford University School of Medicine
Stanford University Medical Center
Stanford, California

Wesley S. Moore, MD
Professor of Surgery
UCLA School of Medicine
Chief, Section of Vascular Surgery
UCLA Center for Health Sciences
Los Angeles, California

Geza Mozes, MD
Fellow in Vascular Surgery
Mayo Medical School
Mayo Clinic and Foundation
Rochester, Minnesota

Albert A. Nemcek, Jr., MD
Associate Professor of Radiology
Northwestern University Medical
  School
Chief, Section of Ultrasonography
Associate, Section of Vascular and
  Interventional Radiology
Northwestern Memorial Hospital
Chicago, Illinois

Takao Ohki, MD
Visiting Clinical Fellow in Vascular
  Surgery
Albert Einstein College of Medicine
Montefiore Medical Center
New York, New York

Kenneth Ouriel, MD
Associate Professor of Surgery
University of Rochester
Attending Surgeon
Strong Memorial Hospital
Rochester, New York

Juan C. Parodi, MD
Chief, Vascular Surgery
Department of Vascular Surgery
Instituto Cardiovascular de Buenos Aires
Buenos Aires, Argentina

Philip S. K. Paty, MD
Associate Professor of Surgery
Albany Medical College
Albany Medical Center Hospital
Albany, New York

William H. Pearce, MD
Professor of Surgery
Division of Vascular Surgery
Department of Surgery
Northwestern University Medical School
Attending Surgeon
Northwestern Memorial Hospital
Chicago, Illinois

Giancarlo Piano, MD
Department of Vascular Surgery
University of Chicago
Chicago, Illinois

John J. Ricotta, MD
Professor of Surgery and Chief of
 Surgery
State University of New York at Buffalo
Chief of Surgery
Millard Filmore Health Systems
Buffalo, New York

Robert D. Riley, MD
Bradshaw Fellow in Surgery
Bowman Gray School of Medicine
North Carolina Baptist Hospital
Winston-Salem, North Carolina

William S. Rilling, MD
Instructor of Radiology
Northwestern University Medical School
Fellow, Vascular and Interventional
 Radiology
Northwestern University Medical School
Chicago, Illinois

Thom W. Rooke, MD
Associate Professor of Surgery
Mayo Medical School
Director, Gonda Vascular Center
Mayo Clinic and Foundation
Rochester, Minnesota

David Rosenthal, MD
Clinical Professor of Surgery
Medical College of Georgia
Chief of Vascular Surgery
Georgia Baptist Medical Center
Atlanta, Georgia

Geoffrey D. Rubin, MD
Department of Surgery
Stanford University School of Medicine
Stanford, California

Darren B. Schneider, MD
Division of Vascular Surgery
University of California, San Francisco
San Francisco, California

Claudio J. Schonholz, MD
Department of Interventional Radiology
Clinica La Sagrada Familia
Buenos Aires, Argentina

Dhiraj M. Shah, MD
Professor of Surgery
Albany Medical College
Chief, Division of General Surgery
Albany Medical Center Hospital
Albany, New York

Philip D. Coleridge Smith, DM, FRCS
Senior Lecturer
Department of Surgery
UCL Medical School
The Middlesex Hospital
London, United Kingdom

James C. Stanley, MD
Professor of Surgery
University of Michigan Medical School
Head, Section of Vascular Surgery
University Hospital
Ann Arbor, Michigan

Anthony W. Stanson, MD
Associate Professor of Surgery
Mayo Medical School
Consultant, Department of Diagnostic
  Radiology
Mayo Clinic and Foundation
Rochester, Minnesota

Michael S. Stephen, FRACS
Clinical Senior Lecturer
University of Sydney
Vascular Surgeon
Royal Prince Albert Hospital
Sydney, Australia

Ronald J. Stoney, MD
Professor of Surgery
Department of Surgery
University of California, San Francisco
San Francisco, California

D. E. Strandness, Jr., MD
Professor of Surgery
Department of Surgery
University of Washington School of
  Medicine
University of Washington
Seattle, Washington

M. David Tilson, MD
Ailson Mellon Bruce Professor of
  Surgery
Columbia College of Physicians and
  Surgeons
Department of Surgery
St. Luke's/Roosevelt Hospital Center
New York, New York

Jonathan B. Towne, MD
Professor of Surgery
Chairman, Vascular Surgery
Medical College of Wisconsin
Department of Vascular Surgery
Milwaukee, Wisconsin

William D. Turnipseed, MD
Professor, Department of Surgery
University of Wisconsin School of
  Medicine
Section Chief, Vascular Surgery
Department of Surgery
University Hospital and Clinics
Madison, Wisconsin

Frank J. Veith, MD
Professor of Surgery
Albert Einstein College of Medicine
Chief of Vascular Surgery
Montefiore Medical Center
New York, New York

Renu Virmani, MD
Professor of Clinical Research
Vanderbilt University
Nashville, Tennessee
Chair, Division of Cardiovascular
  Pathology
Armed Forces Institute of Pathology
Washington, DC

Robert L. Vogelzang, MD
Professor of Radiology
Northwestern University Medical School
Chief of Vascular and Interventional
  Radiology
Northwestern Memorial Hospital
Chicago, Illinois

Richard Waugh, FRACR
Staff Specialist/Interventional
  Radiologist
Department of Radiology
Royal Prince Albert Hospital
Campertown, Australia

Stephen P. Wiet, MD
Vascular Surgeon
Palos Hospital
Orland Park, Illinois

Geoffrey H. White, FRACS
Clinical Associate Professor of Surgery
University of Sydney
Vascular Surgeon
Royal Prince Albert Hospital
Sydney, Australia

Anthony D. Whittemore, MD
Professor of Surgery
Harvard Medical School
Chief, Vascular Surgery
Brigham and Women's Hospital
Boston, Massachusetts

James S. T. Yao, MD, PhD
Magerstadt Professor of Surgery
Division of Vascular Surgery
Department of Surgery
Northwestern University Medical School
Chief, Division of Vascular Surgery
Northwestern Memorial Hospital
Chicago, Illinois

Weiyun Yu, BSc(Med), MB, BS
Research Fellow in Endovascular
  Surgery
University of Sydney
Sydney, Australia

Christopher K. Zarins, MD
Chief of Vascular Surgery
Department of Surgery
Stanford University School of Medicine
Stanford, California

R. Eugene Zierler, MD
Professor of Surgery
Division of Vascular Surgery
University of Washington School of
  Medicine
University of Washington Medical
  Center
Seattle, Washington

Preface

The idea of a vascular symposium devoted to a specific topic was conceived by Dr. John Bergan, formerly Chief, Division of Vascular Surgery, Northwestern University Medical School, Chicago. The first annual symposium was held on December 2–4, 1976, to honor one of the pioneer vascular surgeons, Dr. Geza de Takats of Rush Medical College, Chicago. The topic "Venous Problems" was a subject in which Dr. de Takats had a long and special interest.

The goal of our symposium is to provide state-of-the-art knowledge on a given topic. Accordingly, the faculty consists of world-renowned leaders in a chosen field to provide the participants with a comprehensive review. One of the special features of the symposium has been the completion of a published book at the time of the meeting, a feature not available in other postgraduate courses.

This year marks the twentieth anniversary of the Northwestern University Medical School's vascular symposium. We believe it would be of interest to review the development of vascular surgery as it has progressed through the Northwestern symposia over the past two decades. For the interest of the readers, we list here the topics of the symposia since 1976.

1976 Venous Problems
1977 Correctable Cerebral Ischemia
1978 Gangrene and Severe Ischemia of the Lower Extremities
1979 Surgery of the Aorta and Its Body Branches
1980 Operative Techniques in Vascular Surgery
1981 Aneurysms: Diagnosis and Treatment
1982 Cerebrovascular Insufficiency
1983 Evaluation and Treatment of Upper and Lower Extremity Circulatory Disorders
1984 Surgery of the Veins
1985 Reoperative Arterial Surgery
1986 Vascular Surgical Emergencies
1987 Arterial Surgery: New Diagnostic and Operative Techniques
1988 Aortic Surgery
1989 Techniques in Arterial Surgery
1990 Venous Disorders
1991 Technologies in Vascular Surgery

To keep pace with the rapid developments in vascular surgery, several topics have been repeated. With just a glimpse of the contents of each symposium of the past 20 years, one has to be impressed with the strides that have been made in vascular surgery.

At the beginning of each symposium, a section is dedicated to the basic pathophysiology of vascular disease. The importance of the immune response is being recognized in the atherosclerotic process. T-cells, macrophages, and smooth muscle cells play important roles in plaque hemorrhage, rupture, and symptoms. The review by Renu Virmani, Andrew Farb, and Allen P. Burke (Chapter 1) offers a new understanding of atherosclerotic plaque progression. Gene-based therapy is now used to treat arterial occlusion, modify bypass graft patency, and prevent restenosis. The presentations of James C. Stanley (Chapter 2) and Ulf Hedin and Alexander W. Clowes (Chapter 3) are intended to help practicing vascular surgeons understand this complex field. Although heparin and Coumadin are useful, the need for new antithrombotic drugs is apparent. David Green (Chapter 4) discusses the use of fractionated heparin and hirudin as newer pharmaceutical agents.

Arterial aneurysm formation is an interesting phenomenon. At the 1981 symposium, "Aneurysms: Diagnosis and Treatment," there was very little information on the pathogenesis of aneurysm. With the development of molecular biology, basic science research in aneurysm has proliferated. At the 1993 symposium, "Aneurysms: New Findings and Treatment," there were several articles on pathogenesis, including the genetic basis, the role of enzymes on matrix protein, and the role of inflammatory cells. In this book, M. David Tilson (Chapter 9) provides a comprehensive review of the current concepts of aortic aneurysm pathogenesis. In addition, Jack L. Cronenwett (Chapter 11) provides important clinical data on the size and natural progression of aneurysms, explaining how these data will help in surgical decision making. From plain x-ray to ultrasound and, recently, to CT and MRI scans, our ability to diagnose and size aneurysms accurately has greatly improved. Except in selected instances, arteriography is no longer a prerequisite to surgery. The clinical application of spiral CT and 3-D imaging is described by Christopher K. Zarins, Dainis K. Krievins, and Geoffrey D. Rubin (Chapter 10).

Obviously, the introduction of endovascular grafting technique generates the greatest interest. Wesley S. Moore (Chapter 12) provides an update on the U.S. multicenter trial, which is now entering its second year. James May from Australia and his co-authors (Chapter 13) describe their experience using a different stent-graft. We also welcome the innovators of the endovascular graft, Juan C. Parodi and Claudio J. Schonholz (Chapter 15) from Argentina, who present an overview on stent-graft technology. Jon S. Matsumura and William H. Pearce (Chapter 14) from Northwestern give a follow-up study of the U.S. trial, using CT scan 1 year after the implantation. The findings are both interesting and encouraging.

The diagnosis and treatment of mesenteric ischemia and renovascular problems have significantly changed since the 1979 symposium, "Surgery of the Aorta and Its Body Branches." Refinement of duplex technology has now made duplex scan a standard initial diagnostic or screening test. Contrast arteriography, however, remains the gold standard. In patients with renal failure, an alternate technique is needed to avoid worsening of renal failure. The recent introduction of gadolinium MRA or CO_2 arteriography seems to be useful in these patients. Although many surgical techniques for the treatment of mesenteric ischemia have been described, K. Wayne Johnston and Thomas F. Lindsay (Chapter 17) present the Toronto experience using vein bypass grafts. In renovascular problems, chronic ischemic nephropathy is emerging as a distinct clinical entity, and this challenging surgical problem is presented by Robert D. Riley, Kimberley J. Hansen, and Richard H. Dean (Chapter 18). Edouard Kieffer and Quentin Desiron (Chapter 16) from France have a large series on aortic dissection of descending thoracic aorta and offer new insights into this challenging problem. James I. Fann, R. Scott Mitchell, Michael D. Dake, and D. Craig Miller (Chapter 19) of Stanford University present the most current results of endovascular stent-grafts for the treatment of thoracic aneurysm and aortic dissection.

Perhaps the most significant contribution made by vascular surgeons since the mid-1970s is the use of infrainguinal bypass for limb salvage. In 1978, we examined the treatment of the ischemic extremity in a symposium entitled "Gangrene and Severe Ischemia of the Lower Extremities." Since then, we have repeated this topic on two more occasions: "Evaluation and Treatment of Upper and Lower Extremity Circulatory Disorders" in 1983 and "The Ischemic Extremity: Advances in Treatment" in 1994. With better arteriography to visualize distal arteries, bypass grafting is now extended to pedal arteries. The revitalization of *in situ* graft has extended operability to many patients for whom, formerly, limb salvage was deemed impossible. Currently, we have a better understanding of critical ischemia defined by noninvasive techniques. The long-term result of infrainguinal bypass has now been established and was discussed in the 1992 symposium, "Long-Term Results in Vascular Surgery." In patients who have undergone infrainguinal bypass, especially *in situ* vein graft, wound complication and infection becomes a problem, and these complications prolong hospital stay. Douglas A. Coe and Jonathan B. Towne, who have a long-standing interest in surgical infection, discuss infection control in lower extremity revascularization in Chapter 20. Also, wound complication in *in situ* bypass may be minimized by the endovascular techniques to lysis the valve. David Rosenthal and Giancarlo Piano (Chapter 21) describe this intriguing technique in great detail. One of the recent advances in the treatment of the ischemic extremity is thrombolytic therapy. Kenneth Ouriel (Chapter 22) summarizes his experience with the urokinase trial in occluded native vessels and bypass grafts.

Controversy continues to surround the treatment of intermittent claudication. To fully understand the effectiveness of a given therapeutic scheme, an outcome study is required. Joseph Feinglass and Walter J. McCarthy (Chapter 24), recipients of an Agency for Health Care Policy and Research award, present their work along with recent findings. For upper extremity ischemia, the evaluation of thoracic outlet is often inadequate. CT angiography and 3-D reconstruction provide accurate anatomic detail of this region. The Northwestern vascular surgery–radiology team of William S. Rilling, Albert A. Nemcek, Jr., Robert L. Vogelzang, and Jon S. Matsumura (Chapter 23) describes its findings with this new technology.

Vascular surgical emergencies are a common part of the practice of vascular surgery and were covered in detail in 1986. Since then, several new diagnostic and therapeutic techniques have been introduced. Michael L. Marin, Frank J. Veith, and Takao Ohki (Chapter 25) of Montefiore Medical Center present their experience with stent-grafts in vascular trauma. The diagnosis of aortic dissection is often difficult, and the introduction of transesophageal echography (TEE) as an initial test has revolutionized the diagnostic approach. The Northwestern experience is provided by Stephen P. Wiet and David D. McPherson (Chapter 26). Thrombolytic therapy plays an important role in the treatment of arterial occlusion. Anthony J. Comerota (Chapter 27) provides us with an updated experience on intraoperative and intra-arterial urokinase. Civilian trauma continues to be a problem, especially in patients with extensive soft tissue or multiple organ injuries. Aires A. B. Barros D'Sa (Chapter 28) reviews his experience in Northern Ireland with the use of shunts in the management of arterial injury.

Redo surgery requires special expertise unlike that needed for primary operations, and we examined this subject in our 1985 symposium, "Reoperative Arterial Surgery." With the increased longevity of patients, it is expected that reoperative surgery will become more common in the future. Robert P. Leather and co-authors (Chapter 29) offer a definitive management plan for failing *in situ* grafts detected by surveillance. Anthony D. Whittemore (Chapter 30) reviews the Boston experience with repetitive distal bypasses. Although uncommon, reoperative carotid surgery after carotid endarterectomy either immediately or late is often a challenge. William H. Baker and M. Ashraf Mansour (Chapter 31) elucidate the treatment plan in these patients. Recurrent or metachromous aortic aneurysm is being encountered more often, and the Mayo Clinic experience is summarized by Sunil S. Menawat and Kenneth J. Cherry, Jr. (Chapter 32). Nothing is more challenging then redo surgery for renal and mesenteric arteries, especially following balloon angioplasty or stent placement. The extensive experience of Darren B. Schneider and Ronald J. Stoney (Chapter 33) provides a solution to this difficult surgical problem.

Since the first symposium, "Venous Problems," we have revisited this topic in two other symposia: "Surgery of the Veins" in 1984 and "Venous Disorders" in 1990. Several new developments are important to the practicing surgeon. First, it is now recognized that a uniform classification of venous disorders is necessary. Robert L. Kistner, Bo Eklof, and Elna M. Masuda (Chapter 34) discuss their method of classification. Second, duplex scan has emerged as the standard diagnostic test for deep-vein thrombosis. The technique is also useful for studying the natural progression of the thrombotic process. R. Eugene Zierler and Mark H. Meissner (Chapter 35) give the Seattle experience in the natural history of deep-vein thrombosis. Third, CT or MRI has emerged as a new imaging technique to replace venography. Anthony W. Stanson and Jerome F. Breen (Chapter 36) describe the value of these techniques. Fourth, minimally invasive techniques have been developed, such as endoscopic ligation of perforators and treatment of superior vena cava syndrome using thrombolysis followed by angioplasty and stent placement. These modalities are described by Peter Gloviczki and co-authors (Chapter 37) and Robert L. Volgelzang (Chapter 40), respectively. After treatment of acute axillosubclavian venous thrombosis, the need to remove the first rib remains controversial. Richard M. Green (Chapter 39) provides a rational approach to the management of this disorder. One of the most frequently performed venous surgical procedures is vein stripping. Unfortunately, this procedure often meets with a casual approach. Many surgeons are unaware of the impact of proximal venous valve incompetency in vein stripping. Philip D. Coleridge Smith (Chapter 41) from London summarizes the use of duplex scan as a guide for the proper procedure in vein stripping. Treatment of lymphedema remains most difficult, and surgical treatment has become nearly extinct. Current treatment favors manual physiotherapy and the use of a mechanical pump. Cindy L. Felty and Thom W. Rooke (Chapter 42) of Mayo Clinic give authoritative experience for this often ignored disorder.

In summary, the past two decades have witnessed significant progress in the treatment of many vascular diseases. In addition to standard surgical procedures, emerging technology such as gene-based therapy, endovascular graft, and minimally invasive techniques will continue to evolve and will find a place in the practice of vascular surgery. For diagnosis, 3-D reconstruction of images and tissue characterization of atherosclerotic plaque by noninvasive techniques will add new information. In the assessment of the success of a surgical procedure, graft patency alone is no longer sufficient. Outcome studies taking into consideration the well-being of the patient are the appropriate methods for evaluating the results of surgical procedures. Change is always with us, and we must continue to adjust our practice. It is the sincere hope of the editors that this symposium provides a summary of what we have done in postgraduate education in the past two decades and, most important, what we need to examine in the future.

Acknowledgments

We thank Paula Puntenney and her staff for the organization and preparation of the symposium, and Beryl Dwight and Susan Parmentier for editorial assistance. Without their help, the production of the meeting and this book would not have been possible.

James S. T. Yao
William H. Pearce

I

Basic
Considerations

1

Understanding the Atherosclerotic Plaque

Renu Virmani, MD, Andrew Farb, MD, and Allen P. Burke, MD

Atherosclerosis is a complex, lifelong disease involving cellular and noncellular elements present within the vessel wall and in the circulating blood. The vascular wall elements are the endothelial and smooth muscle cells (SMCs), and the extracellular elements are proteoglycans, collagen, and elastin. The blood constituents are extremely important and can be divided into mobile cellular elements (monocytes, lymphocytes, basophils, platelets, and red blood cells) and circulating noncellular factors (lipids, fibrinogen, coagulation proteins, complement, and immune complexes).[1] Atherosclerosis begins in childhood and affects large elastic and medium-size muscular arteries (e.g., aorta, coronary, carotid, lower limb arteries) and results in the formation of atheroma. The earliest grossly recognizable lesion is the fatty streak that forms and enlarges in selected sites and evolves onto the fibrous plaque, especially in the presence of risk factors.[2-4]

PATHOBIOLOGY OF ATHEROSCLEROSIS

The early and late lesions of atherosclerosis have been classically designated as fatty streak and the fibrous plaque, respectively. The fatty streak is characterized by the accumulation of foam cells and intra- and extracellular lipids (mainly, cholesterol and its esters) in the arterial intima. In the aorta, the intimal lesions appear shortly after birth and increase in size and extent during the second decade of life. Only at selected anatomic sites do fatty streaks develop into fibrous plaque.

In the coronary arteries, fatty streaks appear in adolescence, are less extensive than in the aorta, and occur in all populations. The carotid and vertebral arteries also demonstrate fatty streaks, and the lesions are most prevalent near the bifurcation of the common carotid and in the distal segment of the internal carotid artery, appearing

The opinions and assertions contained herein are the private views of the authors and are not to be construed as official or reflecting the views of the Department of the Army or the Department of Defense.

at the same time as in the aorta. The renal, mesenteric, and pulmonary arteries are less susceptible to atherosclerosis.[5] Severity in one artery does not predict severity in another.

Similar to lesions in the aorta, the coronary, carotid, and vertebral artery fatty streaks may not necessarily be tranformed into the advanced lesion of atherosclerosis. It is now believed that intermediate, transitional lesions occur in areas of fatty streaks before progressing to fibrous plaques. The transitional lesion has been designated as a type III preatheroma in the "Lesions of Atherosclerosis" classification by the American Heart Association (AHA, see below).[6]

The AHA classification further divides the lesions of atherosclerosis into adaptive lesions, fatty streaks, preatheromas, and atheromas. The initial (type I) lesions are adaptive intimal cushions, which are most prominent at branch points. Microscopically, type I lesions consist of SMCs and proteoglycans (Figure 1–1A). The type II lesion is the classic fatty streak, seen grossly as yellow deposits on the intimal surface and as staining red with Sudan III and IV.[7] Microscopically, macrophage foam cells are present in layers, and lipid droplets are seen not only in macrophages but also in SMCs (Figure 1–1B). The lipid consists primarily of cholesterol esters (77%); free cholesterol and phospholipids are also present.[8]

Type III or the intermediate lesions (preatheroma) have microscopically visible extracellular lipid droplets forming pools underneath the layers of macrophages within SMC-rich regions of adaptive intimal thickening (Figure 1–1C). In contrast to the atheroma, a well-formed necrotic core is absent. Evidence that the intermediate lesions progress from fatty streaks is found in the studies in nonhuman primates. Masuda and Ross[9] have shown that in nonhuman primates with low-level hypercholesterolemia induced for 6 months, the first lesion to appear in the fatty streaks consists of monocyte-macrophages, T-lymphocytes, and SMCs. The next stage is the fibrofatty (transitional) lesion, which is characterized by scattered foam cells with large numbers of surrounding SMCs at predilection sites for future fibrous plaque formation (i.e., abdominal aorta, iliac arteries, arterial branch points). The fibrous plaque, seen with prolonged high cholesterol diet from 2 to 3.5 years, consists of increased amounts of fibrous connective tissue, more SMCs, and fewer macrophages. The anatomic sites are similar to fibrofatty lesions and thus support the postulate that fatty streaks convert to fibrous plaques.[10]

The early lesions form by the interaction of lipoproteins and infiltration by circulating white cells. The subendothelial space contains more free cholesterol and fatty acid than the plasma, and trapping of low-density lipoprotein (LDL) particles within the

---

Figure 1–1. Photomicrographs illustrating the American Heart Association classification of atherosclerotic lesions. (**A**) Type I is the adaptive lesion showing intimal smooth muscle cells (SMCs) in a proteoglycan matrix (Movat stain, ×150). (**B**) Type II is the fatty streak showing presence of foamy macrophages close to the lumen with underlying SMCs in proteoglycan collagen matrix (Movat stain, ×150). (**C**) Type III is the preatheroma (intermediate lesion), which illustrates intimal macrophages close to the lumen and deeper small pools of extracellular lipid (*arrows*) (Movat stain, ×120). (**D**) Type IV is the atheroma (fibrous plaque) consisting of a dense, large, extracellular lipid core containing cholesterol crystals in the deep intimal close to the media (*arrows*). Between the lipid core and the lumen, the intima contains macrophages and SMCs and usually lacks extracellular lipid droplets (Movat stain, ×40). (**E**) Type IV lesion showing calcification of the necrotic core (*arrow*) (Movat stain, ×30). (**F**) Type V is the fibroatheroma, consisting of multiple layers of lipid cores (*arrows*), which may have formed at different times. The fibrous cap is thick and is formed by collagen and proteoglycans with interspersed SMCs. Lesions in which the lipid core is absent or small are referred to as type Vc. (**G**) Type VI lesion is essentially a complicated lesion with disruption of the luminal surface (type VIa), hemorrhage (H) into a plaque (type VIb, as shown in this Movat stain, ×20), or thrombosis (type VIc). (**H**) Type VIc lesion showing an occlusive thrombus (T) with rupture of the fibrous cap (*arrow*) and an underlying hemorrhage into a necrotic core.

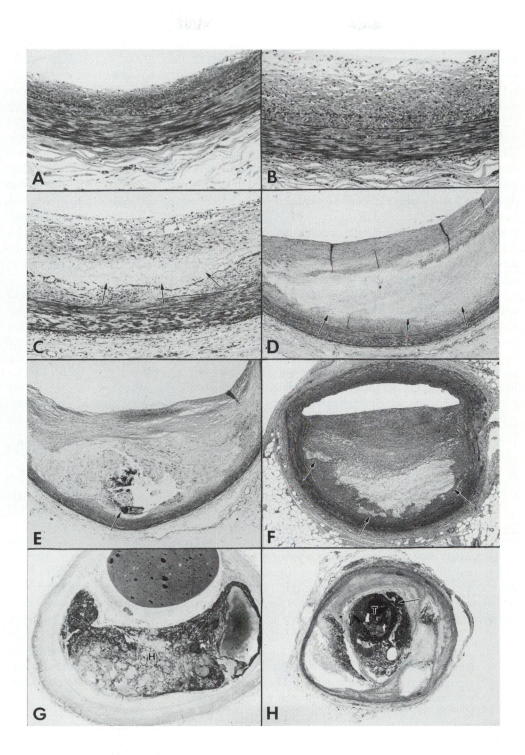

extracellular proteoglycan matrix may explain the higher concentration of apolipoprotein B in the arterial wall than in the plasma.[8,11] Before the monocyte-derived macrophage is transformed into the foam cell within the arterial wall, modification of the protein portion of the LDL particle leads to a loss of recognition by the LDL receptor and a shift to recognition by the scavenger receptor and/or oxidized LDL receptor.[12] Mild oxidation of LDL induces monocytes, but not neutrophils, to adhere to endothelial cells, and this in turn causes endothelial cells to produce potent monocyte activators, monocyte chemoattractant protein 1 (MCP-1), monocyte colony-stimulating factor (M-CSF), and GRO.[12] The mildly oxidized LDL may be "primed" for more and rapid oxidation by reentry into the intima by endothelial cells, macrophages, and SMCs, which have all been shown to cause oxidation in cell culture experiments.[13] Mice that are genetically predisposed to the development of fatty streaks have been shown to have elevated levels of oxidized fatty acids in their arteries, with increased expression of inflammatory genes induced by these oxidized fatty acids.[14] In addition, a genetic link between fatty acid oxidization and an inflammatory response has been hypothesized, suggesting orchestration of aortic lesions in this model by a single major gene.[14] Although there is substantial evidence supporting a role of oxidized lipoproteins in the development of atherosclerotic lesions, the oxidation hypothesis of atherosclerosis in humans remains to be proven.

The type IV fibrous plaque (atheroma) consists of a lipid-rich core with a cap of collagen and proteoglycans (Figure 1–1D). Lymphocytes and mast cells may be present and capillaries, when present, are seen near the base of the lipid core (toward the media) and at the lateral margins. The type IV plaque results in clinical symptoms and can calcify (Figure 1–1E), thrombose, and hemorrhage into the necrotic core. According to Stary et al.,[6] the transformation of the proteoglycan-rich intima above the lipid core into predominantly fibrous tissue (collagen) converts the lesion into type Va (Figure 1–1E). By routine light microscopy of 5-μm-thick sections, it may be difficult to separate type IV from type V lesions and, therefore, these lesions, by the old terminology, are collectively called *fibrous plaques.*

Type V atheromas are subclassified by the presence of calcium and by degree of fibrosis. When the lipid core is calcified, the lesion is designated type Vb, and when there is excessive fibrous tissue and minimal or absent lipid core, the lesion is designated Vc. A multilayered fibroatheroma is called a type Va lesion and is shown in Figure 1–1F.

The type VI lesion has one or more additional features of type IV and V and is called a *complicated lesion.* Type VIa has disruption of the surface. Type VIb has hematoma or hemorrhage (Figure 1–1G), and type VIc has thrombus (Figure 1–1H). The designation "type VIabc" denotes the presence of all three elements—surface disruption, hemorrhage, and thrombosis. In its present form, the AHA classification is most useful in its description of the initial progression of atherosclerotic plaque. However, the morbidity and mortality associated with atherosclerotic disease occurs primarily as a result of complicated plaques, which may occur in both type IV and V lesions. Both the type IV and V lesions and their subclassifications may develop fissures, hematoma, and/or thrombi and, therefore, are of great clinical significance. Because of this overlap, the AHA classification does not appreciably assist in our understanding of an already complex system with too many different basic forms in which calcification, hemorrhage, and thrombosis can occur both separately and simultaneously.

VASCULAR REMODELING

Human coronary arteries enlarge in response to plaque accumulation. Because of this vascular remodeling, first reported by Glagov et al.,[15] functionally significant luminal stenosis does not occur until the lesion occupies 40% of the internal elastic lamina (IEL) area. Clarkson et al.[16] showed a stronger correlation between plaque size and coronary artery size than between plaque area and lumen area (i.e., the arterial enlargement is not reflected in an enlarged lumen). We have also shown that there is compensatory enlargement of coronary arteries with up to 30% luminal stenosis in the left main, left anterior descending, and left circumflex arteries; the lumen then starts to decrease with increasing percent (cross-sectional area luminal) stenosis (Fig. 1–2).[17] In this study, body height and weight were positively associated with coronary artery lumen area but not with intimal plaque area, and plaque area and body surface area were positively correlated with the area within the IEL. There is racial variation that affects remodeling in atherosclerosis; this study[17] showed that blacks had larger coronary arteries and medial area than whites, and that black race, increasing body surface area, and age were independent predictors of larger lumen area. However, percent luminal stenosis is less relevant than absolute lumen area for arterial function, since lumen area is the critical component of overall arterial blood flow.

PLAQUE MORPHOLOGY IN CLINICAL SYNDROMES

There are three major clinical coronary syndromes: angina pectoris (stable and unstable), acute myocardial infarction, and sudden coronary death due to severe coronary athero-sclerosis. Attempts have been made to correlate ischemic syndromes with plaque mor-phology in an effort to evaluate the mechanisms underlying the transformation of

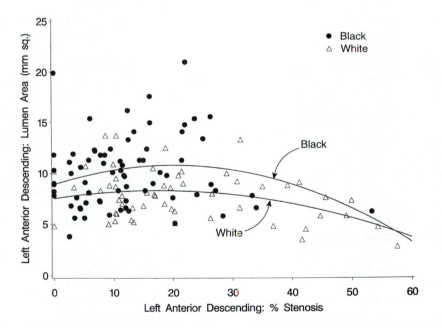

Figure 1–2. The lumen area as a function of the percent stenosis in the left anterior descending coronary artery in both races is depicted. With luminal stenosis of up to 30%, the lumen enlarges; however, greater than 30% stenosis results in a smaller lumen. We believe that a quadratic curve best represents the lumen and percent stenosis relationships. The curves representing the white (lower curve, open triangles) and black (upper curve, solid circles) populations are relatively parallel suggesting that the remodeling process is not significantly different between the races. However, the lumen is larger in blacks than in whites.

stable plaques into active lesions resulting in the clinical presentation of ischemic heart disease.

Stable Angina Pectoris

From the Coronary Artery Surgery Study (CASS), the angiographic extent of severe coronary artery disease (50% to 95% diameter reduction) in patients with stable angina involved one vessel in 16%, two vessels in 33%, and three vessels in 51% of patients. Left main artery disease was an infrequent finding.[18] Because most individuals with only stable coronary plaques do not die from their disease, there are few autopsy studies documenting extent of disease in patients with stable angina. Guthrie et al.[19] reported the extent and type of disease seen in 35 men with stable angina who died after a coronary bypass procedure: 3% had single-vessel disease, 20% had two-vessel disease, and 49% had three-vessel disease; of these, 29% had left main artery disease. Hangartner et al.[20] described coronary atherosclerosis in patients with stable angina who died suddenly within 6 hours of the onset of symptoms and who demonstrated substantial plaque variability. In this study, 76% of segments with >75% cross-sectioned luminal narrowing were concentric lesions, with 48% concentric fibrous plaques and 28% concentric lipid-rich plaques (i.e., >10% of the intimal area occupied by lipid pool). The remaining 24% of severely narrowed segments were eccentric, comprising 12% lipid-rich and 12% fibrous lesions. Recanalized segments were present in 79% of the cases.

Morphologic examination of atherectomy specimens performed in patients shows that the extent of macrophage infiltration in plaques with stable angina is lower than in plaques from patients with unstable angina or myocardial infarction. In one study, the area occupied by macrophages was 11.5 ± 4.1 mm$^2 \times 10^{-2}$ in plaques from patients with stable angina, compared with 55 ± 19 mm$^2 \times 10^{-2}$ in unstable angina ($p < 0.05$) and 87 ± 32 mm$^2 \times 10^{-2}$ in non-Q-wave myocardial infarcts ($p = <0.01$).[21] We have demonstrated that plaques from patients with stable angina pectoris are typically more fibrous and have fewer SMCs as compared with plaques from unstable angina patients.[22]

Unstable Angina Pectoris

Angiographic studies in males with unstable angina pectoris have shown one-vessel disease in 18%, two-vessel disease in 35%, and three-vessel disease in 46% of patients.[23] In the CASS registry, 50% of patients had three-vessel disease, 38% had two-vessel disease, and 14% had significant left main artery disease.[24] At least 10% to 15% of patients have insignificant coronary disease.

In patients with new onset unstable angina in the absence of a history of myocardial infarction or chronic stable angina, the extent of coronary disease is less than in patients with evidence of either of these conditions. In comparing patients with unstable angina to those with chronic stable angina, McCormick et al.[24] found a higher frequency of one-vessel disease (43% versus 27%), and three-vessel disease (23% versus 35%), a lower frequency of left main artery disease (5% versus 10%, respectively), and less well-developed collateral circulation in unstable angina patients. In this study, the most frequent artery affected was the left anterior descending coronary artery, which was involved in 42% of patients with unstable angina, compared to 17% in patients with stable angina.

Patients with unstable angina have a higher incidence of angiographic coronary thrombosis than patients with stable angina.[25] Ambrose et al.[26] found eccentric coronary lesions with irregular borders, suggesting thrombosis, in 71% of patients with unstable angina compared to 16% in patients with stable angina. Angioscopy has demonstrated thrombosis in 67% of patients with unstable angina, with an increased incidence among diabetics.[27]

In autopsy studies, the morphologic extent of coronary atherosclerosis in patients with unstable angina is quite variable and, similar to angiographic data, is greater if there is a history of previous myocardial infarction or preceding chronic stable angina. Most investigators report severe three- or four-vessel disease as the most frequent finding in patients with unstable angina, occurring in 36% and 45% of cases, respectively, with one-vessel disease being infrequent.[28] In unstable angina, the role of thrombus is less well established, but studies by Falk and Davies report a >80% incidence of thrombosis.[29,30]

The typical atherosclerotic plaque associated with thrombus in unstable angina is described as having a large necrotic core (soft atheromatous core) with a thin fibrous cap heavily infiltrated with macrophages and lymphocytes.[21] Richardson et al. reported that the cap is the site of rupture in 83% of cases, and rupture generally occurs where the cap is thinnest.[31] The site of rupture is located at the junction of the fibrous cap with the adjacent normal intima in 49% of cases and is central in 29% of cases.[31] Seventy-five percent of ruptured plaques have foam cell infiltration at the site of the tear.[28] Specimens obtained by coronary atherectomy demonstrate a 45% incidence of thrombosis in patients with crescendo angina, 41% with rest angina, and 69% in acute myocardial infarction. Flugelman et al.[22] reported that >50% of plaques in patients with unstable angina had an abundance of SMCs and that, of these, only one-third demonstrated thrombosis. These data suggest that SMCs may play an important role in unstable angina pectoris and provide an alternative mechanism to plaque rupture and thrombosis.

Acute Myocardial Infarction

The incidence of coronary thrombosis in patients with acute myocardial infarction is >80% in autopsy studies (with the exception of the study by Kragel et al., who report a 69% incidence) and is even higher (90%) by angiography.[33–37] In postmortem coronary angiograms, areas of stenosis with ragged margins and intraluminal translucency have been shown to represent thrombi.[21] In 75% of cases, the area of the plaque underlying the thrombus contains a ruptured or fissured thin fibrous cap that is rich in macrophages and lymphocytes, but poor in SMCs. The underlying necrotic core is a lipid-rich atheromatous "gruel."[21,29,34,38]

Work by Davis and Falk has emphasized plaque rupture as the most important factor in the development of coronary thrombosis in acute myocardial infarction. However, in 25% of cases of coronary thrombosis, the underlying plaque is intact.[39] From our own experience with patients dying with acute myocardial infarction, the incidence of thrombosis is 89%; half of these thrombi are associated with plaque erosion, and half with plaque rupture.[40] Eroded plaques, as described by Davies, are associated with superficial loss of endothelium, an abundance of macrophages, and a severe degree of atherosclerotic stenosis (>80% having 60% diameter reduction).[39] In our study, eroded plaques are characterized by plaque thrombus overlying an eroded intimal surface lacking endothelial cells, with superficial plaques rich in SMCs and proteoglycans. We have not noted large numbers of macrophages and lymphocytes in eroded plaques in cases of acute myocardial infarction.[40] The pathologic findings in atherosclerotic plaques underlying acute coronary thrombi are discussed in further detail in the following paragraphs.

Angiographic studies in patients performed prior to the development of an acute myocardial infarction have demonstrated that the frequency of total occlusion is highest in severely narrowed plaque. However, a greater number of segments of the coronary tree have <50% narrowing (68%) that are eventually involved in total obstruction and myocardial infarction.[41] A pathologic study by Qiao and Fishbein[42] showed a 90 ± 7% obstruction at the site of atherosclerotic plaque rupture, in contradiction to the clinical studies. We have found a greater incidence (48%) of <80% stenosis at site of thrombi in patients dying suddenly, confirming the clinical studies. This difference in pathologic studies may be related to perfusion fixation of the coronary arteries at postmortem and to the study population being younger in our database.[40]

Sudden Coronary Death

At least 15 studies have been published since 1970 describing the incidence of coronary thrombosis in sudden coronary death. The frequency of coronary thrombosis in these studies varies from 11% to 94%.[36,40] Methodologic differences in these studies are reflected in differences in mean age of patients, duration of symptoms before death, use of postmortem angiography, frequency of acute or healed myocardial infarction, and the extent of coronary disease.

The studies that have received the most attention are those of Davies, Falk, and Roberts.[34,43,44] Davies et al.[43] studied 100 sudden coronary deaths in London in individuals with severe coronary atherosclerosis, 40 of whom had myocardial infarctions at autopsy. He identified active arterial lesions, defined as coronary artery thrombi or atherosclerotic plaque fissuring, in 95% of hearts and intraluminal thrombi in 74%. In the 26 cases without luminal thrombi, 21 had intraintimal fibrin and/or platelets within the intima. Therefore, only 5% of cases had neither intraluminal thrombus nor plaque fissuring. The mean percent cross-sectional area luminal narrowing was 79% in arteries with thrombi, 65% of which had >75% luminal stenosis. In their control population who died of noncardiac causes, 3.8% had intraintimal thrombus with plaque fissure, and 6.4% had intraintimal thrombus only.

Falk[30] studied 25 sudden coronary deaths (defined as death within 24 hours of onset of symptoms) in 20 men and 5 women with a mean age of 64 years, 60% of whom had myocardial infarction at autopsy. An acute coronary thrombus was found in all 25 cases. A layered structure of the thrombus was identified in 81%, indicating that the thrombi formed successively by repeated mural deposits. All had ≥75% cross-sectional area luminal narrowing by atherosclerotic plaque.

In contrast to the studies of Davies et al. and Falk et al., in which coronary thrombi were found in the majority of sudden coronary deaths, Warnes and Roberts[44] studied 70 cases of sudden death due to coronary heart disease and found only a 19% incidence of coronary thrombi. In this study, 57 patients were men and 13 women, and none had an acute myocardial infarct at autopsy. The mean age of those with thrombi was 43 years, and 51 years for those without thrombi. A possible technical limitation of this study was the lack of perfusion fixation before coronary dissection. The majority of patients in this study had two- or three-vessel disease and the maximal percent stenosis was ≥75% of all cases.

We have recently studied autopsied hearts of 72 men and 18 women dying suddenly with severe coronary disease. Their mean age was 51 ± 10 years, and all died within 6 hours of onset of symptoms or had been seen in stable condition less than 24 hours prior to death. An acute myocardial infarction was found in 21% of cases.[40] Our method of fixation with postmortem angiography was similar to that used by Davies and Falk. We identified active coronary lesions in 51 cases (57%): acute thrombus plus disrupted plaque in 27, acute thrombus only in 21, and disrupted plaque only in 3. In 19% of hearts, there was neither an infarct (healed or acute) nor an active coronary lesion (Table 1–1). The lower frequency of acute thrombi in our study, as compared to that of Davies and Falk, is probably related to the lower incidence of acute myocardial infarction and to the use of a younger cohort with less severe coronary disease.

A vulnerable plaque has been traditionally defined as a plaque with a large necrotic core and a thin fibrous cap that is heavily infiltrated by macrophages and lymphocytes (Fig. 1–3). We have seen vulnerable plaques at multiple sites in the coronary tree of patients with plaque rupture. However, we have also observed vulnerable plaques in patients dying of unnatural causes. Therefore, it is possible that some plaques progress through the creation of vulnerable plaques, which may be the site of future plaque rupture and thrombosis. Also, it is conceivable that the transformation of stable plaques to vulnerable plaques may be related to the presence of coronary risk factors, especially hypercholesterolemia.

In preliminary studies, we have observed that patients with hypertension have a lower incidence (36%) of acute coronary thrombosis than patients without hypertension (76%). The extent of severe coronary artery disease (luminal narrowing >75% in cross-sectional area) was similar in both hypertensives and normotensives.[45] Left ventricular hypertrophy was more frequent in hypertensives (64%) versus normotensives (33%, $p = 0.007$), and heart weight was greater in patients with plaque rupture (519 ± 109 g) than in eroded plaques (381 ± 92 g, $p = 0.0002$). In normotensives there was a progressive increase in heart weight with one-, two- and three-vessel disease ($p = 0.008$) (Table 1–2).[45]

MORPHOLOGY OF UNDERLYING PLAQUE IN AREAS OF THROMBOSIS

The general consensus appears to be that the majority of thrombi occur in areas of plaque rupture in which there is contact between luminal blood and the necrotic lipid-rich core of the plaque[21,29,38] (Fig. 1–4; see color insert after page 332). Falk reported that in only 20% of thrombi, severe underlying atherosclerotic plaque with superficial intimal injury without a rupture into a lipid core is present.[21]

Plaque Rupture, Cytokines, and Matrix

Atherosclerotic plaques in the aorta with overlying thrombi have been shown to contain a larger necrotic lipid core than plaques that have not ruptured; 90% of ulcerated plaques have lipid cores occupying >40% cross-sectional area.[38] Gertz and Roberts[46] reported that the necrotic core comprises 32% of the plaque area in severely narrowed coronary artery segments with plaque disruption, compared to 12% of severely narrowed segments with an intact surface ($p = 0.02$). In the vast majority of cases with plaque rupture, the fibrous cap overlying the necrotic core has been reported to be thin, richly infiltrated by foam cells and T cells, and poor in SMC content.[38,47] The foam cells occupy a greater proportion of the fibrous cap in ruptured plaques than in intact plaques, and the reverse is true for SMCs.[21,48]

There is an abundance of SMC-derived type I and type III collagen in fibrous caps that have not ruptured.[49] It has been shown that transforming growth factor beta (TGF-β) and platelet-derived growth factor (PDGF) increase the protein synthesis type I and type III collagen by SMCs. In contrast, interferon gamma (IFN-γ) inhibits collagen synthesis.[49] Only T cells can elaborate IFN-γ, and activated T cells have shown

TABLE 1–1. ACTIVE CORONARY LESIONS IN 90 CASES OF SUDDEN CORONARY DEATH WITH DATA SEPARATED BASED ON THE PRESENCE OF MYOCARDIAL INFARCTION

	Active Coronary Lesions (%)			Active Coronary Lesions Present (%)	No Active Coronary Lesion (%)	Large Hemorrhage into Plaque Only (%)	Organized Thrombus (%)
	Acute Thrombus Only	Disrupted Plaque Only	Acute Thrombus with Disrupted Plaque				
All cases (n = 90)	23	3	30	57	43	7	40
Acute MI (n = 19)	42	5	42	89	11	5	47
Healed MI only (n = 37)	19	5	22	46	54	11	59
No acute or healed MI (n = 34)	18	0	32	50	50	3	15
P	.09	NS	NS	.005		NS	.0005

MI, myocardial infarction; NS, not significant.

Reproduced with permission from Farb A, Tang AL, Burke AP, et al. Sudden coronary death frequency of active coronary lesions, inactive coronary lesions, and myocardial infarction. *Circulation.* 1995;92:1701–1705.

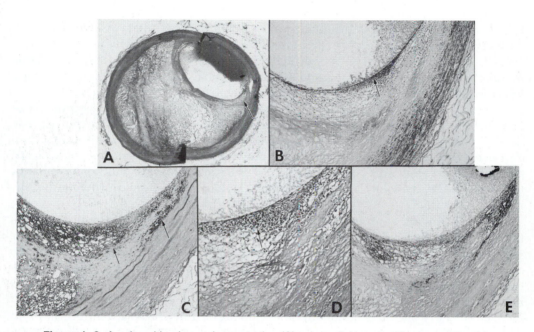

Figure 1–3. A vulnerable plaque demonstrating (**A**) a large lipid core with an overlying thin fibrous cap [hematoxylin-eosin (H&E), ×15]. The dark area in the lumen represents barium gelatin. The area highlighted by the arrow is shown in high power field in **B** (H&E, ×15) to **E** in immunohistochemically stained sections for SMCs, macrophages, T cells, and HLA-DR antigens, respectively. (**B**) The fibrous cap contains few SMCs (*arrow*) as seen by SMC α actin antibody staining (avidin-biotin complex, ×75). (**C**) Note the presence of a large number of macrophages (*arrows*) staining positive for KP-1 antibody close and within the fibrous cap (avidin-biotin complex, ×75). (**D**) The thin fibrous cap focally contains large numbers of T cells (*arrow*) (UCHL positive) (avidin-biotin complex, ×150). (**E**) Few macrophages and T cells stain positive for HLA-DR antigens, representing activated inflammatory cells (avidin-biotin complex, ×75).

TABLE 1–2. SUDDEN CORONARY DEATH: A COMPARISON OF INCIDENCE OF ACUTE THROMBI, HEART WEIGHT, AND HEART WEIGHT AS A FUNCTION OF EXTENT OF DISEASE AND PRESENCE OF HEALED INFARCT, HYPERTENSIVES VERSUS NORMOTENSIVES (WEIGHT VALUES EXPRESSED AS MEAN ± SD, WEIGHT IN GRAMS)

	Hypertensives ($n = 25$)	Nonhypertensives ($n = 46$)	P value
Acute thrombus	9/25 (36%)	35/46 (76%)	0.002
Heart weight/body weight	0.65 ± 0.16	0.52 ± 0.13	0.0007
Left ventricular			0.01
hypertrophy, n[a]	16/25 (64%)	15/46% (33%)	
Heart weight, one vessel	540 ± 158	410 ± 85	
Heart weight, two vessels	504 ± 108	469 ± 125	0.008[a]
Heart weight, three vessels	512 ± 116	573 ± 144	
Heart weight, no infarct	499 ± 114	411 ± 89	0.004[b]
Heart weight, healed infarct	607 ± 157	514 ± 138	0.04[c]

[a]For normotensives, one vessel versus three vessels.
[b]No versus healed infarct, normotensives.
[c]No versus healed infarct, normotensives.

HLA-DR positive staining in the fibrous caps.[40,47,50] Fibrous caps that rupture have fewer SMCs compared to intact fibrous caps; thus, little collagen is being synthesized, possibly because of the production of IFN-γ by activated T cells. Furthermore, there are a large number of activated HLA-DR-positive foam cells that liberate proteolytic enzymes, which could lead to catabolism of extracellular matrix.

These proteolytic enzymes belong to the superfamily of matrix metalloproteinases and include interstitial collagenases, gelatinases, and stromelysins that can degrade fibrillar collagens, collagen fragments, and proteoglycans, respectively.[49] Stromelysin and one of the gelatinases can also break down elastin.[49] These enzymes have to be activated from proenzyme precursors, and SMCs express tissue inhibitors of metalloproteinases (TIMPs) that simultaneously prevent these enzymes from destroying the surrounding tissues.[49]

Certain inflammatory cytokines, such as interleukin 1 (IL-1) and tumor necrosis factor (TNF), induce SMC expression of interstitial collagenase, gelatinase, and stromelysin. These cytokines may produce a net increase in the ability of these enzymes to degrade extracellular matrix.[51] Also, as stated previously, plaque macrophages have been shown to express stromelysin and interstitial collagenase, which can be activated by cytokines such as IFN-γ, TNF, IL-1, or macrophage colony-stimulating factor.[52] Shah et al.[53] have shown that human monocyte-derived macrophages induce collagen degradation of the fibrous caps of human atherosclerotic plaques obtained from the aorta and/or carotid arteries. These cells in culture express MMP1 (interstitial collagenase) and MMP2 (72-kDa gelatinase), which induce the release of hydroxyproline from collagen breakdown of the fibrous plaque. This collagen degradation can be blocked by MMP inhibitor.[53]

Plaque Erosion and Thrombosis

We have recently reported our findings in 50 cases of coronary plaque thrombosis in sudden coronary death.[40] Plaque rupture of a thin fibrous cap occurred in 56% and superficial erosion of a proteoglycan-rich and SMC-rich plaque with thrombosis was seen in 44%. In addition to finding a high incidence of plaque erosion, we noted several differences in cases of plaque erosion as compared to plaque rupture. The mean age was 53 ± 10 years in plaque rupture versus 44 ± 7 years in eroded plaque ($p < 0.02$), and plaque erosion was more frequently seen in women. The mean percent luminal narrowing was $78 \pm 12\%$ in plaque rupture and $70 \pm 11\%$ in superficial erosion ($p < 0.03$). Plaque calcification was present in 69% of rupture versus 23% of erosions ($p < 0.002$). In plaque rupture, the fibrous cap was infiltrated by macrophages and T lymphocytes. In contrast, macrophages and T cells were uncommon in eroded plaques, but SMC in a proteoglycan-rich matrix were almost uniformly seen (Fig. 1–5; see color insert after page 332). HLA-DR expression was more common in plaque rupture and was uncommon in eroded plaques (89% versus 36%, $p = 0.0002$).

The presence of large amounts of proteoglycans in the eroded plaque may be important in the mechanism of thrombosis that occurs at the plaque surface. The SMCs of developing atherosclerotic plaques synthesize and secrete proteoglycans, principally chondroitin sulfate, dermatan sulfate, and to a lesser extent heparan sulfate.[54] Heparan sulfate is an anticoagulant that inhibits thrombin-induced platelet aggregation. Platelet factor 4 (PL-4), a procoagulant, is a heparin antagonist and is complexed to chondroitin sulfate.[55] Heparan sulfate inhibits the binding of PL-4 to endothelial cells *in vitro*.[55] Heparan sulfate has been shown to catalyze the reaction between antithrombin III and thrombin. Thrombin binds to heparan sulfate and to cultured endothelial cells. One could speculate that reduced heparan sulfate and increased chondroitin sulfate as seen in atherosclerotic plaques may contribute to coronary thrombosis via reduced inhibition of the clotting cascade.

Most coronary thrombi are platelet rich and usually form at the site of ruptured plaque or plaque erosion. The fact that platelets play an important role in coronary artery disease is supported by studies showing a 20% reduction in initial and subsequent infarction in patients treated with aspirin. Platelet aggregation requires the binding of fibrinogen and von Willebrand factor to the glycoprotein receptor IIb/IIIa on the platelet surface. Platelet membrane glycoproteins are highly polymorphic: persons positive for P1[A1] and P1[A2] polymorphisms of the glycoprotein IIIa gene are likely to have coronary events before the age of 60 years.[56] Within the plaque itself, the presence of tissue factor and plasminogen activator inhibitor type 1 may also augment the thrombotic potential of an atherosclerotic lesion.[57] Increased circulating levels of hemostatic factors such as fibrinogen, von Willebrand factor, and tissue plasminogen antigen have been shown to be independent predictors of acute coronary syndromes.[58]

Role of Vasa Vasorum in Acute Coronary Syndromes

The adventitia of the aorta, coronary arteries, and peripheral arteries (e.g., carotid and femoral arteries) are rich in vasa vasorum, which most likely serve the nutritional needs of the arterial walls (Fig. 1–6). In some thickened atherosclerotic arteries, the vasa vasorum extend from the adventitia into the media with further extension into the intima. It has been hypothesized that local hypoxia may be the stimulus for growth of vasovasorum.[59]

It has been shown that 70% of intimal vasa vasorum arise from the adventitial vasa vasorum and 30% from the lumen. Most vasa vasorum are thin-walled endothelial lined channels and are therefore prone to compression and rupture. Barger et al. have suggested that vasa vasorum may contribute to plaque hemorrhage, plaque rupture, and thrombosis.[60] Endothelial cells and SMCs express MMP1 (collagenase). Some of the microvessels in the plaques at shoulder regions have been shown to express MMP1, and it is possible that plaque hemorrhage may be related to the disruption of the capillaries caused by MMP1.[61] MMP1 is also present in macrophages, which may surround vasa vasorum and assist in the breakdown of the capillary endothelium (Fig. 1–7). Some vasa vasorum have SMC lining and therefore may regulate the blood flow in plaques. Monkey atherosclerotic coronary arteries have been shown to respond to

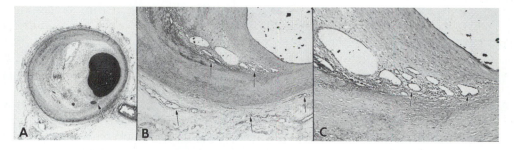

Figure 1–6. (**A**) Note presence of large numbers of thin-walled capillaries within the plaque in the shoulder region of the plaque (*arrow*). (**B**) High magnification showing dilated capillaries within the plaque and in the media after staining for factor VIII (*arrows*). (**C**) The capillary channels lined by endothelial cells are factor VIII positive (*arrows*). In the region of the capillaries there are few SMCs seen as spindle-shaped cells. Most vasa vasorum arise in the adventitia and pass through the media into the intima. (A: Movat stain, ×15; B and C: factor VIII antibody, ×48 and ×120, respectively.)

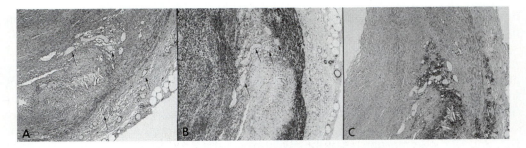

Figure 1–7. At the base of the plaque the vasovasorum (*arrows*) are prominent, traversing the media into the intima. The capillary channels are lined by single factor VIII-positive endothelial cells (**A**) with negative staining for α actin around the capillaries (**B**, *arrows*). These endothelial lined channels are surrounded by macrophages (KP-1 positive)(**C**), which may be responsible for the rupture of the capillaries by the release of metalloproteases. (A: factor VIII antibody, ×75; B: α actin antibody, ×75; and C: KP-1 antibody, ×75.)

vasoconstrictor stimuli, and there is a decrease in vasa vasorum with regression of atherosclerotic plaques.[59]

CONCLUSION

Human atherosclerosis and the consequent ischemic cardiac syndromes are the result of complicated interactions of endogenous and exogenous cellular and noncellular elements. Coronary thrombosis plays a central role in the causation of symptomatic heart disease, but the processes leading to plaque progression and thrombosis are complex and highly variable among individuals. More than 50% of coronary thrombi are associated with plaque rupture, and the remainder are the result of plaque erosion with a base rich in SMCs and proteoglycans. The precipitation of thrombosis involves a complicated balance between the three interrelated protease-protease-inhibitor cascades: thrombosis, fibrinolysis, and the matrix-degrading proteases. Other mechansisms involved in the clinical manifestation of ischemic heart disease include mechanical forces that may result in disruption of the plaque by vasospasm, hemodynamic factors, heart motion, hypoxia-related disruption of vasa vasorum, and many as yet unrecognized factors.

REFERENCES

1. Schwartz CJ, Sprague EA, Valente AJ, et al. Cellular mechanisms in the response of the arterial wall to injury and repair. *Toxicol Pathol.* 1989;17:66–77.
2. Pathobiological Determinants of Atherosclerosis in Youth (PDAY) Research Group. Relationship of atherosclerosis in young men to serum lipoprotein cholesterol concentrations and smoking: a preliminary report from the Pathobiological Determinants of Atherosclerosis in Youth (PDAY) Research Group. *JAMA.* 1990;264:3018–3024.
3. McGill HC Jr, McMahan CA, Malcom GT, et al. Relation of glycohemoglobin and adiposity to atherosclerosis in youth. *Arterioscler Thromb Vasc Biol.* 1995;15:431–440.
4. McGill HC Jr, Strong JP, Tracy RE, et al. Relation of the postmortem renal index of hypertension to atherosclerosis in youth. *Arterioscler Thromb Vasc Biol.* 1995;15:2222–2228.
5. Glagov S, Ozoa AK. Significance of the relatively low incidence of atherosclerosis in the pulmonary, renal and mesenteric arteries. *Am NY Acad Sci.* 1968;149:940–955.

6. Stary HC, Chandler AS, Dinsmore RE, et al. A definition of advanced type of atherosclerosis: a report from the committee on vascular lesions of the council on arteriosclerosis. American Heart Association. *Circulation.* 1995;92:1355–1374.

7. Katz SS, Shipley GG, Small DM. Physical density of the lipids of human atherosclerotic lesions: demonstration of a lesion intermediate between fatty streaks and advanced plaque. *J Clin Invest.* 1976;58:200–211.

8. Kruth HS. Subendothelial accumulation of nonesterified cholesterol: an early event in the atherosclerotic lesion development. *Atherosclerosis.* 1985;57:337–341.

9. Masuda J, Ross R. Atherogenesis during low level hypercholesterolemia in the nonhuman primate. I. Fatty streak formation. *Arteriosclerosis.* 1990;10:164–177.

10. Masuda J, Ross R. Atherogenesis during low level hypercholesterolemia in the nonhuman primate. II. Fatty streak conversion to fibrous plaque. *Arteriosclerosis.* 1990;10:178–187.

11. Hoff HF, Heideman CL, Gotto AM Jr, Ganbatz JW. Apolipoprotein B retention in the grossly normal and atherosclerotic human aorta. *Circ Res.* 1977;41:684–690.

12. Berliner JA, Navab M, Fogelman AM, et al. Atherosclerosis: basic mechanisms. Oxidation, inflammation, and genetics. *Circulation.* 1995;91:2488–2496.

13. Witztum JL. The oxidation hypothesis of atherosclerosis. *Lancet.* 1994;344:793–795.

14. Liao F, Andalipi A, Qiao JH, et al. Genetic evidence for a common pathway mediating oxidative stress, inflammatory gene induction, and aortic fatty streak formation in mice. *J Clin Invest.* 1994;94:877–884.

15. Glagov S, Weisenberg E, Zarins CK, et al. Compensatory enlargement of human atherosclerotic coronary arteries. *N Engl J Med.* 1987;316:1371–1375.

16. Clarkson TB, Prichard RW, Morgan TM, et al. Remodeling of coronary arteries in human and nonhuman primates. *JAMA.* 1994;271:289–294.

17. Litovsky SH, Farb A, Burke AP, et al. Effect of age, race, body surface area, heart weight and atherosclerosis on coronary artery dimensions in young males. *Atherosclerosis.* In press.

18. Detre K, Hultgren H, Takaro T, and the Veterans Administration Cooperative Group. Veterans Administration Cooperative Study of Surgery for Coronary Artery Occlusive Disease. III. Methods and baseline characteristics, including experience with medical treatment. *Am J Cardiol.* 1977;40:212–225.

19. Guthrie RB, Vlodaver Z, Nicoloff DM, Edwards JE. Pathology of stable and unstable angina pectoris. *Circulation.* 1975;51:1059–1063.

20. Hangartner JRW, Charleston AJ, Davies MJ, Thomas AC. Morphological characteristics of clinically significant coronary artery stenosis in stable angina. *Br Heart J.* 1986;56:501–508.

21. Falk E, Shah PK, Fuster V. Coronary plaque disruption. *Circulation.* 1995;92:657-671.

22. Flugelman MY, Virmani R, Correa R, et al. Smooth muscle cell abundance and fibroblast growth factors in coronary lesions of patients with nonfatal unstable angina. A clue to the mechanism of transformation from the stable to the unstable clinical state. *Circulation.* 1993;88:2493–2500.

23. Bugiardini R, Pozzati A, Borghi A, et al. Angiographic morphology in unstable angina and its relation to transient myocardial ischemia and hospital outcome. *Am J Cardiol.* 1991;67:460–464.

24. McCormick JR, Schick EC Jr, McCabe CH, et al. Determinants of operative mortality and long-term survival in patients with unstable angina. The CASS experience. *J Thorac Cardiovasc Surg.* 1985;89:683–688.

25. Roberts KB, Califf RM, Harrell FE Jr, et al. The prognosis for patients with new-onset angina who have undergone cardiac catheterization. *Circulation.* 1983;68:970–978.

26. Ambrose JA, Winters SL, Stern A, et al. Angiographic morphology and the pathogenesis of unstable angina pectoris. *J Am Coll Cardiol.* 1985;5:609–616.

27. Silva JA, Escobar A, Collins TJ, et al. Unstable angina. A comparison of angioscopic findings between diabetic and nondiabetic patients. *Circulation.* 1995;92:1731–1736.

28. Roberts WC, Virmani R. Quantification of coronary artery narrowing in clinically-isolated unstable angina pectoris. An analysis of 22 necropsy patients. *Am J Med.* 1979;67:792–799.

29. Davies MJ, Thomas AC. Plaque fissuring: the cause of acute myocardial infarction, sudden ischaemic death, and crecendo angina. *Br Heart J.* 1985;53:363–373.

30. Falk E. Unstable angina with fatal outcome: dynamic coronary thrombosis leading to infarction and/or sudden death: autopsy evidence of recurrent mural thrombosis with peripheral embolization culminating in total vascular occlusion. *Circulation.* 1985;71:699–708.

31. Richardson PD, Davies MJ, Born GVR. Influence of plaque configuration and stress distribution on fissuring of coronary atherosclerotic plaques. *Lancet.* 1989;2:941–944.
32. DiSciascio G, Cowley MJ, Goudreau E, et al. Histopathologic correlates of unstable ischemic syndromes in patients undergoing directional coronary atherectomy: *in vivo* evidence of thrombosis, ulceration and inflammation. *Am Heart J.* 1994;128:419–426.
33. Davies MJ, Fulton WFM, Robertson WB. The relation of coronary thrombosis to ischemic myocardial necrosis. *J Pathol.* 1979;127:99–110.
34. Falk E. Plaque rupture with severe pre-existing stenosis precipitating coronary thrombosis: characteristics of coronary atherosclerotic plaques underlying focal occlusive thrombi. *Br Heart J.* 1983;50:127–134.
35. Dewood MA, Spores J, Notske, et al. Prevalence of total coronary occlusion during the early hours of transmural myocardial infarction. *N Engl J Med.* 1980;303:897–902.
36. Farb A, Tang AL, Burke AP, et al. Sudden coronary death frequency of active coronary lesions, inactive coronary lesions, and myocardial infarction. *Circulation.* 1995;92:1701–1709.
37. Kragel AH, Gertz SD, Roberts WC. Morphologic comparison of frequency and types of acute lesions in the major epicardial coronary arteries in unstable angina pectoris, sudden coronary death and acute myocardial infarction. *J Am Coll Cardiol.* 1991;18:801–808.
38. Davies MJ, Richardson PD, Woolf N, et al. Risk of thrombosis in human atherosclerotic plaques: role of extracellular lipid, macrophages, and smooth muscle cell content. *Br Heart J.* 1993;69:377–381.
39. Davies MJ. A macro and micro view of coronary vascular insult in ischemic heart disease. *Circulation.* 1990;82(suppl II):II-38–II-46.
40. Farb A, Burke AP, Tang AL, et al. Coronary plaque erosion without rupture into a lipid core. A frequent cause of coronary thrombosis in sudden coronary death. *Circulation.* 1996;93:1354–1363.
41. Ambrose JA, Tannerbaum MA, Alexopoulos D, et al. Angiographic progression of coronary artery disease and the development of myocardial infarction. *J Am Coll Cardiol.* 1988;12:56–62.
42. Qiao J-H, Fishbein MC. The severity of coronary atherosclerosis at sites of plaque rupture and occlusive thrombosis. *J Am Coll Cardiol.* 1991;17:1138–1142.
43. Davies MJ, Thomas A. Thrombosis and acute coronary artery lesions in sudden cardiac ischemic death. *N Engl J Med.* 1984;310:1134–1140.
44. Warnes CA, Roberts WC. Sudden coronary death: comparison of patients with to those without coronary thrombus at necropsy. *Am J Cardiol.* 1984;54:1206–1211.
45. Burke AP, Farb A, Liang Y-H, et al. The effect of hypertension and cardiac hypertrophy on coronary artery morphology in sudden cardiac death. *Circulation.* 1996 (in press).
46. Gertz SD, Roberts WC. Hemodynamic shear force in rupture of coronary arterial atherosclerotic plaques. *Am J Cardiol.* 1990;66:1368–1372.
47. Van der Wal A, Becker AE, van der Loos CM, Das PK. Site of intimal rupture or erosion of thrombosed coronary atherosclerotic plaques is characterized by an inflammatory process—irrespective of the dominant plaque morphology. *Circulation.* 1994;89:36–44.
48. Lendon CL, Davies MJ, Born GVR, Richardson PD. Atherosclerotic plaque caps are locally weakened when macrophage density is increased. *Atherosclerosis.* 1991;87:87–90.
49. Libby P. Molecular basis of the acute coronary syndromes. *Circulation.* 1995;91:2844–2850.
50. Hansson GK, Holm J, Jonasson L. Detection of activated T-lymphocytes in human atherosclerotic plaque. *Am J Pathol.* 1989;135:169–175.
51. Galis Z, Muszynski M, Sukhova G, et al. Cytokine-stimulated human vascular smooth muscle cells synthesize a complement of enzymes required for extracellular matrix digestion. *Circ Res.* 1994;75:181–189.
52. Galis Z, Sukhova G, Kranzhofer R, et al. Macrophage foam cells from experimental atheroma constitutively produce matrix-degrading proteinases. *Proc Natl Acad Sci USA.* 1995;92:402–406.
53. Shah PK, Falk E, Badimon JJ, et al. Human monocyte-derived macrophages induce collagen breakdown in fibrous caps of atherosclerotic plaques. Potential role of matrix-degrading metalloproteinases and implication for plaque rupture. *Circulation.* 1995;92:1565–1569.
54. Wight TN. Cell biology of arterial proteoglycans. *Arteriosclerosis.* 1989;9:1–20.

55. Busch C, Dawes J, Pepper DS, Wasteson A. Binding of platelet factor 4 to cultured human umbilical vein endothelial cells. *Thromb Res.* 1980;19:129–137.
56. Weiss EJ, Bray PF, Tayback M, et al. A polymorphism of a platelet glycoprotein receptor as an inherited risk factor for coronary thrombosis. *N Engl J Med.* 1996;334:1090–1094.
57. Arnman V, Nilsson A, Stemme S, et al. Expression of plasminogen activator inhibitor-1 mRNA in healthy, atherosclerotic and thrombotic human arteries and veins. *Thromb Res.* 1994;76:478–499.
58. Thompson SG, Kienast J, Pyke SDM, et al. Hemostatic factors and the risk of myocardial infarction or sudden death in patients with angina pectoris. *N Engl J Med.* 1995;332:635–641.
59. Williams JK, Heistad DD. Structure and function of vasa vasorum. *Trends Cardiovasc Med.* 1996;6:53–57.
60. Barger AC, Bienwkes R III, Lainey LL, Silverman KS. Hypothesis: vasa vasorum and neovascularization of human coronary arteries. A possible role in the pathophysiology of atherosclerosis. *N Engl J Med.* 1984;310:175–177.
61. Nikkari ST, O'Brien KD, Ferguson M, et al. Interstitial collagenase (MMP-1). Expression in human carotid atherosclerosis. *Circulation.* 1995;92:1393–1398.

2

Gene Therapy for Treatment of Vascular Disease

James C. Stanley, MD

The ability to define molecular mechanisms that control normal physiologic events and cause pathologic states, as well as the ability to manipulate the genetic control of these phenomena by recombinant deoxyribonucleic acid (DNA) technology, represent the basis of a broad, new form of medicine.[1-6] This subject has only recently been introduced to the surgical community.[7-9] The role of molecular genetics in treating arterial and venous disease, by eliminating or modifying certain risk factors such as hypercholesterolemia, as well as altering specific disease states, such as arteriosclerosis and neointimal hyperplasia, is likely to become of practical importance to the vascular surgeon in the next decade.

MOLECULAR GENETICS

Double-stranded DNA is the substance of the 23 chromosomes located in the nucleus of all somatic cells. DNA regulates cell function by controlling protein synthesis. In fact, all heritable information is defined by the specific molecular content of DNA in the chromosomes' genes.

Four molecules (nucleotides) provide the structure of DNA: two purines, adenine and guanine, and two pyrimidines, thymine and cytosine. These four nucleotides are paired on the two strands of DNA such that an adenine and thymine and a guanine and cytosine are always opposite each other. The couplings of these two nucleotides are known as base pairs (bp). The sequence of the bp defines all encoded genetic information. The usual gene is 2,000 to 3,000 bp in length. This may appear to be a rather large structure, but in fact, there are more than 3 billion bp, or 6 billion of the four individual nucleotide molecules, in the nucleus of each human cell. It is estimated that less than one-fifth of these nucleotides has a direct role in the control of cellular activity, the remaining nucleotides representing genetic material acquired through evolution with no known function in contemporary life.

Transcription is the initial process by which genetic information in DNA begins to be expressed in the cell. DNA, under the influence of the enzyme RNA (ribonucleic acid) polymerase, unwinds to facilitate formation of complementary intermediate messenger RNA (mRNA). This unwinding allows complementary molecules, in a paired fashion, to line up alongside the single strand of DNA. Each nucleotide within the DNA has a pairing with a base molecule on the strand of mRNA, except that uracil is substituted for thymine in the mRNA. Further processing of mRNA causes deletion of certain nucleotide segments, called introns, that are believed to be unimportant. This leaves mRNA segments known as exons, which contain the essential genetic information for protein formation.

Translation is the process by which mRNA initiates protein synthesis. Translation occurs in the cytoplasmic ribosomes where mRNA serves as a template to which specific amino acids become aligned. These amino acids are part of a three-dimensional structure known as transfer RNA (tRNA), which has external exposure of three nucleotides that are complementary to the mRNA nucleotides. A genetic code exists such that a given three-segment nucleotide sequence on tRNA, called a codon, causes alignment on mRNA of one of the 20 amino acid protein building blocks. Sixty-four different arrangements of three segment nucleotide sequences (4^3) exist for the 20 amino acids. Thus, some amino acids have more than one codon. The relationship between the codons and amino acids defines the genetic code (Fig. 2–1). These amino acids, two at a time, subsequently merge to form a polypeptide chain (Fig. 2–2). As this process continues, complex proteins are formed within the cell. Knowledge of a protein's amino acid sequence allows one, with some ambiguities, to work backwards in a complementary fashion through tRNA, to mRNA, and then to the DNA nucleotide sequence that represents the gene construct responsible for a given protein's production. Because certain amino acids have multiple codons it should be apparent that the exact gene nucleotide sequence may be difficult to predict for proteins containing hundreds of amino acids.

1st Nucleotide (5' end)	2nd Nucleotide				3rd Nucleotide (3' end)
	U	**C**	**A**	**G**	
U	Phe	Ser	Tyr	Cys	U
	Phe	Ser	Tyr	Cys	C
	Leu	Ser	-	-	A
	Leu	Ser	-	Trp	G
C	Leu	Pro	His	Arg	U
	Leu	Pro	His	Arg	C
	Leu	Pro	Gln	Arg	A
	Leu	Pro	Gln	Arg	G
A	Ile	Thr	Asn	Ser	U
	Ile	Thr	Asn	Ser	C
	Ile	Thr	Lys	Arg	A
	Met	Thr	Lys	Arg	G
G	Val	Ala	Asp	Gly	U
	Val	Ala	Asp	Gly	C
	Val	Ala	Glu	Gly	A
	Val	Ala	Glu	Gly	G

Figure 2–1. The genetic code. Bases are presented as ribonucleotides (U, uracil; C, cytosine; A, adenine; G, guanine). The 64 possible sequences of the three nucleotide molecules (1st, 2nd, 3rd) encode for the 20 amino acids (abbreviated in the central portion of the figure) in a specific manner.

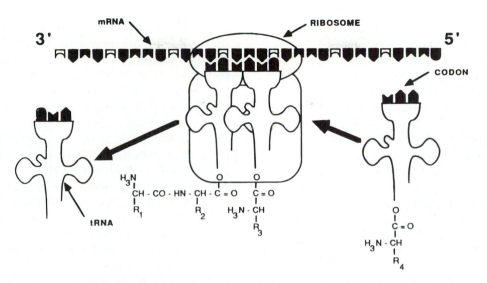

Figure 2–2. Translation. The three-dimensional conformation of the midportion of tRNA specifically provides external exposure of three nucleotides, known collectively as a codon, that associate with mRNA in a complementary fashion. This mRNA–tRNA association occurs on the ribosomes and is restricted to two codons at any one time. This provides approximation of two individual amino acids, and facilitates polymerization and peptide formation. (*Reproduced with permission: Stanley JC, Podrazik RM, Messina LM. Therapeutic potential of genetic engineering on vascular disease. In: Yao JST, Pearce WH, eds. Technologies in Vascular Surgery. Philadelphia: WB Saunders; 1992:57–68.*)

This simple description of cellular protein production, in reality, belies a much more complex process. Regulation of gene expression is under the influence of additional nucleotide sequences of the chromosome called promoters, located proximal to the gene on the DNA, and enhancer regions, located at more remote distances from the gene, both of which bind proteins that facilitate transcription. Furthermore, formation of a transcription complex that positions RNA polymerase at the initiation site of the gene is the result of multiple DNA–protein and protein–protein interaction.

RECOMBINANT DNA TECHNOLOGY

Recombinant DNA technology involves the transfer and recombining of foreign DNA into a host cell's genomic DNA. This allows very small amounts of a specific gene to be removed and inserted into another cell where the cloned gene may be markedly amplified for study or it may produce a protein. Essential to this technology are two important enzymes, restriction endonucleases and ligases, which allow cutting and splicing of nucleotides in a predictable manner. Various agents commonly used in clinical practice, such as insulin, growth hormone, erythropoietin, and tissue-type plasminogen activator (tPA), are produced by recombinant means with gene transfer into prokaryotic cells such as *Escherichia coli* bacteria.

GENE THERAPY

Gene transfer in eukaryotic cells is the basis for human gene therapy. Gene therapy uses a variety of approaches, with most directed toward gene augmentation. This technology has particular application to a subgroup of the nearly 3,500 known genetic diseases having deficiencies in a single specific protein. Gene augmentation may be achieved by placement of genetic material into the cytoplasmic episomes, a process known as gene introduction. The effectiveness of this latter type of gene transfer is limited by the cell's longevity, with cell death terminating any effect of such therapy. A second method of gene augmentation is by placement of foreign genetic material directly into the host chromosome through a process known as gene insertion. This approach has the potential therapeutic effect of being passed on to the progeny of the transduced cell and holds a distinct advantage if stem cells are the recipients of the new genetic material. The current status of gene insertion does not involve specific site-directed insertion, although specific placement of a foreign gene within the host genome is possible and likely to occur as the science of this technology progresses.[10]

Genetic material may be introduced into eukaryotic cells by techniques using physical or chemical means, fusion carriers, and viral transport. Electroporation, for example, uses electrical currents to facilitate transfer across cellular membranes.[11,12] Various agents such as calcium phosphate or diethylaminoethyl dextran achieve a similar transfer of genetic materials into cells.[13,14] Direct microinjection of DNA, with or without its attachment to microprojectiles,[15-17] also permits introduction of DNA.

Genetic material may also be inserted into eukaryotic cells by the process of transfection using a number of viral vectors. An important development was the use of appropriate murine and avian retroviruses for the transfer of genetic material.[18-20] These RNA viruses enter the cell's cytoplasm where they act as a template for reverse transcription of the genetic information within the virus to form complementary viral DNA. This process is initiated by reverse transcriptase that is incorporated within the viral particle. The newly formed viral DNA then is integrated into the host genome as a provirus, where it may be expressed in protein production. Genetic information up to 7,000 base molecules in length may be inserted into the host DNA using retroviral carriers. This usually occurs in dividing cells. Insertion of genes into retroviral carriers has provided the basis for gene transfer in many contemporary experiments.

The nucleotides within the normal wild retrovirus contain sequences essential for the production of core proteins (the *gag* region), reverse transcriptase and ligase (the *pol* region), and other capsule glycoproteins (the *env* region). A ψ segment facilitates later encapsidation of viral RNA into an infective particle. Long terminal repeat (LTR) segments at either end of the central genes within the provirus are necessary for the integration and expression of proviral DNA within the host cell (Fig. 2–3). A virus must be able to replicate itself when used for gene therapy. Thus recombinant retroviral particles are constructed with only enough native sequences to allow encapsidation and later integration. The removal and insertion of this genetic material is undertaken by conventional DNA cutting and splicing techniques. Under most circumstances, there

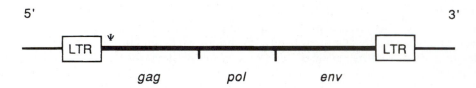

Figure 2–3. Wild retroviral provirus genome. Genes for core proteins (*gag*), reverse transcriptase and ligase (*pol*), and outer capsule glycoproteins (*env*) are preceded by the encapsidation signal ψ and flanked by LTR segments. (*Reproduced with permission: Stanley JC, Podrazik RM, Messina LM. Therapeutic potential of genetic engineering on vascular disease. In: Yao JST, Pearce WH, eds. Technologies in Vascular Surgery. Philadelphia: WB Saunders; 1992:57–68.*)

is a deletion of a considerable portion of native viral genome encoding for the proteins necessary for duplication of the virus. This renders the recombinant viral particles replication incompetent (Fig. 2–4). Most techniques of inserting foreign DNA using retroviruses into host DNA are very inefficient. Insertion of the neomycin resistance gene, a phosphotransferase gene, transmits cellular protection to the cytocidal antimicrobial agent G418. When this gene is inserted individually or in a cassette fashion with other genes, and the cells are exposed to G418 *in vitro*, only those that were successfully transduced survive. This provides a means of selecting only those cells carrying the new genetic material.

Integration of the retrovirus-initiated complementary viral DNA strand as a provirus occurs at random sites within the host genome. Existing technology using retroviral vectors usually leads to insertion of multiple gene copies into the host genome, with their subsequent expression being unregulated. Such unregulated protein production is called constitutive expression. Single copy integration is more likely to occur with use of retroviral carriers. Although random integration and constitutive expression of genetic material represents the current state of recombinant DNA technology involving gene transfer, site-specific insertion and regulated expression are feasible.

Adenoviruses have also proven to be efficient vectors for gene transfer. Adenoviruses can carry up to 30,000 base molecules into a host cell, considerably more than can be transferred by retroviruses. Furthermore, unlike with retroviral vectors, cells need not divide for successful gene transfer with adenoviral vectors to occur. Nevertheless, a number of investigations have documented increased gene transfer and expression in tissues that are in a state of proliferation.[21,22] Similar findings have been observed with simple liposome-mediated gene transfer to arterial tissues.[23,24] A disadvantage of the adenoviruses is that they transport the new genetic material into the cytoplasm and not into the chromosomes of recipient cells. The DNA within the cytoplasm is subject to enzymatic degradation, thus limiting the duration of new gene expression. Similarly, an immune-related inflammatory response may lessen ongoing gene expression, especially after repeated transfections.[25] Schulick and his colleagues[26] demonstrated that certain adenoviral concentrations exist that provide for successful transduction without high-titer viral-related infectious toxicity. Adeno-associated viruses are a third type of viral vector that may be used for integration of new genetic material into the genome of nondividing cells. These small DNA viruses have a predilection to insert in chromosome 19.

Lipofection is a form of gene transfer that involves encapsidation of DNA within a polycationic liposome. The latter fuses with membranes of target cells and allows transfer of the new genetic material into the cytoplasm.[27,28] Although issues of immunity do not accompany liposome-mediated transduction to the same degree as exists with

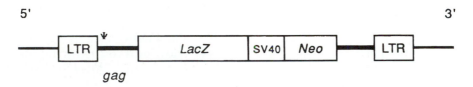

Figure 2–4. Retroviral vector. Replacement of the majority of *gap*, *pol*, and *env* regions by genes for β-galactosidase (*lacZ*), neomycin resistance (Neo), and the simian virus (SV-40) early promoter. This represents the BAG (β-galactosidase at *gag*) vector. (*Reproduced with permission: Stanley JC, Podrazik RM, Messina LM. Therapeutic potential of genetic engineering on vascular disease. In: Yao JST, Pearce WH, eds. Technologies in Vascular Surgery. Philadelphia: WB Saunders; 1992:57–68.*)

adenoviral vectors, liposomes are much less effective than the latter viruses in gene transfer to the arterial wall.[29]

Recombination of foreign DNA into host DNA of humans is the foundation of gene therapy. The conceptual simplicity of molecular genetics, using recombinant DNA technology as a means of producing new cellular proteins, makes it attractive for application in numerous clinical settings. Genetic modification of the vasculature, especially endothelium and smooth muscle, has been successfully accomplished in both *in vitro* and *in vivo* experiments by a number of investigators.

ENDOTHELIAL CELL GENE TRANSFER

Endothelial cells represent an ideal target for transfer of recombinant genes encoding for therapeutic proteins. The target population is enormous, with existence of an estimated 6×10^{13} endothelial cells in adults. Endothelial cells exist in different vascular environments ranging from the major conduits to the microcirculation. Genetically engineered endothelial cells could be placed in either milieu, by seeding the cells onto a vessel or graft, as well as directly into the microcirculation. Two strategies for gene augmentation have been employed: (1) *in vitro* gene transfer, with subsequent reintroduction of the modified endothelial cells by seeding of vessels, vascular grafts, or direct injection into a tissue bed; and (2) *in vivo* site-specific gene transfer using lipofection or viral vectors. A survey of select studies performed by a number of investigators reveals the current state of vascular tissue as a target for gene therapy.

Zwiebel and colleagues[30] at NIH in 1989 were among the first investigators to successfully transfer functioning genes to endothelial cells. They documented expression of gene encoding for neomycin resistance, human adenosine deaminase (ADA), and rat growth hormone in cultured rabbit aortic endothelial cells. In a subset of these experiments, the transduced endothelial cells were grown in culture on silicone-coated polyurethane vascular prostheses. Recombinant growth hormone continued to be secreted by these cells for at least 4 weeks. Zwiebel, in a second study, demonstrated that human umbilical vein endothelial cells were also capable of expressing recombinant genes for neomycin resistance and for human ADA.[31]

In 1989, Nabel and her colleagues[32] documented recombinant gene expression by endothelial cells transduced with the *lacZ* and necomycin resistance genes using a retroviral vector following their placement within iliofemoral arteries of Yucatan minipigs. Arterial tissues examined up to 4 weeks following transplantation of these transduced endothelial cells demonstrated β-galactosidase production, particularly along luminal surface cells. No β-galactosidase activity was observed in control iliac artery segments seeded with nontransduced cells. Conte et al.[33] reported in 1994 similar findings with retroviral-transduced endothelial cells with the *lacZ* gene that were seeded on denuded rabbit carotid arteries.

In a second series of *in vivo* experiments, Nabel and her colleagues[34] documented site-specific gene expression for as long as 21 weeks following direct retroviral-mediated *lacZ* gene transfer in minipig iliac arteries. Optimal expression occurred between 2 and 3 months after transfection, occurring within all three vessel wall layers. Expression was absent from sham-infected control segments. In the same report, they also documented direct DNA transfection using liposomes, with similar site-specific *lacZ* gene expression occurring for up to 6 weeks. Flugelman,[35] in Dichek's laboratory, reported that brief retroviral exposures of 1 minute by balloon-directed delivery to the arterial wall were inadequate to allow therapeutic amounts of gene transfer.

In 1989, Wilson and his colleagues[36] reported on an *in vivo* canine experience with porous carotid artery interposition Dacron grafts that had been seeded with *lac*Z-transduced endothelial cells. Graft examined up to 5 weeks postimplantation revealed β-galactosidase activity in the seeded cells and their progeny. Recently, transfected cells have been seeded on a number of graft substrates, including expanded polytetra-fluoroethylene (PTFE) thoracoabdominal grafts in dogs by Baer[37] and the Michigan group. In the latter studies expression of β-galactosidase was evident in cells harvested from explanted grafts 6 weeks postseeding (Figs. 2–5, 2–6, and 2–7), although the extent of surface area coverage was less with seeding of transduced cells, compared to nontransduced cells. Similar findings of less stable adherence and proliferation of retroviral-transduced endothelial cells seeded on both Dacron and PTFE grafts were reported in 1995 by Sackman and her colleagues.[38]

In 1989, Dichek and his colleagues[39] transferred genes encoding for the production of β-galactosidase and human tPA into cultured sheep endothelial cells that were subsequently seeded onto stainless steel stents. In these studies, β-galactosidase activity was evident in the covering cells. Measurements of tPA in the culture media used to incubate the stents confirmed that the transduced cells were producing the protein at very high levels, up to 400 times the normal rate.

Yao and colleagues[40] in 1991 transduced capillary endothelial cells with a Molony murine leukemia virus-derived retroviral vector that contained the human factor IX cDNA linked to a heterologous promoter and the neomycin resistance gene. These cells expressed recombinant human factor IX that showed full clotting activity. This suggested that capillary endothelial cells were efficient targets for constitutive production of factor IX.

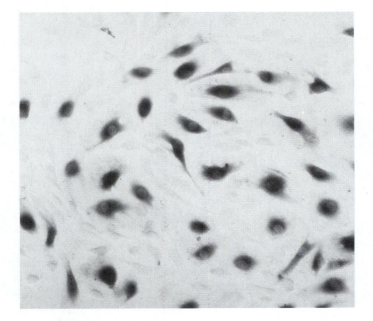

Figure 2–5. Endothelial cells transfected with the *lac*Z gene, recovered from an ePTFE graft 6 weeks after implantation in the dog, expressing β-galactosidase (dark cytoplastic material). (X-gal stain, ×300.) (*Reproduced with permission: Stanley JC, Podrazik RM, Messina LM. Therapeutic potential of genetic engineering on vascular disease. In: Yao JST, Pearce WH, eds. Technologies in Vascular Surgery. Philadelphia: WB Saunders; 1992:57–68.*)

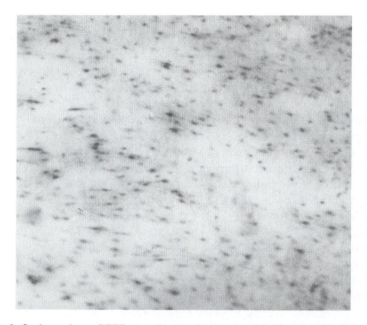

Figure 2–6. Surface of an ePTFE vascular prosthesis removed 6 weeks after being seeded with selected endothelial cells transfected with the *lacZ* and neomycin resistance genes. The dark areas represent cells containing β-galactosidase as a consequence of successful gene transfer. (X-gal stain, ×30.) (*Reproduced with permission: Stanley JC, Podrazik RM, Messina LM. Therapeutic potential of genetic engineering on vascular disease. In: Yao JST, Pearce WH, eds. Technologies in Vascular Surgery. Philadelphia: WB Saunders; 1992:57–68.*)

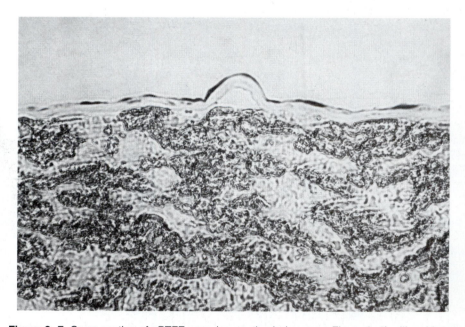

Figure 2–7. Cross-section of ePTFE vascular prosthesis (same as Figure 2–6) with evidence of a luminal monolayer of transduced endothelial cells exhibiting production of β-galactosidase. (X-gal stain, ×200.) (*Reproduced with permission: Stanley JC, Podrazik RM, Messina LM. Therapeutic potential of genetic engineering on vascular disease. In: Yao JST, Pearce WH, eds. Technologies in Vascular Surgery. Philadelphia: WB Saunders; 1992:57–68.*)

Direct liposome-mediated *in vivo* gene transfer into canine carotid and femoral arteries was demonstrated by Lim in 1991.[41] Using a luciferase gene in a lipfectin vector, femoral arterial segments were transfected using a double-balloon catheter technique. Luciferase activity was evident in the exposed vessels. This technology was later demonstrated to be equally effective in the coronary arteries of dogs using a porous percutaneous balloon catheter.

Podrazik and her colleagues[42] in 1992 demonstrated expression of recombinant human tPA in adult canine venous endothelial cells using a highly infective MFG retroviral vector. Longer initially retroviral exposures resulted in greater expression, and confluent cell monolayers expressed more human tPA than those that were in log phase growth. In 1995, Ekhterae and Stanley,[43] using a similar vector, reported successful transfer and expression of the human tPA gene in both human endothelial cells and smooth muscle cells.

Lemarchand and coinvestigators[44] in 1992 used replication-deficient adenoviral vectors containing the *lac*Z and α_1-antitrypsin genes to transduce primary human umbilical vein endothelial cells in cultures, as well as intact human umbilical veins. The first methodology permitted detailed evaluation of *in vitro* gene expression, and the latter represented a model of *in vivo* gene transfer where the vascular architecture was as close to native tissue as possible. These studies demonstrated that gene transfer mediated by replication-deficient adenoviral vectors was feasible in human endothelium. Lemarchand[45] in 1993 reported successful *in vivo* adenoviral-mediated transfer and expression of the *lac*Z and α_1-antitrypsin genes in isolated segments of sheep jugular veins and carotid arteries. Gene products were evident at 14 days in this study, but not as 28 days post-transduction.

Losordo et al.[46] and Takeshita et al.[47] from Isner's group in 1994 noted that gene expression may be of a much greater magnitude than anatomic analysis of transfection efficiency might suggest. Thus, caution should be taken in estimating the potential for a secreted gene product simply based on immunostaining or other means of identifying transfected cells.

Steg et al.[48] in 1994 used a gel containing nuclear-targeted *lac*Z gene adenoviral construct with a balloon delivery device and noted more than a fourfold increase in gene delivery in rabbit iliac arteries when compared to a gene delivery with double balloon catheter systems. In a similar study, March et al.[49] in 1995 reported a tenfold increase in adenoviral-mediated *lac*Z transduction of vascular smooth muscle cells (SMCs) in culture when exposed to a viscous polyol (poloxamer 407).

The potential for gene transfer to diseased arteries has been explored in arteriosclerotic vessels. Landau and associates[21] in 1995 examined adenoviral-mediated *lac*Z gene transfer in arteriosclerotic rabbit iliac arteries using a variety of catheter-based delivery systems, with gene expression being greatest in regions of the vessel contributing most to cellular proliferation. However, Feldman and colleagues[50] reported in 1995 a tenfold decrease in *lac*Z gene expression in adenoviral-transfected arteriosclerotic rabbit iliac arteries compared to normal arteries, raising the question of a potential limitation to adenoviral-based gene therapy in arteriosclerotic vessels. The issue of gene transfer to arteriosclerotic vessels remains ill defined.

The role of gene transfer to capillary endothelium in skeletal muscle and the lung deserves special note. In 1992 Messina and his colleagues[51] demonstrated that the untreated capillary bed of skeletal muscle was a good recipient site into which autologous *ex vivo lac*Z-transduced endothelial cell could be transplanted. They first demonstrated that *lac*Z-transduced, seeded endothelial cells became incorporated into confluent monolayers *in vitro* (Fig. 2–8). In an *in vivo* model, transduced endothelial cells

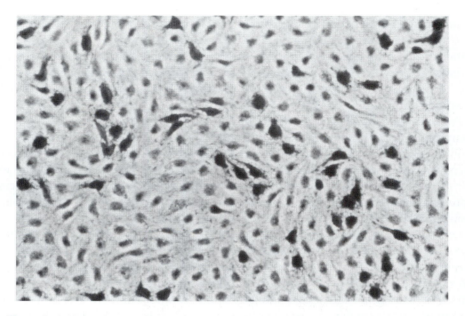

Figure 2–8. Light micrograph of incorporated, *lac*Z-transduced endothelial cells (dark cells) 72 hours after being seeded onto a monolayer of nontransduced cultured endothelium (light cells). (X-gal stain, ×220.) (*Reproduced with permission: Messina LM, Podrazik RM, Whitehill TA, et al. Adhesion and incorporation of lacZ-transduced endothelial cells into the intact capillary wall in the rat. Proc Natl Acad Sci USA. 1992;89:12018–12022.*)

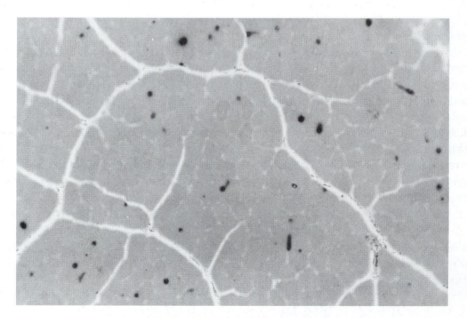

Figure 2–9. Light micrograph of an X-gal–stained cross-section of rat tibialis anterior muscles. Transduced, *lac*Z expressing cells are in numerous capillaries (dark cells) 1 hour after intra-arterial injections (×90.) (*Reproduced with permission: Messina LM, Podrazik RM, Whitehill TA, et al. Adhesion and incorporation of lacZ-transduced endothelial cells into the intact capillary wall in the rat. Proc Natl Acad Sci USA. 1992;89:12018–12022.*)

adhered to, and in certain instances, became incorporated into the capillary wall (Fig. 2–9). This study supported the use of the intact capillary bed as a promising target for transplantation of genetically modified autogenous endothelial cells for human gene therapy. Schachtner et al.[52] in 1994 and Muller et al.[53] in 1995 reported successful adenoviral-mediated gene transfer into the pulmonary arteries, delivering the human placental alkaline phosphatase in a porcine model and nuclear-targeted *lacZ* in a rat model, respectively. The potential applications of this technology relate to therapy of both primary pulmonary pathology as well as thromboembolic diseases.

Isner and his colleagues[54] have undertaken a number of studies using vascular endothelial growth factor (VEGF) to enhance capillary and collateral circulation development. They have been granted approval to pursue this approach in humans with severe extremity ischemia due to nonreconstructable arterial occlusive disease.

VASCULAR SMOOTH MUSCLE CELL GENE TRANSFER

Vascular smooth muscle (VSM) cells play an important role in the pathogenesis of arterial occlusive lesions. Genetic modification of these cells may lead to a decreased incidence of anastomotic neointimal hyperplasia, and possibly a decreased incidence of late atherosclerosis.

In 1991, Plautz and his colleagues[55] described the transfer of genetically modified VSM to localized segments of the arterial wall. Enzymatically derived VSM cells from Yucatan minipigs were transduced with a retroviral vector containing the *lacZ* gene and implanted into denuded iliofemoral arterial segments of pigs using a double balloon catheter. Explanted arterial segments demonstrated β-galactosidase activity throughout the intimal and media up to 11 days postimplantation. This report followed their findings, published in 1990, of site-specific *lacZ* gene expression by direct transfer using lipofection.

In 1992, Lynch et al.[56] used a recombinant retroviral vector to deliver the human ADA gene into rat VSM. Transduced cells were seeded into the distal segment of common carotid arteries. Expression of human ADA in the seeded segments was measured at intervals up to 6 months, but was not evident outside the seeded regions. In a total of 29 test animals, 26 expressed human ADA at levels from 5% to 50% of the total ADA activity. In another study, Lynch and colleagues attempted to carry out direct intraluminal transection using a double balloon catheter technique with retroviruses containing either the *lacZ* or human ADA genes. They were unable to detect direct gene transfer *in situ*, even when the transfection was performed at the time of maximal cellular replication after balloon catheter injury. In 1994, Clowes et al.[57] in the same laboratory, documented that SMCs transfected with the ADA or alkaline phosphatase genes and transplanted into rat carotid arteries did not become transformed and exhibited no ongoing replication.

Lee et al.[58] reported site-specific adenoviral-mediated *lacZ* gene transfer in balloon-injured rat carotid arteries in 1993. β-galactosidase expression was present at 7 days, but declined by 14 days. Approximately 30% of the medial SMCs at the site of injection were transduced. Geary et al.[59] reported in 1994 successful implantation onto ePTFE grafts of SMCs that had been transfected with retroviruses containing the *lacZ* gene. These cells remained in the graft and did not contribute to the neointima or outer capsule tissues. Takeshita et al.,[24] in Isner's laboratory, reported that liposome-mediated transfer of luciferase gene was augmented by the presence of ongoing cellular proliferation, as would be expected to occur in denuded arteries.

In 1994 Ohno et al.[60] from the Nabel laboratory transferred the herpes virus thymidine kinase gene (ADV-tk) using an adenoviral vector to porcine arterial intimal and medial cells that were proliferating following a balloon injury. The thymidine kinase enzyme phosphorylates gancyclovir, which subsequently becomes incorporated into the DNA of dividing cells, inducing chain termination and cell death. The animals were treated with gancyclovir for 6 days, and 3 weeks later a 54% to 87% reduction occurred in intimal hyperplasia that characterized the balloon-injured arteries in nontreated animals. Chang et al.,[61] from the same investigative group, in 1995 reported inhibited smooth muscle proliferation and reduction in neointimal thickening after balloon injury of the rat carotid artery using similar thymidine kinase gene transfer. Similar results had been reported by Guzman et al.[62] in 1994 using an adenoviral vector to transfer the thymidine kinase gene to both SMCs *in vitro* as well as injured rat carotid arteries, followed by treatment with gancyclovir.

Von der Leyen et al.[63] from Dzau's laboratory provided direct evidence in 1995 that transfection of injured rat carotid arteries with the nitric oxide synthetase gene using a Sendai virus–liposome technique decreased neointimal formation 70% by day 14. Morishita et al.,[64] from the same laboratory, a year earlier demonstrated that growth of endothelial cells and VSM cells *in vitro* was inhibited by HVJ viral-mediated transfer of the atrial natiuretic peptide gene.

In 1995 Chang and coworkers[65] from Nabel's laboratory and Leiden's laboratory demonstrated that both *in vitro* proliferation of rat aortic smooth muscle and *in vivo* proliferation of smooth muscle in the injured rat carotid artery and porcine femoral artery were inhibited by adenoviral-mediated transfer of the retinoblastoma gene.

GENE THERAPY AND VASCULAR DISEASE RISK FACTORS

Reduction of risk factors contributing to cardiovascular disease is a relevant goal of molecular genetic and gene therapy. Hyperlipidemic disorders, hypertension, and diabetes mellitus are targets of these efforts. Perhaps the factors best studied relate to elevated cholesterol and accelerated arteriosclerosis.

Familial hypercholesterolemia due to structural and functional low-density lipoprotein (LDL) receptors, especially in homozygotes, contributes to premature cardiovascular disease and death. Genetic engineering with restoration of LDL receptor activity toward normal may lessen the known complications affecting these patients.[66] Wilson and his colleagues[67–69] used a retroviral vector to insert the human LDL receptor gene into hepatocytes with preexisting defective receptors, with a resultant effect of returning cholesterol metabolism toward normal.[69] Similar outcomes in a human with familial hypercholesterolemia were reported in 1994 by the same investigators.[70]

The Human Genome Project, which will map and sequence the entire human genome, will define many heretofore unknown messages encoded in our DNA.[71] Knowledge derived from this monumental task will provide major incentives for human gene therapy. Although considerable progress in vascular gene transfer has occurred, substantial technical issues remain that must be addressed by investigators before this technology enters the clinical arena.[1,72]

REFERENCES

1. Crystal RG. Transfer of genes to humans: early lesions and obstacles to success. *Science.* 1995;270:404–410.

2. Finkel T, Epstein SE. Gene therapy for vascular disease. *FASEB J.* 1995;9:843–851.

3. Friedmann T. Progress toward human gene therapy. *Science.* 1989;244:1275–1281.

4. Hood L. Biotechnology and medicine of the future. *JAMA.* 1988;259:1837–1844.

5. Milligan RC. The basic science of gene therapy. *Science.* 1993;260:926–932.

6. Morsy MA, Mitani K, Clemens P, Caskey CT. Progress toward human gene therapy. *JAMA.* 1993;270:2338–2345.

7. Brown JM, Harken AH, Sharefkin JB. Recombination DNA and surgery. *Ann Surg.* 1990;212:178–186.

8. Rowland RT, Cleveland JC, Meng X, et al. Potential gene therapy strategies in the treatment of cardiovascular disease. *Ann Thorac Surg.* 1995;60:721–728.

9. Wong TS, Passaro E Jr. DNA technology. *Am J Surg.* 1990;159:610–614.

10. Doetschman T, Gregg RG, Maeda N, et al. Targeted correction of a mutant HPRT gene in mouse embryonic stem cells. *Nature.* 1987;330:576–578.

11. Potter H, Weir L, Leder P. Enhancer-dependent expression of human k immunoglobulin genes introduced into mouse pre-B lymphocytes by electroporation. *Proc Natl Acad Sci USA.* 1984;81:7161–7165.

12. Kotnis RA, Thompson MM, Eady SL, et al. Optimisation of gene transfer into vascular endothelial cells using electroporation. *Eur J Vasc Endovasc Surg.* 1995;9:71–79.

13. Graham FL, van der Eb AJ. A new technique for the assay of infectivity of human adenovirus 5 DNA. *Virology.* 1973;52:456–467.

14. Lopata MA, Cleveland DW, Sollner-Webb B. High level transient expression of a chloramphenicol acetyl transferase gene by DEAE-dextran mediated DNA transfection coupled with a dimethyl sulfoxide or glycerol shock treatment. *Nucleic Acids Res.* 1984;12:5707–5717.

15. Capecchi MR. High efficiency transformation by direct microinjection of DNA into cultured mammalian cells. *Cell.* 1980;22:479–488.

16. Klein TM, Wolf ED, Wu R, Sanford JC. High-velocity microprojectiles for delivering nucleic acids into living cells. *Nature.* 1987;327:70–93.

17. Wolff JA, Malone RW, Williams P, et al. Direct gene transfer into mouse muscle *in vivo*. *Science.* 1990;247:1465–1468.

18. Cepko CL, Roberts BE, Mulligan RC. Construction and applications of a highly transmissible murine retrovirus shuttle vector. *Cell.* 1984;37:1053–1062.

19. Danos O, Mulligan RC. Safe and efficient generation of recombinant retroviruses with amphotropic and ecotropic host ranges. *Proc Natl Acad Sci USA.* 1988;85:6460–6464.

20. Tabin CJ, Hoffmann JW, Goff SP, Weinberg RA. Adaptation of a retrovirus as a eucaryotic vector transmitting the herpes simplex virus thymidine kinase gene. *Mol Cell Biol.* 1982;2:426–436.

21. Landau C, Pirwitz MJ, Willard MA, et al. Adenoviral mediated gene therapy transfer to atherosclerotic arteries after balloon angioplasty. *Am Heart J.* 1995;129:1051–1057.

22. Yao A, Wang DH. Heterogeneity of adenovirus-mediated gene transfer in cultured thoracic aorta and renal artery of rats. *Hypertension.* 1995;26:1046–1050.

23. Pickering JG, Jekanowski J, Weir L, et al. Liposome-mediated gene transfer into human vascular smooth cells. *Circulation.* 1994;89:13–21.

24. Takeshita S, Gal D, Leclerc G, et al. Increased gene expression after liposome-mediated arterial gene transfer associated with intimal smooth muscle cell proliferation. *In vitro* and *in vivo* findings in a rabbit model of vascular injury. *J Clin Invest.* 1994;93:652–661.

25. Ueno H, Li JJ, Tomita H, et al. Quantitative analysis of repeat adenovirus-mediated gene transfer into injured canine femoral arteries. *Arterioscler Thromb Vasc Biol.* 1995;15:2246–2253.

26. Schulick AH, Newman KD, Virmani R, Dichek DA. *In vivo* gene transfer into injured carotid arteries. Optimization and evaluation of acute toxicity. *Circulation.* 1995;91:2407–2414.

27. Felger PL, Gadek TR, Holm M, et al. Lipofection: a highly efficient, lipid-mediated DNA-transfection procedure. *Proc Natl Acad Sci USA.* 1987;84:7423.

28. Fraley R, Straubinger RM, Rule G, et al. Liposome-mediated delivery of deoxyribonucleic acid to cells: enhanced efficiency of delivery related to lipid composition and incubation conditions. *Biochemistry.* 1981;20:6978–6987.

29. French BA, Mazur W, Ali NM, et al. Percutaneous transluminal *in vivo* gene transfer by recombinant adenovirus in normal porcine coronary arteries, atherosclerotic arteries, and two models of coronary restenosis. *Circulation.* 1994;90:2402–2413.

30. Zwiebel JA, Freeman SM, Kantoff PW, et al. High-level recombinant gene expression in rabbit endothelial cells transduced by retroviral vectors. *Science.* 1989;243:220–222.

31. Zwiebel JA, Freeman SM, Cornetta K, et al. Recombinant gene expression in human umbilical vein endothelial cells transduced by retroviral vectors. *Biochem Biophys Res Comm.* 1990;170: 209–213.

32. Nabel EG, Plautz G, Boyce FM, et al. Recombinant gene expression *in vivo* within endothelial cells of the arterial wall. *Science.* 1989;244:1342–1344.

33. Conte MS, Birinyi LK, Miyata T, et al. Efficient repopulation of denuded rabbit arteries with autologous genetically modified endothelial cells. *Circulation.* 1994;89:2161–2169.

34. Nabel EG, Plautz G, Nabel GJ. Site-gene expression *in vivo* by direct gene transfer into the arterial wall. *Science.* 1990;249:1285–1288.

35. Flugelman MY, Jaklitsch MT, Newman KD, et al. Low level *in vivo* gene transfer into the arterial wall through a perforated balloon catheter. *Circulation.* 1991;85:1110–1117.

36. Wilson JM, Birinyi LK, Salomon RN, et al. Implantation of vascular grafts lined with genetically modified endothelial cells. *Science.* 1989;244:1344–1346.

37. Baer RP, Whitehill TE, Sarkar R, et al. Retroviral-mediated transduction of endothelial cells with the *lacZ* gene impairs cellular proliferation *in vitro* and graft endothelialization *in vivo.* *J Vas Surg.* 1996 (in press).

38. Sackman JE, Freeman MB, Peterson MG, et al. Synthetic vascular grafts seeded with genetically modified endothelium in the dog: evaluation of the effect of seeding technique and retroviral vector on cell persistence *in vivo. Cell Transplant.* 1995;4:219–235.

39. Dichek DA, Neville RF, Zwiebel JA, et al. Seeding of intravascular stents with genetically engineered endothelial cells. *Circulation.* 1989;80:1347–1353.

40. Yao S, Wilson JM, Nabel EG, et al. Expression of human factor IX in rat capillary endothelial cells: toward somatic gene therapy for hemophilia B. *Proc Natl Acad Sci USA.* 1991;88:8101–8105.

41. Lim CS, Chapman GD, Gammon RS, et al. Direct *in vivo* gene transfer into the coronary and peripheral vasculatures of the intact dog. *Circulation.* 1991;83:2007–2011.

42. Podrazik RM, Whitehill TA, Ekhterae D, et al. High-level expression of recombinant human tPA in cultivated canine endothelial cells under varying conditions of retroviral gene transfer. *Ann Surg.* 1992;216:446–453.

43. Ekhterae D, Stanley JC. Retroviral vector-mediated transfer and expression of human tissue plasminogen activator gene in human endothelial and vascular smooth muscle cells. *J Vasc Surg.* 1995;21:953–962.

44. Lemarchand P, Jaffe HA, Dnel C, et al. Adenovirus-mediated transfer of a recombinant human α_1-antitrypsin cDNA to human endothelial cells. *Proc Natl Acad Sci USA.* 1992;89:6482–6486.

45. Lemarchand P, Jones M, Yamada I, Crystal RG. *In vivo* gene transfer and expression in normal uninjured blood vessels using replication-deficient recombinant adenovirus vectors. *Circ Res.* 1993;72:1132–1138.

46. Losordo DW, Pickering JG, Takeshita S, et al. Use of the rabbit ear artery to serially assess foreign protein secretion after site-specific arterial gene transfer *in vivo.* Evidence that anatomic identification of successful gene transfer may underestimate the potential magnitude of transgene expression. *Circulation.* 1994;89:785–792.

47. Takeshita S, Losordo DW, Kearney M, et al. Time course of recombinant protein secretion after liposome-mediated gene transfer in a rabbit arterial organ culture model. *Lab Invest.* 1994;71:387–391.

48. Steg PG, Feldman LJ, Scoazec JY, et al. Arterial gene transfer to rabbit endothelial and smooth muscle cells using percutaneous delivery of an adenoviral vector. *Circulation.* 1994;90:1648–1656.

49. March KL, Madison JE, Trapnell BC. Pharmacokinetics of adenoviral vector-mediated gene delivery to vascular smooth muscle cells: modulation by poloxamer 407 and implications for cardiovascular gene therapy. *Hum Gene Ther.* 1995;6:41–53.

50. Feldman LJ, Steg PG, Zheng LP, et al. Low-efficiency of percutaneous adenovirus-mediated arterial gene transfer in the arteriosclerotic rabbit. *J Clin Invest.* 1995;95:2662–2671.

51. Messina LM, Podrazik RM, Whitehill TA, et al. Adhesion and incorporation of *lacZ*-transduced endothelial cells into the intact capillary wall in the rat. *Proc Natl Acad Sci USA.* 1992;89:12018–12022.

52. Schachtner SK, Rome JJ, Hoyt RF Jr, et al. *In vivo* adenovirus-mediated gene transfer via the pulmonary artery of rats. *Circ Res.* 1995;76:701–709.

53. Muller DW, Gordon D, San H, et al. Catheter-mediated pulmonary vascular gene transfer and expression. *Circ Res.* 1994;75:1039–1049.

54. Isner JM, Walsh K, Symes J, et al. Arterial gene therapy for therapeutic angiogenesis in patients with peripheral artery disease. *Circulation.* 1995;91:2687–2692.

55. Plautz G, Nabel EG, Nabel GJ. Introduction of vascular smooth muscle cells expressing recombinant genes *in vivo*. *Circulation.* 1991;83:578–583.

56. Lynch CM, Clowes MM, Osborne WRA, et al. Long-term expression of human adenosine deaminase in vascular smooth muscle cells of rats: a model for gene therapy. *Proc Natl Acad Sci USA.* 1992;89:1138–1142.

57. Clowes MM, Lynch CM, Miller AD, et al. Long-term biological response of injured rat carotid artery seeded with smooth muscle cells expressing retrovirally introduced human genes. *J Clin Invest.* 1994;93:644–651.

58. Lee SW, Trapnell BC, Rade JJ, et al. *In vivo* adenoviral vector-mediated gene transfer into balloon-injured rat carotid arteries. *Circ Res.* 1993;73:797–807.

59. Geary RL, Clowes AW, Lau S, et al. Gene transfer in baboons using prosthetic vascular grafts seeded with retrovirally transduced smooth muscle cells: a model for local and systemic gene therapy. *Hum Gene Ther.* 1994;5:1211–1216.

60. Ohno T, Gordon D, San H, et al. Gene therapy for vascular smooth muscle cell proliferation after arterial injury. *Science.* 1994;265:781–784.

61. Chang MW, Ohno T, Gordon D, et al. Adenovirus-mediated transfer of the herpes simplex virus thymidine kinase gene inhibits vascular smooth muscle cell proliferation and neointima formation following balloon angioplasty of the rat carotid artery. *Mol Med.* 1995;1:172–181.

62. Guzman RJ, Hirschowitz EA, Brody SL, et al. *In vivo* suppression of injury-induced vascular smooth muscle cell accumulation using adenovirus-mediated transfer of the herpes simplex virus thymidine kinase gene. *Proc Natl Acad Sci USA.* 1994;91:10732–10736.

63. von der Leyen HE, Gibbons GH, Morishita R, et al. Gene therapy inhibiting neointimal vascular lesion: *in vivo* transfer of endothelial cell nitric oxide synthase gene. *Proc Natl Acad Sci USA.* 1995;92:1137–1141.

64. Morishita R, Gibbons GH, Pratt RE, et al. Autocrine and paracrine effects of atrial natriuretic peptide gene transfer on vascular smooth muscle and endothelial cellular growth. *J Clin Invest.* 1994;94:824–829.

65. Chang MW, Barr E, Seltzer J, et al. Cytostatic gene therapy for vascular proliferative disorders with a constitutively active form of the retinoblastoma gene product. *Science.* 1995;267: 518–522.

66. Wilson JM, Chowdhury JR. Prospects for gene therapy of familial hypercholesterolemia. *Mol Biol Med.* 1990;6:223–232.

67. Wilson JM, Chowdhury NR, Grossman M, et al. Temporary amelioration of hyperlipidemia in LDL receptor-deficient rabbits transplanted with genetically modified hepatocytes. *Proc Natl Acad Sci USA.* 1990;87:8437–8441.

68. Wilson JM, Jefferson DM, Chowdhury JR, et al. Retrovirus-mediated transduction of adult hepatocytes. *Proc Natl Acad Sci USA.* 1988;85:3014–3018.

69. Wilson JM, Johnston DE, Jefferson DM, Mulligan RC. Correction of the genetic defect in hepatocytes from the Watanabe heritable hyperlipidemic rabbit. *Proc Natl Acad Sci USA.* 1988;85:4421–4425.

70. Grossman M, Raper SE, Kozarsky K, et al. Successful *ex vivo* gene therapy directed to liver in a patient with familial hypercholesterolemia. *Nature Genet.* 1994;6:335–341.

71. Watson JD. The Human Genome Project: past, present, and future. *Science.* 1990;248:44–51.

72. Nabel EG. Gene therapy for cardiovascular disease. *Circulation.* 1995;91:541–548.

3

Biology of Vascular Reconstructions

Mechanisms of Intimal Hyperplasia, Stenosis, and Restenosis

Ulf Hedin, MD, PhD, and Alexander W. Clowes, MD

Reconstruction of atherosclerotic arteries by angioplasty, endarterectomy, or by-pass surgery causes vessel injury and induces a healing response in the vessel wall that may lead to luminal narrowing and occlusion of the reconstructed segment. For the past 15 years, the problem of restenosis and vein graft stenosis has been a major challenge to cardiovascular research. Despite significant progress in the understanding of the pathophysiology of vascular repair in animal models, no pharmacologic therapy is available for humans.

Early investigations in this field focused on the pathogenesis of atherosclerosis. One of the first theories about this disease evolved from the assumption that atherosclerosis was an injury response since the advanced fibrotic plaque histologically resembled injury-induced lesions in animal models.[1] These lesions were characterized by the proliferation and deposition of extracellular matrix by smooth muscle cells (SMCs) within the arterial intima. Later, we learned that this vascular repair process was a distinct pathologic phenomenon now known as intimal hyperplasia. It was assumed to contribute not only to atherosclerosis, but also to the development of restenosis after vascular interventions.[2] For many years, intimal hyperplasia was considered the principal cause of restenosis, but today we believe that it is one of many components that contribute to this process in humans.[3] This repair response is not necessarily associated with a restriction in lumen size. In fact, vessels will adjust to the increase in intimal mass caused by intimal hyperplasia by enlargement, a phenomenon called *vascular remodeling*. In spite of this rather complex pathophysiology of human restenosis, the cellular and molecular mechanisms involved in intimal hyperplasia constitute fundamental aspects of vascular biology that must be considered when studying any pathologic process of the vessel wall.

In this chapter, we first summarize the clinical significance of restenosis and vein graft stenosis in vascular surgery. We then describe the observations made in different animal models and consider particular mechanisms that regulate intimal hyperplasia. We focus on how interactions between cells and between cells and the extracellular matrix may control essential parts in this process. The SMCs of the vessel wall do not normally divide and exist in a state that might be actively maintained by growth inhibitors. By disengaging these control mechanisms, for example, by tissue injury or atherogenic factors, SMCs are activated and a disease process such as restenosis or atherosclerosis is initiated.

RESTENOSIS IN VASCULAR SURGERY

Restenosis is a poorly defined term for preocclusive lesions that develop in diseased vessels after reconstructive procedures. Most commonly, these lesions are found where the vessel has been exposed to trauma (angioplasty, endarterectomy, cross-clamping, or anastomotic suture lines). Luminal narrowing, which is a more appropriate term, can occur after injury to a preexisting lesion (angioplasty), after removal of a lesion (endarterectomy), or in a previously normal vessel (vein grafts). This diversity in anatomic location and presumed pathophysiology makes it difficult to envision the restenosis phenomenon as one entity. However, information from animal models indicates that the vessel wall response to trauma is stereotypical and independent of the mode of injury, and it is possible that lesions of diverse origin share common pathophysiologic mechanisms.[4]

The magnitude of the repair response and the anatomy of the reconstructed segment determine the degree of luminal narrowing and symptoms. Thus, angioplasty of iliac arteries is rarely followed by symptomatic restenosis, whereas angioplasty of small-caliber coronary arteries is associated with restenosis and recurrent angina pectoris in 30% to 50% of all patients.[5] Postoperative duplex examinations after carotid endarterectomy have revealed a recurrence of luminal narrowing exceeding 50% in 20% of all cases; however, the recurrence of cerebrovascular ischemic symptoms is lower than 1%.[6] This discrepancy demonstrates the benign features of the lesions with a fibrous, smooth appearance that lacks calcified parts, ruptures, and thrombus in contrast to the original atheroma.

Examinations of restenotic lesions obtained from different reconstructions reveal a similar histologic picture. Most specimens exhibit intimal hyperplasia of the kind observed in animal models and are composed of loose connective tissue rich in SMCs but usually with much less inflammation than the primary lesion (Fig. 3–1).[7,8] In contrast to injured animal arteries, these lesions exhibit little SMC proliferation, which indicates that the mechanisms involved in the formation of intimal hyperplasia in humans may be different for those described in animals.[8] Lesions obtained more than 2 years after surgery are infiltrated with lipids and inflammatory cells and look like atherosclerotic lesions.

Veins that are introduced into the arterial circulation as bypass conduits or venous dialysis fistulas develop intimal hyperplasia and thickening of the media. This response is both related to the injury at the time of implantation (clamp injury, passage of a valvulotome) and to altered hemodynamic forces. The vessel wall structure is modified in response to increased wall shear stress by SMCs that replicate and deposit new extracellular matrix.[9] The response may lead to luminal narrowing and graft occlusion and accounts for the high long-term failure rate of these reconstructions. More than 20% of aortocoronary and between 40% to 50% of peripheral vein grafts require intervention

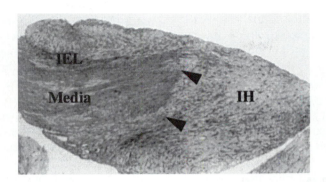

Figure 3–1. Intimal hyperplasia in a restenotic lesion of a coronary artery 6 months after treatment of the primary atherosclerotic lesion by percutaneous directional coronary atherectomy (DCA). Intimal hyperplasia (IH) is seen as a loose connective tissue surrounding the well-organized dense tissue of the media. The cut in the media and in the internal elastic lamina (IEL) by the previous atherectomy is marked by arrowheads. The specimen was obtained by repeated DCA.

within 5 years.[10] In synthetic grafts, stenosis is located at the anastomosis due to a healing response in the traumatized artery.[11]

ANIMAL MODELS OF RESTENOSIS

Most of our understanding of vascular repair comes from studies in animal models. In general, these models involve injury to the vessel by some kind of mechanical trauma, either by the retraction of an inflated Fogarty balloon embolectomy catheter or by intraluminal devices that injure the endothelium and the subendothelial tissue. Other methods of injury have also been used such as drying the endothelium and underlying tissue with a flow of air, removal of the adventitia (which causes ischemia in the media due to loss of blood supply from adventitial capillaries), application of an electrical current along the vessel, or simply application of an outside pressure by cross-clamping with a hemostat.[12] In each situation, the tissue response is remarkably similar within one species, whereas considerable differences may be found between different animal models. Even though these models have greatly improved our understanding of vascular repair, they have failed to predict effective strategies for prevention of restenosis and vein graft stenosis in humans. Most of these studies have been made in nonatherosclerotic animals and there is a need for further work in models with preexisiting advanced atherosclerotic lesions.

Rat Model

The healing response in injured vessels is best characterized in the rat carotid balloon injury model. A small-caliber Fogarty balloon is passed into the common carotid artery via the external carotid. The balloon is inflated and retracted, removing the endothelium and damaging the underlying tissue. Platelet adhesion to the exposed connective tissue follows but is limited to a thin layer and not associated with progressive luminal thrombosis.[13] In the media, SMCs are activated by the injury and several genes are induced.[14] Some cells initiate DNA replication within 24 to 48 hours. The number of cells that synthesize DNA increases from less than 1%/day in normal arteries to 20% to 30%/day.[13] Simultaneously, the morphology of many cells underneath the internal elastic lamina changes. Contractile filaments disappear from the cytoplasm and are replaced by synthetic organelles.[15] After 4 days, migration of SMCs from the media to the intima can be detected. In the intima, these cells replicate several cycles and deposit new extracellular matrix. After 2 weeks, the growth of the intimal mass is mostly due to the formation of extracellular matrix, which occupies 80% of the intima after 3 months and undergoes a structural maturation.[13] Although no typical elastic lamellae are formed, the structure of the intima eventually resembles that of the media. The ultrastructure of the intimal SMCs returns to that of the original medial cells after 4 to 6 weeks. These cells contain abundant contractile filaments in the cytoplasm and a poorly developed secretory apparatus, possibly as a reflection of a return to an inactive, quiescent state.[15]

Regeneration of endothelium takes place from the distal and proximal edges of the vessel segment since the common carotid artery lacks side branches, but generally does not go to completion.[16] Despite the lack of a nonthrombogenic endothelium, the luminal SMCs structurally adapt to the stress forces of flow to form a nonthrombogenic pseudoendothelium.[15] These cells produce nitric oxide (NO) due to an induced expression of nitric oxide synthase (iNOS), which may contribute to the nonthrombogenic properties of the surface in the absence of endothelial cells.[17] The endothelium participates in the control of intima formation and, as these cells regenerate over the surface, SMC growth stops.[16] Thus, intimal hyperplasia is limited in areas of rapid endothelial regeneration.

Mouse Model

A major limitation of studies in small animals is the inherent resistance to vascular disease. Whereas rabbits and larger species can become hyperlipidemic on a high-cholesterol diet, the lipid metabolism is so different in rats and mice that they retain normal lipid levels. In recent years, transgenic and knock-out mice have been engineered with genetic defects relevant for studies of vascular disease. In these animals, single genes can be overexpressed or eliminated, which allows evaluation of the action of individual molecules on different processes in the vessel wall. Animals have been developed with defective lipid metabolism, altered fibrinolytic system, immune defects, and altered expression of matrix degrading enzymes.[18,19] These animals can be used to study the impact of defined molecular defects in the response of vessels to injury.

Lindner et al.[20] have described the vascular repair process in normal mouse carotid arteries subjected to injury with a flexible wire. The response resembles the development of intimal hyperplasia in the rat model. However, the lesion is considerably smaller and the endothelial regeneration more rapid. Other methods of injury have also been used in transgenic mice lacking fibrinolytic components but these have not yet been as well characterized.[21]

Rabbit and Porcine Models

The major advantage of rabbits for the study of restenosis is the tendency of these animals to develop lesions spontaneously either because of a genetic defect or exposure to a high-cholesterol diet. In these animals, vascular segments with preexisting lesions can be injured. These lesions are distinctly different from those found in humans and typically consist of a concentric foam cell infiltration of the intima and inner portions of the media. After injury, thrombosis is common especially in the dissection planes, and the resulting neointima is usually acellular with a lipid-rich extracellular matrix. The most striking difference with the rat model is that these lesions usually contain thrombus, inflammatory cells, and lipid.[12] Similar observations have been made in normal and hypercholesterolemic pigs.

These models have been particularly used to study coronary restenosis.[22] A feature that is more appreciated in both rabbits and pigs than in rats is the remodeling of the vessel structure after injury. In cholesterol-fed Yucatan minipigs and rabbits, the resulting luminal narrowing can be attributed to both vascular remodeling and an increase in intimal mass.[23] Because vascular remodeling seems to be a major component in the human restenosis process,[3] these models can be used to address components of the restenosis process other than intimal hyperplasia. We know little about the mechanisms involved in the injury response of rabbits and pigs in contrast to our understanding of this process in the rat model, and further experimental work is required.

Nonhuman Primate Models

Cholesterol-fed monkeys develop atherosclerotic lesions that are very similar to those of humans. This model has been well characterized in studies of both progression and regression of atherosclerosis.[24] As in humans, these animals first develop fatty streaks with infiltrates of lipid-filled macrophages and later both intermediate and more advanced plaques can be seen. In contrast to humans, monkeys seldom develop stenotic lesions. In a recent study, Geary and coworkers[25] demonstrated a response to balloon injury in the iliac artery of cholesterol-fed cynolmogus monkeys that has features similar to the human process. In this model, the repair response involves intimal hyperplasia, recoil, and remodeling—essentially all the events that are believed to contribute to restenosis in humans. However, because these animals did not have stenotic primary lesions, it is difficult to evaluate how these components actually contribute to restenosis after injury. Nevertheless, this primate model may be useful for elucidating the mechanisms involved in the different components of the human restenosis process. SMC proliferation, which is a key part of the healing response of small animals, is not a prominent feature of the monkey. Since this is also the case in human restenotic lesions, the repair process of humans and monkeys may be similar.[8,25]

MOLECULAR MECHANISMS OF INTIMAL HYPERPLASIA

Intimal hyperplasia occurs in virtually all situations associated with arterial injury. Because of the initial belief that this process caused restenosis in humans, tremendous efforts to characterize the responsible molecular mechanisms with the ultimate goal of finding a successful therapy have taken place.[2] The rat model has been extensively examined and most of our understanding of intimal hyperplasia is derived from studies of this process in normal, nonatherosclerotic arteries. It is worth emphasizing that intimal hyperplasia is not the only factor contributing to restenosis in humans. Furthermore, intimal hyperplasia may also be regulated differently in humans. As mentioned earlier, proliferating SMCs are seldom found in intimal hyperplasia of human restenotic lesions, whereas this is a key feature in the rat.[7,8] Despite these concerns, the rat model has been useful for exploring events and molecules that control essential parts of this process such as growth factors, cytokines, chemotactic agents, proteases, and coagulation factors. These factors can be found also in human lesions.

The response to injury in the rat has been divided into three separate parts. The first part consists of the initial activation of SMCs in the media, the second involves migration of SMCs from the media to the intima, and the third represents the final formation of the intimal mass by intimal SMC proliferation and deposition of extracellular matrix (Fig. 3–2).[7,12]

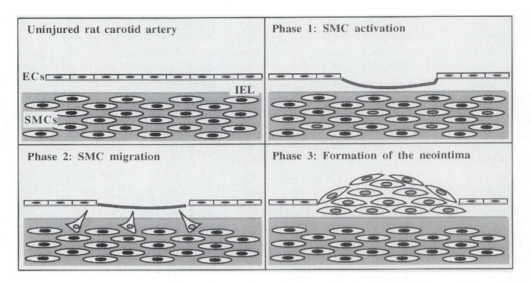

Figure 3–2. Development of intimal hyperplasia in the rat carotid balloon injury model. After injury to the endothelial cells (ECs) with a Fogarty balloon catheter, there is an activation of smooth muscle cells (SMCs) in the media with changes in ultrastructure and the onset of DNA synthesis (phase 1). A few days later, SMCs migrate from the media through and onto the internal elastic lamina (IEL; phase 2). Thereafter, the neointima is formed by proliferation of SMCs and the deposition of large amounts of extracellular matrix by these cells (phase 3).

Phase 1: Medial Replication

At 24 hours after a denuding injury with a Fogarty balloon catheter, DNA synthesis can be detected in medial SMCs. This has been attributed to the release of basic fibroblast growth factor (bFGF) from injured medial cells and stores of growth factor bound to heparan sulfate proteoglycans in the extracellular matrix.[26] Treatment with infusions of heparin at the time of injury have been shown to restrict this response, presumably by displacing the bFGF from the extracellular matrix.[27] SMCs with the ultrastructure usually associated with proliferating, synthetic cells are confined to the inner layers of the media and so are most of the replicating cells.[13,15] There is no strong correlation between the medial replication and later phases of the response. A gentle denuding injury without injury to the media is followed by SMC migration in spite of less medial replication.[7] It is possible that early medial replication is important for repair of the media whereas SMC migration is necessary for intimal repair.

Phase 2: SMC Migration

Migrating cells that exhibit the morphology of activated, synthetic SMCs can be detected above the IEL 4 days after the injury.[15] The factors that contribute to migration are believed to be released from degranulating platelets since SMC migration is reduced in thrombocytopenic rats.[28] Platelet α granules contain potent chemotactic factors for SMCs such as platelet-derived growth factor BB (PDGF BB) and transforming growth factor beta (TGF-β). Although PDGF BB is a very potent mitogen for SMCs *in vitro*, it is primarily a migratory factor *in vivo*. Treatment of injured arteries with infusions of PDGF BB stimulates migration of cells but has little effect on medial replication.[29] Apart from growth factors, proteases are needed for SMC migration from the media to the intima. In the normal media, these cells are encased in a basement membrane and surrounded by a dense extracellular matrix of collagen, elastin, and proteoglycans. Destruction of this environment may not only be necessary for the cells to migrate but may also be an important part of cell activation.[28] Urokinase-like plasminogen activator (uPA) is observed after a couple of hours followed by tissue-type plasminogen activator (tPA) and plasmin a couple of days later.[30] Matrix metalloproteinases (MMPs) have also been detected in the injured rat carotid artery. Whereas the expression of MMP2 occurs in normal arteries, MMP9 is induced during repair.[31] Inhibition of these enzymes using various inhibitors blocks the migration of cells and to various degrees limits lesion growth.[32,33] Matrix proteins that are normally scarce or absent in the normal media such as alternatively spliced variants of fibronectin, thrombospondin, tenascin, osteopontin, and versican are abundant in the rat intima after arterial injury and might affect SMC migration by regulating adhesive and deadhesive events in this process.[34–36] Peptides containing the amino acid sequence arginine-glycine-aspartic acid (RGD) interfere with the binding of integrins, the cellular matrix receptors,[37] to some extracellular matrix molecules. RGD peptides inhibit migration of SMCs *in vitro* and reduce neointima formation in the rat.[38] Integrins that bind this peptide are also expressed in medial and intimal SMCs in this model (Fig. 3–3), and seem to be abundant in normal as well as atherosclerotic human vessels.[39] Inhibition of integrins believed to be involved in cell migration, in particular $\alpha_v\beta_3$,[40,41] may prove to be a good pharmacologic approach for inhibiting intimal hyperplasia.[12]

Phase 3: Formation of the Intima

SMCs that start to accumulate on the luminal side of the IEL continue to replicate for several weeks. The growth factors responsible for this replication are not known. bFGF does not seem to be involved even though it is responsible for medial replication. Growth regulatory molecules such as PDGF A, TGF-β, and angiotensin II (ATII) receptors are expressed by intimal SMCs, especially the luminal cells. These findings indicate that auto- and paracrine mechanisms involving these factors may control intimal replication. In general, there is an elevated responsiveness of the intima to exogenous growth factor stimulation. Thus, addition of ATII but not PDGF to a preexisting neointima will further increase SMC proliferation.[12] The replication takes place primarily in the luminal cells. This replication is associated with the expression of iNOS and NO production by these cells.[17] NO may be important for the antithrombotic properties of the luminal cells and

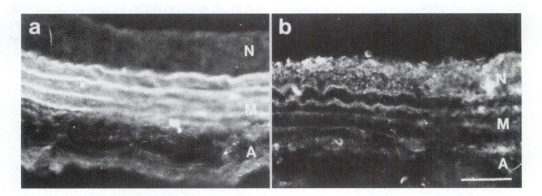

Figure 3–3. Immunohistochemical detection of the integrin subunits α_5 (**a**) and α_v (**b**) in the rat carotid artery 2 weeks after balloon injury. Note the presence of the fibronectin specific α_5 integrin subunit in the media (M) whereas α_v, which is part of integrins that bind a number of different matrix molecules, is confined to the neointima (N). Bar represents 200 μm. A; adventitia.

may also limit growth of SMCs in the intima. In addition, it was recently reported that cell death (apoptosis) is detectable in the luminal layer of intimal SMCs, thus suggesting that both replication and death occur in the same population of cells.[42]

Further increase in intimal mass is obtained by the formation of new extracellular matrix. The intima contains matrix components that are absent from the normal vascular media (mentioned previously). The biologic consequence of this altered composition of the extracellular matrix is not known. Nevertheless, after 4 to 6 weeks, the structure of the intimal matrix changes to a more dense connective tissue with increased content and organization of collagen and elastin. Along with the cessation of growth, the intimal SMCs adopt an ultrastructure similar to normal medial cells.[15] These cells also behave like medial cells when put in culture, whereas those obtained from the intima at earlier time points have different features *in vitro*.[43] Whether the intima is composed of different cell populations or the phenotype of intimal SMCs is stably expressed when these cells are put into culture at different times during intimal development is not known.

Control of SMC Function

The medial SMCs control vascular tone by contraction and relaxation in response to a variety of physiologic stimuli. However, in contrast to differentiated cells in many other tissues, SMCs seem to be easily activated and undertake functions that are intended to restore vascular structure. What makes this tissue so special and why are we faced with a biologic process that apparently counteracts the desired result, which is to restore vessel structure and blood flow in the region exposed to injury? Perhaps we should instead ask how vessel integrity is normally maintained under the constant exposure to harmful, atherogenic stimuli and the physiologic stress of the flow of blood?

The control of SMC function after injury to the vessel is intimately associated with the presence or absence of endothelial cells. Most animal models involve some kind of destruction of the luminal endothelium. Later, as the endothelium regenerates and covers the intima, SMC replication and further growth of the intima stops. Stimulation of endothelial regeneration with selected growth factors has been used to inhibit intimal hyperplasia in animal models.[44] By stimulating endothelial regrowth over the injured surface, SMC replication is inhibited. Although the mechanisms are not completely understood, the ability of the endothelium to suppress SMC replication may be explained by the secretion of growth inhibitory substances such as TGF-β, heparan sulfate, or NO.[45] *In vitro* studies have shown that NO can efficiently inhibit SMC growth, and *in vivo* transfection of SMCs with the endothelial form of NOS (ecNOS) has been shown to restrict SMC growth after injury in the rat model.[46] In addition, administration of NO analogues inhibits neointima formation.[47] In atherosclerotic vessels, NO metabolism is severely disturbed. The release of NO by constitutive ecNOS in endothelial cells is compromised, whereas inflammatory cells such as macrophages express high levels of iNOS.[48] The net production of NO in this environment may influence SMC growth and explain the limited SMC proliferation seen in human restenosis. Human lesions are rich in capillaries and macrophages and in animals lacking these components, SMC proliferation is a prominent feature.

Although these examples point to the importance of an intact endothelium for SMC quiescence, SMC replication may under some circumstances take place underneath an endothelial monolayer. Endothelial cells constitutively express NOS and the level of NO production is regulated by flow forces. During increased flow and shear stress, NO production goes up and vessels dilate. In a baboon model of intimal hyperplasia, a porous polytetrafluorethylene (PTFE) graft is inserted between the infrarenal aorta and the iliac artery. High flow is achieved by a downstream fistula between the femoral artery and vein. In these large-pore-size grafts, capillaries and SMC-like mesenchymal cells grow through the pores and a neointima covered by an intact endothelium develops on the graft surface. Under high flow, the thickness of this tissue and SMC replication is moderate, but if the graft is exposed to low flow by ligation of the downstream fistula, SMC replication is enhanced and the intima thickens even though the endothelium is intact and thrombosis is absent.[49,50] These grafts cannot contract or expand and luminal size instead depends on the thickness of the intima in order to maintain wall shear stress constant under different flow conditions. The changes might be regulated by the endothelium, which can sense shear stress and regulate SMC growth by NO. Similar factors are also involved in the pathogenesis of vein graft stenosis where the combined actions of endothelial denudation, vessel wall trauma, and abnormal flow conditions have to be considered.[10] Taken together, the influence of endothelial cells on SMCs appears to be designed to suppress the activated, proliferating state of SMCs and keep these cells in a state of quiescence. The disruption of this balance, either by altered flow conditions or trauma to the vessel with loss of endothelium, will tip the balance in favor of vasoconstriction and cell proliferation.

This relationship is probably not the only mechanism involved in control of SMC function. SMCs in the media of normal vessels are embedded in a basement membrane-like matrix. This matrix may be essential to maintain the contractile and quiescent function of SMCs. In embryos, SMCs proliferate in a matrix devoid of basement membrane components, but in the mature media, laminin, type IV collagen, and heparan sulfate proteoglycans surround the cells.[51,52] *In vitro*, SMCs that are cultured on or within reconstituted basement membrane also retain their contractile features and do not respond to exogenous growth factors.[53,54] If the cells are exposed to matrix proteins that promote cytoskeletal rearrangement such as fibronectin, they will start proliferating and lose their contractile apparatus.[55] These interactions are integrin mediated.[56] Although the main function of integrins is to anchor cells in the extracellular matrix, they also mediate intracellular signals through tyrosine kinases linked to the cytoplasmic portion of the receptor that influence migration, growth, and differentiation of cells.[57] If these interactions are altered by changes in the composition of the extracellular matrix or changes in integrin expression, SMC function may be affected. This can occur by increased expression of matrix molecules not normally associated with SMCs, such as fibronectin,[58] or by digestion of the matrix by proteases. By creating new contacts between integrins and matrix components, SMCs may become susceptible to stimuli to which they would not normally respond. This process may be the reason why stimulation of arteries with growth factors is not followed by SMC replication in the media, unless the vessel is injured.[59] Like the endothelium, the extracellular matrix seems to restrict the proliferative capacity of SMCs by keeping them in a contractile, quiescent state. Perhaps this state is also influenced by integrin function. Modulation of integrin β_1 avidity regulates the affinity of this receptor to its ligand; the active form can be induced by certain antibodies and ECMs. In baboons, the active conformational state was detected in SMCs of the normal media, but decreased after balloon injury.[60] *In vitro*, there is also a correlation between the expression of the active state and quiescence.[61] In addition, the expression of integrins is altered both in proliferating SMCs *in vitro* and in lesions.[62] These results indicate that integrin function and expression may be involved in the control of SMC activation.

To summarize, we can distinguish at least two mechanisms whereby SMC function is controlled and the cells kept in a quiescent state through interactions with soluble factors secreted by the endothelium and interactions with the surrounding extracellular matrix through integrins (Fig. 3–4). A better understanding of the exact mechanisms whereby both the endothelium and the extracellular matrix control SMC function may ultimately lead to the development of new treatment strategies in restenosis prevention.

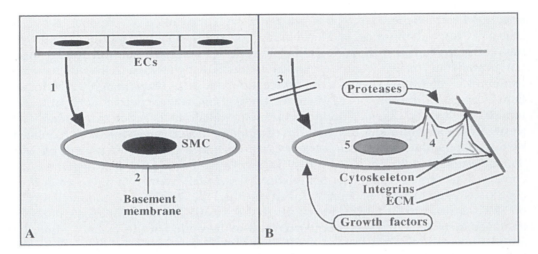

Figure 3–4. Hypothetical model for the maintenance of SMC function by the principle of "negative growth control." (**A**) Normally, these cells are in a quiescent and contractile state controlled by endothelial cells, most likely by the action of NO (1), and by the surrounding basement membrane, which maintain the contractile structure of the cells (2). (**B**) After injury and loss of endothelium, the inhibitory influence of NO is lost (3), and by the action of proteases released from injured SMCs, new interactions between extracellular matrix components (ECMs) and integrins promote cytoskeletal reorganization (4). Together, these changes make the cells responsive to the actions of growth factors such as bFGF (5).

FEATURES OF THE HUMAN RESTENOSIS PROCESS

Although studies in the rat model of arterial injury have improved our understanding of the principles of vascular repair and the mechanisms involved in intimal hyperplasia, several drugs that efficiently inhibit this process in the rat do not inhibit restenosis in humans. The failure of pharmacologic responses in the rat to predict outcome in humans might reflect the differences between an intimal repair process in a normal vessel of an atherosclerosis-resistant species and the complex response in the diseased vessels of humans. Intimal hyperplasia, although present in most examined human lesions, is not necessarily associated with restriction in lumen size. Even in the rat, the increase in intimal mass is only partially linked to the decrease in luminal area. The loss of lumen 2 weeks after balloon injury is greater than after 6 weeks despite a similar intimal thickness; vasoconstriction accounts for much of the early luminal loss.[63] Examinations of coronary and carotid atherosclerotic lesions have shown that the increase in intimal mass due to lesion progression is accompanied by vessel enlargement, thus compensating the restriction in luminal area.[3] This phenomenon, vascular remodeling, is a normal response of the vessel to maintain wall shear stress and a constant blood flow and is probably involved in restenosis development in humans. Postangioplasty restenosis in rabbits, atherosclerotic pigs, and monkeys consists of both an increase in intimal mass and arterial remodeling.[23,25] Investigations with intracoronary ultrasound indicate that these events may contribute to postangioplasty restenosis in humans also.[12] It appears that neither intimal hyperplasia nor one of the central events in this process, SMC replication, is a prominent feature of restenosis in humans. Thus, what was believed to be an elegant target for intervention either by drugs or gene therapy may no longer be the best choice.[64]

Perhaps we should not even interfere with this repair response.[65] Most interventions, especially in coronary arteries, address complex atherosclerotic lesions that may

Chows Talk.

There is new stuff. Relating Restruins and
Compaction - VSMC dilatation. They used aortic
wall Explants & look at smc migration.
They then used things like endokuns, growth
Factors etc To modify This also ICa. Nittous oxide
HBse can effect as well. It seems To inhibit The
migration. I don't know if This stuff is in the
Chapter or Reference or not.

eventually fracture, thrombose, and lead to occlusion of the vessel. This instability of the plaque may be attributed to weaknesses, particularly at the shoulder regions where the fibrous cap composed of SMCs and extracellular matrix is thin. MMPs produced by inflammatory cells at these sites may destabilize the plaque and cause plaque rupture.[66] What we achieve when such lesions are dilated by balloon angioplasty, is indeed a fracture of the plaque and controlled plaque thrombosis.[67] Under appropriate conditions, these events are not followed by thrombotic occlusion. Instead, a healing response takes place that contributes structural integrity and stability to the plaque. Thus, the healing response may actually do what the biology intended, namely, repair the damaged tissue. Under such circumstances, inhibition of SMC function might not be desirable.

So, if intimal hyperplasia is not the process we should interfere with, what other components of the restenosis process can we target? The mechanisms behind arterial remodeling have yet to be determined. In the rat, vasorelaxing agents are able to inhibit the contraction seen early after arterial injury but not at later time points. The vessel apparently has two phases of remodeling. One is due to contraction and another involves a structural rearrangement of the tissue. We can expect that events involved in intimal hyperplasia, such as deposition of extracellular matrix molecules and expression of proteases, are also involved in the structural reorganization of the injured vessel. Thrombosis may also contribute to human restenosis. Complex atherosclerotic lesions contain elevated levels of tissue factor, expressed by SMCs and macrophages.[14] In addition, thrombin activity, thrombin receptor, and large amounts of fibrin are found in plaques and restenotic lesions together with components of the fibrinolytic system.[68,69] Thus, the plaque is in a prothrombotic state, which predisposes lesions to thrombotic events in association with injury. These events probably contribute to the healing process and the following structural reorganization of the vessel. This is an important aspect to consider when new strategies to target restenosis are developed.

CONCLUSION

Despite the tremendous progress of vascular biology in recent years, the solution to the restenosis problem remains a major challenge in cardiovascular research. We know more about cellular and molecular mechanisms involved in the development of intimal hyperplasia in normal arteries than any other process in the vessel wall, but we still need to understand fundamental aspects of how diseased atherosclerotic vessels respond to the physical trauma associated with a reconstructive procedure. In the future, detailed studies in more relevant animal models such as the atherosclerotic monkey should provide essential information. When combined with our detailed knowledge about the pathophysiology of intimal hyperplasia, we may come up with appealing new strategies to target this annoying process.

Acknowledgments
Ulf Hedin was supported by funds from the Swedish Medical Research Council (11387), The Swedish Society for Medicine, Karolinska Institutet, Astra Hässle AB, and Hoffmann La Roche, Inc.

REFERENCES

1. Ross R, Glomset J. The pathogenesis of atherosclerosis: part 1. *N Engl J Med.* 1976;295:369–377.
2. McBride W, Lange RA, Hillis LD. Restenosis after successful coronary angioplasty: pathophysiology and prevention. *N Engl J Med.* 1988;318:1734–1737.

3. Glagov S. Intimal hyperplasia, vascular modeling, and the restenosis problem. *Circulation.* 1994;89:2888–2891.

4. Clowes AW. Prevention and management of recurrent disease after arterial reconstruction: new prospects for pharmacological control. *Thromb Haemost.* 1991;66:62–66.

5. Berk BC, Harris K. Restenosis after percutaneous transluminal coronary angioplasty: new therapeutic insights from pathogenic mechanisms. *Adv Intern Med.* 1995;40:445–501.

6. Clagett GP, Robinowitz, Youkey JR, et al. Morphogenesis and clinicopathologic characteristics of recurrent carotid disease. *J Vasc Surg.* 1986;3:10–23.

7. Clowes AW, Reidy MA. Prevention of stenosis after vascular reconstruction: pharmacologic control of intimal hyperplasia—a review. *J Vasc Surg.* 1991;13:885–891.

8. O'Brien ER, Alpers CE, Stetwart DK, et al. Proliferation in primary and restenotic coronary atherectomy tissue: implications for antiproliferative therapy. *Circ Res.* 1993;73:223–231.

9. Clowes AW. Intimal hyperplasia and graft failure. *Cardiovasc Pathol.* 1993;2:179S–186S.

10. Davies MG, Hagen PO. Structural and functional consequences of bypass grafting with autologous vein. *Cryobiology.* 1994;31:63–70.

11. Swedberg SH, Brown BG, Sigley R, et al. Intimal fibromuscular hyperplasia at the venous anastomosis of PTFE grafts in hemodialysis patients. *Circulation.* 1989;80:1726–1736.

12. Schwartz SM, deBlois D, O'Brien ERM. The intima: soil for atherosclerosis and restenosis. *Circ Res.* 1995;77:445–465.

13. Clowes AW, Reidy ME, Clowes MM. Kinetics of cellular proliferation after arterial injury, I. Smooth muscle cell growth in the absence of the endothelium. *Lab Invest.* 1983;3:10–23.

14. Taubman MB. Gene induction in vessel wall injury. *Thromb Haemost.* 1993;70:180–183.

15. Thyberg J, Blomgren K, Hedin U, Dryjski M. Phenotypic modulation of smooth muscle cells during the formation of neointimal thickenings in the rat carotid artery after balloon injury: an electronic–microscopic and stereological study. *Cell Tissue Res.* 1995;281:421–428.

16. Reidy ME, Clowes AW, Schwartz SM. Endothelial regeneration. V. Inhibition of endothelial regrowth in arteries of rat and rabbit. *Lab Invest.* 1983;49:569–575.

17. Hansson GK, Geng YJ, Holm J, et al. Arterial smooth muscle cells express nitric oxide synthase in response to endothelial injury. *J Exp Med.* 1994;180:733–738.

18. Breslow JL. Transgenic mouse models of lipoprotein metabolism and atherosclerosis. *Proc Natl Acad Sci USA.* 1993;90:8314–8318.

19. Dzau VJ, Gibbons GH, Kobilka BK, et al. Genetic models of vascular disease. *Circulation.* 1995;91:521–531.

20. Lindner V, Fingerle J, Reidy MA. Mouse model of arterial injury. *Circ Res.* 1993;73:792–796.

21. Carmeliet P, Collen D. Gene targeting and gene transfer studies of the plasminogen/plasmin system: implications in thrombosis, hemostasis, neointima formation, and atherosclerosis. *FASEB J.* 1995;9:934–938.

22. Schwartz RS, Edwards WD, Huber KC, et al. Coronary restenosis: prospects for solution and new perspectives from a porcine model. *Mayo Clin Proc.* 1993;68:54–62.

23. Post MJ, Borst C, Kuntz RE. The relative importance of arterial remodeling compared with intimal hyperplasia in lumen renarrowing after balloon angioplasty: a study in the normal rabbit and the hypercholesterolemic Yucatan minipig. *Circulation.* 1994;89:2816–2821.

24. Clarkson TB, Bond MG, Bullock BC, et al. A study of atherosclerosis regression in Macaca mulatta, V: changes in abdominal aorta and carotid and coronary arteries from animals with atherosclerosis induced for 38 months and then regressed for 24 or 48 months at plasma cholesterol concentrations of 300 or 200 mg/dl. *Exp Mol Pathol.* 1984;41:96–118

25. Geary RL, Williams JK, Golden D, et al. Time course of cellular proliferation, intimal hyperplasia, and remodeling following angioplasty in monkeys with established atherosclerosis. A nonhuman primate model of restenosis. *Arterioscl Thromb Vasc Biol.* 1996;16:34–43.

26. Lindner V, Reidy MA. Proliferation of smooth muscle cells after vascular injury is inhibited by an antibody against basic fibroblast growth factor. *Proc Natl Acad Sci USA.* 1991;88:3739–3743.

27. Lindner V, Olson NE, Clowes AW, et al. Inhibition of smooth muscle cell proliferation in injured rat arteries. Interaction of heparin with basic fibroblast growth factor. *J Clin Invest.* 1992;90:2044–2049.

28. Fingerle J, Johnson R, Clowes AW, et al. Role of platelets in smooth muscle cell migration and proliferation after vascular injury in rat carotid artery. *Proc Natl Acad Sci USA.* 1989;86:8412–8416.

29. Jawien A, Bowen-Pope DF, Lindner V, et al. Platelet-derived growth factor promotes smooth muscle migration and intimal thickening in a rat model of balloon angioplasty. *J Clin Invest.* 1992;89:507–511.

30. Reidy MA, Irvin C, Lindner V. Migration of arterial wall cells. Expression of plasminogen activators and inhibitors in injured rat arteries. *Circ Res.* 1996;78:405–414.

31. Zempo N, Kenagy RD, Au YP, et al. Matrix metalloproteinases of vascular wall cells are increased in balloon-injured rat carotid artery. *J Vasc Surg.* 1994;20:209–217.

32. Bendeck MP, Irvin C, Reidy MA. Inhibition of matrix metalloproteinase activity inhibits smooth muscle cell migration but not neointimal thickening after arterial injury. *Circ Res.* 1996;78:38–43.

33. Zempo N, Koyama N, Kenagy RD, et al. Regulation of vascular smooth muscle cell migration and proliferation *in vitro* and in injured rat arteries by a synthetic matrix metalloproteinase inhibitor. *Arterioscler Thromb Vasc Biol.* 1996;16:28–33.

34. Majesky MW. Neointima formation after acute vascular injury. Role of counteradhesive extracellular matrix proteins. *Texas Heart Inst J.* 1994;21:78–85.

35. Hedin U, Holm J, Hansson GK. Induction of tenascin in rat arterial injury: relationship to altered smooth muscle cell phenotype. *Am J Pathol.* 1991;139:649–656.

36. Giachelli C, Bae N, Almeida M, et al. Osteopontin is elevated during neointima formation in rat arteries and is a novel component of human atherosclerotic plaques. *J Clin Invest.* 1993;92:1686–1696.

37. Hynes RO. Integrins: versatility, modulation, and signaling in cell adhesion. *Cell.* 1992;69:11–25.

38. Choi ET, Engel L, Callow AD, et al. Inhibition of neointimal hyperplasia by blocking $\alpha_v\beta_3$ integrin with a small peptide antagonist GpenGRGDSPCA. *J Vasc Surg.* 1994;19:125–134.

39. Hoshiga M, Alpers CE, Smith LL, et al. $\alpha_v\beta_3$ integrin expression in normal and atherosclerotic artery. *Circ Res.* 1995;77:1129–1135.

40. Clyman RI, Mauray F, Kramer RH. β_1 and β_3 integrins have different roles in the adhesion and migration of vascular smooth muscle cells on extracellular matrix. *Exp Cell Res.* 1992;200:272–284.

41. Liaw L, Skinner MP, Raines EW, et al. The adhesive and migratory effects of osteopontin are mediated via distinct cell surface integrins: role of $a_v\beta_3$ in smooth muscle cell migration to osteopontin *in vitro. J Clin Invest.* 1995;95:713–724.

42. Bochaton-Piallat M-L, Gabbiani F, Redard M, et al. Apoptosis participates in cellularity regulation during rat aortic intimal thickening. *Am J Pathol.* 1995;146:1059–1064.

43. Orlandi A, Ehrlich HP, Ropraz P, et al. Rat aortic smooth muscle cells isolated from different layers and at different times after endothelial denudation shows distinct biological features *in vitro. Arterioscler Thromb.* 1994;14:982–989.

44. Cascells W. Growth factor therapies for vascular injury and ischemia. *Circulation.* 1995;91:2699–2702.

45. Scott-Burden T, Vanhoutte PM. The endothelium as a regulator of vascular smooth muscle proliferation. *Circulation.* 1993;87:V51–V55.

46. von der Leyen HE, Gibbons GH, Morishita R, et al. Gene therapy inhibiting neointimal vascular lesion: *in vivo* transfer of endothelial cell nitric oxide synthase gene. *Proc Natl Acad Sci USA.* 1995;92:1137–1141.

47. Groves PH, Banning AP, Penny WJ, et al. The effects of exogenous nitric oxide on smooth muscle cell proliferation following porcine carotid angioplasty. *Cardiovasc Res.* 1995;30:87–96.

48. Dusting GJ. Nitric oxide in cardiovascular disorders. *J Vasc Res.* 1995;32:143–161.

49. Kohler TR, Kirkman TR, Kraiss LW, et al. Increased blood flow inhibits neointimal hyperplasia in endothelialized vascular grafts. *Circ Res.* 1991;69:1557–1565.

50. Geary RL, Kohler TR, Vergel S, et al. Time course of flow-induced smooth muscle cell proliferation and intimal thickening in endothelialized baboon vascular grafts. *Circ Res.* 1994;74:14–23.

51. Risau W, Lemmon V. Changes of the vascular extracellular matrix during embryonic angiogenesis and vasculogenesis. *Dev Biol.* 1988;125:441–450.

52. Clowes AW, Clowes MM, Gown AM, et al. Localization of proteoheparansulphate in rat aorta. *Histochemistry.* 1984;80:379–384.

53. Hedin U, Bottger BA, Forsberg E, et al. Diverse effects of fibronectin and laminin on phenotypic properties of cultured arterial smooth muscle cells. *J Cell Biol*. 1988;107:307–319.

54. Li X, Tsai P, Wieder ED, et al. Vascular smooth muscle cells grown on matrigel: a model of the contractile phenotype with decreased activation of mitogen-activated protein kinase. *J Biol Chem*. 1994;269:19653–19658.

55. Hedin U, Thyberg J. Plasma fibronectin promotes modulation of arterial smooth muscle cells from contractile to synthetic phenotype. *Differentiation*. 1987;33:239–246.

56. Bottger BA, Hedin U, Johansson S, Thyberg J. Integrin-like fibronectin receptors in rat arterial smooth muscle cells. Isolation, partial characterization and role in cytoskeletal organization and control of differentiated properties. *Differentiation*. 1989;41:158–167.

57. Clark EA, Brugge JS. Integrins and signal transduction pathways: the road taken. *Science*. 1995;268:233–239.

58. Bardy N, Karillon GJ, Merval R, et al. Differential effects of pressure and flow on DNA and protein synthesis and on fibronectin expression by arteries in a novel organ culture system. *Circ Res*. 1995;77:684–694.

59. Lindner V, Lappi DA, Baird A, et al. Role of basic fibroblast growth factor in vascular lesion formation. *Circ Res*. 1991;68:106–113.

60. Koyama N, Seki J, Vergel S, et al. Regulation and function of an activation-dependent epitope of β_1-integrins in vascular cells *in vitro* and following balloon injury in baboon arteries. *Am J Pathol*. 1996;148:749–761.

61. Seki J, Koyama N, Kovach N, et al. Regulation of β_1-integrin function in cultured human vascular smooth muscle cells. *Circ Res*. 1996;78:596–605.

62. Skinner MP, Raines EW, Ross R. Dynamic expression of $\alpha_1\beta_1$ and $\alpha_2\beta_1$ integrin receptors by human vascular smooth muscle cells. *Am J Pathol*. 1994;145:1070–1081.

63. Clowes AW, Reidy MA, Clowes MM. Mechanisms of stenosis after arterial injury. *Lab Invest*. 1983;49:208–215.

64. Currier JW, Faxon DP. Restenosis after percutaneous transluminal coronary angioplasty. Have we been aiming at the wrong target? *J Am Coll Cardiol*. 1995;25:516–520.

65. Weissberg PL, Clesham GJ, Bennett MR. Is vascular smooth muscle cell proliferation beneficial? *Lancet*. 1996;347:305–307.

66. Nikkari ST, O'Brien KD, Ferguson M, et al. Interstitial collagenase (MMP-1) expression in human carotid atherosclerosis. *Circulation*. 1995;92:1393–1398.

67. Losordo DW, Rosenfield K, Pieczek A, et al. How does angioplasty work? Serial analysis of human iliac arteries using intravascular ultrasound. *Circulation*. 1992;86:1845–1858.

68. Baykal D, Schmedtje, Runge MS. Role of thrombin receptor in restenosis and atherosclerosis. *Am J Cardiol*. 1995;75:82B–87B.

69. Lupu F, Heim DA, Bachmann F, et al. Plasminogen activator expression in human atherosclerotic lesions. *Arterioscler Thromb Vasc Biol*. 1995;15:1444–1455.

4

New Pharmaceutical Agents in Antithrombotic Therapy

David Green, MD, PhD

Prior to discussing the new pharmaceutical agents being introduced for the management of thrombotic disease, it is logical to ask why these drugs are needed. After all, the current anticoagulants, warfarin and heparin, have been in clinical use for 50 years. However, the initiation of heparin therapy usually requires hospitalization and careful laboratory monitoring. Warfarin therapy must also be closely monitored with repeated prothrombin times. Treatment failures with either drug are often encountered, and the therapeutic index for each is relatively narrow. Adverse events in the form of bleeding, thrombocytopenia and osteoporosis with heparin, and skin necrosis with warfarin are serious and cause considerable morbidity and mortality. Thus, safer and more effective antithrombotic agents that do not require a hospital setting or repeated monitoring have been sought.

A vast array of antithrombotic drugs is being readied for clinical use; some are listed in Table 4–1. Rather than briefly discussing every new agent, this review instead focuses on a class of drugs currently approved for thromboprophylaxis and now also being used for thrombus treatment: the low-molecular-weight heparins (LMWHs). The interested reader is referred to several recent review articles that describe antiplatelet and other antithrombotic agents.[1–3]

LOW-MOLECULAR-WEIGHT HEPARINS

Preparation and Properties

Low-molecular-weight heparins are prepared by the depolymerization of standard heparin (SH). A particular method leads to the production of a specific drug; for example, nitrous acid depolymerization is used to prepare nadroparin and dalteparin; benzylation followed by alkaline depolymerization yields enoxaparin; peroxidative depolymerization gives ardeparin; and enzymatic treatment with heparinase yields tinzaparin.[4] Each drug differs from the others in molecular weight, and there are also differences in their pharmacokinetics,[5] but whether these influence their clinical characteristics is unclear. The U.S. Food and Drug Administration (FDA) has taken the

TABLE 4–1. NEW PHARMACEUTICAL AGENTS FOR ANTITHROMBOTIC THERAPY

Antiplatelet agents
Cyclooxygenase inhibitors and prostacyclin analogues
Antibodies to glycoprotein (Gp) IIb/IIIa
Antagonists of the Gp IIb/IIIa receptor
Inhibitors of adenosine diphosphate-induced platelet aggregation
Anticoagulants
Activated protein C
Activators of antithrombin III and heparin cofactor II
   Heparin, low-molecular-weight heparins, heparinoids, pentasaccharide
Inhibitors of activated factor VII, X, and tissue factor
   Factor VIIai, Xa ($Asn^{322}Ala^{419}$), anticoagulant peptides derived from ticks, hookworms, and
   leeches; hementins from *Haementeria officinalis* (antistasin) and *ghilianii*
Specific thrombin inhibitors
   Chloromethyl-ketone peptides, agrotroban, thrombin aptamers (single-stranded
   deoxynucleotides), peptides from *Hirudo medicinalis,* hirudin, hirulog
Defibrinating agents (ancrod)
Fibrinolytic agents
Plasminogen activators (PA)
   Urokinase (UK), pro- and single-chain UK, tissue PA; vampire bat PA, streptokinase,
   anistreplase, staphylokinase
Activators of PA receptors
Plasmin and plasmin analogues
Binders of plasminogen activator inhibitors

position that the safety and efficacy of each preparation must be established as a condition for licensure. At this writing, only enoxaparin and dalteparin are licensed in the United States, although some of the other drugs are licensed elsewhere.

SH consists of a mixture of sulfated polysaccharides with chain lengths ranging from 12 to more than 100 saccharide units and having a mean molecular weight of 13 kDa.[6] The LMWHs have molecular weights of 4 to 6 kDa, and average chain lengths of only 18 saccharide units. This difference in chain lengths is important, because thrombin is unable to bind to heparin molecules consisting of less than 18 saccharides. Thus, the antithrombin activity of LMWHs is low compared to SH. However, the antifactor Xa activity of heparins depends on their ability to bind and activate antithrombin III. Antithrombin III binds to a specific pentasaccharide sequence present on approximately one-third of either SH or LMWH saccharide chains, so that both SH and LMWH have similar antifactor Xa activity. The inhibition of factor Xa accounts for much of the antithrombotic activity of LMWHs, but bleeding may be less because of a relative lack of antithrombin activity as compared to SH.

SH and LMWH differ in a variety of characteristics including absorption, half-life, and effects on platelets, endothelial cells, and osteoclasts. After a single subcutaneous injection, the bioavailability of a LMWH (CY216) was 100% as compared to 24% for SH.[7] Similar excellent bioavailability was observed for dalteparin (87%),[8] enoxaparin (100%),[9] and tinzaparin (90%).[10] Thus, peak anti-Xa activity is higher after subcutaneous injections of LMWH than after equivalent doses of SH. The virtually complete absorption of LMWH renders the need for monitoring unnecessary. Frydman et al.[9] demonstrated that there was a linear relationship between the dose injected and plasma anti-Xa activity. Since the anticoagulant effect of a particular dose is predictable, verification of anticoagulation by testing of the patient's plasma usually is not required. Another desirable property of LMWH is its longer half-life. The half-life of SH is dose dependent, because SH binds to plasma proteins, endothelial cells, and platelets, and the half-life is dependent on saturation of these binding sites.[4] LMWHs have a much lower affinity for these binding sites, which probably contributes to their longer half-life, ranging from 3 to 4 hours after subcutaneous injection.[6]

SH promotes bleeding not only by its inhibition of thrombin, but also by its effects on von Willebrand factor, platelets, and endothelial cells. SH alters von Willebrand factor-dependent platelet function, inhibits collagen-induced platelet aggregation, and increases vascular permeability;[4] LMWH does not have these effects and therefore might induce less bleeding at equivalent antithrombotic doses.

Heparin-induced thrombocytopenia appears to be due to heparin binding to platelet factor 4 (PF-4) on the surface of activated platelets.[11] The heparin–PF-4 complexes stimulate antibody formation; antibody that binds to these complexes also binds to platelet F_c receptors. Cross-linking of these bound antibodies results in platelet granule release, platelet aggregation, thrombocytopenia, and thrombosis. Since LMWHs show less affinity for platelet binding than does SH, the incidence of heparin-induced thrombocytopenia with LMWHs is lower than with SH.[12]

Osteoporosis is a serious complication of prolonged SH administration. SH has a number of effects on bone metabolism, including stimulation of the process of bone resorption. As compared with SH, LMWH has significantly less effect on bone resorption.[13] Small studies in pregnant women have shown no change in bone density during LMWH administration[14] and significantly fewer spinal fractures.[15]

Prevention of Thrombosis

Measures to prevent thrombosis are needed for patients with acute medical or surgical illnesses, as well as for pregnant women with a previous history of thrombosis. The medical conditions associated with thrombosis are those in which patients are considered "hypercoagulable," and include vascular defects (artificial heart valves, unstable atheromatous plaques, aneurysms, vascular grafts), metabolic disturbances (diabetes, hyperlipidemias, hyperhomocysteinemia), antiphospholipid antibody syndrome, paralysis, certain infections, neoplasms and chemotherapeutic agents, exposure to cyclosporine and oral contraceptive agents, and a variety of other disorders.

In some of these conditions, the use of low-dose SH, 5,000 U every 12 hours while the patient is hospitalized, will suffice to prevent venous thrombosis. However, in others such as distal vascular grafts, mechanical prosthetic valves, metastatic malignancies, and spinal cord injury, low-dose heparin has been found to be inadequate, and treatment with either dose-adjusted SH, warfarin, or LMWH is required.

ACUTE SPINAL CORD INJURY, STROKE, AND NEUROSURGERY

We have studied the use of LMWH in patients with acute spinal cord injury and complete motor paralysis.[16] Prophylaxis was initiated within 72 hours of the spinal cord injury. The LMWHs, either tinzaparin, 50 anti-Xa units per kilogram once daily, or enoxaparin, 30 mg twice daily, were given subcutaneously, and no coagulation monitoring was performed. As compared with SH, LMWH prophylaxis was associated with a significant reduction in thromboembolic episodes, and with fewer bleeding complications. Treatment was generally continued until hospital discharge.

Heparinoids have also been evaluated in thrombus prevention in patients with acute stroke. In two trials, Turpie et al.[17,18] showed that a heparinoid, danaproid, was significantly more effective than either placebo or SH (5,000 U every 12 hours) in preventing deep-vein thrombosis in acute thrombotic stroke, and the risk of bleeding was low (2%).

The use of anticoagulants to prevent thromboembolism in patients undergoing neurologic surgery is problematic, because intracranial bleeding may have dire consequences. However, in a recently reported trial in which all subjects wore compression stockings, a LMWH (nadroparin) was compared with placebo.[19] The addition of the LMWH, 7,500 U given 18 to 24 hours postoperatively, resulted in a significant decrease in deep-vein thrombosis (29% total and 40% proximal) with only a modest increase in major bleeding events (LMWH, 2.5%; placebo, 0.8%; $p = 0.09$). There were more deaths in the LMWH group, but these were due to neurologic and not anticoagulant causes. Additional trials, using other LMWHs and perhaps lower doses, are justified by this pilot study.

VASCULAR GRAFTS

There have been few studies evaluating LMWH in the prevention of occlusion of vascular grafts.[20] In one trial, enoxaparin, 40 mg once daily, was compared with SH, 7,500 U twice daily, in patients having aortic aneurysmectomy, aortoiliac repair, and lower limb revascularization.[21] No differences in the rate of bypass graft thrombosis were observed. In another study, patients having femorodistal reconstructive surgery were randomized to enoxaparin, 75 anti-Xa U/kg or SH 150 U/kg given twice daily.[22] Graft thrombosis occurred in 8% of the enoxaparin group and 22% of the SH group ($p < 0.009$). There were no differences in bleeding rates or mortality between the two groups. A third study compared dalteparin, 2,500 U given once daily, with 300 mg aspirin and 100 mg dipyridamole given 8 hourly in patients having femoropopliteal bypass grafting.[23] The use of LMWH resulted in superior graft patency in patients having salvage surgery, but not in those having primary procedures. In the 93 patients having salvage surgery, at 1 year the graft failure rate was 18% with LMWH versus 55% with aspirin/dipyridamole, and bleeding was infrequent in both groups. In summary, although only a few small trials have been conducted in patients undergoing reconstructive vascular surgery, the results suggest that in selected situations LMWH may improve limb salvage.

PROSTHETIC JOINT REPLACEMENT

In contrast to the paucity of studies of LMWH in vascular surgery, there have been a number of trials of LMWH in patients undergoing prosthetic joint replacement (reviewed in Ref. 24). Clagett et al.[25] analyzed a dozen studies of LMWH in hip replacement and concluded that postoperative subcutaneous twice-daily fixed-dose unmonitored LMWH was a satisfactory strategy for prevention of thromboembolism in these patients. Also recommended were warfarin (target international normalized ratio (INR): 2 to 3) or adjusted-dose SH started preoperatively. In patients undergoing knee replacement surgery, LMWH is also effective. In studies directly comparing LMWH with warfarin, efficacy is greater with LMWH, but bleeding occurs more often.[26,27] Bleeding frequency is decreased by beginning prophylaxis 18 hours or more after surgery. Whether efficacy may be improved by giving a small dose of LMWH preoperatively is still unclear. Another area of uncertainty is the optimal duration of treatment postoperatively. Current data suggest 10 to 14 days is the minimal length of time for continuing therapy.

TREATMENT OF THROMBOEMBOLISM

Rapid and complete absorption by the subcutaneous route, a relatively long half-disappearance time, and few adverse reactions commend LMWHs for the treatment of thrombotic disorders. As long ago as 1988, home treatment for deep-vein thrombosis was reported using dalteparin, 120 U/kg twice daily, as initial treatment followed by oral anticoagulation.[28] Subsequently, randomized trials were conducted comparing subcutaneous LMWH with intravenous SH. An open trial in patients with submassive pulmonary embolism found no differences between the two drugs,[29] and a large (more than 400 patient) double-blind randomized study found that LMWH (tinzaparin, 175 U/kg, once daily subcutaneously) was at least as effective and incurred significantly less bleeding than intravenous SH.[30] Similar conclusions have been reported by studies using other LMWHs and open designs.[31,32] An unexpected finding in many of these trials was a decrease in mortality in patients randomized to receive LMWH.[33] A meta-analysis of five trials encompassing more than 1,000 patients found a 47% reduction in risk of death in the LMWH group as compared with the SH group ($p < 0.04$). Most of this decrease in mortality was in cancer patients, whose risk reduction was 64% ($p < 0.01$). This striking decrease in mortality has not been apparent in the more recent trials.[34,35]

Recently, two trials have specifically addressed home treatment with LMWH as compared to in-hospital therapy with SH.[34,35] Both studies showed that LMWH at home was feasible, safe, and effective. However, not every patient who presents with a thrombosis is suitable for home treatment; in the Levine study,[34] 67% of patients were excluded because of coexistent medical conditions, concurrent symptomatic pulmonary embolism, previous thromboembolism, and other reasons. Similarly, in the Koopman investigation,[35] 31% of patients had exclusion criteria and 16% refused to give consent. These two studies were performed outside the United States; at the time of this writing, the FDA has not approved LMWH for the treatment of thrombosis. Until such approval is given, only carefully selected patients should be considered for outpatient thrombosis management; for example, persons who are familiar with the signs and symptoms of thrombosis, knowledgeable in the use of anticoagulants, and willing to take the risk of an adverse event occurring at home (recurrent thrombosis, pulmonary embolus, or bleeding).

COST EFFECTIVENESS

The concept of cost effectiveness goes beyond the cost of a particular drug to include the total expense of managing an illness and its complications. LMWHs are considerably more expensive than SH and warfarin; if the condition being addressed is associated with a low risk of treatment failure, then the use of a LMWH will probably not be cost effective. An example would be the prevention of thrombosis in major abdominal surgery, where the risks of thrombosis are only 0.6% with SH prophylaxis.[36] However, prosthetic joint replacement may be complicated by thromboembolism in up to 50% of patients. Studies comparing the costs of LMWH, warfarin, and placebo in patients having hip and knee replacement surgery demonstrate that both LMWH and warfarin are more cost effective than placebo, and that LMWH and warfarin are roughly equivalent in terms of cost.[37,38] Formal cost-effectiveness analyses of treatment studies are in progress, but both trials assessing home treatment with LMWH concluded that this approach is likely to be more cost effective than inpatient treatment. However, the need to provide caregivers in the home setting also must be considered in the overall assessment of cost. Nevertheless, home treatment of thrombophlebitis with LMWH is likely to become the standard of care in the very near future.

HIRUDIN

Although it was recognized for many years that secretions of the medicinal leech, *Hirudo medicinalis,* had anticoagulant properties, the isolation, characterization, and preparation of hirudin by recombinant (r) DNA technology occurred only recently.[39] In addition, it became possible to prepare hirudin derivatives, such as hirulog (the C-terminal peptide fragment of hirudin linked to a synthetic thrombin inhibitor) with potent anticoagulant activity.[40] Interest in these agents as replacements for heparin is based on several unique properties of these drugs. First, they are potent inhibitors of thrombin and have no requirement for antithrombin III as a cofactor. Therefore, they may be useful in inherited or acquired disorders characterized by low antithrombin III levels, such as congenital antithrombin III deficiency, nephrotic syndrome, or L-asparaginase therapy. Second, they inhibit clot-bound thrombin; neither heparin nor LMWHs are capable of preventing clot-bound thrombin from continuing to generate fibrin from fibrinogen.[41,42] Third, they do not bind to PF-4, and therefore do not cause heparin-induced thrombocytopenia. Their disadvantages include a narrow therapeutic index; serious bleeding led to the early closure of a trial comparing hirudin with heparin as adjunctive therapy to tissue-type plasminogen activator and aspirin in patients with acute myocardial infarction.[43] When compared with LMWHs and dermatan sulfate in an animal model, r-hirudin was found to produce the most bleeding.[44] This may be because r-hirudin, but not LMWH, inhibits platelet activation.[45] Lastly, there is no readily available antidote should the anticoagulant effect require rapid reversal.

A number of clinical trials have confirmed the effectiveness of r-hirudin and hirulog as antithrombotic agents. Two papers in the *New England Journal of Medicine*[46,47] studied patients with coronary artery disease. When given immediately after angioplasty, there were fewer early cardiac events with hirudin as compared to heparin, but restenosis at 7 months was similar.[46] Bleeding events occurred with equal frequency in both groups. In the second study, hirulog or heparin was given immediately prior to angioplasty, and subsequent ischemic and hemorrhagic events were recorded.[47] While there were no differences in ischemic complications overall, a decrease in such events was reported in the subgroup of patients with postinfarction angina assigned to hirulog and, for all patients, bleeding was significantly less common with hirulog than heparin. A third study examined the safety and efficacy of r-hirudin in the prevention of deep-vein thrombosis after total hip replacement.[48] Hirudin at all three dose levels tested was significantly more effective than heparin in decreasing the frequency of venous thromboembolism. Surgical blood loss was increased in the group receiving the highest dose of hirudin, but there was no increase in bleeding complications or requirements for transfusion.

In summary, hirudin and its derivatives may find an important application in patients with arterial thrombosis, because of their ability to inhibit clot-bound thrombin and platelet function. For the same reasons, they may also be valuable in the management of other thrombotic disease resistant to treatment with heparin or LMWH. Lastly, they would be very useful in patients with heparin-induced thrombocytopenia or antithrombin III deficiency.

REFERENCES

1. Lefkovits J, Plow EF, Topol EJ. Platelet glycoprotein IIb/IIIa receptors in cardiovascular medicine. *N Engl J Med.* 1995;332:1553–1559.
2. Weitz J. New anticoagulant strategies: current status and future potential. *Drugs.* 1994;48:485–497.
3. Lahav J, Vermylen J, eds. 1995 state of the art. *Thromb Haemost.* 1995;74:302–308; 360–368; 373–381; 464–481; 493–505; 565–571.
4. Hirsh J, Levine MN. Low molecular weight heparin. *Blood.* 1992;79:1–17.
5. Collignon F, Frydman A, Caplain H, et al. Comparison of the pharmacokinetic profiles of three low molecular mass heparins—dalteparin, enoxaparin and nadroparin—administered subcutaneously in healthy volunteers (doses for prevention of thromboembolism). *Thromb Haemost.* 1995;73:630–640.
6. Barrowcliffe TW, Johnson EA, Thomas DP. Low Molecular Weight Heparin. New York: John Wiley & Sons; 1992:209.
7. Harenberg J, Wurzner B, Zimmermann R, Schettler G. Bioavailability and antagonization of the low molecular weight heparin CY216 in man. *Thromb Res.* 1986;44:549–554.
8. Bratt G, Tornebohm E, Widlund L, Lockner D. Low molecular weight heparin (Kabi 2165, Fragmin): pharmacokinetics after intravenous and subcutaneous administration in human volunteers. *Thromb Res.* 1986;42:613–619.
9. Frydman AM, Bara L, Le Roux Y, et al. The antithrombotic activity and pharmacokinetics of enoxaparine, a low molecular weight heparin, in humans given single subcutaneous doses of 20 to 80 mg. *J Clin Pharmacol.* 1988;28:609–618.
10. Pedersen PC, Ostergaard PB, Hedner U, et al. Pharmacokinetics of a low molecular weight heparin, Logiparin, after intravenous and subcutaneous administration to healthy volunteers. *Thromb Res.* 1991;61:477–487.
11. Aster RH. Heparin-induced thrombocytopenia and thrombosis. *N Engl J Med.* 1995;332:1374–1376.
12. Warkentin TE, Levine MN, Hirsh J, et al. Heparin-induced thrombocytopenia in patients treated with low molecular-weight heparin or unfractionated heparin. *N Engl J Med.* 1995;332:1330–1335.
13. Shaughnessy SG, Young E, Deschamps P, Hirsh J. The effects of low molecular weight and standard heparin on calcium loss from fetal rat calvaria. *Blood.* 1995;85:1368–1373.
14. Melissari E, Parker CH, Wilson NV, et al. Use of low molecular weight heparin in pregnancy. *Thromb Haemost.* 1992;68:652–656.
15. Monreal M, Lafoz E, Olive A, et al. Comparison of subcutaneous unfractioned heparin with a low molecular weight heparin (Fragmin) in patients with venous thromboembolism and contraindications to coumarin. *Thromb Haemost.* 1994;71:7–11.
16. Green D, Chen D. Spinal cord injury: pathophysiology of hypercoagulability and clinical management. In: Seghatchan MJ, Samama MM, Hecker SP, eds. *Hypercoagulable States.* Boca Raton, FL: CRC Press; 1996:293–302.
17. Turpie AGG, Hirsh J, Levine MN, et al. Double-blind randomised trial of ORG 10172 low molecular weight heparinoid in prevention of deep vein thrombosis in thrombotic stroke. *Lancet.* 1987;i:523–526.
18. Turpie AGG, Gent M, Cote R, et al. A low molecular weight heparinoid compared with unfractionated heparin in the prevention of deep vein thrombosis in patients with acute ischemic stroke. *Ann Intern Med.* 1992;117:353–357.
19. Nurmohamed MT, van Riel AM, Henkens MA, et al. Low molecular weight heparin and compression stockings in the prevention of venous thromboembolism in neurosurgery. *Thromb Haemost.* 1996;75:233–238.
20. Samama CM, Combe S, Ill P, et al. Are low-molecular-weight heparins useful for the prophylaxis and treatment of arterial thrombi? *Haemost.* 1996;26(suppl 2):57–64.
21. Farkas JC, Chapuis C, Combe S, et al. A randomized controlled trial of a low-molecular-weight heparin (enoxaparin) to prevent deep-vein thrombosis in patients undergoing vascular surgery. *Eur J Vasc Surg.* 1993;7:554–560.

22. Samama CM, Gigou F, Ill P, for the ENOXART Study Group. Low-molecular-weight heparin in femorodistal reconstructive surgery: a multicenter open randomized study. *Ann Vasc Surg.* 1995;9(suppl):S45–S53.

23. Edmondson RA, Cohen AT, Das SK, et al. Low-molecular weight heparin versus aspirin and dipyridamole after femoropopliteal bypass grafting. *Lancet.* 1994;344:914–918.

24. Green D, Hirsh J, Heit J, et al. Low molecular weight heparin: a critical analysis of clinical trials. *Pharmacol Rev.* 1994;46:89–109.

25. Clagett GP, Anderson FA Jr, Heit J, et al. Prevention of venous thromboembolism. *Chest.* 1995;108(suppl):312S–334S.

26. Hull R, Raskob G, Pineo G, et al. A comparison of subcutaneous low-molecular-weight heparin with warfarin sodium for prophylaxis against deep-vein thrombosis after hip or knee implantation. *N Engl J Med.* 1993;329:1370–1376.

27. Leclerc JR, Geerts WH, Desjardins L, et al. Prevention of venous thromboembolism after knee arthroplasty. *Ann Intern Med.* 1996;124:619–626.

28. Bakker M, Dekker PJ, Knot EAR, et al. Home treatment for deep venous thrombosis with low-molecular-weight heparin. *Lancet.* 1988;ii:1142. Letter.

29. Meyer G, Brenot F, Pacouret G, et al. Subcutaneous low-molecular-weight heparin Fragmin versus intravenous unfractioned heparin in the treatment of acute nonmassive pulmonary embolism: an open randomized pilot study. *Thromb Haemost.* 1995;74:1432–1435.

30. Hull RD, Raskob GE, Pineo GF, et al. Subcutaneous low-molecular-weight heparin compared with continuous intravenous heparin in the treatment of proximal-vein thrombosis. *N Engl J Med.* 1992;326:975–982.

31. Prandoni P, Lensing AWA, Buller HR, et al. Comparison of subcutaneous low-molecular-weight heparin with intravenous standard heparin in proximal deep-vein thrombosis. *Lancet.* 1992;339:441–445.

32. de Valk HW, Banga JD, Wester JWJ, et al. Comparing subcutaneous danaparoid with intravenous unfractionated heparin for the treatment of venous thromboembolism. *Ann Intern Med.* 1995;123:1–9.

33. Lensing AWA, Prins MH, Davidson BL, et al. Treatment of deep venous thrombosis with low-molecular-weight heparins: a meta-analysis. *Arch Intern Med.* 1995;155:601–607.

34. Levine M, Gent M, Hirsh J, et al. A comparison of low-molecular-weight heparin administered primarily at home with unfractionated heparin administered in the hospital for proximal deep-vein thrombosis. *N Engl J Med.* 1996;334:677–681.

35. Koopman MMW, Prandoni P, Piovella F, et al. Treatment of venous thrombosis with intravenous unfractionated heparin administered in the hospital as compared with subcutaneous low-molecular-weight heparin administered at home. *N Engl J Med.* 1996;334:682–687.

36. Kakkar VV, Cohen AT, Edmonson RA, et al. Low molecular weight versus standard heparin for prevention of venous thromboembolism after major abdominal surgery. *Lancet.* 1993;341:259–265.

37. Menzin J, Colditz GA, Regan MM, et al. Cost-effectiveness of enoxaparin vs low-dose warfarin in the prevention of deep-vein thrombosis after total hip replacement surgery. *Arch Intern Med.* 1995;155:757–764.

38. Hull RD, Raskob G, Pineo GE, et al. Subcutaneous low-molecular-weight heparin (LMWH) versus warfarin sodium (WS) for prophylaxis of deep-vein thrombosis (DVT) after total hip or total knee replacment (THR/TKR): an economic perspective. *Blood.* 1994;84:70a. Abstract.

39. Markwardt F. Hirudin and derivatives as anticoagulant agents. *Thromb Haemost.* 1991;66:141–152.

40. Fox I, Dawson A, Loynds P, et al. Anticoagulant activity of Hirulog™, a direct thrombin inhibitor, in humans. *Thromb Haemost.* 1993;69:157–163.

41. Weitz JI, Hudoba M, Massel D, et al. Clot-bound thrombin is protected from inhibition by heparin-antithrombin III but is susceptible to inactivation by antithrombin III-independent inhibitors. *J Clin Invest.* 1992;86:385–391.

42. Agnelli G, Renga C, Weitz JI, et al. Sustained antithrombotic activity of hirudin after its plasma clearance: comparison with heparin. *Blood.* 1992;80:960–965.

43. Neuhaus KL, von Essen R, Tebbe U, et al. Safety observations from the pilot phase of the randomized r-hirudin for improvement of thrombolysis (HIT-III) study. *Circulation.* 1994;90:1638–1642.

44. Matthiasson SE, Linblad B, Stjernquist U, et al. The haemorrhagic effect of low molecular weight heparins, dermatan sulphate and hirudin. *Haemostasis.* 1995;25:203–211.
45. Eichinger S, Wolzt M, Schneider B, et al. Effects of recombinant hirudin (r-hirudin, HBW 023) on coagulation and platelet activation in vivo. *Arterioscler Thromb Vasc Biol.* 1995;15:886–892.
46. Serruys PW, Herrman J-PR, Simon R, et al. A comparison of hirudin with heparin in the prevention of restenosis after coronary angioplasty. *N Engl J Med.* 1995;333:757–763.
47. Bittl JA, Strony J, Brinker JA, et al. Treatment with bivalirudin (hirulog) as compared with heparin during coronary angioplasty for unstable or postinfarction angina. *N Engl J Med.* 1995;333:764–769.
48. Eriksson BI, Ekman S, Kalebo P, et al. Prevention of deep-vein thrombosis after total hip replacement: direct thrombin inhibition with recombinant hirudin, CGP 39393. *Lancet.* 1996;347:635–639.

II

Cerebrovascular Insufficiency

5

Diagnosis of Carotid Stenosis

Magnetic Resonance Arteriography, Duplex Scan, or Angiography?

William D. Turnipseed, MD

Stroke is one of the major health care problems in the United States today. Stroke disables more than 500,000 people annually and, as the third leading cause of mortality, accounts for more than 150,000 deaths each year. Furthermore, current estimates suggest that there are now more than 3 million stroke survivors in our country who require ongoing supportive care. This puts an estimated $200 million drain on health care resources and incurs indirect costs of more than $30 billion each year. To moderate the adverse consequences of stroke, risk factors that predispose to ischemic neurologic injury must be identified: High-risk individuals within any given population must be detected and preventive medical and/or surgical care provided whenever possible.

Our current knowledge about risk factors associated with carotid artery disease has emerged from a formidable database derived from surveillance and screening studies performed since the mid-1970s. Associated risk factors include presence of systolic hypertension, diabetes, hyperlipidemias, presence of carotid occlusive disease, cervical bruits, and a previous history of transient cerebral ischemia. The early clinical correlation between the presence of carotid occlusive disease and the development of ipsilateral ischemic brain injury has resulted in a proliferation of vascular imaging techniques, which have made it possible to understand better the natural history of this disease.

With the advent of contrast arteriography, it became possible to evaluate the cervical and intracranial circulation directly and to correlate disease distribution, configuration, and severity with the development of focal hemispheric ischemic symptoms. Meticulous clinical observation and the results of contrast arteriography established and confirmed the strong correlation between the presence of ipsilateral carotid occlusive disease and the development of hemispheric strokes. These studies also suggested that prevalence of carotid occlusive disease in individuals without cervical bruits or cerebrovascular symptoms was low (less than 5%) and confirmed that the prevalence and severity of carotid disease increased with age and with the presence of arthrosclerotic risk factors such as coronary artery and peripheral vascular disease.[1]

Although contrast arteriography made it possible to identify the surface features of plaque, degree of stenosis, and occlusive changes in the cervical carotid vessels, and to identify intracranial vascular abnormalities such as aneurysms, arteriovenous fistulae, and cerebral hemorrhage in symptomatic patients, it soon became evident that interventional arteriography had limited value as a global screening technique because of its associated risks, cost, and poor patient acceptance. Early carotid arteriograms were performed by injecting contrast agent through a needle placed directly into the cervical carotid artery. Morbidity was significant (>6%), ARCH lesions usually overlooked, intracranial vessels poorly visualized, and the severity of disease often underestimated because biplane imaging was difficult to obtain. Significant technical modifications, developed during the past 20 years, have improved image quality and safety of interventional contrast arteriography. The use of fluoroscopy, development of overwire retrograde catheterization, use of controlled-volume power injection of nonionic contrast agents, and the development of digital subtraction image enhancement have reduced morbid risks (0.5% to 3%) and improved patient acceptance of this technique.[2]

The need to more precisely evaluate asymptomatic, high-risk patient groups, to better select symptomatic candidates for contrast arteriography, and to avoid risk exposure and escalated cost created the impetus for developing noninvasive cerebrovascular screening tests. Advances in medical technology created an opportunity to evaluate physiologic changes in cerebrovascular circulation and to correlate these changes with changes in vessel wall anatomy. Noninvasive tests can be classified as indirect or direct. Indirect tests such as directional Doppler assessment, oculoplethysmography, phonoangiography, and ocular dynomometry helped to characterize regional changes in blood flow dynamics through internal carotid artery and collateral communications between the external carotid and periorbital vessels; to assess differences in systolic pulse arrival time between the right and left internal carotid, or between the ipsilateral carotid and its external branch; and to measure retinal perfusion pressures in each eye. Reversal in the direction of blood flow through periorbital collaterals, asymmetric pulse arrival time, or differential retinal perfusion pressures suggested significant alterations in normal carotid artery blood flow.[3-5] These indirect tests were useful for diagnostic screening but were quickly replaced by techniques that allowed direct assessment of the carotid bifurcation and vertebral artery origins. These included Doppler ultrasonography (continuous-wave or pulse-gated), spectral frequency fast Fourier analysis, and high-resolution B-mode imaging. These tests made it possible to analyze regional blood flow dynamics more accurately through the carotid branch vessels, to evaluate plaque morphology, to determine flow surface characteristics of the carotid lumen, and to correlate these changes with clinically and angiographically defined risk factors. [6,7]

ULTRASOUND

The continuous-wave Doppler assessment was performed using a 5- or 10-MHz directional sensitive transducer, whereas pulse-gated Doppler testing utilized a multielement annular array transducer with frequencies ranging from 6 to 10 MHz. These transducers coupled to a position sensing arm could be used to produce crude two-dimensional flow maps of the carotid bifurcation as the artery was interrogated. Blood flow signals were obtained using a 45- to 60-degree angle of insonation, and were usually displayed online using fast Fourier analysis of spectral frequencies measured in kilohertz versus time. Continuous-wave transducers sampled all frequencies transmitted from the spectral scan window, whereas pulse-gated transducers made it possible to sample flow frequencies more precisely from the central portion of the artery lumen. Doppler ultrasonography made it possible to identify monophasic systolic and diastolic flow disturbances within the internal carotid branch and to distinguish these changes from multiphasic flow in the external carotid branch. Doppler flow characteristics associated with higher grades of stenosis included progressive spectral frequency broadening and increases in peak systolic and diastolic frequencies. Doppler ultrasonography has established itself as an important noninvasive diagnostic test because of its capacity to display visually and numerically flow frequency and velocity changes that predictably occur with increasing severity of carotid occlusive disease. Major limitations of Doppler ultrasound include its inability to subclassify minor levels of occlusive disease, to evaluate flow through calcified arteries, to distinguish preocclusive stenosis precisely from complete arterial occlusion, and to grade categories of disease precisely when contralateral occlusion or severe stenosis is present.[8-11]

The development of real-time B-mode imaging and its coupling with Doppler ultrasound analysis of carotid artery flow resulted in (duplex) testing, which made it possible to evaluate physiologic characteristics of arterial flow across the carotid bifurcation and to assess morphologic changes in the blood vessel wall that occur with the development of artherosclerotic plaques. B-mode imaging analyzes sound-wave reflection from tissues of different acoustic density using an 8-MHz transducer with variable depth focus. By using variations in time gain control, it is possible to enhance contrast differences between thrombus, plaque, and flowing blood. This technique provided a noninterventional method for dynamic assessment of arterial wall anatomy and calculation of arterial lumen reduction at sites of stenosis; identification of internal flow surface abnormalities such ulceration, dissection, and flap formation; and sonographic characterization of arthrosclerotic plaque.

These capabilities enabled clinicians to understand more clearly the natural history of stroke by establishing a relationship between temporal and qualitative changes in plaque morphology, the development of hemodynamic alteration in regional carotid blood flow, and the development of cerebrovascular symptoms.[12,13] This is borne out by the work of Lusby, who was one of the first to demonstrate that echolucent sonographic changes in carotid plaques correlated with the presence of intraplaque hemorrhage in surgical specimens removed from the carotid arteries of patients with focal hemispheric cerebrovascular symptoms. He developed a pathologic grading system for carotid plaques based on the visual ratio of echolucency (hemorrhage) and echogenicity (fibrosis). He used this grading system to evaluate prospectively a group of symptomatic postendarterectomy patients with contralateral asymptomatic carotid disease and an unoperated group of patients with asymptomatic carotid lesions. He demonstrated a statistically significant increase in the development of new neurologic symptoms in patients with echolucent or complex heterogeneous plaques and in patients who demonstrated a significant change in grading category over the course of clinical surveillance. He also documented a higher incidence of new neurologic symptoms in patients that had hemodynamically significant stenoses, exceeding 75% lumen reduction.[14]

The correlation between the presence of high-grade carotid artery occlusive disease and the development of cerebrovascular symptoms has been clearly documented in clinical trials where arteriography was used to document disease severity in surgically treated patients. The ability of duplex ultrasonography to document flow abnormalities in the region of arterial stenoses and to distinguish lesions of hemodynamic significance from complete occlusions has established this test as a useful screening tool for evaluation of asymptomatic patients and as a useful method of triage in individuals with hemispheric symptoms.[15-17]

Recent innovations in duplex scanning, including the use of two-dimensional real-time imaging, color flow imaging of the patent arterial lumen, use of peak systolic and diastolic flow velocities, and/or systolic flow velocity ratios between the internal carotid and common carotid artery, have improved its capacity to detect hemodynamically significant disease and to distinguish critical levels of stenosis from complete arterial occlusion (Table 5–1). Despite this fact, duplex imaging is incapable of precisely characterizing occlusive lesions in the borderline zone between moderate and severe occlusive disease, nor can it with absolute certainty distinguish complete occlusion from preocclusive stenosis. For this reason, the practice of using duplex ultrasonography as the only test for determining therapeutic management in asymptomatic patients might easily be challenged.[18] In contrast, duplex testing in patients with focal cerebrovascular symptoms has proven to be an effective triage technique. Duplex testing is effective in discriminating between normal and diseased carotid vessels; it can distinguish hemodynamically insignificant disease from high grades of stenosis; and it allows for morphologic assessment of carotid plaque. This noninvasive test is probably the most effective means for determining which symptomatic patients are candidates for arteriography and for determining what arterial imaging techniques should be used.

In some health care systems, duplex ultrasonography is the only preoperative diagnostic test used to evaluate patients with cerebrovascular symptoms and to determine who should be candidates for carotid endarterectomy. For this practice to be safe and effective, noninvasive testing should be performed by experienced certified technicians using high-quality imaging machines in accredited diagnostic facilities. On-site comparison testing between duplex ultrasonography and contrast arteriograms is required to determine institutional diagnostic accuracy, and periodic quality assurance should be performed to maintain high standards.[19]

ARTERIOGRAPHY

The traditional role of contrast arteriography in the preoperative evaluation of patients with cerebrovascular symptoms has changed considerably as less invasive methods of arteriography have become available. Traditional x-ray arteriograms obtained by intra-arterial injection of ionic contrast agents remains the most accurate method of obtaining high-quality imaging of the cerebrovascular system. However, despite better fluor-

TABLE 5-1. CAROTID DUPLEX VELOCITY CRITERIA NASCET CATEGORY SEVERE INTERNAL CAROTID STENOSIS (70%–99%)

Reference	Velocity (cm/s) Peak Systolic	Accuracy (%)
Faught WE et al. *J Vasc Surg.* 1994;19:818–828	≥130	88
Turnipseed WD. Unpublished	≥225	91
Monet A et al. *J Vasc Surg.* 1993;17:152–159	≥325	88
	$\dfrac{ICA}{CCA} = 4.0$	88
Patel MR et al. *Stroke.* 1995;26:1753–1758	230	86
	$\dfrac{ICA}{CCA} = 4.0$	93

Trends in end diastolic flow can be helpful in selective identification of patients where peak systolic velocities may underestimate true level of stenosis.
ICA, internal carotid artery; CCA, common carotid artery.

oscopy, use of smaller catheters, and digital computer image enhancement, contrast arteriography is still not completely safe. Although postangiographic risks for death or stroke remain quite low (0.1% to 1.0%), transient morbidity is not uncommon, and is most frequently associated with catheter-induced hemorrhage (2%), embolization (2%), or allergic reactions to injected contrast media (1%). Furthermore, x-ray arteriography is expensive ($5,000 = technical + professional charges + ambulatory surgery). It costs almost as much as carotid endarterectomy and increases the potential for morbid injury as much as 25%. Despite these facts, x-ray arteriography has been one of our most important diagnostic tools, because of its ability to define precisely the severity and distribution of disease within the cerebrovascular system. Furthermore, prospective randomized clinical trials evaluating indications and outcomes for carotid endarterectomy in both symptomatic and asymptomatic patients have based their conclusions on angiographically defined categories of disease.[20-22] Although methods for calculating disease severity differ somewhat between the NASCET and the ECST trials, conclusions from both studies strongly suggested that carotid surgery reduces the risk for death and stroke by as much as 71% in patients with severe ispilateral carotid artery stenosis (>70% lumen reduction). The major argument against continued routine use of x-ray arteriography in the assessment of cerebrovascular symptoms continues to be risk exposure, cost, and poor patient acceptance.

The use of arteriography in the diagnosis and management of cerebrovascular disease has been significantly influenced by the development of digital subtraction and magnetic resonance imaging (MRI) techniques.

Digital subtraction arteriography (DSA) uses computerized enhancement to amplify signals obtained from small quantities of intravascularly administered contrast agent. The capacity of DSA to detect minute quantities of contrast, to store and summate multiple contrast image signals, and to subtract background soft tissue densities by digital video processing made it possible to obtain arterial pictures by intravenous or by a small-volume intra-arterial injections of contrast. Intravenous DSA (IVDSA) was attractive because it made arteriography less invasive by avoiding the risks of intra-arterial catheterization. It was cheaper than standard x-ray arteriography; it could be performed without hospitalization; it had better patient acceptance; and like noninvasive duplex testing, it was best suited for detection of complete arterial occlusions and high-grade stenotic lesions of the cervical or proximal intracranial carotid artery segments.

To obtain arterial images with the IVDSA technique, rapid injection of large contrast volumes were required for each image projection (60 mL contrast; injection rate of 12 to 14 mL/s). Diabetics, renal failure patients, and individuals with congestive heart failure were not well suited for IVDSA testing. Simultaneous bilateral imaging of the carotid and vertebral system made interpretation difficult because of image overlap and an inability to profile the carotid bifurcations predictably. Furthermore, image clarity and spatial resolution was not as good as x-ray arteriography, making IVDSA more likely to miss short segment high-grade strictures, minor stenotic lesions, ulcerations, and small vessel intracranial pathology.[23-25]

Intra-arterial (IADSA) instead of intravenous DSA is now routinely performed in most interventional diagnostic radiology units. The image quality of IADSA has improved despite limitations in spatial resolution (2 line pairs/mm for DSA versus 10 line pairs/mm for x-ray arteriography) because of greatly amplified contrast density in the arterial circulation. As a consequence, contrast volume requirements for IADSA are significantly smaller than those required for IVDSA or standard x-ray angiography. The ability to detect small amounts of contrast with digital processing decreases the need for selective catheterization, thus reducing risk for cerebral embolization and ischemic brain injury. Additional advantages of IADSA include shortened examination time, reduced film costs, and the ability to obtain road map images for selective branch vessel catheterization.[26] In general, IADSA is used for evaluation of the arch and cervical carotid vessels because of its high sensitivity and specificity for detection of hemodynamically significant stenoses and complete occlusions. Standard x-ray arteriograms should be performed when a high degree of spatial resolution is required, as is commonly the case when intracranial arterial or venous pathology is suspected.

MAGNETIC RESONANCE ARTERIOGRAPHY

More recent experience with MRI suggests that physiologic characterization and anatomic display of the cerebrovascular circulation can be obtained without necessity of vascular catheters or injection of contrast agents. Magnetic resonance angiography (MRA) uses a combination of time-of-flight (TOF) and phase contrast (PC) techniques to image the extra- and intracranial circulation, respectively. Two- and three-dimensional TOF images of the carotid bifurcation can be constructed from a stack of 80 or more consecutive axial 1.0- to 1.5-mm-thick flow-compensated, gradient recall echo scans. A targeted maximum intensity projection ray-tracing algorithm is used to create projection images of each carotid bifurcation at 30-degree increments over 180-degree rotation. Two-dimensional PC images of the distal cervical and intracranial circulation are obtained in coronal and sagittal planes using a two-dimensional PC localizer scan with velocity encoding of 30 cm/s. Coronal image slabs are usually 70 mm thick and sagittal slabs are 50 to 60 mm thick.

Unlike x-ray arteriography, MRA has a tendency to overestimate the severity of occlusive disease because of flow void artifacts that result from intravoxel dephasing in areas of turbulent flow, in-plane flow, or proximity of the artery to metallic clips or orthopedic instrumentation. The use of three-dimensional TOF imaging and timed intravenous injection of gadolinium (a nonionic, nontoxic contrast agent) has effectively eliminated many of the problems related to flow void's overestimation of disease status. Adequate screening of MRA candidates will ensure good-quality arterial imaging in most cases. Patients with cardiac pacers, orthopedic instrumentation, severe claustrophobia, unstable pulmonary or cardiac insufficiency, and disoriented individuals unable to follow oral commands should not have MRA performed. Contrast arteriography is an appropriate evaluation for these patients.

MRA has demonstrated the capacity to accurately identify complete arterial occlusion and to distinguish occlusions from severe stenoses with an overall accuracy greater than 95%. Sensitivity and specificity for detection of high-grade stenoses are 100% and 93%, respectively. The capacity of MRA to confirm duplex findings in symptomatic patients has made it possible in many cases to avoid the cost and additional risk exposure associated with routine preoperative contrast arteriography. Like duplex imaging, MRA is noninvasive, safe, and can be done on an outpatient basis. It is also cheaper than standard x-ray arteriography. Unlike duplex imaging, the combination of MRI and MRA can be used to image the brain and screen for pathologic conditions such as ischemia, hemorrhage, tumor, or aneurysm. An additional advantage over duplex imaging is the fact that MRA can determine intracranial directional blood flow patterns through intracranial collateral communications between the carotid and vertebral system, and it can be used to quantitate regional hemispheric blood flow.[27,28]

CONCLUSION

In summary, the most appropriate algorithm for pretreatment evaluation of patients with symptomatic or high-risk carotid occlusive disease will vary somewhat based on available diagnostic resources. In health care centers where Doppler ultrasonography and high-quality MRA are available, it is possible to avoid routine use of contrast arteriography in up to 85% of all symptomatic patients. Doppler ultrasonography should be the first test that is performed in patients with cervical bruits or symptoms suggestive of cerebral ischemia. Doppler ultrasound can be used to establish the presence or absence of significant cervical carotid disease, and to differentiate moderate grades of carotid stenosis (30% to 69%), from severe disease (70% to 99%), or complete occlusion.

In symptomatic patients with negative duplex tests, computed tomography (CT) or an MRI of the head should be performed to rule out hemorrhage, tumor, or focal intracerebral ischemia. If the original head scan is negative, it should be repeated within 3 to 5 days if neurologic symptoms persist. In those patients with focal cerebral symptoms, a negative head scan, and a duplex test that is negative for significant occlusive disease but demonstrates evidence of diffuse echolucent or complex heterogeneous plaque, three-dimensional TOF MRA and MR spectroscopy may be helpful in further evaluation of plaque chemistry and morphology.[29] Three-dimensional TOF MRA should be used to evaluate all symptomatic patients with duplex evidence of moderate and/or high-grade carotid occlusive disease. Those individuals that have flow void artifacts that cannot be successfully interrogated with three-dimensional TOF imaging, should have IV gadolinium for contrast enhancement of this stenosis. A combination of two-dimensional and three-dimensional TOF evaluations of cervical carotid vessels and coronal PC imaging of the intracranial circulation is most effective for distinguishing high-grade stenosis from complete internal carotid artery inclusion. Intra-arterial contrast arteriography should be reserved for use in situations where concordance between Doppler ultrasound and MRA cannot be established, or when intracranial vascular pathology is suspected. One of the most common sources for Doppler ultrasound overestimation of stenosis is accelerated ipsilateral flow that occurs with coexistent contralateral carotid occlusion.[30,31]

Asymptomatic patients with cervical bruits and duplex evidence of borderline high-grade stenoses (65% to 75%) [peak systolic velocity (PSV)>200 cm/s] should have three-dimensional TOF with gadolinium contrast, because clinical management decisions in these patients depend on the most accurate grading of stenosis severity. Doppler alone cannot clearly distinguish borderline intermediate stenoses from high-grade lesions (Fig. 5–1).

Diagnostic strategies may vary in centers where MRA is not available or where institutional standards for the diagnostic accuracy of MRA have not been established. In this setting, preliminary diagnostic testing for patients with bruits or ischemic symptoms should be Doppler ultrasonography. Symptomatic patients with duplex evidence of ipsilateral high-grade carotid stenosis or possible occlusion should have intra-arterial contrast arteriography. (IDSA is now performed in most diagnostic facilities.) The practice of using duplex as a sole preoperative diagnostic test in symptomatic patients may be acceptable when good-quality images are obtained by skilled technicians in certified diagnostic facilities. Head CT or MRI should be performed in these patients to rule out significant intracranial pathology. When intermediate-grade disease is detected by ultrasonography (PSV of 180 to 210 cm/s) in patients with focal symptoms, contrast arteriography is appropriate to establish disease severity and to determine

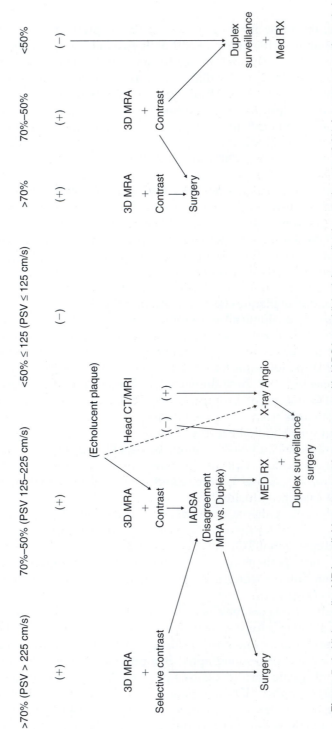

Figure 5–1. High-quality MRA available—comparative accuracy with IADSA established (complication stroke rate<2.0% for contrast angiography). (*Duplex PSU data from The University of Wisconsin–Madison.*)

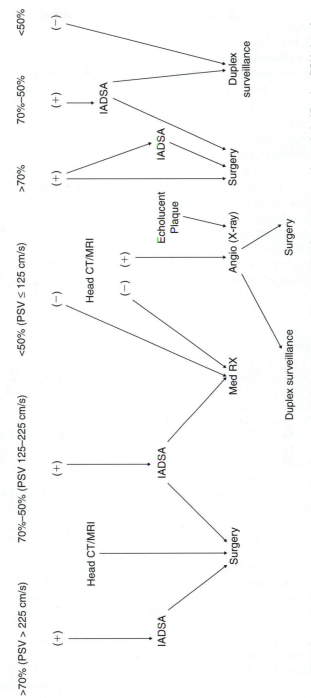

Figure 5–2. MRA not available or accuracy standards not established (complication stroke rate<2.0% for contrast angiography). (*Duplex PSU data from The University of Wisconsin–Madison.*)

whether surgical or medical management is indicated. In asymptomatic patients with high-grade occlusive disease (PSV of >225 cm/s), institutional policy should dictate whether arteriography should be performed or not. Surveillance duplex imaging should be established for those asymptomatic patients with duplex evidence of moderate-grade occlusive disease (Fig. 5–2).

What does the future hold for MRA? Those involved in its research and development are convinced that it will become one of the most important diagnostic imaging tests for evaluating carotid disease. Technical modifications continue to improve the imaging product rapidly. Unfortunately, the current technical evolution of MRA has created a serious "quality gap" between MRA performed in developmental centers and that performed in community-based imaging systems. Standardized protocols for MRA imaging of the carotid system currently do not exist. It is essential to conduct institutional quality controls to determine comparative accuracy with x-ray arteriograms and other noninvasive diagnostic tests and to repeat these studies when new techniques are adapted. It is quite likely that MRA will replace routine diagnostic conventional x-ray arteriography to a large extent. However, MRA will not be able to compete with traditional arteriographic methods, in any significant way, when therapeutic intervention such as endovascular graft or stent placement, balloon angioplastry, thrombolytic therapy, or intraoperative imaging is required.[32]

REFERENCES

1. Lefkowitz D. Asymptomatic carotid artery disease in the elderly: diagnosis and management strategies. *Clin Geriatr Med.* 1991;7:417–428.
2. Fenright E, Trader SD, Hanna GR. Cerebral complications of angioscopy for transient ischemia and stroke: predictions of risk. *Neurology.* 1979;29:4–15.
3. O'Hara PJ, Brewster DC, Darling C, Hallett JW Jr. Oculopneumoplethysmography: its relationship to intraoperative cerebrovascular hemodynamics. *Arch Surg.* 1980;115:1156–1158.
4. Kartchner MM, McRae LP. Noninvasive evaluation and management of the "asymptomatic" carotid bruit. *Surgery.* 1997;82:840–847.
5. Satiani B, Cooperman M, Clark M, Evans WE. An assessment of carotid phonoangiography and oculoplethysmography in the detection of carotid artery stenosis. *Am J Surg.* 1978;136:618–621.
6. Spencer MP, Reid JM. Quantitation of carotid stenosis with continuous-wave (C-W) Doppler ultrasound. *Stroke.* 1979;10:326–330.
7. Barnes RW, Bone GE, Reinertson J, et al. Noninvasive ultrasonic carotid angiography: prospective validation by contrast arteriography. *Surgery.* 1976;80:328–335.
8. Johnston KW, Baker WH, Burnham SJ, et al. Quantitative analysis of continuous-wave Doppler spectral broadening for the diagnosis of carotid disease: results of a multicenter study. *J Vasc Surg.* 1986;4:493–504.
9. Zwiebel WJ, Zagzebski JA, Crummy AB, Hirscher M. Correlation of peak Doppler frequency with lumen narrowing in carotid stenosis. *Stroke.* 1982;13:386–391.
10. Moore DJ, Miles RD, Ohgi S, et al. Relative accuracy of the diagnostic components of noninvasive carotid arterial tests: a comparison of pulsed Doppler arteriography and spectrum analysis. *J Vasc Surg.* 1986;3:502–506.
11. Bandyk DF, Levine AW, Pohl L, Towne JB. Classification of carotid bifurcation disease using quantitative Doppler spectrum analysis. *Arch Surg.* 1985;120:306–314.
12. Ricotta JJ, Bryan FA, Bond MG, et al. Multicenter validation study of real-time (B-mode) ultrasound, arteriography, and pathologic examination. *J Vasc Surg.* 1987;6:512–520.
13. Comerota AJ, Cranley JJ, Katz ML, et al. Real-time B-mode carotid imaging: a three-year multicenter experience. *J Vasc Surg.* 1984;1:84–95.

14. Langsfeld M, Gray-Weale AC, Lusby RJ. The role of plaque morphology and diameter reduction in the development of new symptoms in asymptomatic carotid arteries. *J Vasc Surg.* 1989;9:548–557.
15. Zwiebel WJ, Austin CW, Sackett JF, Strother CM. Correlation of high-resolution, B-mode and continuous-wave Doppler sonography with arteriography in the diagnosis of carotid stenosis. *Radiology.* 1983;149:523–532.
16. Harward TRS, Bernstein EF, Fronek A. Continuous-wave versus range-gated pulsed Doppler power frequency spectrum analysis in the detection of carotid arterial occlusive disease. *Ann Surg.* 1986;204:31–37.
17. Blakeley DD, Oddone EZ, Hasselblad V, et al. Noninvasive carotid artery testing: a meta-analytic review. *Ann Intern Med.* 1995;122:360–367.
18. Goodson SF, Flanigan DP, Bishara RA, et al. Can carotid duplex scanning supplant arteriography in patients with focal carotid territory symptoms? *J Vasc Surg.* 1987;5:551–557.
19. Chervu A, Moore WS. Carotid endarterectomy without certeriography. *Ann Vasc Surg.* 1984;8:296–302.
20. North American Symptomatic Carotid Endarterectomy Trial Collaborators. Beneficial effect of carotid end certerectomy patients with high grade stenosis. *N Engl J Med.* 1991;325:445–453.
21. European Carotid Surgery Trialists' Collaborative Group. MRC European carotid surgery trial: interim results for symptomatic patients with severe (70–90%) or with mild (0–29%) carotid stenosis. *Lancet.* 1991;337:1235–1243.
22. Executive Committee for the Asymptomatic Carotid Atherosclerosis Study. End ostectomy for asymptomatic carotid artery stenosis. *JAMA.* 1995;273:1421–1428.
23. Eikelboom BC, Ackerstaff GA, Ludwig JW, et al. Digital video subtraction angiography and duplex scanning in assessment of carotid artery disease: comparison with conventional angiography. *Surgery.* 1983;94:821–825.
24. Acher CW, Turnipseed WD, Sackett JF, et al. Digital subtraction angiography and continuous-wave Doppler studies. Their use in postoperative study of patients with carotid endarterectomy. *Arch Surg.* 1983;118:462–464.
25. Turnipseed WD, Acher CW. The diagnostic interface between noninvasive cerebral vascular testing and digital arteriography. *J Vasc Res.* 1986;3:486–492.
26. Crummy AB, Stieghorst MF, Turski PA, et al. Digital subtraction angiography: current status and use of intra-arterial injection. *Radiology.* 1982;145:303–307.
27. Turnipseed WD, Kennell TW, Turski PA, et al. Combined use of duplex imaging and magnetic resonance angiography for evaluation of patients with symptomatic ipsilateral high-grade carotid stenosis. *J Vasc Surg.* 1993;17:832–840.
28. Turnipseed WD, Kennell TW, Turski PA, et al. Magnetic resonance angiography and duplex imaging: noninvasive tests for selecting symptomatic carotid endarterectomy candidates. *Surgery.* 1993;114:643–649.
29. Wasserman BA, Haacke EM, Li D. Carotid plaque formation and its evaluation with angiography, ultrasound, and MR angiography. *J Magn Res Imag.* 1994;4:515–517.
30. Kent KC, Kuntz KM, Patel MR, et al. Perioperative imaging strategies for carotid endarterectomy: an analysis of morbidity and cost-effectiveness in symptomatic patients. *JAMA.* 1995;274:888–893.
31. Patel MR, Kuntz KM, Klufas RA, et al. Preoperative assessment of the carotid bifurcation: can magnetic resonance angiography and duplex ultrasonography replace contrast arteriography? *Stroke.* 1995;26:1753–1758.
32. Turnipseed WD, Grist TM. Can magnetic resonance angiography replace contrast arteriography? *Vasc Surg.* 1996;30:177–178.

6

Carotid Endarterectomy

Lessons Learned from Randomized Trials

Jerry Goldstone, MD

Stroke continues to be a major health problem in the United States. According to American Heart Association data, about 500,000 new strokes per year cause nearly 150,000 deaths, making stroke the third leading cause of death in the United States. Perhaps more significant is the fact that strokes render 40% of victims in need of some type of special services and 10% in need of total care. Although the incidence of stroke and the death rate from stroke appear to be declining, the economic impact is still enormous with an estimated $16.7 billion being expended annually for both direct and indirect costs. It is not surprising that the federal government and third-party payers have become increasingly interested in stroke and its prevention.

It has been also estimated that carotid artery bifurcation atherosclerosis is responsible for 20% to 30% of all strokes. One of the most effective means of stroke prevention is carotid endarterectomy. Introduced into clinical practice more than 40 years ago, its use increased rapidly in the United States. In 1970, 7.4 carotid endarterectomies were performed per 100,000 population. By 1980, the incidence had increased to 24 per 100,000 population. By 1985, 105,000 carotid endarterectomies were performed in non-federal U.S. hospitals. Enthusiastic use of this procedure was supported by countless published reports of clinical experiences from both large and small medical centers and hospitals, which reported excellent results with low rates of morbidity and mortality. However, when analyzed carefully, most of these were retrospective reviews with imprecise and nonuniform classifications of patients, outcome criteria, and follow-up. In many of the series, up to 50% of the patients were operated on for asymptomatic carotid stenosis. In still other reviews, even by the standards of 20 to 25 years ago, unacceptably high rates of perioperative morbidity and mortality were associated with this surgical procedure. In the mid-1980s, several leading neurologists began to express their concern about the widespread and increasing use of this operation.[1-3] Part of the concern was based on the belief that aspirin had been demonstrated to be an effective therapy for patients with transient cerebral ischemic attacks. A vigorous debate ensued between those who challenged the efficacy of carotid endarterectomy (mostly neurologists) and those who believed in its efficacy (mostly surgeons).[4,5] This debate took place not only in scientific journals and symposia but also in the lay media, and led several groups to propose and organize randomized prospective clinical trials of carotid endarterectomy for both symptomatic and asymptomatic patients. Arguments put forth in support of the need for these trials included the following:

1. Contemporary prospective randomized trials comparing surgical and nonsurgical treatment of hemispheric transient ischemic attacks did not exist at that time. Recent improvements in the methodology for conducting randomized prospective clinical trials made the few previous efforts in this area obsolete.
2. There was in fact, no definite evidence that surgery was superior to medical treatment in these patients in spite of the many publications with excellent results, almost all of which, as noted above, were nonrandomized retrospective reviews.
3. The surgical morbidity and mortality of carotid endarterectomy were believed to be excessive, especially in community hospitals where the vast majority of these operations were performed, thus negating whatever benefits might be derived from surgical treatment. In some community-wide surveys, the combined morbidity and mortality of carotid endarterectomy exceeded 10%, an alarming figure even in 1985.
4. The indications for the rapidly increasing number of carotid endarterectomies were not well defined, especially in asymptomatic patients, on whom more than 50% of the procedures were being performed in some centers. Furthermore, the natural history of asymptomatic carotid bifurcation atherosclerosis was largely unknown.
5. The economic cost of the large number of carotid endarterectomies being performed was also becoming a major concern, with the costs approximating $1.2 billion in 1985.

In fact, two randomized clinical trials of carotid endarterectomy had been performed by 1980. These included a small British trial of 41 patients conducted in 1965 but not reported until 1984[6] and the more widely known Joint Study of Extra-Cranial Arterial Occlusion, which was a large multicenter trial conducted between 1962 and 1972.[7] It included one cohort of 316 patients with transient ischemic attacks (TIAs) and an ipsilateral carotid stenosis. In spite of the fact that the surgically treated patients in this group seemed to have an improved outcome, this outcome was largely negated by a high surgical complication rate. These two studies were not conclusive and did not meet the design criteria that have evolved for scientifically valid randomized prospective clinical trials of this type. Since 1983, seven contemporary trials have been initiated, three comparing carotid endarterectomy plus medical therapy with the best medical therapy alone in patients with symptomatic carotid stenosis and four in patients with asymptomatic carotid stenosis. The final or interim results have been published for six of these trials.

ASYMPTOMATIC PATIENTS

U.S. Department of Veterans Affairs Asymptomatic Carotid Endarterectomy Trial (VAACET) (Cooperative Study #167)

VAACET was the first of the contemporary prospective randomized trials on carotid endarterectomy. Initially planned in the late 1970s, this trial was conducted in 11 U.S.

TABLE 6–1. RANDOMIZED TRIALS OF CAROTID ENDARTERECTOMY: ASYMPTOMATIC

	CASANOVA	VAACET	ACAS
Patients	410	444	1662
Institutions	10	11	39
Countries	1	1	2
Follow-up (months)	43	48	32.4
Primary outcomes	Stroke and death	Ipsilateral TIA or stroke/ipsilateral stroke	Ipsilateral stroke, TIA, death
Control	11.3%	20.6/9.4	11.0
Surgical	10.7%	8.0/4.7	5.1
Perioperative stroke/death	6.9%	4.3%	2.3%
Relative risk reduction	5%*	61%/50%*	53%

CASANOVA, Carotid Artery Stenosis, Asymptomatic Narrowing Operation vs. Aspirin; VAACET, Veterans Affairs Asymptomatic Carotid Endarterectomy Trial; ACAS, Asymptomatic Carotid Atherosclerosis Study.
* = Nonsignificant.

Veterans Affairs medical centers from 1983 to 1991.[8] The results were published in January 1993.[9]

The primary objective of VAACET was to determine the efficacy of carotid endarterectomy combined with optimal medical management that included aspirin therapy in reducing the incidence of neurologic outcome events (TIAs, transient monocular blindness, and stroke) in comparison to optimal medical management plus aspirin alone in patients with stenosis of one internal carotid artery producing 50% or greater diameter reduction. Although noninvasive modalities were used for screening patients, degree of stenosis was determined angiographically and computed by comparing the smallest residual lumen diameter to that of the distal extra cranial internal carotid artery. Of the 444 randomized male patients, 211 underwent carotid endarterectomy (Table 6–1).

Average follow-up was 47.9 months. All patients initially received 1300 mg of aspirin per day; however, by the conclusion of the trial only 57% were taking the full dose and 16% had discontinued aspirin therapy because of intolerance. The perioperative, 30-day mortality was 1.9% and the operative stroke rate was 2.4% (4.3% total). The incidence of ipsilateral neurologic end points was reduced from 20.6% in the medical group to 8.0% in the surgical group ($p < 0.001$) representing a relative risk reduction of 61% (Table 6–1). Ipsilateral stroke was reduced from 9.4% in the medical group to 4.7% in the surgical group ($p = 0.06$), a relative risk reduction of 50%. The lack of statistical significance for stroke reduction alone has been attributed to an inadequate sample size and this failure to demonstrate a significant benefit of carotid endarterectomy in reducing the incidence of stroke alone has made the results of this trial somewhat controversial. However, it should be remembered that the trial was designed to examine the combined end points of both TIA and stroke and it was only at the insistence of the editorial reviewers that a separate analysis for stroke alone was performed and included in the published results.

Carotid Artery Stenosis Asymptomatic Narrowing Operation Versus Aspirin (CASANOVA)

The CASANOVA trial was conducted in 10 German medical centers under the direction of H. C. Diener.[10] It included 410 patients with internal carotid artery stenosis of between 50% and 90% determined angiographically in a manner similar to that described previously for VAACET. Patients were randomized into one of two groups: Those in group A with unilateral stenosis underwent unilateral endarterectomy and those with bilateral stenosis underwent bilateral endarterectomy. Patients assigned to group B with unilateral stenosis did not undergo operations but those in group B with bilateral stenosis underwent endarterectomy for the most severely stenotic lesion. All patients received 350 mg aspirin per day plus 75 mg dipyridamole three times per day. The primary end points were stroke and death, but not TIA. After an average follow-up of 43 months, the incidence of primary end points was 10.7% in group A compared with 11.3% in group B, a difference that was not statistically significant (Table 6–1). This led the authors to conclude that endarterectomy was not appropriate for asymptomatic internal carotid artery stenosis of less than 90%. However, serious errors in the design and statistical analysis of this study limit its value. First, patients with stenosis of 90% or greater were deemed to be unsuitable for randomization because of the severity of the stenosis and were preferentially operated on and thereby excluded from the trial. These patients probably represent the highest risk group for neurologic events. In addition, more than 50% (118/206) of patients in the control group actually underwent endarterectomy but because of an "intention to treat" design analysis they were statistically treated as nonsurgical patients. Some of these patients had bilateral carotid stenosis and underwent carotid endarterectomy for the most severe lesion and observation for the lesser lesion. Lesions that progressed to more than 90% stenosis during the course of the study were also subjected to endarterectomy. Furthermore, if control patients with unilateral stenosis developed bilateral stenosis (greater than 50% diameter reduction), unilateral endarterectomy was performed. Finally, endarterectomy was performed if patients developed TIAs. None of these events, which caused patients originally randomized to medical therapy to be operated on, were considered as end points or considered as treatment failures for the purpose of statistical analysis, and this explains the lack of difference in the outcomes. Fortunately, these problems have caused most reviewers to attribute relatively little importance to this study.

Asymptomatic Carotid Atherosclerosis Study (ACAS)

This National Institutes of Health (NIH)-funded prospective randomized trial with Dr. James Toole as principal investigator, included 1,662 patients with asymptomatic carotid artery stenosis of 60% or greater diameter reduction who were randomly assigned to either medical treatment (325 mg per day of aspirin plus risk factor reduction) or surgical treatment (carotid endarterectomy plus medical treatment). Randomization occurred from December 1987 through December 1993.[11] The results were published in May 1995.[12]

The degree of stenosis was determined by carefully calibrated duplex ultrasound and/or arteriography but arteriography was mandatory only for patients undergoing endarterectomy. Angiographic stenosis was calculated by comparing the minimal residual lumen diameter with the distal lumen diameter at the first point of the internal carotid beyond the stenosis where the arterial walls became parallel. Primary end points were initially TIA or cerebral infarction in the distribution of the study artery or any TIA, stroke, or death occurring in the perioperative period. During the last year of the trial the primary end points were changed to include cerebral infarction occurring in the distribution of the study artery or any stroke or death occurring in the perioperative period. After a median follow-up of 2.7 years the aggregate risk over 5 years for ipsilateral stroke or any perioperative stroke or death was 5.1% for the surgical patients compared with 11.0% for patients treated medically ($p = 0.004$) (Table 6–1). This yielded an aggregate risk reduction of 53%, but women faired less well than men with a relative risk reduction of only 17% compared with 66% for men. Among the 825 surgical patients, 2.3% had a stroke or died in the perioperative period. This includes 5 patients (1.2%) who suffered strokes as an arteriographic complication. There was no statistically significant difference in the risk of stroke between deciles of stenosis of 60% to 69%, 70% to 79%, or 80% to 99%. The large size of this trial combined with the care with which it was designed and conducted has led many reviewers to consider this the most significant of the published studies on asymptomatic stenosis to date.

Asymptomatic Carotid Surgery Trial (ACST)

This randomized prospective trial is being conducted in 17 European countries and New Zealand under the direction of Alison Halliday, Averil Mansfield, and Dafydd Thomas of London.[13] Randomization began in April 1993, and is ongoing. As of August 1996, 1,316 patients had been entered into the trial. The aim of ACST is to determine whether carotid endarterectomy and best medical treatment improve stroke-free survival time when compared with best medical treatment alone. Entry criteria include the presence of unilateral or bilateral carotid artery stenosis but the severity of stenosis is not specifically defined and can range from greater than 90% to about 50% with soft plaque. Patients may be entered into ACST if the surgeon is satisfied that the lesion is clinically and technically appropriate to operate on if randomized to the surgical option. As with the European (Symptomatic) Carotid Surgery Trial to be described in the next section, in order to be randomized there must be substantial uncertainty about whether a patient is better treated by surgery and appropriate medical treatment or by medical treatment alone (uncertainty principle). The best medical treatment is directed toward smoking, hypertension, diabetes, ischemic heart disease, and hyperlipidemia. Either anticoagulant or antiplatelet therapy may be included but neither is mandatory. Preoperative angiography is not mandatory. Participating surgeons are required to submit a record of their 50 previous endarterectomies in order to ensure that each surgeon's results compare favorably with standards in Europe and the United States. The main study end points are stroke and death. It is hoped that by randomizing a very large number of patients, there will be sufficient data to answer the question "Does carotid endarterectomy prevent disabling stroke or death in patients with asymptomatic carotid artery stenosis?"

Other Trials

A trial was initiated at the Mayo Clinic in 1989 that compared aspirin with surgery. Because of an unacceptably high myocardial infarction rate in the surgically treated group, the trial was terminated after only 71 patients had been randomized.[14]

SYMPTOMATIC PATIENTS

North American Symptomatic Carotid Endarterectomy Trial (NASCET)

This was a large multi-institutional randomized clinical NIH-funded trial and directed by Henry Barnett and his group in New London, Ontario. The study design called for the enrollment of 3,000 patients who had had hemispheric or retinal TIAs or nondisabling strokes within 120 days and who had at least 30% stenosis of the ipsilateral internal carotid artery by biplane angiogram. The patients were divided into two groups, both of which would receive the best available medical treatment with special attention to control of serum lipids, hypertension, and diabetes (risk factor modification). In addition, all patients were to receive 1,300 mg of aspirin per day. In addition, one group underwent carotid endarterectomy. Patients were further stratified into two groups based on the degree stenosis, 30% to 69% and 70% to 99%. All patients were less than 80 years of age. NASCET used strict criteria to define and measure the degree of carotid stenosis (see earlier discussion). The outcome criteria were nonfatal strokes, fatal strokes, and deaths. Within 18 months of this anticipated 5-year study, the results between the two groups exceeded the stopping rules established by the investigators, and in February 1991, the preliminary data were released by the issuance of a clinical alert from the NIH. For patients with greater than 70% stenosis of the appropriate internal carotid artery as determined by the reduction in diameter of the artery relative to the distal internal carotid artery, the surgically treated patients had statistically significant improved outcomes in all of the end point categories: any stroke, any ipsilateral stroke, major ipsilateral stroke, and any major stroke. After less than 2 years of follow-up, patients with a greater than 70% stenosis had a 65% relative risk reduction for these combined neurologic outcomes[15] (Table 6–2). This part of the trial was stopped and no additional patients with 70% or greater carotid stenosis have been randomized.

Secondary analyses of the NASCET data were stratified for decile decrements in percent carotid stenosis (i.e., 70% to 79%, 80% to 89%, 90% to 99%). The investigators documented a decreasing benefit of endarterectomy with each 10% decrement in degree of stenosis. For example, patients with 90% to 99% stenosis achieved a 26% absolute risk reduction, which decreased to 18% for 80% to 89% stenosis, and to 12% for stenosis of 70% to 79%. The data for lesions for less than 70% diameter reduction were not and to date are still not sufficiently different between surgically and nonsurgically treated patients to cause cessation of the study and release of the results. Patient accrual has now ceased for this group of patients, that is, 30% to 69% stenosis, but follow-up is ongoing.

Several interesting subgroup analyses have more recently become available from the high-grade stenosis groups. Amaurosis fugax (retinal TIAs) carried a considerable risk of ipsilateral strokes; however, in comparison with hemispheric TIAs, patients with retinal TIAs had a better prognosis. The risk of subsequent ipsilateral stroke at 2 years was estimated at 16.6% for patients with retinal TIAs as their first ever event compared with 43.5% for patients with hemispheric TIAs.[16] More than half of the 2-year risk of stroke in each group was realized within the first 2 months of randomization. Surgical treatment benefited both groups equally. Carotid plaque ulceration was also examined as an independent risk factor. There was a poor correlation between ulceration, as identified by the preoperative arteriogram, and ulceration as identified intraoperatively by the surgeon. Nevertheless, plaque ulceration was associated with a worse prognosis in the nonsurgically treated group but surgical treatment benefited those with ulceration equally as well as it did those without ulceration. The presence of a contralateral carotid occlusion or severe stenosis was also associated with a worse

TABLE 6–2. NASCET RESULTS: HIGH-GRADE STENOSIS (70% to 99%)

	Treatment		
	Medical	*Surgical*	**Absolute Risk Reduction**
Patients	331	328	
Ipsilateral stroke	26%	9%	17%
Major/fatal stroke	13.1%	2.5%	10.6%

prognosis in both the surgically and medically treated groups, but again patients treated surgically were still benefited by endarterectomy. Advanced age, defined as greater than 65 years, was also associated with a poorer prognosis in the medically treated group but endarterectomy benefited these patients as much as it did younger patients. The presence of intraluminal thrombus was also associated with a worse prognosis in both the medically and surgically treated groups. There was nearly a 25% stroke risk with either surgical or nonsurgical treatment when intraluminal thrombus was present. This was the only subgroup in the original data analysis of the NASCET trial that was not benefited by surgical treatment.

The NASCET trial did not attempt to answer all the questions relative to carotid endarterectomy. As noted previously, data have still not been provided on which to decide what the best management is for patients with moderate degrees of stenosis (30% to 69%). This may represent the largest potential group of patients. Similarly, the long-term prognosis for both the medically and surgically treated patients is not yet known since the data were published after only 2 years of follow-up. For this reason, careful and complete follow-up of all patients is ongoing. The study design allowed inclusion of patients whose events occurred no more than 120 days prior to randomization. NASCET therefore provides no data regarding the benefit of surgical treatment in patients with symptoms of more than a 120-day duration. In spite of these uncertainties, NASCET is a landmark clinical trial that has had a profound effect on the treatment of carotid artery disease.

European Carotid Surgery Trial (ECST)

The ECST trial was a multinational randomized trial conducted in 80 medical centers in 14 European countries under the direction of Charles Warlow of Edinburgh. Funded largely by the Medical Research Council of Great Britain, it extended from 1981 to 1991.[17] Although similar to NASCET in many ways, there were several important differences between the two studies. First, the study design was different in that the European trialists wanted to study a heterogeneous patient population in order for their results to be more widely generalized. Therefore, they needed a large number of patients, eventually randomizing more than 2,500. It was, in fact, at the time of publication, the largest ever randomized clinical trial involving a surgical procedure. Second, ECST was based on the "uncertainty principle," which allowed a patient to be randomized *only* if the physician who was caring for the patient was substantially uncertain whether to recommend endarterectomy or not. Thus, a patient was not eligible for randomization if his or her physician was either reasonably certain that carotid endarterectomy was indicated or reasonably certain that carotid endarterectomy was not indicated. Third, by design, 60% of the patients were randomized to surgical treatment and 40% to medical treatment.

All patients received aspirin at a nonspecified dose and appropriate medical treatment for hypertension as well as efforts to ensure smoking cessation. Eligibility criteria included carotid territory nondisabling ischemic stroke, retinal or hemispheric transient attack, or retinal infarction during the previous 6 months. The degree of carotid stenosis was determined by comparing the minimum residual lumen diameter to the estimated diameter of the carotid bulb, which is different from the NASCET method, which uses the distal cervical internal carotid artery as the denominator. In ECST, 2,518 patients were randomized and stratified into three groups according to the degree of carotid stenosis: mild (0% to 29%), moderate (30% to 69%), or severe (70% to 99%). In May 1991, shortly after release of the NASCET data, the interim results of ECST were published. After an average follow-up interval of 3 years, the late stroke rate was

TABLE 6–3. EUROPEAN CAROTID SURGERY TRIAL SURGICAL RESULTS

	Percent Stenosis	
	0% to 30%	*70% to 99%*
Number of patients	219/374*	455/788*
Death	3	4
Death or severe stroke	5 (2.3%)	17 (3.7%)
Death or any stroke >7 days	10 (4.6%)	34 (7.5%)

* Total randomized in this category.

2.8% in the surgically treated group with severe stenosis compared with 16.8% in the nonsurgical group (Table 6–3). This represented an 85% relative risk reduction for the primary end points of fatal or disabling stroke and nondisabling strokes lasting more than 7 days and occurred in spite of a 7.5% perioperative risk of significant stroke or death. For patients with mild stenosis (less than 30%), there were no statistically significant differences between the medically treated and surgically treated groups. This has been attributed to the relatively high surgically induced stroke morbidity and mortality. As with NASCET, no data were published by the European trialists on patients with moderate stenosis (30% to 69%) and randomization in this group is ongoing.

Department of Veterans Affairs Symptomatic Carotid Stenosis Trial (VA Cooperative Study #309)

The third and final trial in symptomatic patients was conducted in 16 university-affiliated Department of Veterans Affairs medical centers and was directed by Mark Mayberg, Eric Wilson, and Frank Yatsu.[18] It was a much smaller trial than either NASCET or ECST with only 189 patients, all males, randomized (Table 6–4). The reason that this trial was so small is that when the results of the North American and European trials were made public, the VA trialists believed that it would have been unethical to continue to randomize patients. Inclusion criteria included hemispheric or retinal TIAs or small or completed strokes occurring less than 120 days prior to randomization, associated with greater than 50% stenosis of the ipsilateral internal carotid artery as

TABLE 6–4. RANDOMIZED TRIALS OF CAROTID ENDARTERECTOMY: SYMPTOMATIC

	NASCET	ECST	VASCET
Patients	1,360	2,518	192
Institutions	50	80	16
Countries	4	14	1
Follow-up (months) (avg)	18	36	11.9
Primary outcomes	Ipsilateral stroke/major or fatal ipsilateral stroke	Surgical death or disabling or fatal stroke	Crescendo TIA and/or ipsilateral stroke
Control	26%/13%	11.0%	25.6%
Surgical	9%/2.5%	6.0%	7.9%
Perioperative stroke/death	5.8%	7.5%	6.7%
Relative risk reduction*	65%/80%	85%	70%

NASCET, North American Symptomatic Carotid Endarterectomy Trial; ECST, European Carotid Surgery Trial; VASCET, Veteran Affairs Symptomatic Carotid Endarterectomy Trial.
* For >70% stenosis.

determined angiographically. The method of measurement of the degree of carotid stenosis was similar to that employed by NASCET. Patients received either 325 mg of aspirin per day or carotid endarterectomy plus 325 mg of aspirin per day. Primary end points were ipsilateral cerebral infarction or crescendo TIAs and death within 30 days of operation. After a median follow-up of only 11.9 months, the surgically treated group had a statistically significant better outcome with a 70% relative risk reduction in combined end points. Surgical results included a 4.4% risk of major stroke or death and a 6.7% risk of any stroke or death within 30 days of the operation. Thus, these results are nearly identical to those reported by the other two trials in symptomatic patients.

LESSONS LEARNED AND QUESTIONS UNANSWERED

The recently completed carotid endarterectomy trials have reaffirmed the value of large, multi-institutional randomized clinical trials to answer important clinical questions. Many surgeons had become skeptical of randomized trials for surgical procedures because many previous ones had failed to show the benefits of operations.

We have come to appreciate that randomized clinical trials of this type are extremely complex and time-consuming experiments. They are also very expensive. NASCET for example, had a budget of nearly $17 million for direct costs for the first 5 years and more than $20 million for the current phase. Nevertheless, randomized trials remain the most reliable method for comparisons of treatments.[19]

We have also learned, or perhaps relearned, that the fine print must be read; knowing only the results of one or more trials does not give one sufficient information to apply these results to future patients who are not similar to those studied. The inclusion/exclusion criteria must be appreciated, the nature of tests, procedures, and medications must be understood, the length of follow-up known, etc. Without this knowledge, the results of randomized trials cannot be generalized.

Although the overall relative risk reduction of endarterectomy in ACAS was 66% for men, it was only 17% for women. However, this difference was not statistically significant. With an overall 5-year stroke risk of only 11%, is carotid endarterectomy really beneficial in asymptomatic women? For symptomatic patients, endarterectomy provides similar benefit for men and women.[20]

Does the degree of stenosis really matter once it is above a certain level? NASCET demonstrated an increasing benefit from endarterectomy as the degree of carotid stenosis increased. None of the other studies showed this relationship. Perhaps it was an artifact introduced by the use of different methods for quantifying the degree of carotid stenosis used in the different trials. The so-called NASCET method (% ICA stenosis = $(1 - $ [narrowest ICA diameter/diameter normal distal ICA] $) \times 100$ differs from the method used in ECST, which compares the narrowest residual lumen diameter with the estimated diameter of the carotid bulb, which is larger. When ECST arteriograms were remeasured by the NASCET formula, this difference in technique resulted in 48% of ECST patients who were originally classified as severe (>70% stenosis) becoming moderate (<70% stenosis).[21,22] Fortunately, the NASCET and ECST measurements of stenosis are equally good predictions of stroke. But ACAS used 60% stenosis as the lower limit for randomization while the VA asymptomatic trial used 50% stenosis (both of these trials used the NASCET formula for determining stenosis). This leaves us with the seeming paradox that a less severe degree of stenosis has been shown to warrant endarterectomy in asymptomatic patients than for symptomatic patients. These seemingly small differences may be important because very often the decision to perform endarterectomy is based on a single measurement of stenosis. And, as clinicians, we still don't know, based on these studies, if more severe lesions are really more dangerous than less severe lesions once some threshold is exceeded.

The randomized trials discussed here have all shown that carotid endarterectomy can be performed with acceptably low rates of surgically induced morbidity and mortality but not as low in some cases as most surgeons would deem ideal, reaching 7.5% in the largest of the trials. Clearly this operation must be done expertly if its potential benefit is to be achieved and maintained.

It is still unknown what the optimum dose of aspirin is for cerebrovascular protection. Dosages used in these trials varied from 325 to 1,300 mg/day. What should individual practitioners recommend for their patients? The answer is not clear.

Neither NASCET nor ECST demonstrated benefit of endarterectomy for patients with mild (<30% to 40%) carotid stenosis. Surgeons who believe that carotid operations are beneficial for symptomatic patients with nonstenotic but ulcerated lesions must now reassess those beliefs in light of these results.

NASCET and ECST have also shown that whatever the ultimate outcomes are for patients with moderate stenosis, the differences between surgically and nonsurgically treated groups are not likely to be large even if they are statistically significant. With the large number of patients and lengthy follow-up now accumulated in both trials, one would expect that striking differences would have led to publication of results by now.

Finally, trials such as these do not establish permanency of endarterectomy's role as the best therapy for severe carotid stenosis. As new therapeutic agents and procedures are introduced, new comparative trials will be needed. Endarterectomy is best today but something else may be better in the future. Carotid balloon angioplasty with intraluminal stenting is currently being advocated by an enthusiast group of interventionists who have performed this procedure. Hopefully, its rightful place in the treatment of carotid artery disease will be determined by carefully designed, scientifically sound, meticulously conducted clinical trials.

CONCLUSION

The clinical trials on carotid endarterectomy reviewed herein were all multicenter, prospective, and randomized and collectively show an unequivocal benefit of carotid endarterectomy for high-grade stenosis of the internal carotid artery in both symptomatic and asymptomatic patients. The trials vary significantly in a number of important aspects and conclusions drawn must be limited to matching circumstances. Much remains to be learned about cerebrovascular disease. Hopefully, future lessons learned will be the result of scientifically conducted studies like those reviewed here. For these trials, we should be grateful to the dedicated physicians, scientists, and patients who have contributed so much to our knowledge.

REFERENCES

1. Barnett HJM, Plum F, Walton JN. Carotid endarterectomy—an expression of concern. *Stroke*. 1984;15:941–943. Editorial.
2. Chambers BR, Norris JW. The case against surgery for asymptomatic carotid stenosis. *Stroke*. 1984;15:964–967.

3. Dyken ML, Pokras R. The performance of endarterectomy for disease of the extracranial arteries of the head. *Stroke.* 1984;15:948–950.

4. Goldstone, J. Arguments against the need for a randomized trial of carotid endarterectomy in symptomatic patients. In Powers WJ, Raichel ME, eds. *Cerebrovascular Diseases: Fifteenth Research (Princeton) Conference.* New York: Raven Press; 1987:223–231.

5. Plum F. Introduction: should the efficacy of carotid endarterectomy in symptomatic patients be examined in a controlled clinical trial? In: Powers WJ, Raichle ME, eds. *Cerebrovascular Diseases: Fifteenth Research (Princeton) Conference.* New York: Raven Press; 1987:205–206.

6. Shaw DA, Venables GS, Cartlidge NEF, et al. Carotid endarterectomy in patients with transient cerebral ischemia. *J Neurol Sci.* 1984;64:45–53.

7. Fields WS, Maslenikovv V, Meyers JS, et al. Joint study of extracranial arterial occlusion. V. Progesss report on prognosis following surgery or non-surgical treatment for transient cerebral ischemic attacks and carotid artery lesions. *JAMA.* 1970;211:1993–2003.

8. Veterans' Administration Cooperative Study: Role of carotid endarterectomy in asymptomatic carotid stenosis. *Stroke.* 1986;17:534–539.

9. Hobson RW II, Weiss DG, Goldstone J, et al. Efficacy of carotid endarterectomy for asymptomatic carotid stenosis. *N Engl J Med.* 1993;328:221–227.

10. CASANOVA Study Group. Carotid surgery vs. medical therapy in asymptomatic carotid stenosis. *Stroke.* 1991;22:1229–1235.

11. Asymptomatic Carotid Artery Stenosis Group. Study design for randomized prospective trial of carotid endarterctomy for asymptomatic atherosclerosis. *Stroke.* 1989;20:844–849.

12. Executive Committee for the Asymptomatic Carotid Atherosclerosis Study. Endarterectomy for asymptomatic carotid artery stenosis. *JAMA.* 1995;273:1421–1428.

13. Halliday AW, Thomas D, Mansfield A, et al. The Asymptomatic Carotid Surgery Trial. *Eur J Vasc Surg.* 1994;8:703–710.

14. Mayo Asymptomatic Carotid Endarterectomy Study Group. Effectiveness of carotid endarterectomy for asymptomatic carotid stenosis: design of a clinical trial. *Mayo Clin Proc.* 1989;64:897–904.

15. North American Symptomatic Carotid Endarterectomy Trial Collaborators. Beneficial effect of carotid endarterectomy in symptomatic patients with high-grade carotid stenosis. *N Engl J Med.* 1991;325:445–453.

16. Streifler JY, Eliasziw M, Benavente OR, et al. The risk of stroke in patients with first-ever retinal vs hemispheric transient ischemic attacks and high-grade carotid stenosis. *Arch Neurol.* 1995;52:246–249.

17. European Carotid Surgery Trialists' Collaborative Group. MRC European Carotid Surgery Trial: interim results for symptomatic patients with severe (70–99%) or with mild (0–29%) carotid stenosis. *Lancet.* 1991;337:1235–1243.

18. Mayberg MR, Wilson SE, Yatsu F, et al. for the Veterans Affairs Cooperative Studies Program 309 Trialist Group. Carotid endarterectomy and prevention of cerebral ischemia in symptomatic carotid stenosis. *JAMA.* 1991;266:3289–3295.

19. Byar DP, Simon RM, Friedewald WT, et al. Randomized clinical trials: perspectives on some recent ideas. *N Engl J Med.* 1976;95:74–80.

20. Goldstein LB, Hasselblad V, Matchar DB, et al. Comparison and meta-analysis of randomized trials of endarterectomy for symptomatic carotid artery stenosis. *Neurology.* 1995;45:1965–1970.

21. Barnett HJM, Warlow CP. Carotid endarterectomy and the measurement of stenosis. *Stroke.* 1993;24:1281–1284.

22. Eliasziw M, Smith RF, Singh N, et al. Further comments on the measurement of carotid stenosis from angiograms. *Stroke.* 1994;25:2445–2449.

7

Carotid Endarterectomy and Coronary Bypass

John J. Ricotta, MD

The management of atherosclerosis coexisting in the coronary and carotid circulations has been a subject of controversy since Bernhard et al.'s report in 1972.[1] Recently, attention has been refocused on this issue for a number of reasons. As the coronary bypass population ages, the coexistence of significant carotid bifurcation stenosis has become more frequent. Furthermore, availability of carotid duplex ultrasound has provided a simple mechanism to screen for carotid bifurcation disease and increased its detection in the coronary population. Finally, after a decade of controversy, large prospective randomized trials[2–5] have clearly established the efficacy of carotid endarterectomy in management of hemodynamically significant carotid stenosis. Renewed focus on overall reduction of cardiovascular morbidity in patients with atherosclerosis has encouraged clinicians to readdress the problem of combined coronary and carotid disease.

Stroke remains one of the major noncardiac sources of morbidity and mortality after coronary surgery. In the Coronary Artery Surgery Study (CASS), stroke occurred in 1.9% of bypass patients during their hospital stay and in a total of 3.4% within 1 year of coronary artery bypass graft (CABG).[6] It represents a devastating and costly complication for the patient, surgeon, and the health care system alike. While the causes of post-CABG stroke are multiple, a significant minority are associated with carotid bifurcation stenosis and there has been a persistent effort to refine this association and determine the impact of carotid endarterectomy (CEA) on post-CABG stroke. This chapter attempts to review the rationale for considering these problems in concert, summarize the literature on carotid stenosis and post-CABG stroke, and define the areas of current controversy and investigation.

INCIDENCE OF CAROTID STENOSIS IN CABG POPULATION

Atherosclerosis is known to be a systemic disease, therefore it should come as little surprise that carotid stenosis is associated with coronary artery disease. Vascular surgeons have known for years that coronary disease was present in 30% to 50% of patients with carotid stenosis and that myocardial infarction is the major cause of late death in patients after carotid endarterectomy. These observations were first made by DeWeese et al.,[7] later by Callow et al.,[8] and most recently reaffirmed by Chimowitz et al.[9] in the Veterans Administration (VA) asymptomatic carotid stenosis trial. In the latter, an extraordinary number (approximately 40%) of patients suffered late cardiac complications during follow-up after CEA. In a landmark study, Hertzer et al.[10] found 26% incidence of coronary disease in patients who underwent screening coronary angiography prior to CEA. More recently, Love et al.[11] have found abnormalities in 50% of nuclear cardiograms in patients being evaluated for carotid stenosis. In a review of our own experience,[12] 18% of patients with no history of cardiac events experienced a myocardial infarction (MI) within 3 years of CEA.

There has not been as great an appreciation of the prevalence of carotid stenosis in the coronary population. Brener et al.'s[13,14] early reports on CABG patients suggested that operable carotid disease was present in less than 5% of patients. However, more recent studies indicate that this percentage may have increased. Faggioli et al.[15] screened 529 patients prior to CABG and found carotid stenosis >75% in 8.7%. Furthermore, when patient age was considered, the incidence increased from 3.8% in patients <60 years old to 11.3% in patients >60 years old. The increasing frequency of carotid stenosis in older patients undergoing CABG has also been seen by Berens et al.[16] and Schwarz et al.[17] There are indications that by using selective screening of patients at high risk (e.g., peripheral vascular disease, neck bruit) one might increase the yield of significant carotid lesions to >20%. A summary of studies reporting the incidence of carotid stenosis in patients screened prior to CABG is presented in Table 7–1.[14–26] Two series from the Buffalo VA[21,23] serve to emphasize the increasing frequency of carotid stenosis in CABG patients. Using the same screening techniques in the same hospital, the more recent series found that the incidence of significant carotid stenosis in CABG patients

TABLE 7–1. PREVALENCE OF SIGNIFICANT CAROTID STENOSIS IN CABG POPULATION

Author	Year	Number of Patients	% Stenosis	Method	% Positive
Mehigan[18]	1977	874	>50	OPG-K OPG-G	5.6
Turnipseed[19]	1980	170	>50	Doppler	11.8
Barnes[20]	1986	324	>50	Doppler	12.3
Balderman[a21]	1983	500	>50	OPG	3.4
Brener[14]	1987	4,047	>50	OPG Duplex	3.4
Faggioli[15]	1990	539	>50	Duplex	19.9
			>75	Duplex	8.7
Berens[16]	1992	1,087	>50	Duplex	17.0
			>80		5.9
Ricotta[22]	1994	1,179	>50	Duplex	15.7
Pillai[a23]	1994	1,603	>70	+OPG	7.6
Matano[24]	1994	1,780	>70	+OPG	5.6
Schwartz[17]	1995	582	>50	Duplex	22.0
			>80		12.0
Gerraty[25]	1993	358	>50	Duplex	17.6
			>80		9.8
Salisidis[26]	1995	387	>80	Duplex	8.5

a From the same institution but including later patients.

TABLE 7–2. DISTRIBUTION OF STENOSIS IN CABG PATIENTS SCREENED PROSPECTIVELY BY CAROTID DUPLEX—SUNY AT BUFFALO EXPERIENCE

<50%	1,332 pts (84%)
50–75%	144 pts (9%)
>75%	104 pts (7%)

N=1,580.

doubled over a decade. Our cumulative experience with screening 1,580 patients is presented in Table 7–2. Clearly, as the coronary bypass population ages, the number of patients with carotid stenosis who are candidates for CABG will continue to increase. We estimate that this may include 7% to 12% of the current CABG population.

SIGNIFICANCE OF CAROTID STENOSIS IN CABG PATIENTS

The vast majority of carotid stenoses in CABG patients are asymptomatic. As such, they have received relatively little attention until the publication of the Asymptomatic Carotid Atherosclerosis Study (ACAS)[2] and VA trials[3] on asymptomatic carotid stenosis. It is now clear that these asymptomatic carotid lesions will put survivors of CABG at increased long-term risk of stroke. Indeed, some might argue on the strength of the asymptomatic randomized trials that CABG patients should all be screened for carotid disease. Whether this is addressed before or after treatment of their coronary disease is a matter of debate.

For 25 years surgeons have asked the questions of whether (1) carotid stenosis leads to post-CABG neurologic deficits and (2) whether prophylactic CEA before or with CABG is efficacious in stroke prevention. These questions, first raised by Bernhard et al. in 1972[1] remain unanswered. However, while one cannot be dogmatic about a cause-and-effect relationship between carotid stenosis and post-CABG stroke, there is clear evidence that the presence of carotid stenosis is associated with an increased post-CABG stroke rate.

Stroke occurs in 1% to 3% of patients after coronary bypass.[6] Interestingly, in the CASS study, more than 50% of post-CABG strokes occurred more than 24 hours after surgery.[6] These observations have been confirmed by others,[15] although the implication of these findings is unclear at present. Only a few articles in the literature address stroke incidence after CABG in patients with known unoperated carotid stenosis. These reports are summarized in Table 7–3.[14,15,17,20,24,26–30] Studies by Barnes et al.[20] and Schultz et al.[29] suggest that the risk of post-CABG stroke is low in patients with carotid stenosis, although both series report a high perioperative mortality. However, a number of other studies indicate that stroke risk is significantly increased in such patients. In our initial report, we noted a 14% post-CABG stroke rate in patients in whom the asymptomatic carotid stenosis is ignored.[15] This association has been confirmed by Pillai et al.[23] in a report on the VA CABG population and in a later larger report from our own institution in which carotid stenosis was the most powerful predictor of post-CABG stroke, increasing the odds ratio of stroke sixfold.[22]

Despite these data, a cause-and-effect relationship remains difficult to establish for multiple reasons. Foremost among these is the multifactorial nature of post-CABG stroke where risk factors include prior stroke,[31–33] pump time,[32–34] aortic atherosclerosis,[35–37] arrhythmias,[32] intracardiac thrombus, and intra- or postoperative hypotension, to name a few. Fully half of the strokes that occur after CABG do so in patients without

TABLE 7–3. INCIDENCE OF ADVERSE EVENTS IN PATIENTS UNDERGOING ISOLATED CABG WITH KNOWN CAROTID STENOSIS

Author	Number of Patients	Incidence of Adverse Events (%)		
		MI	*CVA*	*Death*
Barnes[20]	40	—	2.5	10.0
Ivey[27]	19	—	15.8	—
Furlan[28]	29	—	15.8	—
Brener[14]	64	—	6.3	15.7
Schultz[29]	50	—	2.0	6.0
Faggioli[15]	28	—	14.3	7.1
Matano[24]	73	—	4.0	1.0
Schwartz[17]	75	—	5.3	—
Salisidis[26]	33	—	18.2	—
VanCauwelaert[30]	61	—	6.6	—

carotid stenosis[6,38,39] (although the size of this group is much larger than those with carotid disease). Furthermore, in patients with carotid stenosis, only about two-thirds of the postoperative neurologic events are in the distribution of the stenotic artery. The situation is made more confusing by the fact that these data are drawn in a large part from small series that were retrospectively reviewed and analyzed.

Given the clear association between carotid stenosis and post-CABG stroke, what possible mechanisms can tie the two together? Intraoperative change in blood flow was initially the most attractive theory. Although this is likely to be operative in some cases, those cases are the minority. Johnsson et al.[40] have shown that cerebral blood flow does not drop significantly in most patients during cardiopulmonary bypass even in the face of a proximal carotid stenosis. This should not be surprising, given the brain's ability to autoregulate cerebral flow. However, failure of autoregulation or intracerebral collateral flow, particularly combined with hypotension or arrhythmia, clearly contributes to postoperative deficits in some patients with carotid stenosis. It is also possible that carotid bifurcation stenosis is merely a marker for more proximal or distal disease, which itself may be critical to post-CABG stroke. The association of bifurcation and intracranial disease is well known. Davila-Roman et al.[41] have pointed out a similar association between carotid bifurcation disease and proximal aortic athero-sclerosis. Atheroemboli from proximal disease have become increasingly recognized as a source of stroke and have been documented using transesophageal echocardiography at the time of aortic cannulation and decannulation.[42–45] This is likely to be one of several reasons for the linkage between carotid stenosis and stroke in CABG patients. Finally, the carotid bifurcation may thrombose or serve as a source of postoperative embolization in CABG patients. Coronary bypass is associated with changes in complement, platelets, fibrinogen, and likely other undescribed alterations in the hemostatic and fibrinolytic system. As such, an irregular stenotic carotid bifurcation might well accumulate additional thrombus, which could then embolize or cause occlusion in the post-CABG period. This theory is particularly attractive when one attempts to explain the delayed strokes seen after CABG.

The most convincing evidence of a direct relationship between carotid stenosis and post-CABG stroke is the results from series in which prophylactic CEA has been performed before or concomitant with coronary bypass. In his early reports, Brener

TABLE 7–4. SELECTED RECENT AND/OR LARGE SERIES OF STAGED AND COMBINED CEA/CABG

Name	Number of Patients	Deaths	Staged/Combined	CVA
Faggioli[22]	17	0	Staged	0
Curl[60]	34	0.117	Combined	0.062
Curl[60]	64	0.03	Staged	0.03
Cambria[46]	71	0.028	Combined	0.042
Akins[48]	200	0.035	Combined	0.03
Chang[47]	189	0.02	Combined	0.03
Minami[56]	114	0.018	Combined	0.044
Halpin[49]	133	0.015	Combined	0.023
Hertzer[51]	170	0.053	Combined	0.053
Hertzer[51]	24	0.04	Staged	0.04
Rosenthal[63]	14	0.071	Staged	0
Reule[53]	164	0.049	Staged	0.024
Newman[62]	28	0	Staged	0
Babu[52]	57	0.048	Combined	0.016
Rizzo[54]	127	0.055	Combined	0.063
Vermeulen[55]	230	0.035	Combined	0.061
Freddy[57]	230	0.035	Combined	0.061
Pome[61]	52	0	Combined	0.019
Pillai[23]	44		Combined/Staged	0.023
Carrel[59]	2	0.38	Combined	0
Klima[58]	89	0.022	Combined	0.056
Carrel[59]	45	0.044	Staged	0
Reule[53]	143	0.042	Combined	0.028
Brener[14]	57	0.105	Combined	0.07

was unable to show decreased overall morbidity with combined coronary and carotid surgery compared to coronary surgery alone in patients with carotid and coronary lesions. More recent data, from Cambria et al.,[46] Chang et al.,[47] Akins et al.,[48] and Halpin et al.[49] have reported significantly lower overall complication rates in combined procedures (range 2% to 4%). Most interesting, is that the *stroke rate* has been much lower than patients with carotid stenosis in whom CEA has not been performed and in many cases approach the stroke rates seen in CABG patients as a whole. Patients in whom a prophylactic CEA can be performed prior to coronary bypass have the lowest overall stroke risk (although their cardiac risk is increased).[50] In our own experience, prophylactic CEA reduces overall periprocedural neurologic morbidity to 3%. Our data, and that of selected series, is presented in Table 7–4.[14,22,23,46–49,51–63] The observation that removing the carotid stenosis reduces stroke risk, while anecdotal, represents the strongest argument for a cause-and-effect relationship between carotid stenosis and post-CABG stroke.

DILEMMA OF COMBINED CAROTID AND CORONARY DISEASE

Data have been presented that surgical lesions in the coronary and carotid systems coexist in 5% to 20% of CABG patients depending on the characteristics of the group of interest. This represents at least 15,000 and as many as 60,000 patients of the >300,000 undergoing CABG each year. There are two arguments for addressing the carotid stenosis in these patients: (1) the increased long-term stroke risk associated with stenotic carotid bifurcation disease (as shown in the VA and ACAS trials) and (2) the possibility that carotid surgery may reduce perioperative stroke risk. These arguments become more compelling in the case of symptomatic carotid lesions. Three approaches to this problem have been developed: (1) prophylactic CEA prior to coronary bypass (staged); (2) operation under the same anesthetic; and (3) delayed CEA until after CABG ("reverse staged"). Each of these is discussed separately.

"Staged" Prophylactic Carotid Endarterectomy Prior to Coronary Surgery

In this approach, the carotid surgery is done under a separate anesthesia with CABG following anywhere from 24 hours to several weeks later. There are several advantages in practice to this alternative, the chief being surgeon comfort and familiarity. Each surgical team can proceed independently in an unhurried manner and in their customary fashion. The neurologic risk should not exceed that of CEA alone followed by a 1% to 2% stroke risk associated with subsequent coronary surgery. The major drawback of this approach is the cardiac risk associated with CEA in patients in need of CABG. Concern over this risk has resulted in Hertzer et al.'s[51] conclusion that it is applicable in no more than one-third of patients. However, in our experience, surgeons who are committed to this approach have been able to apply it in two-thirds to three-quarters of cases. We have successfully used staged procedures in patients with unstable angina who have required medical therapy including heparin and nitroglycerin for stabilization, some of whom have remained on heparin for their coronary disease through the CEA. While surgery can be performed under a general anesthetic, we find that an effective cervical block will simplify perioperative management of blood pressure. In most patients, CABG can follow within 24 to 48 hours. In our experience, this approach is associated with a *combined* neurologic and cardiac complication rate of 6% in staged patients. In no patient was the carotid procedure associated with stroke, MI, or death (Table 7–5).

TABLE 7–5. SUNY BUFFALO EXPERIENCE WITH STAGED AND COMBINED CAROTID/ CORONARY SURGERY

	Staged (N = 64)	Combined (N = 34)	P Value
Age	65.3 ± 8.5	67.5 ± 9.1	NS[b]
Cerebral symptoms	16 (25%)	10 (29%)	NS
Bilat carotid disease	27 (42%)	17 (50%)	NS
% ejection fraction	55.3 ± 13.7	47.8 ± 11.6	NS
Redo CABG	10 (15.6%)	4 (13.3%)	NS
Atrial fibrillation	8 (12.5%)	3 (10%)	NS
Prior MI	34 (53%)	22 (64%)	NS
Urgent or emergency CABG	8 (12%)	14 (41%)	P < .005
Unstable angina	25 (39%)	29 (85%)	P < .0005
Stroke[a]	2 (3.1%)	2 (6.25%)	NS
Death[a]	2 (3.1%)	4 (11.7%)	0.1 > P > .05

[a] All events related to CABG, no MI, death, or stroke after CEA.
[b] NS, not significant.

Staged surgery is not applicable to all patients, particularly those with left main stenosis, large masses of myocardium at risk, hemodynamic lability, or failure to respond to medical management. Unfortunately, no standard definition of the "unstable" patient exists, and most decisions are made based on a clinical gestalt. Nonetheless, this option is useful and may be preferred in patients with elective or urgent, but not emergent, coronary disease, particularly if the carotid disease is critical (i.e., symptomatic or bilateral).

Combined Carotid Endarterectomy and Coronary Bypass

This option appears the most popular among groups who believe that the treatment of the carotid lesion should not be deferred. It presents some logistic difficulties when two teams are used and extends operative times, both of which factors surely contributed to high complication rates in early series. More recently, several large series have appeared with overall mortality and neurologic morbidity less than 5%.[46–49] Clearly, individual centers have developed a successful protocol to address these complex issues. Combined surgery has the advantage of being most widely applicable to patients of all degrees of cardiac and carotid risk, as well as requiring a single anesthetic. The Achilles heel of this approach is the perceived difficulty when it is not applied with regularity. Many individual surgeons find combined surgery inconvenient and have had poor personal experience. When neurologic events do occur, it is often difficult to determine whether they were related to the CEA, more proximal embolization, or central changes in hemostasis or cerebral autoregulation. With the exception of the series mentioned earlier, most series continue to report overall complication rates in the 6% to 12% range (see Table 7–4). Whether or not this is the result of limiting the approach to the most severely ill patients remains unclear.

A variety of approaches have been advocated for single-stage surgery, including CEA prior to cannulation, endarterectomy under hypothermia, with or without arrest, and the use of sidearm perfusion through the bypass circuit to maintain prograde perfusion during carotid clamping. No one technique has proven clearly superior. Regardless of how it is performed, combined surgery remains the preferred approach to patients at high cardiac risk with symptomatic or severe bilateral carotid lesions.

Deferred ("Reverse Staged") Carotid Surgery

This is probably the most widely practiced approach by virtue of the fact that in many centers the carotid arteries are not evaluated prior to CABG. In this approach, asymptomatic carotid stenoses are ignored prior to CABG based on the reported complication rates of combined surgery and the perceived or real increased cardiac risk of staged procedures. If the patient recovers from CABG, the carotid lesion is addressed on its own merits at a later time. This approach ignores the data presented earlier on the increased stroke risk after CABG in patients with known unoperated carotid stenosis. However, in daily practice, this stroke risk is hard for an individual practitioner to appreciate since only 5% to 10% of CABG patients have carotid stenosis and only 10% to 15% of them will have a stroke. It is only by retrospective analysis of a large series that the potential impact of carotid disease becomes apparent. For many practitioners then, the issue is easily ignored.

There has been one randomized study of combined versus reverse staged procedures.[51] In it, Hertzer and colleagues found a very high rate of neurologic deficits in the deferred ("reverse staged") strategy. Half of these were associated with the deferred CEA, most of which were done within 10 days of CABG. This may relate to alterations in hemostasis postoperatively since the author's stroke rate in reverse staging (7%) was two to three times that reported by them for elective CEA. No control (i.e., CABG alone) patients were included in this series.

Reverse staging minimizes cardiac risk in patients with combined disease.[50] It is likely to be most appropriate in patients with high cardiac risk or those with unilateral asymptomatic stenosis. It is certainly less attractive in patients with symptomatic or bilateral carotid disease. In cases of reverse staging, endarterectomy should be deferred for >2 weeks and probably until the patient has completely recovered from CABG.

SOME GUIDELINES FOR MANAGEMENT OF COMBINED DISEASE

While there currently are no clear guidelines on the management of combined coronary and carotid disease, a few general statements can be made. These should be interpreted as personal clinical opinion supported by experience, but as yet, unconfirmed by clinical trials. These guidelines are as follows:

1. In patients with surgical lesions of the carotid bifurcation and stable cardiac disease, these lesions should be addressed prior to CABG, if possible. This position is based on the premises that CEA will eventually be required and that prophylactic endarterectomy may decrease post-CABG stroke. Patients who might qualify for this approach include patients with normal or moderate cardiac risk and high-grade or symptomatic carotid stenosis. Normal cardiac risk is difficult to quantify, but would imply a stable anginal pattern (or one stabilized on medical therapy), adequate ventricular function, and absence of severe left main disease, without large ventricular mass at risk.
2. Patients with critical carotid lesions should have these corrected before or at the time of CABG. Critical carotid lesions include those that are symptomatic and individuals with bilateral severe stenosis (or severe stenosis with contralateral occlusion). When the cardiac condition is stable we prefer the staged approach; when unstable, a combined approach is preferred. In patients with bilateral disease, the most severe operable lesion should be fixed. We have avoided bilateral synchronous carotid endarterectomy with CABG, although this has been reported by Chang et al.[47] from Albany with good results in a limited series. In most cases, we have been satisfied with reconstruction of one carotid artery or used a combination of a staged and combined approach.
3. Patients at high cardiac risk with symptomatic or bilateral carotid disease should have a combined procedure. Ideally, this should be done by an experienced team with a record of close collaboration and good results.
4. Patients with asymptomatic unilateral stenosis and high cardiac risk can be treated by either combined or reverse staged procedures. This decision should be based on local experience. In institutions where the overall complication rate (death and stroke) is less than or equal to 8%, combined surgery would appear most efficacious and should be considered. If reverse staging is done, this should be deferred for 4 to 6 weeks.

No data are currently available on stratifying stroke risk other than on the basis of symptomatology and bilaterality. It is clear that both bilateral lesions and those which are asymptomatic have roughly double the stroke rate of unilateral asymptomatic stenoses after CABG.[52] Whether positron emission tomography, xenon computed tomography, or transcranial Doppler can be used to further stratify cerebral risk is

Smelters CABG Cost ?

	CVA	MI	Death
Smelters			5.6
Coated Then CABg	3%?		9.0
CABg Then CEA	10%		4.5

When to do

   unilat Symplmatic $\geq 70\%$ Stenos

   Bilat Asympt $\geq 70\%$ "

   unilat Asym $\geq 80\%$ "

STRANDNESS

Parech

Assumptions:
  UA Trial - ? Addison -
  Boorg AsA - 250% STens

  A = AS -
      60% STens.
    1600 pts.
      325 ASA.
    2-3 Prin op. Stats/Darth. (1-2% from sign).
    4.8 Studies vs 10.8 formal.
    But not on good in $ or $

Question left
  ? Long Term Follow up Data?
  ? what is best for 30-69% Asymptotic Stens.

Read His chapter.

ZicsTTA
  We should look up & report on own combined/r
  Staged costs / carve pts.

II Cerebrovascular Disease –

Turnipseed.

MRI Angio –

Disadvantage – claustrophobia, pacers, otico implants, clips,

may over estimate.

Therapeutic ~$500 $1500
Duplex, MRI MRA – if agree → done – go to OR.
If not add contrast angiogram –
$4500

Goldstone – Trials

Symptomatic · NASCET.

ASA 1300 mg : Angio be med.

Symptomatic VA Study –
use ASA – Study Terminated Due to
Same Data as NASCET

European Study – ECST (Symptomatic)
only E Tard + randomized pt That Doctor Did not know
what to do ā –
Even ā ~7.5% peri op Stroke Rate ō Surgery
it was Still 6 fold better Than Medicine.

unclear. Certainly, these techniques have been used to identify patients with limited cerebrovascular reserve, which theoretically might correlate with higher post-CABG stroke risk, but this remains to be evaluated. Finally, as with other operations, it is imperative that surgeons review and update their experience on a continuous basis with the management of these difficult patients. This is particularly important since no single institution is likely to accumulate a large experience. It seems unlikely that prophylactic or combined surgery will be superior to reverse staging if combined death and stroke rates significantly exceed 10% and rates >14% are likely to be detrimental. While these numbers are approximate, they should serve as appropriate guidelines.

There has been recent interest in applying carotid bifurcation angioplasty to this group of patients. There is no doubt that this technique, if successfully applied prior to CABG, could relieve carotid stenosis without the need for staged or combined endarterectomy. However, claims by some authors that this is a clear indication for balloon angioplasty are premature. Current complication rates from the best series of balloon angioplasties are 6% to 9%,[64,65] and this is not significantly different from reported series of staged or combined endarterectomy and CABG. Furthermore, there is no evidence to support or refute the contention that balloon angioplasty would reduce post-CABG stroke, since the lesion itself will remain in the carotid circulation and may become even more prone to embolization after CABG. Finally, without long-term data on efficacy of carotid balloon angioplasty, with or without stent, it would be unwise to choose this option preferentially over CEA because of a theoretical, but yet unproven, potential to reduce periprocedural complications. The temptation to perform prophylactic balloon angioplasty at or subsequent to coronary angiography, but prior to CABG, should be resisted until such time as data are available on which to base sound clinical decisions. It is certainly possible, however, that balloon angioplasty, if it proves safe and effective, may eventually play a significant role in the treatment of patients with combined disease.

Finally, the issue of proper management of surgical lesions of the carotid and coronary circulation will not be resolved without prospective standardized comparisons. These will need to compare different strategies in similar patients and eventually are likely to include carotid angioplasty and stenting as one treatment option. As such, they will require standard definitions of cardiac and neurologic risk, objective standards or perioperative evaluation, and detailed analysis of postoperative events (including stroke mechanism). Such trials are currently being planned.

REFERENCES

1. Bernhard VM, Johnson WD, Peterson JJ. Carotid artery stenosis: association with surgery for coronary artery disease. *Arch Surg.* 1972;105:837–840.
2. Executive Committee for the Asymptomatic Carotid Atherosclerosis Study. Endarterectomy for asymptomatic carotid artery stenosis. *JAMA.* 1995;273(18):1421–1428.
3. A Veterans Administration Cooperative Study. Role of carotid endarterectomy in asymptomatic carotid stenosis. *Stroke.* 1986;17:534–539.
4. Barnett HJM, and the North American Symptomatic Carotid Endarterectomy Trial Collaborators. Beneficial effects of carotid endarterectomy in symptomatic patients with high grade stenosis. *N Engl J Med.* 1991;325:445.
5. European Carotid Surgery Trialists Collaborative Group. MRC European carotid surgery trial—interim results for symptomatic patients with severe (70%–99%), or mild (0%–29%) carotid stenosis. *Lancet.* 1991;437:1235–1243.
6. Frye RL, Knonmal R, Schaff HV, et al. Stroke in CABG surgery: an analysis of the CASS experience. The participants in the CASS trial. *Int J Cardiol.* 1992;36(2):213–221.

7. DeWeese JA, Rob CG, Satran R, et al. Results of carotid endarterectomies for transient ischemic attacks—five years later. *Ann Surg.* 1973;178(3):258–264.

8. Callow AD, Mackey WC. Long-term follow-up of surgically managed carotid bifurcation atherosclerosis. *Ann Surg.* 1989;210:308–316.

9. Chimowitz MI, Weiss DG, Cohen SL, et al. Cardiac prognosis of patients with carotid stenosis and a history of coronary artery disease. *Stroke.* 1994;25:759–765.

10. Hertzer NR, Beven EG, Young JR, et al. Coronary artery disease in peripheral vascular patients. *Ann Surg.* 1984;199(2):223–233.

11. Love BB, Grover-McKay M, Biller J, et al. Coronary artery disease and cardiac events with asymptomatic and symptomatic cerebrovascular disease. *Stroke.* 1992;23:939–945.

12. Ricotta JJ, O'Brien MS. Late cardiac events after carotid endarterectomy. *Stroke.* 1996;27(1):4. Abstract.

13. Brener BJ, Brief DK, Alpert J, et al. A four-year experience with preoperative noninvasive carotid evaluation or two thousand twenty-six patients undergoing cardiac surgery. *J Vasc Surg.* 1984;2:326–338.

14. Brener BJ, Brief DK, Alpert J, et al. The risk of stroke in patients with asymptomatic carotid stenosis undergoing cardiac surgery: a follow-up study. *J Vasc Surg.* 1987;5:269–279.

15. Faggioli GL, Curl GR, Ricotta JJ. The role of carotid screening before coronary artery bypass. *J Vasc Surg.* 1990;12:722–729.

16. Berens ES, Kouchoukos NT, Murphy SF, Wareing TH. Preoperative carotid artery screening in elderly patients undergoing cardiac surgery. *J Vasc Surg.* 1992;15:313–323.

17. Schwartz LB, Bridgman AH, Kieffer RW, et al. Asymptomatic carotid artery stenosis and stroke in patients undergoing cardiopulmonary bypass. *J Vasc Surg.* 1995;21(1):146–153.

18. Mehigan JT, Buch WS, Pipkin ED, Fogarty TJ. A planned approach to coexistent cerebrovascular disease in coronary artery bypass candidates. *Arch Surg.* 1977;112:1403–1409.

19. Turnipseed WE, Berkoff HA, Belzer FD. Postoperative stroke in cardiac and peripheral vascular disease. *Ann Surg.* 1980;192:365–368.

20. Barnes RW, Nix ML, Sansonetti D, et al. Late outcome of untreated asymptomatic carotid disease following cardiovascular operations. *J Vasc Surg.* 1985;2:843–849.

21. Balderman SC, Guiterrez IZ, Makula P, et al. Noninvasive screening for asymptomatic carotid artery disease prior to cardiac operation. Experience with 500 patients. *J Thorac Cardiovasc Surg.* 1983;85:427–433.

22. Ricotta JJ, Faggioli GL, Castilone A, Hassett JM. Risk factors for stroke after cardiac surgery: Buffalo Cardiac-Cerebral Study Group. *J Vasc Surg.* 1995;21(2):359–364.

23. Pillai L, Guttierez I, Curl GR, et al. Evaluation and treatment of carotid stenosis in open heart surgery patients. *J Surg Res.* 1994;57:312–315.

24. Matano R, Ascer E, Gennaro M, et al. Outcome of patients with abnormal ocular pneumoplethysmographic measurements undergoing coronary artery bypass grafting. *Cardiovasc Surg.* 1994;2:266–269.

25. Gerraty RP, Gates PC, Doyle JC. Carotid stenosis and perioperative stroke risk in symptomatic and asymptomatic patients undergoing vascular or coronary surgery. *Stroke.* 1993;24(8):1115–1118.

26. Salisidis GC, Latter DA, Steinmetz OK, et al. Carotid duplex scanning in preoperative assessment for coronary artery revascularization: the association between peripheral vascular disease, carotid artery stenosis and stroke. *J Vasc Surg.* 1995;21:154–162.

27. Ivey TD, Strandness E, Williams DB, et al. Management of patients with carotid bruit undergoing cardiopulmonary bypass. *J Thorac Cardiovasc Surg.* 1984;87:183–189.

28. Furlan AC, Craciun AR. Risk of stroke during coronary artery bypass graft surgery in patients with internal carotid artery disease documented by angiography. *Stroke.* 1985;16:797–799.

29. Schultz RD, Sterpetti AV, Feldhaus RJ. Early and late results in patients with carotid disease undergoing myocardial revascularization. *Ann Thorac Surg.* 1988;45:603–609.

30. VanCauwelaert P, Muylaert P, Tombeur J, et al. The cerebrovascular problem in coronary bypass surgery. *Acta Chirurgica Belgica.* 1988;88(2):97–103.

31. Rorick MB, Furlan AJ. Risk of cardiac surgery in patients with prior stroke. *Neurology.* 1990;40:835–837.

32. Reed GL, Singer DE, Picard EH, DeSanctis RW. Stroke following coronary artery bypass surgery: a case-control estimate of the risk of carotid bruits. *N Engl J Med.* 1988;319:1246–1250.

33. Gardner TJ, Horneffer PJ, Manolio TA, et al. Major stroke after coronary artery bypass surgery: changing magnitude of the problem. *J Vasc Surg.* 1986;684–687.

34. Kuroda Y, Uchimoto R, Kaieda R, et al. Central nervous system complications after cardiac surgery: a comparison between coronary artery bypass grafting and valve surgery. *Anesth Analg.* 1993;76:222–227.

35. Bar-El Y, Goor DA. Clamping of the atherosclerotic ascending aorta during coronary artery bypass surgery. Its cost in strokes. *J Thorac Cardiovasc Surg.* 1992;104:469–474.

36. Wareing TH, Davila A, Roman VG, et al. Strategy for the reduction of stroke incidence in cardiac surgical patients. *Ann Thor Surg.* 1993;55:1400–1408.

37. Marschall K, Kanchuger M, Kessler K, et al. Superiority of transesophageal echocardiography in detecting aortic arch atheromatous disease: identification of patients at increased risk of stroke during cardiac surgery. *J Cardiothorac Vasc Anesth.* 1994;8(1):5–13.

38. Opie JC. Cardiac surgery and acute neurological injury. In: Willner A, ed. *Cerebral Damage Before and After Cardiac Surgery.* Dordrecht: Kluwer Academic Publishers; 1993:15–36.

39. Hornick P, Smith PL, Taylor KM. Cerebral complications after coronary bypass grafting. *Curr Opin Cardiol.* 1994;9:670–679. Review.

40. Johnsson P, Algotsson L, Ryding E, et al. Cardiopulmonary perfusion and cerebral blood flow in bilateral carotid artery disease. *Ann Thorac Surg.* 1991;51:579–584.

41. Davila-Roman V, Barzilai B, Wareing T, et al. Atherosclerosis of the ascending aorta—prevalence and role as an independent predictor of cerebrovascular events in cardiac patients. *Stroke.* 1994;25:2010–2016.

42. Hosoda Y, Watanabe M, Hirooka Y, et al. Significance of atherosclerotic changes of ascending aorta in coronary bypass surgery and its intraoperative detection using echography. *J Cardiothorac Surg.* 1989;30:2.

43. Kouchoukos NT, Wareing TH, Daily BB, Murphy SF. Management of the severely atherosclerotic aorta during cardiac operations. *J Cardiac Surg.* 1994;9(5):490–494.

44. Barbut D, Hinton RB, Szatrowski TP, et al. Cerebral emboli detected during bypass surgery are associated with clamp removal. *Stroke.* 1994;25(12):2398–2402.

45. Aranki SF, Rizzo RJ, Adams JH, et al. Single-clamp technique: an important adjunct to myocardial and cerebral protection in coronary operations. *Ann Thor Surg.* 1994;58(2):296–302.

46. Cambria RP, Ivarsson BL, Akins CW, et al. Simultaneous carotid and coronary disease: safety of the combined approach. *J Vasc Surg.* 1989;9:56–64.

47. Chang BB, Darling RC III, Shah DM, et al. Carotid endarterectomy can be safely performed with acceptable mortality and morbidity in patients requiring coronary artery bypass grafts. *Am J Surg.* 1994;168(2):94–96.

48. Akins CW, Moncure AC, Daggett WM, et al. Safety and efficacy of concomitant carotid and coronary artery operations. *Ann Thorac Surg.* 1995;60:311–318.

49. Halpin D, Riggins S, Carmichael J, et al. Management of coexistent carotid and coronary artery disease. *South Med J.* 1992;87(2):187–189.

50. Moore WS, Barnett HJM, Beebe HG, et al. Guidelines for carotid endarterectomy. *Circulation.* 1995;91(2):566–579.

51. Hertzer NR, Loop FD, Beven EG, et al. Surgical staging for simultaneous coronary and carotid disease: a study including prospective randomization. *J Vasc Surg.* 1989;9:455,463.

52. Babu SC, Shah PM, Singh BM, et al. Coexisting carotid stenosis in patients undergoing cardiac surgery: indications and guidelines for simultaneous operations. *Am J Surg.* 1985;150:207–211.

53. Reule GJ Jr, Cooley DA, Duncan JM, et al. The effect of coronary bypass on the outcome of peripheral vascular operations in 1093 patients. *J Vasc Surg.* 1986;3:788–798.

54. Rizzo RJ, Whittemore AD, Couper GS, et al. Combined carotid and coronary revascularization: the preferred approach to the severe vasculopath. *Ann Thorac Surg.* 1992;54:1099–1109.

55. Vermeulen F, Hamerlijnck R, Defaun J, Ernst S. Synchronous operation for ischemic cardiac and cerebrovascular disease: early results and long-term follow-up. *Ann Thorac Surg.* 1992;53:381–390.

56. Minami K, Sagoo KS, Breymann T, et al. Operative strategy in combined coronary and carotid artery disease. *J Thorac Surg.* 1988;95:303–309.

57. Freddy EE, Vermeulen MD, Ruben PH, et al. Synchronous operation for ischemic cardiac and cerebrovascular disease: early results and long-term follow-up. *Ann Thorac Surg.* 1992;53:381–390.
58. Klima V, Wimmer-Greinecker G, Harringer W, et al. Surgical management of coronary heart disease and simultaneous carotid artery stenosis. *Wiener Klinische Wo Chenschriff.* 1993;105(3):76–78.
59. Carrel T, Stillhard G, Turina M. Combined carotid and coronary artery surgery: early and late results. *Cardiology.* 1992;80:118–125.
60. Curl GR, Pillai L, Raza ST, et al. Staged versus combined carotid endarterectomy in coronary bypass patients. Abstract presented at Eastern Vascular Society, May 5–7, 1995 Buffalo, NY.
61. Pome G, Passini L, Colucci V, et al. Combined surgical approach to coexistent carotid and coronary artery disease. *J Cardiovasc Surg.* 1991;32(6):787–793.
62. Newman DC, Hicks R, Horton DA. Coexistent carotid and coronary artery disease. *J Cardiovasc Surg.* 1987;28:599–606.
63. Rosenthal D, Caudill DR, Lamis PA, et al. Carotid and coronary artery disease: a rational approach. *Am Surg.* 1984;50:233–235.
64. NACPTAR Investigators. Update of the immediate angiographic results and in-hospital CNS complications of cerebral percutaneous transluminal angioplasty. *Circulation.* 1995;92 (suppl): 1–383.
65. Dietrich EB, Ndiaye M, Reid DB. Stenting in the carotid artery: initial experience in 110 patients. *J Endovasc Surg.* 1996;3:42–62.

8

Carotid Endarterectomy without Angiography

D. E. Strandness, Jr., MD

The past 20 years have shown tremendous progress in the diagnosis and treatment of carotid artery disease. The parallel development of its surgical management combined with advances in diagnostic techniques has been remarkable. For example, the first reports on the feasibility of combining imaging with Doppler appeared in 1974 with the first usable systems for evaluating the carotid artery appearing about the time of the first symposium held by the Division of Vascular Surgery at Northwestern University.[1–3] Arteriography also continued to evolve during this time frame with the introduction of digital methods. This was also a period of increasing uncertainty for vascular surgeons who were coming under increasing attack by neurologists for proposing carotid endarterectomy as a method of stroke prevention. The neurologists' concerns centered on the risks and the poor results from the operation reported from some centers combined with the uncertainties of its role in the prevention of stroke.[4] Barnett was one of our most prominent critics.[5] His criticisms finally paid off with a sharp reduction in the numbers of these procedures being done and the mounting of randomized clinical trials to study the outcome for both symptomatic and asymptomatic patients with carotid bifurcation disease.[6,7]

It was believed by many neurologists that the data from historical controls were inadequate and that the reporting of surgical series could not be trusted. This led to four major clinical trials, which have now reported their results. Each of these trials, although positive, has led to new disputes and controversies some of which are the subject of this chapter.

CLINICAL TRIALS

To consider the topic at hand, it is necessary to consider briefly these trials and their contribution both to our knowledge and confusion over this topic. The important trials are as follows:

1. The North American Symptomatic Carotid Endarterectomy Trial (NASCET). This trial reported its interim results in 1991.[8] The trials had been under way

for only 2 years when a stopping rule had been reached for the >70% diameter reducing stenoses. The stroke rate in the surgical arm of the trial was 7% as compared to 25% in the medical arm of the trial at 24 months. The diagnostic tests used in the protocol included ultrasound but the final testing done prior to randomization was arteriography. The internal carotid artery distal to the bulb was taken as the normal reference artery in the estimation of the degree of stenosis.

2. The European Carotid Surgery Trial (ECST) came to very similar conclusions at the same time NASCET did.[6] They reported a beneficial effect of endarterectomy over medical therapy within the same time interval. At the time of this report, not many people realized that all arteriographic measurements in ECST were made at the level of the carotid bulb. Thus while ECST also found the cutoff point to be a 70% diameter reduction, it was not the same 70% for the two trials. This fact has caused considerable confusion, which continues up to the time of this writing.

3. The U.S. Department of Veterans Affairs Asymptomatic Carotid Endarterectomy Trial (VAACET) reported a significant reduction of strokes, transient ischemic attacks (TIAs) and death in patients treated surgically with a >50% diameter reducing lesion of the carotid bulb.[9] They used the NASCET form of measurement for the estimation of the degree of diameter reduction.

4. The National Institutes of Health (NIH)-supported Asymptomatic Carotid Artery Surgery (ACAS) trial reported a beneficial effect of endarterectomy in patients with a >60% diameter reducing stenosis.[10,11] It is important to remember that the screening tests used were OPG (oculopneumoplethysmography) and a variety of ultrasound methods. Arteriography was done only on those patients randomized to the surgical arm of the trial. Again the results of endarterectomy were found superior to those with conventional medical therapy.

The debates that have ensued since publication of these trial results have centered in part on the role of arteriography and the use of ultrasound both as a screening test and its possible role as the sole diagnostic test prior to operation. The first issue of importance is the type of arteriography employed, its risks, and the variability associated with its use.

ARTERIOGRAPHY

Methods of Measurement

Arteriography permitted the successful application of surgical methods for the treatment of vascular disease wherever it occurs. It has also undergone an evolution both in how the dye is introduced into the circulation and in how the image information is handled. In my lifetime, the evolution proceeded from single injections at the level of the aortic arch to selective catheterization of the carotid and vertebral arteries. The views of the carotid bulb varied by the method used. When selective injections were used it was common to employ cut-film with multiple views of the bulb.[12] One of the most promising developments occurred with the development of digital methods for handling the image data. This led to the development of intravenous angiography, which when first introduced appeared to offer a simple and safe approach to carotid studies. Initial enthusiasm for the method was rapidly dampened by the realization that the pictures were often "fuzzy" and frequently inadequate. In addition, the need for large volumes of contrast materials limited the application to patients with normal renal function. However, this new technology permitted the use of digital subtraction methods with intra-arterial injection of smaller volumes of contrast material.

What is being measured and how is it done? There is no doubt that the most important item is the "load" of the plaque in the carotid bifurcation. One of the difficult aspects of this problem is the anatomy of the bulb itself. It constitutes a "wide" spot in the road, which makes it unique in the arterial system. Another important consideration is that the disease atherosclerosis confines itself nearly entirely to the bulb. While there have been a variety of methods devised to document the extent of involvement in the bulb, the degree of diameter reduction is the one that has been most widely applied by physicians, and it is unlikely that any other measurement will find widespread acceptance by the medical community.

If the artery at the site of measurement was perfectly circular in its configuration, there would be no dispute as to what would represent a normal "reference" diameter. However, since the bulb is so unique, there are several problems. It is clear that the internal carotid artery distal to the bulb does not constitute the normal "reference" artery for the bulb. Yet this is the point of measurement used in NASCET, VAACET and ACAS[8,9,11] but not used in ECST.[6] In fact, the use of the bulb is more logical since it produces a value for the degree of diameter reduction that is the closest to reality. The problems with using the bulb are that its outer margins may not always be seen well, making its position one of estimation. Nonetheless, the use of the bulb in ECST and the distal internal carotid artery in NASCET has led to some interesting conclusions. While they both claim that a 70% diameter reduction is the cutoff point where endarterectomy is warranted, the 70% lesions are not the same for the two studies. For example, a 50% stenosis in ECST is a 0% stenosis in NASCET! This is obviously nonsense. To make the matter even worse, it is possible to have a negative stenosis in NASCET when one considers the amount of diameter reduction at the level of the bulb!

The situation has not improved but gotten worse. The European group, which is cognizant of the problems, has proposed another method of assessing the degree of diameter reduction in the bulb.[13] They have suggested that the common carotid artery be used as the reference artery. This view has been rejected by NASCET who insist that their imperfect method of assessment must remain in place.[14]

Costs

With the increasing interests in the costs of health care, it is only natural that the total price to the patient and his or her carrier be taken into account. In my own institution, the University of Washington School of Medicine, I was alarmed to find that the total cost for a carotid arteriogram was approximately $6,000. I did an informal survey of various institutions around the United States and found the price to range from $3,000 to $6,000! If $4,500 were taken as the median cost, the total cost to the health care system would be approximately 450 million dollars for every 100,000 studies done!

Safety

It is common practice to refer to the "best" reported figures to support the use of arteriography. Barnett, for example, stated that a 0.4% and 0.5% persistent neurologic complication rate reported from the two institutions within 72 hours should be considered acceptable.[15,16] With these low rates, there would still be between 400 and 500 patients in the United States with a permanent deficit for every 100,000 done. However, this is not the entire story and this may not represent reality. Davies and Humphrey in 1993 reported their complication rates in 200 consecutive digital subtraction studies.[17] Their mortality rate was 1% with a 4% major neurologic event rate. They also noted that the risk of a complication increased with the degree of stenosis with the tighter lesions being the more dangerous. With these figures, for every 100,000 studies done there would be 1,000 deaths and 4,000 neurologic events. Is this an isolated example? It is not, as evidenced by the report of Riles et al.[18] who also had a 4.4% stroke rate following arteriography. In fact their results led Riles to conclude that in spite of all the advances with arteriography, it still remains the most dangerous diagnostic test performed in medicine. To further confirm the results of these more recent series, the published results with the ACAS trial showed that arteriography was as dangerous as carotid endarterectomy. In this trial, the stroke rate for arteriography was 1.2% and accounted for nearly one-half of the strokes that were reported for the entire study (2.3%).[11]

ULTRASOUND

Historically, ultrasound is in its infancy when compared to arteriography. At the University of Washington, our first publication on the clinical use of duplex scanning appeared in 1979![19] It must also be remembered that this was in the very early stages of the use of the method and was done without the benefit of the many advances that are now so commonplace. The first papers to examine in depth the role of duplex scanning for the classification of the degree of stenosis of the carotid arteries began to appear in 1980 to 1982, which is a relatively short time ago.[3,20] All our efforts to document outcome were achieved in steps as our understanding of the problems became evident. The period from 1980 until the present has represented a period of extensive growth both in technology and in our ability to handle it intelligently.

Since physicians were used to the classification of arterial disease by the degree of diameter reduction, all our efforts with duplex ultrasound were in this direction as well. In collaboration with our neuroradiologic colleagues, we began with a classification scheme that would apply to all arterial beds. This was as follows[21-23]:

1. The critical stenosis was defined as a 50% diameter reduction. It was at this level that there was a drop in pressure and flow across the stenosis.
2. So the initial classification was <50% and >50%. Our neuroradiologist noted that there were patients whose disease was so minimal that the degree of diameter reduction could not be measured. These formed a category of 1% to 15%.
3. This resulted in the following categories
   a. normal
   b. 1% to 15%
   c. 16% to 49%
   d. 50% to 99%
   e. occlusion.

Very early in our experience, it became clear that for the carotid bifurcation, the 50% to 99% category was much too broad. For this reason, we divided it into two separate groups—50% to 79% and 80% to 99% stenosis. As history has shown, this turned out to be an important separation since it is the very tight lesions that are most likely to get patients into trouble.

Accuracy

One of the key questions that needed to be answered was how accurate duplex scanning was in relationship to the gold standard of arteriography. We carried out several validation studies to document this.[21] For each step, we used cut-film with selective injections of the bulb using three views of the bulb itself. There are several ways of looking at the accuracy of a diagnostic test. The first is to examine it against the gold standard, which is considered to be 100% accurate. However, this becomes very suspect when no one agrees on what the best method of measuring the end point might be. For example, the end point with the ECST method would be considerably different than the values obtained when the NASCET approach is used.

In our case, all our validation studies were done using the carotid bulb as the reference vessel. The patients had plain films of their neck subtracted looking for the telltale calcification that can often be seen in the lateral aspect of the bulb itself.[24] When this was identified, it was then possible to make a reasonable estimate of the outer boundary of the bulb. We then carried out the following studies[21]:

1. We compared the duplex method with arteriography.
2. For intraobserver variability, we had the same radiologist reread the same films at a later date.
3. For interobserver variability, we employed two neuroradiologists to read the same films.
4. The radiologists used calipers and from three views of the bulb measured the degree of diameter reduction.
5. From these data we were able to calculate what is referred to as a kappa statistic. If there is perfect agreement between the two tests or two readers, the kappa statistic is 1.0. If the values are randomly distributed the kappa value is 0.00. For our studies, the following results were obtained:
   a. intraobserver kappa was 0.711 ± 0.039
   b. interobserver kappa was 0.568 ± 0.058
   c. duplex scanning against a single neuroradiologist gave a kappa value of 0.769 ± 0.039.

This is fine but it is not enough to satisfy most physicians' curiosity when given a single set of figures from a single measurement either by duplex or arteriography. The physician wants to know to what extent the measurement will provide the necessary assurance that proper therapy is or will be applied. Barnett insists that precision is the name of the game.[24] For example, a 69% diameter reducing stenosis in a symptomatic patient is sufficient to provide medical therapy alone and thus avoid the surgeon's knife. For me this is ridiculous since the precision is simply not there in the assessment. I have adopted the rule that for any single estimate of the degree of diameter reduction a value that is either greater or less than that by ±20% is not unreasonable.

What about duplex? Since our studies do not in general refer to a specific degree of diameter reduction but rather by categories that are rather large, we face a different type of problem. In our validation studies, it is rather easy to examine to what extent misclassification errors can occur for each category of narrowing.[21] Let's examine this in more detail:

1. Fifty-six bulbs were normal by arteriography. By duplex, 47 (84%) were so identified. The remaining 9 were classified in the 1% to 15% category. The 1% to 15% category is not significant clinically.
2. For the 1% to 15% category, there were 61 sides. In 49 (87%), the lesions were accurately classified. Eight (13%) were classified into the 16% to 49% category.

Four (7%) were classified as normal. The patient with a 16% to 49% stenosis is generally treated conservatively so this would not be a serious misclassification if it were in fact such.

3. For the 16% to 49% group, there were a total of 80 sides. Perfect agreement was achieved in 78%. Four (5%) were placed into a higher category and 14 (18%) placed into a lower category.

4. For the 50% to 79% category, 1 (1.4%) was classified in the 1% to 15% group. Another 7 (10%) were placed in the 16% to 49% group with 56 (78%) being perfectly categorized. Eight (11%) were placed in the 80% to 99% category. This degree of disease would result in a surgical correction regardless of the symptomatic status of the patient.

5. In the 80% to 99% category, 5 (18%) were placed in the 50% to 79% category with 1 (4%) labeled as an occlusion. Perfect agreement was obtained in 22 (79%).

6. For the total occlusion, there were 39 so identified with 38 (97%) correctly labeled. There was one total occlusion labeled as an 80% to 99% stenosis.

7. Given these kinds of results what might one expect if the duplex alone were used to take the patient to the operating room? For the 80 patients with a 16% to 49% stenosis, 4 (5%) were placed in the next higher category and might be subject to operation if they were symptomatic. For the 50% to 79% group, 8 would have been placed in the 80% to 99% category and subjected to operation. The one total occlusion that was called an 80% to 99% stenosis might well have been subjected to a futile operation if an arteriogram had not been ordered. However, I must point out that these were all based on the assumption that the arteriogram was correct, which is not necessarily the case.

STUDIES OF DUPLEX SCANNING ALONE PRIOR TO OPERATION

Regardless of the validation studies, it is necessary to prospectively examine the role of duplex as a stand-alone method for taking the patient to the operating room. In order to be clear, I want to make the following points with regard to indications for operation:

1. At the present time the only factor that has been consistently shown to be predictive of outcome is the degree of stenosis. It is the high-grade lesions that are the most dangerous. For example, in 1984, we showed that the >80% diameter reducing lesions were the most dangerous and this remains true today.[25]

2. While there is no doubt that ulceration of a plaque is important in the genesis of TIAs and stroke, it is not possible as yet to detect ulceration accurately by any means.

3. Although Barnett's group keeps insisting on precision in measurement, they have not been able to achieve this in their own studies. The 70% cutoff point did not come out as significant due to the precision of the arteriographic measurement.

4. There remains and will remain an element of judgment in decision making for this disease. Let me give some examples:
   a. Is a 50% stenosis in a patient with a stroke enough to warrant operation?
   b. Is the patient with a contralateral occlusion and a 60% stenosis the same as one with disease confined to one side only?

Why arteriography? When it was first widely applied there were certain guidelines that were proposed and remain with us to some extent even today. There was the belief that all studies should include the arch, the bifurcation, the siphon and the intracranial circulation, and the available collateral pathways. It was also considered essential in order to not miss lesions within the skull that might modify one's approach to the patient. Aneurysms, tumors, and arteriovenous malformations (AVMs) are but a few examples of what were considered important. Many of these concerns preceded the development of computed tomography (CT) scanning, which could certainly detect many of the lesions of concern. Yet even today with the availability of magnetic resonance imaging (MRI) as well, it is not clear what role they play in the preoperative evaluation of patients being considered for endarterectomy. There is no evidence that arteriography should be considered an alternative to other imaging studies to detect pathology within the skull. The key question we need to address is whether elimination of arteriography for most patients places them at any increased risk for an adverse outcome. This has to be considered in two separate phases:

1. *The screening phase*: It is here where duplex scanning is first done and will provide the direction that one might need to take. I reject Barnett's statements that the invasive studies must be done at this stage.[26] This is not reasonable and would subject thousands of patients to unnecessary risks and cost.
2. *The planning phase*: This is the most critical time since it is here that a decision must be made relative to therapy. I have divided this into several steps each of which is critical to the decision-making process. These are as follows:
   a. Is the patient symptomatic or asymptomatic?
   b. Is the disease confined to the bulb?
   c. Are there additional lesions found on duplex study?
   d. Is the disease unilateral or bilateral?
   e. Was the study difficult?

To determine if such an approach is safe for the patient, the studies must be done prospectively to assess the validity of the method. In our center we prospectively studied 111 carotid arteries in 103 patients over a period of 29 months.[27] In each case the surgeon had to record his or her plan of management prior to the performance of the arteriogram. The outcome was then assessed based on patient course and the type of therapy that was finally recommended. Seventeen patients were excluded since arteriography was not done or had been performed prior to our duplex study. The findings of our study can be summarized as follows:

1. The duplex scan was considered diagnostic in 87 (93%) of the patients.
2. The factors responsible for a nondiagnostic scan were as follows:
   a. Disease was not confined to the bulb in 4 cases.
   b. Anatomic or pathologic factors interfered with the study in 1 case.
   c. An internal carotid occlusion could not with certainty be distinguished from a high-grade stenosis in 2 cases.
3. Arteriography provided information that affected management in one case. This patient was found to have an occlusion of the middle cerebral artery distal to a high-grade stenosis at the bifurcation. Operation was not performed because of this finding. Five months later, the patient died of a massive stroke secondary to thrombosis of the carotid artery at the level of the bulb.

DISCUSSION

Since our study is not the only one to propose this approach, it is important to review other studies as well as our knowledge concerning the disease we are treating. It is important to review those circumstances in which the duplex scan might lead to the wrong operation or an adverse outcome.[28–32] At this point it is necessary to point out that the operation itself is well standardized with very few significant differences between surgeons with experience in the field. The situations of concern are as follows:

1. High-grade stenosis versus total occlusion. Clearly, one would not want to miss a high-grade stenosis by calling the internal carotid occluded since this would deprive the patient of a chance for stroke prevention. However, one would not want to perform a neck exploration under the assumption that the artery was open when in fact it was occluded. This latter concern can often be avoided if the duplex study is done in proximity to the timing of the operation. We would not object to the performance of an arteriogram when these situations arise. However, the accuracy of this distinction now approaches 95%, providing confidence in most situations where this consideration might come into play.

2. Missing an arch lesion. If one were to miss a high-grade lesion of the arch it could be a serious problem from a surgical standpoint. It might well set the stage for thrombosis to occur at the site of plaque removal from the bifurcation. How often does this occur? In the study by Akers et al.,[33] intrathoracic abnormalities were found in only 1.8% of 1,000 arteriograms. In two-thirds their presence was suggested by the finding of unequal arm pressures. With the improvements in transducer design, it is now possible to "look" down at the arch to detect flow abnormalities from high-grade stenoses at this level. It is important to remember that not all arch lesions are a problem and that there are ways of determining their hemodynamic significance prior to operation. For example, peak systolic velocities in the common carotid artery are good indicators of the significance of proximal lesions.

3. The presence of concurrent lesions either in the siphon or inside the skull.[34] This has always been a concern and one reason for suggesting the necessity of an arteriogram. In a study done by Roederer et al.[34] of 282 siphons studied arteriographically, some degree of narrowing was found in 84% but this did not correlate with the presenting symptoms or the outcome after endarterectomy.

A criticism of this approach by Barnett is that the method is not accurate enough to make the necessary distinctions.[35,36] He makes that statement based on the poor performance of some of the centers in the NASCET trial. However, what he fails to mention are the following:

1. A wide variety of ultrasound devices and methods were used in NASCET.
2. No attempt was made at standardization or quality control.
3. The protocol for ultrasound studies was not followed.
4. The NASCET investigators failed to heed the requests of the Data Monitoring Committee.[37]
5. In essence, the views expressed by Barnett have to be taken with a grain of salt.[35,36] Several of the centers in NASCET did good ultrasound studies and in fact, have subsequently helped in the development of the ultrasonic criteria for the definition of a >70% stenosis.

Finally, we note that the Intersocietal Commission for the Voluntary Accreditation of Vascular Laboratories is in place providing a critically important accreditation process for those laboratories who carry out these studies. This accreditation process, which is well under way, can provide some assurance that the protocols and outcome have been developed and followed to the satisfaction of the commission.

REFERENCES

1. Barber FE, Baker DW, Nation AWC, et al. Ultrasonic duplex echo Doppler scanner. *IEEE Trans Biomed Eng.* 1974;21:109–113.
2. Barber FE, Baker DW, Strandness DE Jr. Duplex scanner II for simultaneous imaging of artery tissues and flow. *Ultrasonics Symp Proc IEEE.* 1974;74CH0896-ISU.
3. Phillips DJ, Powers JE, Eyer MK, et al. Detection of peripheral vascular disease using duplex scanner III. *Ultrasound Med Biol.* 1980;6:205–218.
4. Easton JD, Sherman DG. Stroke and mortality rate in carotid endarterectomy: 228 consecutive operations. *Stroke.* 1977;8:565–568.
5. Barnett HJM, Plum F, Walton JN. Carotid endarterectomy: an expression of concern. *Stroke.* 1984;15:941–943.
6. European Carotid Surgery Trialists' Collaborative Group. MRC European Carotid Surgery Trial: interim results for symptomatic patients with severe (70–99%) or with mild (0–29%) stenosis. *Lancet.* 1991;337:1235–1243.
7. Pokras R, Dyken M. Dramatic changes in the performance of endarterectomy for diseases of the extracranial arteries of the head. *Stroke.* 1988;10:1289–1290.
8. North American Symptomatic Carotid Endarterectomy Trial Collaborators. Beneficial effect of carotid endarterectomy in symptomatic patients with high-grade carotid stenosis. *N Engl J Med.* 1991;325:445–463.
9. Hobson RW, Weiss DG, Fields WS, et al. Efficacy of carotid endarterectomy for asymptomatic carotid stenosis. *N Engl J Med.* 1993;328:221–227.
10. Clinical advisory: carotid endarterectomy for patients with asymptomatic carotid artery stenosis. *Stroke.* 1994;25:2523–2524.
11. Executive Committee, Asymptomatic Carotid Atherosclerosis Study. Endarterectomy for asymptomatic carotid artery stenosis. *JAMA.* 1995;273:1421–1428.
12. Chikos PM, Fisher LD, Hirsch JH, et al. Observer variability in evaluating extracranial arterial stenosis. *Stroke.* 1983;14:885–892.
13. Rothwell PM, Gibson RJ, Slattery J, et al. Equivalence of measurements of carotid stenosis: a comparison of three methods on 1001 angiograms. *Stroke.* 1994;25:2435–2439.
14. Eliasziw M, Smith RF, Singh N, et al. Further comments on the measurement of carotid stenosis from angiograms. *Stroke.* 1994;25:2445–2449.
15. Dion JE, Gates PC, Fox AJ, et al. Clinical events following neuroangiography: a prospective study. *Stroke.* 1987;18:997–1004.
16. Earnest FI, Forbes G, Sandok BA, et al. Complications of cerebral angiography. *AJR.* 1984;142:247–253.
17. Davies KN, Humphrey PR. Complications of cerebral angiography in patients with symptomatic carotid territory ischaemia screened by carotid ultrasound. *J Neurol Neurosurg Psychiatry.* 1993;56:967–972.
18. Riles TS, Eidelman EM, Litt AW, et al. Comparison of magnetic resonance arteriography, conventional arteriography and duplex scanning. *Stroke.* 1992;23:333–341.
19. Blackshear WM, Phillips DJ, Thiele BL, et al. Detection of carotid occlusive disease by ultrasonic imaging and pulsed Doppler spectral analysis. *Surgery.* 1979;86:698.
20. Knox R, Phillips DJ, Breslau PJ, et al. Empirical findings relating sample volume size to diagnostic accuracy in pulsed Doppler cerebrovascular studies. *J Clin Ultrasound.* 1982;227–232.
21. Langlois YE, Roederer GO, Chan ATW, et al. Evaluating carotid artery disease: the concordance between pulsed Doppler/spectrum analysis and angiography. *Ultrasound Med Biol.* 1983;9:51–63.
22. Roederer GO, Langlois YE, Jager KS, et al. A simple parameter for accurate classification of severe carotid disease. *Bruit.* 1989;3:174–178.
23. Thiele BL, Young JV, Chikos PM, et al. Correlation of arteriographic findings and symptoms in cerebrovascular disease. *Neurology.* 1980;30:1041–1046.
24. Barnett HJM, Eliasziw M, Meldrum HE. The identification by imaging methods of patients who might benefit from carotid endarterectomy. *Arch Neurol.* 1995;52:827–831.

25. Roederer GO, Langlois YE, Jager KA, et al. The natural history of carotid arterial disease in asymptomatic patients with cervical bruits. *Stroke*. 1984;15:605–613.
26. Strandness DE Jr. Angiography before carotid endarterectomy—no. *Arch Neurol*. 1995;52: 832–833.
27. Dawson DL, Zierler RE, Strandness DE Jr, et al. The role of duplex scanning and arteriography before carotid endarterectomy: a prospective study. *J Vasc Surg*. 1993;18:673–683.
28. Mattos MA, Hodgson KJ, Faught WE, et al. Carotid endarterectomy without angiography: is color-flow duplex scanning sufficient? *Surgery*. 1994;116:776–783.
29. Moore WS, Ziomek S, Quinones-Baldrich WJ, et al. Can clinical evaluation and noninvasive testing substitute for arteriography in the evaluation of carotid artery disease? *Ann Surg*. 1988;208:91–94.
30. Ricotta JJ, Holen J, Schenk E, et al. Is routine arteriography necessary prior to carotid endarterectomy? *J Vasc Surg*. 1984;1:96–102.
31. Cartier R, Cartier P, Fontaine A. Carotid endartectomy without angiography. The reliability of Doppler ultrasonography and duplex assessment in preoperative assessment. *Can J Surg*. 1993;36:411–416.
32. Turnipseed WD, Kennell TW, Turski PA, et al. Magnetic resonance angiography and duplex imaging: Noninvasive tests for selecting symptomatic carotid endarterectomy candidates. *Surgery*. 1993;114:643–649.
33. Akers D, Bell W, Kerstein M. Does intracranial dye study contribute to evaluation of carotid artery disease? *Am J Surg*. 1988;156:87–90.
34. Roederer GO, Langlois YE, Chan RTW, et al. Is siphon disease important in predicting the outcome of carotid endarterectomy? *Arch Surg*. 1983;118:1177–1181.
35. Haynes RB, Taylor DW, Sackett DL, et al. Poor performance of Doppler detecting high-grade carotid stenosis. *Clin Res*. 1992;40:184A.
36. Barnett HJM, Eliasziw M, Meldrum HE. The identification by imaging methods of patients who might benefit from carotid endarterectomy. *Arch Neurol*. 1995;52:827–831.
37. Strandness DE Jr. What you didn't know about the North American Symptomatic Carotid Endarterectomy Trial (NASCET). *J Vasc Surg*. 1995;21:163–165.

III

Aortic Aneurysm

9

Molecular Mimicry and the Etiology of the Nonspecific Abdominal Aortic Aneurysm

M. David Tilson, MD

The last several years of our laboratory work have led to the conclusion that the abdominal aortic aneurysm (AAA) is an autoimmune disease of maturity, like rheumatoid arthritis. One of the first clues pointing in this direction was discovered by one of my former students, Bob Rizzo, who was working in Chicago with Dr. William H. Pearce and Dr. James S. T. Yao, doing a research year as part of his vascular surgical fellowship. When I was visiting to give a lecture, Bob showed me some AAA histology that revealed a conspicuous infiltration of inflammatory cells in routine non-specific AAAs. Bob briefly described these observations in his paper on the biochemistry of AAA matrix in 1989,[1] and they were subsequently reported in more detail by Koch et al.[2]

Before Rizzo and Koch had published their papers, I had an invitation from Cal Ernst and Jim Stanley to contribute a chapter on the pathology of AAA for one of their books,[3] and I put one of my all-time best students, Colleen Brophy, on the assignment. She reported soon that she couldn't find more than one original scientific paper on the subject in decades.[4] I said that proved what I had always said about writing chapters (paraphrasing J. Frank Dobe): that it's like moving bones around from one graveyard to another. I suggested that we write an original scientific paper of our own, and Colleen organized a seance with a Yale pathologist, Walker Smith, at one of those now-obsolete teaching microscopes with multiple viewing heads. Walker had been reporting about AAAs for many years, but when we started through a tray of AAAs from a dozen or so patients, with a similar number of atherosclerotic aortic controls, Walker commented that the extent of inflammatory changes in the adventitia of the aneurysms was most impressive, even "reminiscent of syphilis." Then he spotted some Russell bodies, which are B cells that have made so much IgG that they have choked on it, becoming the eosinophilic inclusions that are typical of autoimmune diseases such as Hashimoto's thyroiditis.[5]

PURIFICATION OF AAA IgG AND IDENTIFICATION OF AN 80-kDa AUTOANTIGEN

Brophy also deserves credit for the next important observation. After seeing the Russell bodies in the AAA specimens, she extracted soluble proteins from AAA and control specimens. Western blots probed with protein A displayed substantially more IgG from the AAA specimens, normalized to controls for total protein extracted.[5] She saw the scientific problem clearly and said that if we purified the autoantigen against which the AAA IgG was immunoreactive, as had been done by others in systemic lupus erythematosis, we would have an important clue to the underlying pathobiology of the disease.

Brophy moved on to her vascular surgical fellowship in Boston, focusing thereafter on the biology of the smooth muscle cell; and I moved to New York. I neglected the question of autoimmunity in AAA for several years, because I thought there would be a better chance of getting funding from the National Institutes of Health (NIH) to do the relatively safe science of working out the issue of the origin of the ''killer'' elastase in AAA and related problems dealing with the matrix metalloproteinases.[6–10] I lost my grant anyway, so I went back to work on the question of autoimmunity.

Another talented student, Anita Gregory, focused on the problem of whether an autoantigen could be detected with IgG extracted from AAA aortas. During her year in laboratory, she accomplished two important objectives. First, she showed that AAA IgG localized immunohistochemically with the elastin-associated microfibril in the aortic adventitia.[11] Second, using AAA IgG as a probe on Western immunoblots, she found that the putative autoantigen had a molecular weight of ~80 kDa.[11]

So, what was it, this ~80-kDa autoantigen? My research assistant during 1994 to 1995, Nancy X. Yin, purified the protein for amino acid sequencing, and although our yields were miniscule, we identified a motif that had been reported in a bovine aortic elastin microfibril-associated glycoprotein (MW = 36 kDa, thus, MAGP-36).[12] MAGP-36 occurs in nature as a dimer, so our 80-kDa protein was a candidate for the human version in dimeric form. Unlike the other known MAGPs, which are distributed ubiquitously with elastin, the tissue distribution of MAGP-36 was reported to be limited to the aorta.[13] This unique localization might explain why autoimmunity to a MAGP could have consequences more or less limited to the aorta and its branches.

THE DISCOVERY OF ANEURYSM-ASSOCIATED ANTIGENIC PROTEIN, 40 kDa (AAAP-40)

My present research assistant, Simon Xia, picked up where Nancy left off in the summer of 1995, and since we now knew that the autoantigen could be a disulfide-bonded dimer, we carried out the extractions of aortic tissue under reducing conditions. A 40-kDa protein was recovered as predicted, and it was immunoreactive with AAA IgG. Before the end of the year, we had sufficient sequence information to submit a follow-up report on the identification of AAAP-40.[14] Among several interesting features, AAAP-40 shares sequence motifs with MAGP-36 that are also seen in vitronectin (VN) and fibrinogen (FB). Also, both AAAP-40 and MAGP-36 may have a calcium-binding motif. Curiously, there is a similarity (FQ.T = FQ.S) with a sequence in the uveitopathic peptide of retinal photoreceptor retinoid-binding protein (Behçet's syndrome). The same sequence occurs in cytomegalovirus and herpes virus 6.

THE CONCEPT OF MOLECULAR MIMICRY

The notion of molecular mimicry is that epitopes of microbial pathogens may so closely resemble some of the normal proteins of the host that infection with the organism may trigger an autoimmune disease.[15] This concept has provided an explanation for numerous previous observations that had been poorly understood until the hypothesis of the shared epitope. An interesting example occurred when the Faeroe Islands were occupied by British soldiers during World War II. The natives were exposed to numerous Western viruses, and many contracted influenza. An outbreak of multiple sclerosis then occurred. Myelin basic protein is the target of autoimmunity in multiple sclerosis, and susceptibility to the disease is linked to the major histocompatibility complex (MHC) Class II locus DRB1*1501. Taking advantage of knowing how one of the immunodominant epitopes of myelin basic protein binds to DRB1*1501, Wucherpfennig and Strominger[16] recently identified seven viral proteins that are effective mimics, including a peptide from influenza type A.

The hypothesis of molecular mimicry has also been a subject of interest in the field of rheumatology. In 1983, 10 cases resembling rheumatoid arthritis were reported among 159 cancer patients receiving immunotherapy with bacille Calmette-Guérin (BCG).[17] Thereafter, it was found that mycobacterial antigens are cross-reactive with proteoglycans of cartilage.[18] It was also shown in the adjuvant rat arthritis model (*Mycobacterium tuberculosis* in oil) that autoreactive T cells triggered by mycobacterial antigens mediate persistent disease activity (or, under some experimental conditions, confer protection).[19]

Herpes simplex virus has recently been implicated in the AAA. By polymerase chain reaction, Tanaka et al.[20] detected herpes virus DNA in 10 of 37 AAA specimens, versus 1 of 16 normal aortas. Considering the present hypothesis that herpes may exert its influence on the pathogenesis of the aortic aneurysm by the mechanism of molecular mimicry, the observations of DePalma et al.[21] about an outbreak of ruptured aneurysms in a colony of Capuchin monkeys are quite extraordinary. Several years prior to the manifestations of aneurysmal disease in the monkeys, they had been experimentally infected at NIH with herpes virus.

Tanaka et al. also found cytomegalovirus in 65% of the AAAs, versus 31% of the normal aortas. If one-third of us harbor cytomegalovirus in our aortas, and if cytomegalovirus exerts its effect as a molecular mimic, the following question must be considered.

WHY DOESN'T EVERYONE WITH CYTOMEGALOVIRUS GET AN ANEURYSM?

The capacity of the immune system of an individual to recognize a peptide as an antigen depends on the inheritance of a personal repertoire of MHC Class II genes. The association of rheumatoid arthritis (RA) and Class II major histocompatibility locus DR4 was first reported by Stastny in 1978.[22] Weynand and colleagues[23] have reported that 98 of 102 (96%) patients express one of the major North American disease-linked polymorphisms (*04, *0101, or *1402). Forty-seven patients carried a double dose of the relevant sequence stretch. Nodular disease was expressed in 100% of the patients typed as HLA-DRB1*04/04. Patients with a double dose of the shared sequence tended to have more severe manifestations of rheumatoid disease. Thus, at least in this rather homogeneous population seen by the arthritis group at the Mayo Clinic, DR4 appears to be required to recognize the autoantigen of cartilage responsible for triggering RA.

As a pilot study we have to date tissue typed 31 patients with AAAs. Since AAAs are less common in African Americans than Caucasians, it has been one of my hypotheses for years that Americans of color might have a double dose of the susceptibility allele. Because of the demographics of the patient population of our hospital system, we have five Americans of color in the sample. Only 3 DR types occurred among the 10 black AAA haplotypes: 02, 12, and 13. By comparison to the expected frequencies,[24] we have calculated that this result would occur by chance alone at $p = 7 \times 10^{-5}$.

Inspection of the amino acid sequences of the most common alleles of 02, 12, and 13 revealed that the residues that they have in common are at positions 31 and 47 of the second hypervariable region; specifically, both residues are phenylalanines.[25] The other DRB1 alleles that have phenylalanine at positions 31 and 47 are DR3 and DR11. Revisiting the data on all 31 patients, 24 (77%) have an allele with phenylalanine at positions 31 and 47; and 9 (23%) have a double dose of one of the putative "aneurysmogenic" alleles. If the requirement for a phe at position 47 is relaxed to permit a phe at position 37 as a substitute, 30 of 31 (97%) of the AAAs have at least one dose, and 18 of 31 (58%) have a double dose.

This preliminary study is small, and the notion that alleles of DRB1 are the long-sought genetic susceptibility factors in AAA remains to be proven by a larger study. But, at least, there is now a testable hypothesis to evaluate prospectively.

CLONING THE GENE FOR AAAP-40: DIAGNOSTIC AND THERAPEUTIC IMPLICATIONS

The production of recombinant AAAP-40 would open the door to exploring the potential practical consequences of identifying the putative autoantigen. If there were an abundant resource of the protein, development of an enzyme-linked immunosorbent assay (ELISA) to titer serum anti-AAAP-40 IgG would enable a screening tool that might detect susceptibility to AAA disease before the aneurysm even develops. Then, the availability of r-AAAP-40 would facilitate experiments to evaluate whether tolerance to the antigen could be induced, with the goal of preventing the disease in susceptible persons. Simon Xia, and my students this year, Kathleen Ozsvath and Gene Hirose, have been making considerable progress.

As a first step, a cDNA library was prepared from mRNA purified from human aortic adventitia. Since AAAP-40 has sequences that occur in VN and FB, and since VN and FB are not synthesized in aorta, we screened the library with polyclonal antibodies to VN and FB. As of this writing, we have not identified a clone of AAAP-40 among the first five, but the hypothetical proteins encoded by our first clones No. 1 and No. 5 may lead to new insights into the potential complexity of the situation, as they also have motifs that occur in cytomegalovirus.

Clones 1 and 5 are so similar in domain structure, that the hypothetical proteins can be aligned in eight regions beginning with the N-terminus. The domain structure is novel and perhaps represents a new family of mammalian genes. Region 1 is a lengthy sequence highly homologous to Ig kappa V (88 to 120 residues). Region 2 is a 44 to 63 residue sequence, which in the case of clone 5 has a 6 residue sequence that also occurs in cytomegalovirus. Region 3 is a 9 to 12 residue sequence that is conserved from Ig kappa. Region 4 is a possible calcium-binding motif in clone 1, while clone 5 has a gly/pro rich sequence. Region 5 is an aromatic-rich sequence (FFFFSPF in clone 5), which resembles the FFFS sequence in VN, the FFYS sequence in AAAP-40, and the FFFSP sequence in cytomegalovirus. Region 6 is a gly/pro rich sequence in both clones. Region 7 returns to a conserved sequence from Ig kappa, which in clone 1 contains an RGE motif (potential cell-binding site). Region 8 is a second aromatic-rich sequence, which occurs near the C-terminus of both hypothetical proteins. The use of an immuno-globulin domain as a specificity determinant has been described in the fibroblast growth factor receptor, but the use of Ig kappa sequences in proteins that have features of matrix peptides has not been described. The findings also raise the question of whether, in addition to AAAP-40, there are additional shared epitopes of cytomegalovirus and aortic matrix that are involved in aneurysm autoimmunity.

LOOKING TOWARD THE FUTURE

The notion that aneurysmal disease has features in common with autoimmune diseases like rheumatoid arthritis opens the way for many new approaches to the issues of treatment and prevention. If specific antibodies are detectable in serum, as preliminary results suggest, it may be possible to detect susceptibility to the disease before significant aortic degeneration has occurred. If tolerance for the aortic autoantigen can be induced, it may be possible to down-modulate progression of aortic degeneration (as has been reported for symptoms of rheumatoid arthritis[26]). I believe that we are at the threshold of a radically new conception of AAA disease, which may possibly save many persons from sudden death.

REFERENCES

1. Rizzo RJ, McCarthy WJ, Dixit SN, et al. Collagen types and matrix protein content in human abdominal aortic aneurysms. *J Vasc Surg.* 1989;10:365–373.
2. Koch AE, Haines GK, Rizzo RJ, et al. Human abdominal aortic aneurysms: immunopheno-typic analysis suggesting an immune-mediated response. *Am J Pathol.* 1990;137:1199–1219.
3. Brophy CM, Smith GJW, Tilson MD. Pathology of nonspecific abdominal aortic aneurysm disease. In: Ernst CB, Stanley JC, eds. *Current Therapy in Vascular Surgery.* 2nd ed. Philadelphia: BC Decker; 1991:238–241.
4. Beckman EN. Plasma cell infiltrates in abdominal aortic aneurysm. *Am J Clin Pathol.* 1986;85:21–24.
5. Brophy CM, Reilly JM, Smith GJW, Tilson MD. The role of inflammation in nonspecific abdominal aortic aneurysm disease. *Ann Vasc Surg.* 1991;5:229–233.
6. Tilson MD, Newman KM. Proteolytic mechanisms in the pathogenesis of aortic aneurysms. In: Yao JST, Pearce WH, eds. *Aneurysms: New Findings and Treatments.* Norwalk, CT: Apple-ton & Lange; 1994:3–10.
7. Irizarry E, Newman KM, Gandhi RH, et al. Demonstration of interstitial collagenase in abdominal aortic aneurysm disease. *J Surg Res.* 1993;54:571–574.
8. Jean-Claude J, Newman KM, Li H, Tilson MD. Possible key role for plasmin in the pathogene-sis of abdominal aortic aneurysms. *Surgery.* 1994;116:472–478.
9. Newman KM, Malon AM, Shin RD, et al. Matrixmetalloproteinases in abdominal aortic aneurysm: characterization, purification, and their possible sources. *Connective Tissue Res.* 1994,30:265–276.
10. Newman KM, Jean-Claude J, Li H, et al. Cellular localization of matrix metalloproteinases in the abdominal aortic aneurysm wall. *J Vasc Sur.* 1994;20:814–820.
11. Gregory AK, Yin NX, Capella J, et al. Features of autoimmunity in the abdominal aortic aneurysm. *Arch Surg.* 1996;131:85–88.

12. Tilson MD. Similarities of an autoantigen in aneurysmal disease of the human aorta to a 36-kDa microfibril-associated bovine aortic glycoprotein. *Biochem Biophys Res Comm.* 1995; 213:40–43.

13. Kobayashi R, Tashima Y, Masuda H, et al. Isolation and characterization of a new 36-kDa microfibrile-associated glycoprotein from porcine aorta. *J Biol Chem.* 1989;264:17437–17444.

14. Xia S, Ozsvath K, Hirose H, Tilson MD. Partial amino acid sequence of a novel 40 kDa human aortic protein, with vitronectin-like, fibrinogen-like, and calcium binding domains: aortic aneurysm associated protein-40 (AAAP-40) [human MAGP-3, proposed]. *Biochem Biophys Res Comm.* 1996:219:26–39.

15. Fujinami RS, Oldstone MB. Molecular mimicry as a mechanism for virus-induced autoimmunity. *Immunol Res.* 1989;8:3–15.

16. Wucherpfenning KW, Strominger JL. Molecular mimicry in T cell mediated autoimmunity: viral peptides activate human T cell clones specific for myelin basic protein. *Cell.* 1995;80:695–705.

17. Torisu M, Miyahara T, Shinohara N, et al. A new side-effect of BCG immunotherapy: BCG-induced arthritis in man. *Cancer Immunol Immunother.* 1983;5:77–83.

18. Holoshitz J, Druker I, Yaretzky A, et al. T-lymphocytes of rheumatoid arthritis patients show augmented reactivity to a fraction of mycobacteria cross-reactive with cartilage. *Lancet.* 1986;2:305–309.

19. Cohen IR, Holoshitz J, Van Eden W, Frenkel A. T lymphocyte clones illuminate pathogenesis and affect therapy of experimental arthritis. *Arthritis Rheum.* 1985;28:841–845.

20. Tanaka S, Komori K, Okadome K, et al. Detection of active cytomegalovirus infection in inflammatory aortic aneurysms with RNA polymerase chain reaction. *J Vasc Surg.* 1994;20:235–243.

21. DePalma RG, Sidaway AN, Giordana JM. Associated aetiological and atherosclerotic risk factors in abdominal aneurysms. In: Greenhalgh RM, Mannick JA, Powell JT, eds. *The Cause and Management of Aneurysms.* London: WB Saunders; 1990:97–104.

22. Stastny P. Association of the B-cell alloantigen DRw4 with rheumatoid arthritis. *N Engl J Med.* 1978;298:869–871.

23. Weynand CM, Hicok KC, Conn DL, Goronzy JJ. The influence of HLA-DRB1 genes on disease severity in rheumatoid arthritis. *Ann Intern Med.* 1992;117:801–806.

24. Tsuji K, Aizawa M, Sasazuki T. *HLA 1991: Proceedings of the Eleventh International Histocompatibility Workshop and Conference;* November 6–13, 1991; Yokohama, Japan. Oxford University Press; 1992;1:Table 12:W15.1.

25. Lechler RI, Simpson E, Bach FH. Major and minor histocompatibility antigens: an introduction. In: Bach FH, Auchincloss H Jr, eds., *Transplantation Immunology.* New York: Wiley-Liss; 1995:1–34.

26. Trentham DE, Dynesium-Trentham RA, Oran EJ, et al. Effects of oral administration of type II collagen on rheumatoid arthritis. *Science.* 1993;261:1727–1730.

10

Spiral Computed Tomography and Three-Dimensional Reconstruction in the Evaluation of Aortic Aneurysm

Christopher K. Zarins, MD, Dainis K. Krievins, MD, and Geoffrey D. Rubin, MD

Abdominal aortic aneurysms can be diagnosed by physical examination or abdominal ultrasound. Proper planning for operative treatment requires further evaluation and imaging. This is usually accomplished with computed tomography (CT) and/or contrast angiography in order to develop a precise operative plan. The introduction of new endovascular approaches to the treatment of aneurysms with stent grafts has created a need for even more precise vascular imaging in the evaluation of aortic aneurysms. Newly developed techniques of three-dimensional (3-D) spiral CT-angiography can provide increased information on aortic aneurysms and branch vessel morphology in a cost-effective manner and will allow the continued development of new interventional techniques to treat aneurysms.

CONVENTIONAL COMPUTED TOMOGRAPHY

Conventional CT provides intermittent transaxial slices of the aorta and provides information on aneurysm size, location, and relationship to branch vessels. Both the thoracic and abdominal aorta can be well visualized with identification of common and internal iliac artery aneurysms, contained retroperitoneal ruptures, periaortic fibrosis, and inflammatory aneurysms.[1] Associated intra-abdominal conditions and anomalies of venous structures can readily be identified. Intravenous contrast infusion allows CT evaluation of the aortic lumen and mural thrombus. This allows the identification of aortic dissections with differentiation between the true and the false lumen. However, renal and visceral artery stenosis cannot be reliably identified. Accessory renal arteries may be missed and associated iliac occlusive disease cannot be accurately described. These conditions often require further evaluation with contrast angiography.

CONTRAST ANGIOGRAPHY

Contrast angiography provides important information for preoperative planning including definition of the extent of the aneurysm, especially suprarenal and iliac involvement, and demonstration of the degree of associated renal or visceral artery stenosis and identification of accessory renal arteries. The proximal and distal neck of the aneurysm and iliac artery size, tortuousity, and stenosis can be evaluated to determine the potential for introduction of intraluminal stent-grafts. However, contrast arteriography provides only information regarding the lumen and provides no visualization of the artery wall or mural thrombus. Thus, the true character of the proximal and distal neck of the aneurysm may not be accurately depicted by angiography. Furthermore, angiography exposes the patient to the risk of arterial puncture and intra-arterial manipulation. Contrast arteriography is also considerably more expensive than CT scanning.

SPIRAL CT-ANGIOGRAPHY

Spiral CT-angiography provides the imaging advantages of both conventional CT and contrast arteriography. Spiral CT data acquisition differs from conventional CT in that continuous data acquisition is coupled with continuous longitudinal patient transport. Thus, the table moves the patient continuously through the x-ray gantry while scanning, which results in the collection of volumetric imaging data instead of intermittent stationary transaxial sections. Iodinated contrast material is introduced into an antecubital vein and a test dose administered in order to determine the injection bolus arrival time to the region of interest. The iodinated contrast is injected at a rate of 4 to 5 mL/s and the spiral data are collected during a single 30- to 40-second breath hold. Typical acquisition parameters include a collimator of 3 mm and table speed of 3 to 6 mm/s.[2-6] Thus a high-resolution, spiral examination of the abdominal aorta can be acquired in 30 to 40 seconds with transaxial images available within 5 to 10 minutes and 3-D reconstructions available in less than an hour.

Transaxial Images

Conventional transaxial cross-sectional images of the body are displayed at 3- to 5-mm intervals. These images provide precise information on the aortic aneurysm, lumen contour, mural thrombus, branch vessels, and the relationship to surrounding structures (Fig. 10–1A). However, the aorta is often tortuous and the axis of the lumen is oblique to the axis of the section. This results in an oval, rather than normal, lumen contour and can provide misleading information regarding the true lumen dimensions.

Three-Dimensional Reconstruction

Three-dimensional images of the aorta may be produced by processing of the volumetric data set in two main reconstruction formats: maximum intensity projection and shaded surface displays.

Maximum Intensity Projection

Maximum intensity projections (MIPs) are generated by passing an imaginary ray through the volume of interest and determining the maximum pixel value encountered along the path of each ray. This highlights the contrast-filled vessel because contrast material has higher attenuation than all structures except bone. As a result, the skeletal structures must be removed in order to prevent them from obscuring the vasculature.

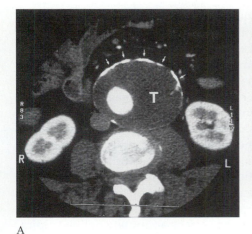

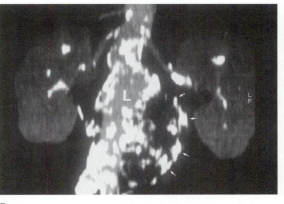

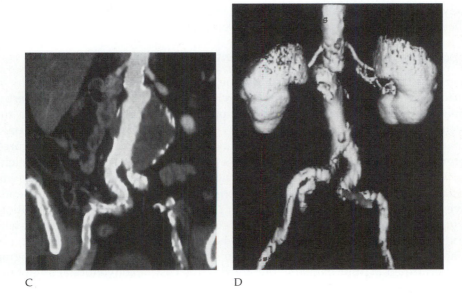

Figure 10–1. Spiral CT angiogram of a patient with an 8.3-cm infrarenal aortic aneurysm. Four imaging modalities are demonstrated. (**A**) Transaxial cross-sectional image demonstrating aneurysm lumen, mural thrombus (T), and calcified wall (*arrows*). (**B**) Maximum intensity projection (MIP) differentiates patent aortic lumen (L) and mural calcium (*arrows*). (**C**) Curved planar reformation (CPR) demonstrates arterial lumen, aortic wall, and mural thrombus. Left iliac artery is out of image plane and therefore not fully visible. (**D**) Shaded surface display (SSD) of lumen contrast shows 3-D relationships well, but does not demonstrate aneurysm size and shape or thrombus.

A cine loop created from multiple projections about an axis of rotation allows a display of the anatomy rotating in three dimensions. Calcifications and vessel lumina are differentiated with MIPs (Fig. 10–1B). Curved planar reformation (CPR) images clearly outline the aortic lumen, aneurysm wall, and mural thrombus (Fig. 10–1C).

Shaded Surface Displays

Shaded surface displays (SSDs) are created by selecting a threshold CT number to extract a surface. Depth is based on a computer-calculated degree of reflected light that would be expected from an imaginary light source. This provides 3-D models of the vasculature and organs but does not provide information regarding relative CT attenuation and significant information such as the true size and shape of the aneurysm may be lost (Fig. 10–1D). Thus, contrast-filled vessels, contrast-enhanced parenchyma, and calcified plaque all appear to have the same brightness when viewed in SSD, if their attenuation is greater than the threshold selected. While attractive images can be obtained with SSD, examination of the transaxial sections and MIP images are additionally needed in order to fully evaluate the lesion.[6,7]

Three-dimensional rendering provides a useful depiction of aortic branches and associated structures. The image may be rotated and viewed from arbitrary directions and visceral/renal artery stenoses and the aortic aneurysm neck can be evaluated. Spiral CT scanning is particularly useful in evaluating aortic dissections. Multiple aortic dissection flaps and differentiation of true and false lumens can be obtained.[8] Spiral CT reliably depicts second- to fourth-order aortic branches[4] and the surgical neck and length of the aneurysm are easily appreciated. Renal artery stenosis can be accurately defined. Spiral CT was 92% sensitive and 83% specific for detecting renal artery stenosis considered hemodynamically significant (>70% diameter stenosis).[6] Demonstration of ostial lesions may be superior with CT-angiography compared to conventional arteriography.

Preoperative Evaluation of Patients with Aneurysms

Preoperative evaluation of patients undergoing standard aortic aneurysm repair may be performed rapidly and cost effectively with spiral CT-angiography. All pertinent information necessary for planning of the operation can be obtained with a timed intravenous contrast bolus injection and a 30- to 40-second data acquisition time. It is thus particularly useful in the rapid evaluation of patients with suspected ruptured or symptomatic aneurysms. The image set always includes transaxial images, which are available almost immediately. Three-dimensional reconstructions require some image processing time and are not essential in emergent situations. In evaluating patients for elective aneurysm repair 3-D reconstruction provides clinically useful information on aneurysm size and tortuousity, relationship to the renal arteries, patency or stenosis of the visceral and renal arteries and the presence or absence of renal and iliac aneurysms or stenosis in an easy-to-read format[8,9] (Figs. 10–2 and 10–3). Spiral CT-angiography can be performed at approximately one-third of the cost of conventional angiography

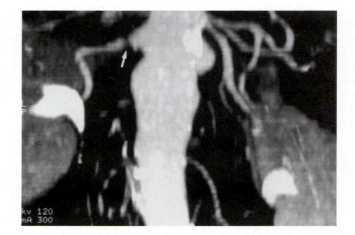

Figure 10–2. MIP of a spiral CT angiogram demonstrates proximal right renal artery stenosis (*arrow*).

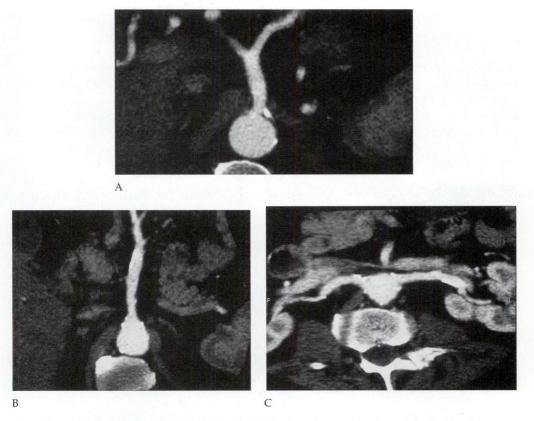

Figure 10–3. Curved planar reformation (CPR) images demonstrate visceral artery branches clearly: (**A**) celiac trunk, (**B**) superior mesenteric artery (SMA), and (**C**) renal arteries.

and would provide even greater cost savings over combined imaging modalities of conventional CT plus contrast angiography. In most instances, it is unnecessary to obtain contrast arteriography in order to obtain precise and complete preoperative imaging for infrarenal abdominal aneurysms, juxtarenal and suprarenal aortic aneurysms, and thoracic aortic aneurysms.[8,10]

Evaluation and Planning for Stent Graft Repair

Endovascular repair of aortic aneurysms requires precise information on aneurysm morphology and the proximal and distal neck of the aneurysm. Precise characterization of the infrarenal aortic segment is needed with characterization of its lumenal diameter, tortuosity, calcification, and composition (Fig. 10–1). The length and tortuosity of the aneurysm must be determined as well as the tortuosity and dimensions of the iliac arteries. The presence of accessory renal arteries, patent inferior mesenteric artery, and characteristics of the mural thrombus are critical factors in planning endovascular repair. Characteristics of spiral CT image analysis include thin slice axial CT images, 3-D reconstructions, oblique CT sections cut perpendicular to the center line of flow, calculation of eccentricities of the flow channel, tortuosity and length of the aorta and iliac arteries, the true axial cross-sectional area of the iliac arteries, volume calculation of the thrombus, and evaluation of the visceral branches and stenoses.

Thoracic aortic aneurysms similarly must be evaluated in relation to the left subclavian artery and celiac artery in order to determine anchoring sites for stent graft repair of thoracic aortic aneurysms (Figs. 10–4A–C).

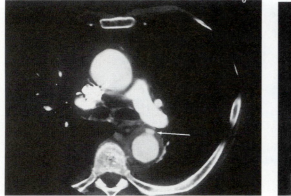

A

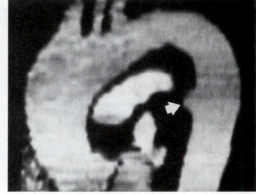

B

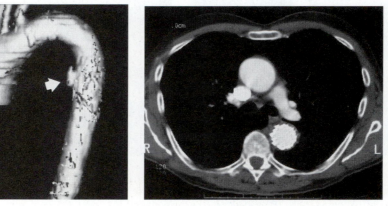

C   D

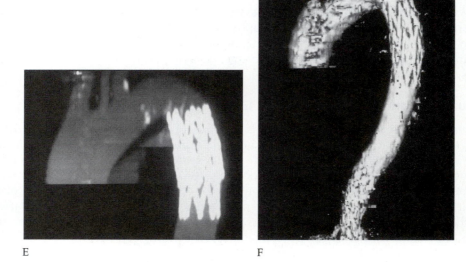

E   F

Figure 10–4. Spiral CT-angiography in a patient with chest pain and a penetrating aortic ulceration with mural hematoma. (**A**) Transaxial image of aortic ulceration (*arrow*). (**B**) MIP demonstrates ulcer (*arrow*). (**C**) SSD of ulcer (*arrow*). (**D**) Transaxial image with no fill of ulcer. (**E**) MIP demonstrates stent. (**F**) SSD demonstrates contrast-filled lumen stent graft in place with no fill of ulcer.

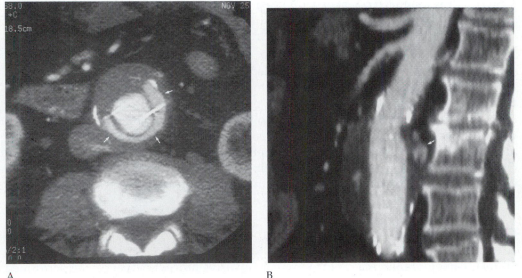

A   B

Figure 10–5. Postoperative evaluation of patient following stent-graft repair of infrarenal aneurysm. Arrows show perigraft leak into aneurysmal sac on (**A**) transaxial cross-sectional image and (**B**) MIP 3-D reconstruction.

Postoperative Evaluation of Aneurysms

Spiral CT-angiography is an important component of postoperative evaluation of aneurysms treated with stent-graft repairs. Incomplete exclusion of the aneurysm with stent-graft repairs continue to expose the patient to risk of aneurysm rupture and death. Spiral CT can clearly depict the position and location of the proximal and distal extent of the stent graft.[11] It can demonstrate visceral vessel patency and determine whether or not the aneurysm continues to fill (Figs. 10–4D–F). Perivascular extravasations can be identified (Fig. 10–5) as well as iliac flow and kinking of the stent graft. Imaging of vascular stents, vascular grafts, and stents with spiral CT-angiography offers detailed information that is useful in graft or stent surveillance. Metallic stainless steel stents can be well visualized with spiral CT.[6]

SPIRAL CT-ANGIOGRAPHY VERSUS CONTRAST ANGIOGRAPHY

Both spiral CT-angiography and contrast angiography require administration of iodinated contrast media. Thus patients with severe contrast allergies, renal failure, or other contraindications to intravenous contrast cannot undergo either imaging modality. Contrast angiography has superior spatial and contrast resolution, particularly in selective branch imaging.[12] However, contrast arteriography requires an arterial puncture, and the operator must angle the tube and inject contrast for each different projection. In contrast, spiral CT requires an intravenous contrast injection, and data can be acquired rapidly in 30 seconds. Since data are acquired volumetrically, images can be produced through an innumerable number of projection angles, and a video loop can be created to display the vasculature dynamically. Thus despite a lower resolution, spiral CTA provides more information that is clinically useful.

SPIRAL CT-ANGIOGRAPHY VERSUS MAGNETIC RESONANCE ANGIOGRAPHY

Magnetic resonance angiography (MRA) is superior to spiral CT-angiography in that it does not require the injection of iodinated contrast agents and does not expose the patient to radiation. It thus can be used to image aneurysms in patients with renal failure and contrast allergy. In addition, magnetic resonance can provide not only spatial morphometric information, but also blood flow information in the aorta, vena cava, and branch vessels.[13] But magnetic resonance scans are relatively time consuming and may be distorted by motion artifact, extensive calcified plaque, and metallic surgical clips. MRA cannot be used in patients with pacemakers or with metallic intra-arterial stents.[14] It thus is not useful for postoperative evaluation of patients with stent-grafts.

CONCLUSION

Spiral CT-angiography is a rapid, minimally invasive procedure that can be performed on out-patients for the preoperative assessment of aortic aneurysms. Three-dimensional reconstruction may provide more clinically useful information than conventional CT or contrast angiography. CT-angiography is less invasive, less expensive, faster, and easier to perform than conventional angiography. Its cost is approximately one-third that of conventional angiography, and the risks of arterial catheterization can be avoided. Spiral CT-angiography provides the tools necessary to select patients and plan for endovascular repair of aneurysm using stent-grafts and will be useful for post stent-graft evaluation and follow-up. Spiral CT-angiography is becoming the diagnostic imaging modality of choice in the preoperative assessment of patients with aortic aneurysms. In most cases, it will eliminate the need for preoperative contrast angiography.

REFERENCES

1. Papanicolaou N, Wittenberg J, Ferrucci JT, et al. Preoperative evaluation of abdominal aortic aneurysms by computed tomography. *AJR.* 1986;146:711–715.
2. Kalender WA, Seissler W, Klotz E, Vock P. Spiral volumetric CT with single-breath-hold technique, continuous transport, and continuous scanner rotation. *Radiology.* 1990;176:181–183.
3. Vock P, Soucek M, Daepp M, Kalender WA. Lung: spiral volumetric CT with single-breath-hold technique. *Radiology.* 1990;176:864–867.
4. Rubin GD, Walker PJ, Dake MD, et al. Three-dimensional spiral computed tomographic angiography: an alternative imaging modality for the abdominal aorta and its branches. *J Vasc Surg.* 1993;18:656–665.
5. Rubin GD, Dake MD, Napel S, et al. Three-dimensional spiral CT angiography of the abdomen: initial clinical experience. *Radiology.* 1993;186:147–152.
6. Rubin GD, Dake MD, Napel S, et al. Spiral CT of renal artery stenosis: comparison of three-dimensional rendering techniques. *Radiology.* 1994;190:181–189.
7. Rubin GD, Dake MD, Semba CB. Current status of three-dimensional spiral CT scanning for imaging the vasculature. *Radiol Clin North Am.* 1995;33:51–70.
8. Balm R, Eikelboom BC, van Leeuwen MS, Noordzij J. Spiral CT-angiography of the aorta. *Eur J Vasc Surg.* 1994;8:544–551.
9. Galanski M, Prokop M, Chavan A, et al. Renal arterial stenoses: spiral CT angiography. *Radiology.* 1993;189:185–192.

10. Hoe LV, Baert AL, Gryspeerdt S, et al. Supra- and juxtarenal aneurysms of the abdominal aorta: preoperative assessment with thin-section spiral CT. *Radiology.* 1996;198:443–448.
11. Rozenblit A, Marin ML, Veith FJ, et al. Endovascular repair of abdominal aortic aneurysm: value of postoperative follow-up with helical CT. *AJR.* 1995;165:1473–1479.
12. Napel S, Marks MP, Rubin GD, et al. CT angiography with spiral CT and maximum intensity projection. *Radiology.* 1992;185:607–610.
13. Kaufman JA, Yucel EK, Waltman AC, et al. MR angiography in the preoperative evaluation of abdominal aortic aneurysms: a preliminary study. *JVIR.* 1994;5:489–496.
14. Sardelic MB, Fletcher JP, Ho D, Simmons K. Assessment of abdominal aortic aneurysm with magnetic resonance imaging. *Austral Radiol.* 1995;39:107–111.

11

Abdominal Aortic Aneurysms

Predicting the Natural History

Jack L. Cronenwett, MD

The natural history of an abdominal aortic aneurysm (AAA) is to expand gradually and ultimately rupture unless the patient dies of other causes. Fortunately, elective surgical repair can prevent rupture and prolong life in properly selected patients. Appropriate decision making requires knowledge of the natural history of untreated AAAs, both in terms of rupture risk and expansion rate. The fact that AAAs occur in elderly patients substantially complicates these decisions. AAA repair is designed to prolong life, and thus has maximal potential impact in younger patients. Many elderly patients with low-risk AAAs die from other causes before rupture, and would not benefit from elective AAA repair. Thus, careful evaluation of the risk factors for AAA rupture and future expansion is required, especially in more elderly patients. Finally, economic restraints for health care delivery require that AAA repair should be performed only when it is cost effective compared with other common medical practices. This chapter describes our current knowledge of the risk factors that determine the rupture rate and expansion rate of AAAs, and demonstrates that these factors determine the cost effectiveness of AAA repair.

AAA RUPTURE RISK

Theory

La Place's law indicates that the wall tension of an ideal cylinder is proportional to the radius and intraluminal pressure, and inversely proportional to wall thickness. Although AAAs are not ideal cylinders, this concept predicts that increasing diameter and blood pressure should increase AAA wall tension, and thus rupture risk. Although AAA wall thickness and strength have not been quantifiable from a clinical perspective, basic research concerning the cellular and molecular mechanisms of AAA formation may allow us to incorporate this concept in future prediction of natural history.

To define the natural history (expansion rate and rupture risk) of AAAs, one would ideally follow a large cohort of carefully analyzed patients until the AAAs ruptured.

Given the effectiveness of AAA repair, however, this approach would be unethical for most AAAs. Thus, appropriate surgical intervention has thwarted a precise knowledge of the natural history of AAAs, since most large and many small AAAs are selectively repaired. This leads to an underestimate of rupture risk in most "natural history" studies, which are really studies of selective surgical management. There are currently two randomized prospective studies comparing early surgery with watchful waiting for small, low-risk AAAs, which should provide useful natural history information in the future. For large AAAs, the best information is derived from historical data before the era of surgical reconstruction, or from high-risk patients who have large AAAs but are not surgical candidates. Although we cannot precisely define the rupture risk for a given AAA, sufficient studies have been performed to delineate factors that influence both rupture and expansion rate, which are described in the following paragraphs.

Size, Hypertension, and COPD

Size, measured by diameter, is the best recognized predictor of AAA rupture, especially for large AAAs. In an early clinical study, Szilagyi et al.[1] demonstrated that patients managed nonoperatively with AAAs of >6 cm in diameter had a 5-year survival of only 6%, compared with 48% survival in patients with smaller aneurysms. Autopsy studies have also demonstrated that larger AAAs are more prone to rupture. Among consecutive AAAs noted during postmortem examinations, Darling et al.[2] observed that 75% of AAAs of >7 cm in diameter had ruptured, compared with only 19% rupture in AAAs of ≤7 cm in diameter. These and other studies have produced general agreement that AAA rupture risk increases exponentially with size even though precise size–risk estimates are difficult (Fig. 11–1).

To determine which risk factors were associated with rupture of 4- to 6-cm-diameter AAAs, we analyzed 67 patients who were followed nonoperatively for a mean interval of 3 years.[3] During this time, the AAAs expanded from a mean maximal diameter of 3.9 cm to a final diameter of 4.7 cm and only 3% underwent elective surgical repair, making this a relatively "pure" natural history study. During follow-up, 12 patients

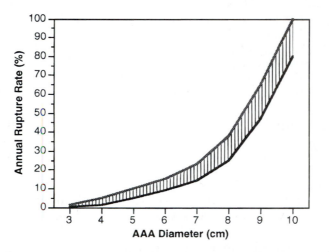

Figure 11–1. Estimated annual rupture rate based on AAA diameter. The range at each size is based on different published estimates and likely reflects other variables such as hypertension and COPD that also influence rupture risk. (*From Sampson LN, Cronenwett JL. Abdominal aortic aneurysms. In: Zelenock GB, ed. Problems in General Surgery in Vascular Surgery. Philadelphia: JB Lippincott; 1995;II:385–417.*)

(18%) required emergent AAA repair for rupture ($n = 8$) or acute symptomatic expansion ($n = 4$); of these, 8 patients died. This yielded an annual rupture rate of 6%, with an annual mortality rate caused by rupture of 5%. Multivariate analysis indicated that initial AAA size ($p < 0.01$), hypertension ($p < 0.02$), and chronic obstructive pulmonary disease (COPD, $p < 0.001$) were independently predictive of future AAA rupture. Diastolic blood pressure was a more accurate predictor of rupture than systolic blood pressure. COPD was the most influential risk factor, a somewhat unexpected finding, which we attributed to a possible increase in systemic proteinase activity affecting both pulmonary and aortic connective tissue.[3]

Other studies have confirmed the influence of size, hypertension, and COPD on AAA rupture risk. Using multivariate analysis, Sterpetti et al.[4] compared 220 patients who died with an intact aneurysm versus 77 patients who died from AAA rupture. These investigators found that AAA size ($p < 0.001$), hypertension ($p < 0.001$), and bronchiectasis ($p < 0.025$) were independent predictors of rupture. Patients with ruptured AAAs had significantly larger aneurysms (8.0 versus 5.1 cm), more frequently had hypertension (54% versus 28%), and more frequently had both emphysema (67% versus 42%), and bronchiectasis (29% versus 15%). These results also suggested a generalized connective tissue defect as the unifying hypothesis to explain the association between COPD and AAA rupture. Other studies have confirmed the influence of hypertension on AAA rupture risk. Among 75 patients with AAAs managed nonoperatively, Foster et al.[5] noted that death from rupture occurred in 72% of patients with diastolic hypertension, but in only 29% of patients with diastolic blood pressure <100 mm Hg. In a similar analysis of patients with AAAs managed nonoperatively, Szilagyi et al.[1] also emphasized that diastolic hypertension was associated with rupture. They found that diastolic hypertension (>150/100 mm Hg) was present in 67% of patients who experienced AAA rupture, but in only 23% of those without rupture. Thus, AAA diameter, hypertension, and COPD have been confirmed to be independent risk factors for AAA rupture in at least two different studies, using both clinical results and autopsy data.

Other Risk Factors for Rupture

Several other risk factors for AAA rupture have been suggested and await confirmation by additional studies. A positive family history of AAA is known to increase the prevalence of AAAs in other first-degree relatives (FDRs).[6] It is less clear, however, whether familial AAAs have a higher rupture risk per se. In one study of 86 families with 209 FDRs with AAAs, Darling et al.[7] found that the likelihood of AAA rupture increased with the number of FDRs with AAAs: 14.8% rupture with 2 FDRs, 29% with 3 FDRs, and 36% with ≥4 FDRs. Furthermore, these investigators found that women with familial aneurysms had a higher incidence of rupture (30%) than men with familial aneurysms (17%). These results suggest that a strong family history of AAA may be an additional risk factor for rupture, especially if the patient is female. This study was not able to consider many other potential confounding variables such as AAA size, however, which might have been different in the familial group. Thus, whether a positive family history is an independent predictor of increased AAA rupture risk has not yet been established.

It is commonly believed that comparably sized AAAs in patients with smaller diameter aortas are at higher risk for rupture. In our analysis of patients with 4- to 6-cm-diameter AAAs, we found that absolute AAA diameter was a more accurate predictor of future rupture than AAA/aortic diameter ratio.[3] However, this study was not large enough to exclude the AAA/aortic ratio as a possible additional risk factor for rupture, which should be considered by future studies. In another comparison of AAA size, Ouriel et al.[8] have suggested that relative aneurysm size compared with vertebral body size may be a better predictor of rupture. These investigators compared CT scans in patients undergoing elective AAA repair with those who presented with a ruptured AAA, and found that none of the ruptured AAAs had a diameter smaller than the transverse diameter of the L-3 vertebral body. However, only 29% of the electively repaired AAAs were smaller than the L-3 vertebral diameter, and by ROC analysis, the aortic–vertebral ratio was only slightly more accurate (68%) than the absolute AAA diameter alone (60%) to discriminate the future likelihood of AAA rupture. Thus, additional studies are required to determine whether the ratio of AAA diameter to the aorta or vertebral diameter is a better predictor of rupture than absolute diameter alone.

The potential interaction between smoking, COPD, and AAA rupture risk is also not settled. Based on a large study of men in England, Strachen[9] found that the relative risk of death from AAA rupture increased 2.4-fold for pipe/cigar smokers, 4.6-fold for cigarette smokers, and 14.6-fold for smokers of hand-rolled cigarettes. However, in this epidemiologic study it was not possible to analyze many other individual risk factors, including COPD, which might have been the actual causative variable. In smaller studies that have identified COPD as an independent risk factor for rupture, smoking was not found to be independently predictive of rupture.[3,4] However, from a case management standpoint, the possibly independent role of cigarette smoking to increase AAA rupture risk should not be overlooked.

The shape of AAAs ranges from cylindrical to saccular, and general clinical opinion holds that eccentric, saccular aneurysms are at greater rupture risk than diffuse cylindrical aneurysms of the same size. This belief, however, has not been proven. In fact, Wolf et al.[10] were unable to associate AAA configuration with either rupture risk or expansion rate. Furthermore, Veldenz et al.[11] found that relative flattening of the arc of an AAA was associated with greater rupture risk, which they attributed to an effective increase in radius, and thus tension, by La Place's law. This would predict that diffuse cylindrical enlargement would be more likely to rupture than sacular AAAs. Thus, the potential impact of AAA shape on rupture risk remains undetermined.

Analogous to AAA shape, the potential of contained thrombus within an AAA to alter rupture risk has been speculated on, but not proven. One study suggested that thrombus was less thick (9 mm) in patients with ruptured AAAs compared with nonruptured AAAs (19 mm thick).[12] This observation requires further investigation, since the mechanism by which contained thrombus would reduce rupture risk is not clear. In fact, it is believed that thrombus continues to transmit pressure to the aneurysm wall, as demonstrated by the subsequent rupture of previously thrombosed AAAs.[13]

Finally, rapid AAA expansion rate is generally considered to increase AAA rupture risk and is often considered an indication for repair of small AAAs. It is difficult to separate a direct effect of expansion rate from the influence of expansion rate on absolute diameter, however, which alone could influence rupture. In our study we found that absolute AAA size, rather than expansion rate, was a better predictor of rupture.[3] Nevitt et al.[14] also found that absolute size, but not expansion rate, was associated with increased rupture risk. Other studies, however, have found that expansion rate was greater in patients with ruptured rather than nonruptured AAAs. For example, Schewe et al.[15] found that both AAA size (7.3 versus 6.1 cm) and expansion rate (0.47 versus 0.23 cm/year) were greater in patients with ruptured ($n = 8$) versus nonruptured ($n = 191$) AAAs. However, since AAAs with more rapid expansion also had larger diameter in these series, it is impossible to determine whether expansion rate is an independent predictor of rupture, or only of increased absolute diameter. This question may be moot, however, since more rapid AAA expansion obviously increases future size, which increases rupture risk.

AAA EXPANSION RATE

Size

Numerous studies using ultrasound or computed tomography (CT) scans have sequentially measured the size of small AAAs in patients initially selected for watchful waiting. Few studies have been able to characterize the expansion rate of larger AAAs, since nearly all of these undergo elective repair. Thus, the analysis of factors that influence the expansion rate of AAAs is largely derived from smaller aneurysms, and assumed to apply to all sizes. To determine which factors increase AAA expansion rate, we reviewed patients with AAAs of <6 cm in diameter who were followed with serial ultrasound measurements for a mean interval of 3 years.[16] Using multivariate analysis, we found that initial AAA diameter and hypertension (see the next section) predicted AAA expansion rate. We calculated that 3- to 6-cm AAAs expand on average at 10% of their diameter per year, which implies an exponential function. Thus, in 1 year, a 3-cm-diameter AAA would be expected to expand 0.3 cm, while a 6-cm-diameter AAA would be expected to expand 0.6 cm. This result is nearly identical to a more sophisticated mathematical analysis by Limet et al.,[17] which demonstrated that AAAs expand at an exponential rate, equivalent to an 11% diameter increase per year for small AAAs. At least three additional studies have confirmed that AAAs expand as an exponential function of their initial diameter.[18–20] Increased accuracy of an exponential model for predicting future AAA size increases as the time interval increases. For practical purposes, it is sufficient to estimate the expected annual expansion of a small AAA as 10% of the current diameter/year.

Blood Pressure

In our multivariate analysis, we found that AAA expansion rate is a function not only of initial size, but also of blood pressure.[16] Specifically, we found a positive correlation with systolic blood pressure and a negative correlation with diastolic pressure, suggesting that increased pulse pressure (systolic minus diastolic pressure) is associated with increased AAA expansion rate. Our regression model predicted that expansion rate would increase from 0% to 18% of AAA diameter/year, as the pulse pressure increased from 10 to 120 mm Hg (Fig. 11–2). Since most elderly patients with AAAs have a relatively high pulse pressure, this accounts for the 10% diameter increase per year that we found for an "average" AAA. A second study has also shown that AAA

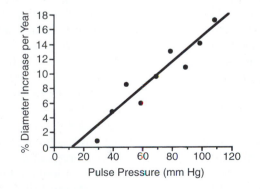

Figure 11–2. Predicted annual increase in AAA diameter based on varying pulse pressure. [*From Cronenwett JL. Variables that affect the expansion rate and rupture of abdominal aortic aneurysms. In: Tilson DA, ed. The Abdominal Aortic Aneurysm: Genetics, Pathophysiology, and Molecular Biology. Annals of the New York Academy of Sciences (in press).*]

expansion rate is increased by hypertension. Schewe et al.[15] found that both systolic and diastolic blood pressure were positively correlated with expansion. By multivariate analysis, they found that diameter and diastolic blood pressure were the best predictors of expansion rate. Using this model, however, they were only able to account for 40% of the variance in AAA expansion rate, while we were able to account for 74% of the variation observed in expansion rate using initial size and pulse pressure. Thus, the influence of both size and hypertension on increased AAA expansion rate has been confirmed in several studies, and there is a suggestion that pulse pressure may help predict future expansion more accurately.

Other Factors Influencing Expansion Rate

In an analysis of 80 small AAAs followed with CT scans for an average of 2 years, Wolf et al.[10] found that thrombus content was an important predictor of AAA expansion rate. Using multivariate analysis, these investigators found that the portion of the circumference of the AAA covered by thrombus was the best predictor of expansion rate, although the correlation was relatively low ($r = 0.43$). In their study, carotid artery disease was the only clinical factor associated with increased expansion rate. Rapid expansion, defined as >0.5 cm/year occurred in 19% of their patients. If the portion of the arc of the AAA covered by thrombus (TARC) was $>120°$, 34% of patients demonstrated rapid expansion, compared with only 7% of patients with a TARC $<120°$ ($p < 0.001$). Experimental studies suggest a possible role for plasmin derived from thrombus in the activation of metalloproteinases in the AAA wall, which could translate into more rapid expansion, and thus explain the relationship between AAA thrombus and increased expansion rate.[21]

Cigarette smoking has also been suggested to be a risk factor for increased AAA expansion rate. In a small group of patients, MacSweeney et al.[22] found a higher median expansion rate of 0.16 cm/year in patients who continued to smoke, than in patients who no longer smoked (0.09 cm/year, $p < 0.04$).[22] This observation has not yet been corroborated by other investigators.

Finally, two studies have suggested that propranolol may reduce AAA expansion rate. Potential mechanisms include not only a reduction in blood pressure and cardiac contractility, but also a potential direct effect on aortic wall connective tissue strength. In a small series of 27 patients with AAAs, Leach et al.[23] found that the expansion rate in patients treated with β-blockade was 0.17 cm/year, compared with 0.4 cm/year in patients not on β-blockade. While this difference was not statistically significant, the proportion of AAAs expanding at a rate exceeding the mean was higher (53%) in patients not taking β-blockers than in the β-blockade group (8%, $p = 0.013$). In this series, only half the patients receiving β-blockade were treated with propranolol, which is relevant, since it has been observed that β_1-selective agents do not have beneficial effects on AAA expansion in animal models.[24] In a larger clinical study, Gadowski et al.[25] found that patients not receiving β-blockade had an expansion rate of 0.44 cm/year, versus 0.3 cm/year in patients receiving β-blockers ($p = 0.07$).[25] Furthermore, in patients not receiving β-blockade, 60% demonstrated an expansion rate greater than the mean, while only 19% of patients treated with β-blockers had rapid expansion ($p = 0.03$). This was especially significant in patients with AAAs ≥ 5 cm. In the subgroup of patients treated with β-blockade who received propranolol, the expansion rate was only 0.2 cm/year, compared with 0.42 cm/year for patients receiving β_1-selective blockers (atenolol or metoprolol, $p = 0.03$).[25] Although significant blood pressure reduction in the propranolol-treated group was not observed in this study, cardiac contractility could not be measured. Furthermore, there is ongoing debate concerning the primary mechanism of propranolol in animal models (hemodynamic effects versus connective tissue effects).[26] Nonetheless, there is suggestive clinical information that propranolol reduces the expansion rate of small AAAs, an observation that deserves further attention.

CLINICAL APPLICATION

Estimating Rupture Risk

There is general agreement that AAAs of <4 cm in diameter have negligible rupture risk. For AAAs in the 4- to 5-cm-diameter range, however, there is less agreement concerning rupture risk. In a population-based study of selective AAA management, Brown et al.[27] found that none of the AAAs of <5 cm in diameter ruptured, although a large proportion expanded to a greater diameter and required elective surgery during follow-up.[27] Nevitt et al.[14] noted that none of the 4- to 5-cm-diameter AAAs ruptured during follow-up, although many of these AAAs were electively repaired, potentially reducing the opportunity for rupture. In contrast to these studies, Limet et al.[17] found that 5.4% of 4- to 5-cm-diameter AAAs ruptured each year during watchful waiting, even though 38% underwent elective repair during 2-year follow-up. In our study of small AAAs managed nonoperatively, we calculated the rupture risk to be 3.3%/year for AAAs that remain 4 to 5 cm in diameter.[3,28] Thus, the estimates for rupture risk of 4- to 5-cm-diameter AAAs range from 0% to 5%/year. This relatively large range in estimates probably relates to differences in patient selection and rate of elective repair during follow-up. More important, however, it strongly suggests that factors other than size have an important influence on the risk of individual AAAs.

Several studies have suggested a relatively abrupt increase in the rupture risk for AAAs of ≥5 cm in diameter. Nevitt et al.[14] found the annual rupture risk of ≥5-cm-diameter AAAs to be 6.3%/year, while Limet et al.[17] estimated this annual rupture risk to be 15.8%/year, despite the fact that approximately one-third of these patients underwent elective repair during follow-up. Based on these and other studies, the annual rupture rate for AAAs of ≥5 cm in diameter is estimated to be 5% to 15%/year, increasing with increased size and other factors such as COPD or hypertension.

In summary, for AAAs of <4 cm in diameter, we estimate the rupture risk to be negligible. For 4- to 5-cm-diameter AAAs, we estimate the rupture risk to be 0% to 2%/year if no other risk factors for rupture are present, but as much as 5%/year if the patient has coexistent hypertension, COPD, and a positive family history. For AAAs of 5 to 7 cm, we estimate the annual rupture risk to be 5% to 15%/year, with the specific risk within this range again dependent on the presence of other risk factors for rupture. For AAAs >7 cm in diameter, the rupture risk likely exceeds 15%/year.

Cost-Effectiveness Analysis

To place the variables that influence rupture risk and expansion rate into an appropriate clinical context, we have developed a decision analysis model, and a cost-effectiveness analysis for small AAAs.[28,29] This model compares early surgery when an AAA is identified versus watchful waiting, with subsequent repair only if a specific size threshold is reached during follow-up. We have focused our attention on AAAs in the 4- to 5-cm-diameter range, where most current controversy exists. The decision analysis model calculates the projected life expectancy for the initial decision of early surgery versus watchful waiting, depending on the specific patient variables that are entered into the simulation. Life expectancy is measured in quality-adjusted life years (QALYs), by reducing the value of survival in the presence of morbidity. To construct this model, we estimated the probabilities of each possible outcome from a literature review, and then tested the impact of these variables on the final decision by examining them over their expected range. To perform a cost-effectiveness analysis, we determined the actual costs for all the treatments involved in the strategies of early surgery and watchful waiting in our hospital. As has previously been observed by others, we found that the cost of caring for a patient with a ruptured AAA was twice that of patients undergoing elective repair.[29,30] The cost effectiveness of any procedure that improves life expectancy depends on the incremental cost and improved survival of that procedure relative to the alternative strategy. The measure of cost effectiveness is the ratio of this incremental cost divided by the improved survival (dollars per QALYs). Thus, a strategy is considered to be more "cost effective" as the cost-effectiveness ratio decreases. We included all direct hospital costs in our model, adjusted to 1992 dollars, and employed a discount rate of 5% to reduce the future value of costs and benefits.

For purposes of illustration, we considered the cost effectiveness of early AAA repair in a 60-year-old man with a 4-cm-diameter AAA compared with watchful waiting, where subsequent repair is performed only if a 5-cm-diameter threshold is reached.[28,29] At an elective operative mortality rate of 4.6% and an estimated annual rupture risk of 3.3%/year, we calculated that early surgery would improve survival of a 60-year-old man by 0.34 QALYs, at an additional cost of $5,858 compared with watchful waiting. This yielded an incremental cost-effectiveness ratio of $17,404/QALY saved by early surgery compared with the strategy of watchful waiting. In this scenario, initial cost of early surgery for all patients makes this strategy more expensive than watchful waiting, in which only 70% of such patients are ultimately predicted to undergo elective surgery, since 22% of these patients are predicted to die from other causes before their AAA reaches the 5-cm-diameter threshold for elective repair. However, the additional cost of elective AAA repair is narrowed by the increased cost of treating the estimated 8% of patients whose AAAs rupture during watchful waiting, as well as the greater incidence of high cost and chronic complications following ruptured AAA surgery, such as stroke and renal failure. The impact of the significantly greater cost for ruptured AAA repair and its complications results in a relatively low incremental cost of early surgery for this hypothetical 4-cm-diameter AAA, at approximately $17,000/QALY saved. This compares favorably with other commonly accepted health care strategies, such as coronary artery surgery and screening and treating hypertension.[29]

By examining the impact of different clinical variables in our cost-effectiveness model, we determined which variables could change the correct initial decision between early surgery and watchful waiting for any given AAA. We found that the key variables that determine cost effectiveness of AAA repair are patient age, elective operative mortality rate, and AAA rupture risk.[29] Importantly, the influence of these key variables on cost effectiveness is an exponential rather than a linear function. For example, as patient age increases beyond 70 to 80 years, the cost of early surgery rises exponentially. This is not surprising given the difficulty (and thus expense) of increasing life expectancy in the elderly. A conservative definition of "cost-effective" health care is that which has a cost-effectiveness ratio ≤$40,000/QALY. Using this criterion, if a patient has a 4-cm-diameter AAA with a rupture risk estimated to be 3.3%/year, and an elective mortality rate of 5%, it can be seen that early AAA repair (versus watchful waiting until a size of 5 cm is reached) remains cost effective for patients younger than approximately 70 years of age (Fig. 11–3). Above this age threshold, however, the cost of early

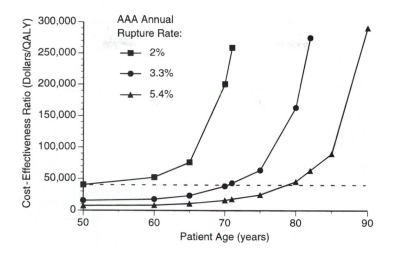

Figure 11–3. The cost effectiveness of early surgery compared with watchful waiting as a function of initial patient age for three different AAA annual rupture rates. The dotted line indicates the cost-effectiveness ratio of $40,000/QALY below which health care interventions are generally regarded as "cost effective." (*From Katz DA, Cronenwett JL. The cost-effectiveness of early surgery versus watchful waiting in the management of small abdominal aortic aneurysms. J Vasc Surg. 1994;19:980–991.*)

repair increases dramatically, and would not compare favorably with other health care measures competing for these same resources. In the same patient with a larger aneurysm, or with more risk factors for rupture, where the estimated rupture is as high as 5.5%/year, early repair would remain cost effective until approximately age 80 (Fig. 11–3). For patients above age 80, however, AAA repair would not be cost

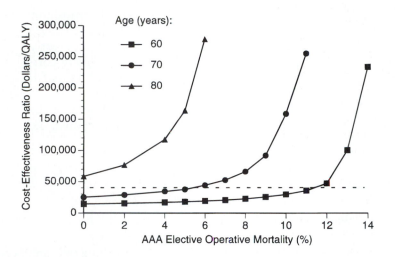

Figure 11–4. The cost effectiveness of early surgery compared with watchful waiting as a function of elective operative mortality in three age groups. The dotted line indicates the cost-effectiveness ratio of $40,000/QALY below which health care interventions are generally regarded as "cost effective." (*From Katz DA, Cronenwett JL. The cost-effectiveness of early surgery versus watchful waiting in the management of small abdominal aortic aneurysms. J Vasc Surg. 1994;19:980–991.*)

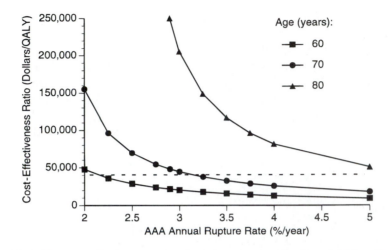

Figure 11–5. The cost effectiveness of early surgery compared with watchful waiting as a function of average annual rate of AAA rupture or acute expansion in three age groups. The dotted line indicates the cost-effectiveness ratio of $40,000/QALY below which health care interventions are generally regarded as "cost effective." (*From Katz DA, Cronenwett JL. The cost-effectiveness of early surgery versus watchful waiting in the management of small abdominal aortic aneurysms. J Vasc Surg. 1994;19:980–991.*)

effective unless the rupture risk were even higher, such as for an AAA of >6 cm in diameter, or when many other risk factors for rupture are also present.

The same nonlinear influence on cost effectiveness is observed for the key variables of elective operative mortality and annual rupture rate. For a 70-year-old patient, early repair of a 4-cm-diameter AAA with a 3.3% annual rupture risk remains cost effective until the elective operative mortality rate exceeds 6% (Fig. 11–4). In a younger, 60-year-old patient, early surgery remains cost effective even if the elective operative mortality is as high as 12% (Fig. 11–4). Finally, the effect of the most important variable on cost effectiveness, namely, AAA rupture risk, is illustrated in Figure 11–5. For a 70-year-old patient with an elective operative mortality rate of 5%, early repair remains cost effective for AAAs with rupture risk >3%/year. This likely corresponds to any AAA of ≥5 cm in diameter and those 4- to 5-cm-diameter AAAs that are accompanied by other risk factors for rupture, such as hypertension, COPD, or a positive family history. At lower rupture risk (<2%/year), however, such as in 4- to 5-cm-diameter AAAs without other risk factors for rupture, early AAA repair is not cost effective compared with watchful waiting.

CONCLUSION

Our analysis indicates that AAA rupture risk is increased by increasing AAA diameter, hypertension, and COPD. A positive family history, rapid AAA expansion rate, and cigarette smoking may also be influential factors. AAA expansion rate increases as an exponential function of current size, with an expected annual diameter increase of 10%/year. This is also increased by hypertension, with pulse pressure a potentially important predictor. Cigarette smoking and increased thrombus within an AAA are additional factors that appear to increase expansion rate, while propranolol may reduce expansion rate. For AAAs of <4 cm in diameter, the rupture risk appears to be negligible.

For AAAs of 4 to 5 cm in diameter, the estimated rupture risk varies from 0% to 5%/year, and for AAAs of ≥5 cm in diameter, the rupture risk increases to 5% to 15%/year. The precise rupture risk of a given AAA within these range estimates depends on a synthesis of the other risk factors described previously for AAA rupture. Appropriate, cost-effective decision making for AAA repair requires an understanding of these risk factors, taken in the context of patient age and life expectancy, in addition to an accurate assessment of elective operative risk. Thus, appropriate decision making for AAA repair requires considerable surgical judgment to customize the management strategy for individual patients.

REFERENCES

1. Szilagyi DE, Elliot JP, Smith RF. Clinical fate of the patient with asymptomatic abdominal aortic aneurysm and unfit for surgical treatment. *Arch Surg.* 1972;104:600–606.
2. Darling PC, Messina CR, Brewster DC, et al. Autopsy study of unoperated abdominal aortic aneurysm: the case for early resection. *Circulation.* 1977;56:161–164.
3. Cronenwett JL, Murphy TF, Zelenock GB, et al. Actuarial analysis of variables associated with rupture of small abdominal aortic aneurysms. *Surgery.* 1985;98:472–483.
4. Sterpetti AV, Cavallaro A, Cavallari N, et al. Factors influencing the rupture of abdominal aortic aneurysms. *Surg Gynecol Obstet.* 1991;173:175–178.
5. Foster JH, Bolasny BL, Gobbel WG Jr, Scott HW Jr. Comparative study of elective resection and expectant treatment of abdominal aortic aneurysm. *Surg Gynecol Obstet.* 1969;129:1–9.
6. Johansen K, Koepsell T. Familial tendency for abdominal aortic aneurysms. *JAMA.* 1986;14:1934–1936.
7. Darling RC III, Brewster DC, Darling RC, et al. Are familial abdominal aortic aneurysms different? *J Vasc Surg.* 1989;10:39–43.
8. Ouriel K, Green RM, Donayre C, et al. An evaluation of new methods of expressing aortic aneurysm size: relationship to rupture. *J Vasc Surg.* 1992;15:12–20.
9. Strachan DP. Predictors of death from aortic aneurysm among middle-aged men: the Whitehall study. *Br J Surg.* 1991;78:401–404.
10. Wolf YG, Thomas WS, Brennan FJ, et al. Computed tomography scanning findings associated with rapid expansion of abdominal aortic aneurysms. *J Vasc Surg.* 1994;20:529–538.
11. Veldenz HC, Schwarcz TH, Endean ED, et al. Morphology predicts rapid growth of small abdominal aortic aneurysms. *Ann Vasc Surg.* 1994;8:10–13.
12. Kushihashi T, Munechika H, Matsui S, et al. CT of abdominal aortic aneurysms—aneurysmal size and thickness of intraaneurysmal thrombus as risk factors or rupture. *Nippon Igaku Hoshasen Gakkai Zasshi.* 1991;51(3):219–227.
13. Inahara T, Geary GL, Mukherjee D, Egan JM. The contrary position to the nonresective treatment for abdominal aortic aneurysm. *J Vasc Surg.* 1985;2:42–48.
14. Nevitt MP, Ballard DJ, Hallett JW Jr. Prognosis of abdominal aortic aneurysms: a population-based study. *N Engl J Med.* 1989;321:1009–1013.
15. Schewe CK, Schweikart HP, Hammel G, et al. Influence of selective management on the prognosis and the risk of rupture of abdominal aortic aneurysms. *Clin Invest.* 1994;72:585–591.
16. Cronenwett JL, Sargent SK, Wall MH, et al. Variables that affect the expansion rate and outcome of small abdominal aortic aneurysms. *J Vasc Surg.* 1990;11:260–269.
17. Limet R, Sakalihassan N, Albert A. Determination of the expansion rate and incidence of rupture of abdominal aortic aneurysms. *J Vasc Surg.* 1991;14:540–548.
18. Hirose Y, Hamada S, Takamiya M. Predicting the growth of aortic aneurysms: a comparison of linear versus exponential models. *Angiology.* 1995;46:413–419.
19. Bengtsson H, Nilsson P, Bergqvist D. Natural history of abdominal aortic aneurysm detected by screening. *Br J Surg.* 1993;80:718–720.

20. Grimshaw GM, Thompson JM. The abdominal aorta: a statistical definition and strategy for monitoring change. *Eur J Endovasc Surg.* 1995;10:95–100.

21. Jean-Claude J, Newman KM, Li H, et al. Possible key role for plasmin in the pathogenesis of abdominal aortic aneurysms. *Surgery.* 1994;116:472–478.

22. MacSweeney STR, Ellis M, Worrell PC, et al. Smoking and growth rate of small abdominal aortic aneurysms. *Lancet.* 1994;344:651–652.

23. Leach SD, Toole AL, Stern H, et al. Effect of β-adrenergic blockade on the growth rate of abdominal aortic aneurysms. *Arch Surg.* 1988;123:606–609.

24. Boucek RJ, Gunja-Smith Z, Noble NL, et al. Modulation by propranolol of the lysyl cross-links in aortic elastin and collagen of the aneurysm-prone turkey. *Biochem Pharmacol.* 1983;32:275–280.

25. Gadowski GR, Pilcher DB, Ricci MA. Abdominal aortic aneurysm expansion rate: effect of size and beta-adrenergic blockade. *J Vasc Surg.* 1994;19:727–731.

26. Moursi MM, Beebe HG, Messina LM, et al. Inhibition of aortic aneurysm development in blotchy mice by beta adrenergic blockade independent of altered lysyl oxidase activity. *J Vasc Surg.* 1995;21:792–800.

27. Brown PM, Pattenden R, Vernooy C, et al. Selective management of abdominal aortic aneurysms in a prospective measurement program. *J Vasc Surg.* 1996;23:213–222.

28. Katz DA, Littenberg BL, Cronenwett JL. Management of small abdominal aortic aneurysm: early surgery versus watchful waiting. *JAMA.* 1992;268:2678–2686.

29. Katz DA, Cronenwett JL. The cost-effectiveness of early surgery versus watchful waiting in the management of small abdominal aortic aneurysms. *J Vasc Surg.* 1994;19:980–991.

30. Brechwoldt WL, Mackey WC, O'Donnell TF Jr. Economic implications of high-risk abdominal aortic aneurysms. *J Vasc Surg.* 1991;13:798–804.

IV

Endovascular Treatment of Aortic Aneurysm

12

Endovascular Repair of Abdominal Aortic Aneurysm

An Update on the Multicenter Endovascular Graft System Trial

Wesley S. Moore, MD

Direct repair of abdominal aortic aneurysm (AAA) represented one of the important milestones in the evolution of vascular surgery. For the first time, an otherwise fatal disease condition could be successfully managed with surgical repair. Countless thousands of lives have been saved with the repair of AAAs. Through the years, the morbidity and mortality associated with direct repair of AAA has steadily gone down so that centers of excellence are now reporting combined morbidity and mortality of less than 3.0%.[1] In spite of this, community-based studies continue to show a morbidity and mortality with conventional repair in the range of 10%.[2] Furthermore, in the index year of 1988, in spite of the fact that there were 40,000 elective repairs of AAA in the United States, approximately 15,000 patients died that same year from rupture. This represents the tenth leading cause of death in humans older than the age of 55.[3] The reasons that patients went on to die from ruptured AAAs in the age of available direct surgical repair are probably varied. However, they no doubt include patients whose aneurysms were unrecognized because of the absence of effective screening programs as well as patients who had, in the minds of their clinicians, relatively small aneurysms whose benefit from repair might be outweighed by the risk of operation.

The opportunity to repair an AAA without subjecting the patient to a laparotomy, utilizing an endovascular approach through a femoral artery, offers some exciting possibilities and potential solutions to the above-mentioned problems. First of all, it is highly likely that the morbidity and mortality from operation will be reduced considerably. If this is the case, it will ultimately lead to offering patients with smaller aneurysms the opportunity for endovascular repair and, if successful, may well lead to more effective ultrasound screening programs in order to identify patients at an earlier stage and thus hopefully reduce the incidence of fatal rupture.

While there are several early experimental reports dealing with endovascular grafting from a remote site,[4-7] Parodi and colleagues[8] reported the first successful clinical repair in 1991. The objective of this chapter is to update a multicenter clinical trial being carried out in the United States by Endovascular Technologies, Inc. (EVT).

At the present time, this represents the only FDA-approved multicenter trial designed to determine the safety, efficacy, and long-term results of endovascular repair of AAAs.

THE EGS TUBE GRAFT SYSTEM

The description of the endovascular graft system (EGS) as well as the technique of insertion have been well described in the literature.[9–14] In order for a patient to be considered a candidate for endovascular repair with a tube graft, several anatomic criteria must be fulfilled. Preoperative imaging includes a computed tomography (CT) scan, usually with a spiral reconstruction, followed by a contrast angiogram using marker catheter in order to finalize size characteristics of a proposed graft. The patient must have a proximal neck of abdominal aorta, between the renal arteries and the beginning of the aneurysm, that is at least 1.5 cm in length and no larger than 28 mm in diameter. A distal neck (cuff) must also be present with similar size characteristics. Finally, at least one iliac artery must be large enough to accommodate the catheter delivery system and sheath and optimally should be at least 8.0 mm in diameter. Other factors, noted on angiography, that would potentially eliminate patients from consideration include severe angulation of the aneurysm on the proximal neck, excessive tortuosity or occlusive lesions within the iliac arteries, dependence on the inferior mesenteric artery for collateral circulation to the gastrointestinal tract in the presence of occlusive lesions in the celiac or superior mesenteric artery, and aberrant take-off of renal arteries that might be compromised with the placement of an endovascular graft. Using these selection criteria, we have previously reported that only one out of seven patients with abdominal aortic aneurysm is a candidate for tube graft repair using an endovascular technique.[10]

For patients who are satisfactory candidates for tube graft repair, the procedure is performed in an operating room setting under general anesthesia. The patient is positioned on an operating table with a marker board under the patient's back. The marker board contains movable horizontal cursors that permit delineation of the proximal and distal sites of graft attachment using fluoroscopic control. The patient's abdomen and both groins are surgically prepared and draped. This permits the opportunity to convert to open repair should that be required, particularly under emergent circumstance. One femoral artery is selected as being the optimum side for instrumentation. This is usually the right side, for a right-handed surgeon. A vertical incision is made over the common femoral artery, and that vessel is exposed at the level of the inguinal ligament. The median and lateral circumflex branches are divided between ligature, and sufficient length of the retroperitoneal portion of the external iliac artery as well as the common femoral artery are mobilized. A 7 French angiogram sheath is then inserted into the femoral artery, and a guide wire is advanced under fluoroscopic control to the suprarenal portion of the aorta. A marker catheter is then passed over the guide wire into position, and an on-table angiogram using a digital fluoroscopic imaging system is obtained. It is recommended that this system have road-mapping capability. This provides the team with the opportunity to once again measure the length of the graft that is required to confirm the preoperative measurement. The horizontal cursors in the marker board are then adjusted, with the proximal cursor being placed just below the lowest renal artery and the distal cursor being placed immediately above the flow divider at the level of the aortic bifurcation. The patient is then systemically heparinized. The angiogram sheath is removed, leaving the guide wire in position.

The femoral artery is clamped proximally and distally, and a fishmouth, oblique transverse incision is made in the femoral artery through the guide wire puncture site. The EVT expandable introducer sheath is then loaded over the guide wire and advanced under fluoroscopic control up the iliac system and into the aorta. The endovascular deployment assembly containing the endograft endovascular prosthesis is then loaded over the guide wire and advanced up the sheath into anatomic position. This is positioned under fluoroscopic control such that the proximal and distal attachment systems are positioned opposite the horizontal cursor markers. The proximal attachment system is then deployed. The self-expanding attachment system springs open, with the radial hooks engaging the wall of the aorta. These hooks are then driven into the aortic wall by the expansion of an intrinsic balloon catheter that is positioned across the attachment system. A similar maneuver is then carried out distally. Finally, a completion angiogram is obtained to demonstrate the position of the graft, its function, and to determine whether or not there is any evidence of perigraft leak into the aneurysm sac. The guide wire and introducer sheath are then removed. The arteriotomy is repaired in the standard fashion, and the femoral incision is closed. The patient is observed briefly in the recovery room and then transferred to a regular hospital bed. The patient is usually ready for discharge the following morning. Periodic follow-up examinations including physical examination, noninvasive laboratory testing including duplex scanning, plain films of the abdomen, and contrast-enhanced CT scanning are performed to document the subsequent result of endovascular grafting.

THE EGS BIFURCATED GRAFT SYSTEM

The technical considerations of the bifurcated system, in an experimental setting, have previously been reported.[15] Selection of patients for a bifurcated graft involves the same preoperative imaging as for the tube graft. Patients are candidates for a bifurcated prosthesis if they have a proximal neck of appropriate length and diameter but fail to have a distal neck. The iliac arteries cannot be aneurysmal, and the ratio between the iliac artery diameter and neck of the aneurysm cannot exceed 1:2.

The operating room setting for the bifurcated graft is identical to that of the tube graft. However, both femoral arteries must be surgically exposed. One femoral artery is designated as the ipsilateral side. It is on that side that the EVT expandable introducer sheath will be placed, and through which the catheter delivery system containing the graft will be inserted. The other side is designated as the contralateral side. The preliminary steps including angiography with road-mapping and positioning of the horizontal cursors are similar to that described for the tube graft. The contralateral femoral artery is then accessed with an 11 French sheath. Through that sheath, an Amplatz snare catheter system is then advanced, initially over a guide wire, into the terminal aorta at the bifurcation. The catheter delivery system, containing the bifurcated graft, has a "pull wire" that emerges from the superior end of the jacket covering the bifurcated graft. This pull wire is attached to the contralateral limb of the graft. It is the objective to insert the pull wire up the ipsilateral side to pass it through the loop of the snare catheter and to draw the pullwire into the contralateral side in order to make preparation for deployment of the bifurcated graft. Once the pullwire is drawn into the contralateral side, the catheter delivery system is then loaded over the ipsilateral guide wire and passed up the EVT expandable sheath into the aorta. It is then advanced into a suprarenal position while the jacket is retracted. As the jacket is retracted, the pull wire unfolds and the limbs of the bifurcated graft separate. The contralateral limb, attached to the pull wire, is then directed toward the contralateral iliac artery. The whole assembly is then drawn down into the proposed anatomic position with the proximal attachment system being positioned opposite the superior cursor immediately below the lowest renal artery. The ipsilateral iliac limb and the contralateral iliac limb are then positioned opposite the distal cursor in the common iliac arteries. Sequentially, the proximal attachment system, the contralateral iliac attachment system, and the ipsilateral iliac attachment system are then deployed. Each attachment system has a series of radially placed pins that engage the aorta and iliac arteries, respectively. These pins are then driven into position with the inflation of balloon catheters. Upon completion of deployment, an angiogram is then obtained to document the anatomic result and to determine whether or not there is evidence of proximal or distal periattachment system leak into the aneurysm sac. The introducer sheaths are then removed, and the femoral arteries are repaired. The femoral incisions are closed, and the patient is returned to the recovery room and to a regular hospital room for overnight observation. Hospital discharge is possible the following day. Follow-up imaging follows a similar schedule to that of the tube graft.

TRIAL DESIGN

The EGS system is the only multicenter trial for endovascular repair of AAAs to have been approved by the FDA. The trial design includes three phases for the tube graft as well as the bifurcated graft.

Phase 1

Phase 1 is designed to determine the feasibility, safety, and efficacy of endovascular repair. A series of patients who are candidates for either a tube or bifurcated graft is identified at each of the participating centers, and a series of implantations is carried out. The cumulative results with respect to 30-day morbidity and mortality and short-term follow-up are then reviewed and reported to the FDA. If the investigators, the company consultants, and finally the FDA are satisfied with the results, authority is then granted to proceed with phase 2.

Phase 2

The objective of phase 2 is to carry out a comparative study of endovascular repair with conventional surgical repair in order to document any differences with regard to morbidity, mortality, and cost. Patient selection is based on a nonrandomized, concurrent control series. Control patients receiving conventional repair include those patients who, for a variety of reasons, would not have been candidates for endovascular repair but in whom the conventional repair utilizes a comparable surgical procedure and graft configuration. That is, patients in the tube graft series are candidates for tube graft repair by conventional means, and patients in the bifurcated graft series would require a bifurcated prosthesis when undergoing conventional surgical repair.

When the phase 2 series is completed, a request will be made to the FDA to approve endovascular repair as a clinically accepted technique. However, the continued follow-up of patients who have undergone endovascular repair in phase 1 and phase 2 will continue in phase 3.

Phase 3

The objective of phase 3 is to carry out a long-term follow-up of patients undergoing abdominal aneurysm repair by endovascular grafting in order to determine whether or not there are any late problems with respect to the protection of patients against aneurysm enlargement and rupture. It will also be the opportunity to determine whether or not any mechanical problems develop over the course of the patient's lifetime.

EGS TUBE GRAFT PHASE 1 RESULTS

Phase 1 was started in 3 centers. Following initial experience in those centers, and in anticipation of moving on to phase 2, an additional 10 centers were added, bringing it to a total of 13 centers participating in the phase 1 protocol.

The first implantation took place on February 10, 1993, at UCLA Medical Center. Between that date and December 6, 1994, a total of 46 patients underwent endovascular repair using the EGS system.[14] The number of implants varied from 1 to 13 per center. Fifteen implants were performed with the original EGS system, and 31 implants were performed with the newer, improved EGS-II device.

Thirty-nine of the 46 implants (85%) were deemed to be initially successful. Seven patients required conversion to conventional repair. The majority of these occurred early in the series, with 5 conversions out of 15 EGS-I implants and only 2 conversions out of 31 EGS-II implants. The reasons for conversion included iliac stenosis in 4 patients, subintimal deployment in 1 patient, proximal attachment system displacement in 1 patient, and short or inadequate distal neck in 1 patient.

There were no postoperative deaths either in hospital or within 30 days of operation. Complications included one mild myocardial infarction as manifested by ECG and enzyme changes, which did not prolong hospitalization. There were no amputations, major emboli, or episodes of mesenteric ischemia.

Contrast enhancement outside the graft, as seen on CT scan, was detected initially in 17 implants (44%). These represented either incomplete seal of the attachment system, thus permitting some blood flow into the aneurysm sac, or back bleeding from a lumbar or inferior mesenteric artery. Nine of 17 (53%) resolved spontaneously. Of the 8 patients who manifest persistent contrast enhancement in the aneurysm sac, 1 was successfully controlled with a transluminal balloon angioplasty of the attachment system. One patient underwent surgical explantation because of aneurysm enlargement. Six patients continued to be observed, and so far have had no evidence of aneurysm enlargement with follow-up ranging from 6 to 27 months following operation and follow-up complete through May 1995. There have been no aneurysm ruptures.

On January 28, 1995, a metallic attachment system fracture was identified in a patient on plain abdominal film. Retrospective review of all abdominal films in all patients, looking specifically for attachment fracture, was then carried out. Simultaneously, the device malfunction was reported to the FDA, and the implant program was placed on temporary hold. Retrospective review identified a total of nine implants (23%) with attachment system fracture. One patient, with a good functioning implant without leak, underwent explantation because it was apparent that the proximal attachment system, which had fractured, was beginning to migrate. The remaining eight patients continue to function normally in spite of identifiable attachment system fracture, and these patients continue to be followed closely.

EGS TUBE GRAFT PHASE 2 STATUS

A total of 19 experimental and 13 control patients were entered into the phase 2 study before the trial was temporarily suspended due to the attachment system fracture problem. The engineers at Endovascular Technologies then undertook a very extensive program of analysis to determine the mechanism of attachment system fracture and to reengineer the attachment systems so as to avoid the problem. Following the redesign, and prolonged bench testing, the data were resubmitted to the FDA and subsequently approved by the FDA to resume implantation in October 1995. To date, a total of 24 implants have been performed in the phase 2 trial and 25 control patients have undergone operation.

Phase 2 is ongoing and the results are currently not available since the complete study has not been analyzed or published.

EGS BIFURCATED GRAFT PHASE 1 STATUS

Phase 1 of the EGS bifurcated graft program began on September 14, 1994, with the first two implantations at UCLA Medical Center. Both of these were successful, and a third graft was added to our group prior to recognition of an attachment system fracture problem, which mandated placing the implant program on temporary hold. The hold was lifted in October 1995. Nine implants were placed in United States participating centers. Phase 1 is still in progress, and the study has not been analyzed or published, and therefore the results are not available at the time of this writing.

REFERENCES

1. Ernst CB. Abdominal aortic aneurysm. *N Engl J Med.* 1993;328:1169–1172.
2. Taylor LM, Porter JM. Basic data related to clinical decision-making in abdominal aortic aneurysm. *Ann Vasc Surg.* 1980;1:502–504.
3. Goldstone J. Aneurysms of the aorta and iliac arteries. In: Moore WS, ed. *Vascular Surgery: A Comprehensive Review.* 4th ed. Philadelphia: WB Saunders; 1993:401–423.
4. Dotter CT. Transluminally-placed coil spring endarterial tube grafts: long term patency in canine popliteal artery. *Invest Radiol.* 1969;4:329–332.
5. Cragg A, Lund G, Rysavy J, et al. Non-surgical placement of arterial endoprosthesis: a new technique using nitinol wire. *Radiology.* 1983;147:261–263.
6. Balko A, Piasecki GJ, Shah DM, et al. Transfemoral placement of intraluminal polyurethane prosthesis for abdominal aortic aneurysm. *J Surg Res.* 1986;40:305–309.
7. Mirich D, Wright KC, Wallace S, et al. Percutaneously placed endovascular grafts for aortic aneurysms: feasibility study. *Radiology.* 1989;170:1033–1037.
8. Parodi JC, Palmaz JC, Barone HD. Transfemoral intraluminal graft implantation for abdominal aortic aneurysms. *Ann Vasc Surg.* 1991;5:491–499.
9. Lazarus HM. Endovascular grafting for the treatment of abdominal aortic aneurysms. *Surg Clin North Am.* 1992;72:959–968.
10. Moore WS, Vescera CL. Repair of abdominal aortic aneurysm by transfemoral endovascular graft placement. *Ann Surg.* 1994;220:331–341.
11. Moore WS. Endovascular grafting technique: a feasibility study. In: Yao JST, Pearce WH, eds. *Aneurysms: New Findings and Treatments.* Norwalk, CT: Appleton and Lange; 1993:333–340.
12. Moore WS. Transfemoral endovascular repair of abdominal aortic aneurysm using the endovascular graft system device. In: Greenhalgh RM, ed. *Vascular and Endovascular Surgical Techniques: An Atlas.* 3rd ed. Philadelphia: WB Saunders; 1994:78–91.

13. Moore WS. The role of endovascular grafting technique in the treatment of infrarenal abdominal aortic aneurysm. *Cardiovasc Surg.* 1995;3:109–114.
14. Moore WS, Rutherford RB, for the EVT Investigators. Transfemoral endovascular repair of abdominal aortic aneurysm: results of the North American EVT phase 1 trial. *J Vasc Surg.* 1996;23:543–553.
15. Quiñones-Baldrich WJ, Deaton DH, Mitchell RS, et al. Preliminary experience with the Endovascular Technologies bifurcated endovascular aortic prosthesis in a calf model. *J Vasc Surg.* 1995;22:370–381.

13

Endoluminal Repair of Abdominal Aortic Aneurysms

The Sydney Experience

James May, MS, FRACS, FACS, Geoffrey H. White, FRACS, Weiyun Yu, BSc(Med)MB, BS, Richard Waugh, FRACR, Michael Stephen, FRACS, and John P. Harris, MS, FRACS, FACS

The endoluminal method of abdominal aortic aneurysm (AAA) repair has attracted much attention following the demonstration of the feasibility of the technique by Parodi et al.[1] After their report the authors followed the pioneering work of Parodi and, as of April 1996, have experience with 133 aneurysms in which the endoluminal method has been used for repair. In 113 of these, the aneurysm was situated in the abdominal aorta and these form the basis of this report. The minimally invasive nature of the endoluminal method has always been attractive but the limitation has been the unknown outcome of the procedure. With the aim of overcoming this deficiency, at least in part, we present the clinical outcome of our patients and a computed tomography (CT) study of the fate of AAA treated by the endoluminal method.

MATERIAL AND METHODS

Between May 1992 and April 1996, the endoluminal method was used to repair AAA in 113 patients at the Royal Prince Alfred Hospital. There were 8 females and 105 males with a mean age of 70 years. Comorbidities leading to rejection for conventional open repair at other centers were present in 48 patients (Table 13–1). The mean diameter of the AAA was 5.8 cm with a range of 3.5 to 8 cm. Those aneurysms with the smallest diameter were saccular and considered to be at greater risk of rupture than a similar sized fusiform aneurysm. The criterion for selection was a proximal neck of thrombus-free aorta between the renal arteries and an aneurysm of length 1.5 cm or greater with a diameter of 28 mm or less. Patients were divided into two subgroups.[2] Those with a proximal neck as described and a distal neck of thrombus-free aorta between the aneurysm and the aortic bifurcation of 1.5 cm or greater and nontortuous iliac arteries

TABLE 13–1. COMORBIDITIES

Poor left ventricular function (and renal impairment in three)	25
Renal failure	
On dialysis	1
Successfully transplanted	1
Chronic obstructive airways disease	7
Bilateral thoracoplasties	1
Chronic liver disease	4
Hostile abdomen	9
TOTAL	48

of diameter 8 mm or greater. These aneurysms were suited for endoluminal repair using a tube endoprosthesis and were designated type I. Type II aneurysms were those with proximal neck as described but lacking one or more of the criteria for inclusion in type I. These aneurysms were suited for endoluminal repair using either a tapered iliac/aortofemoral graft or a bifurcated graft.

Endoprostheses

The endoprostheses used were the modified Parodi, the Sydney (White/Yu), the Endovascular Technologies (EVT), and the Mintech stentor (Miahle). Table 13–2 indicates the number of patients receiving the different devices and the configuration of the prostheses. The design of the different delivery systems and the endoprostheses used have been reported previously.[3-10] Our largest experience is with the Sydney endograft developed by White and Yu in our own endovascular laboratory. This is a balloon-expandable device constructed of commercially available woven Dacron of thickness 0.24 mm (Fig. 13–1). The endoprosthesis is anchored by means of metallic graft attachment devices that are incorporated into the fabric of the graft. The endoprosthesis is mounted on an 8-cm-long, noncompliant balloon (William Cook, Eight Mile Plains, Australia) (Fig. 13–2). This is the longest balloon of the required diameter available and limits the size of the endograft to 8 cm. Because the entire length of abdominal aorta between the renal arteries and the aortic bifurcation has the potential to become aneurysmal, it is desirable that any endoprosthesis used should cover this segment in its entirety, irrespective of the length of the aneurysm. In some cases the 8-cm-long Sydney endograft can achieve this aim. In the majority of patients, however, a second endograft has to be introduced using the overlapping double prosthesis or

TABLE 13–2. TYPES OF ENDOPROSTHESES

	Graft Configuration			
System	**Tube**	**Aortoiliac/Aortofemoral**	**Bifurcated**	**Total**
Modified Parodi	3	6	1	10
Sydney (White/Yu)	41	19	13	73
EVT	11		4	15
Chuter			1	1
Stentor	—	—	14	14
TOTAL	55	25	33	113

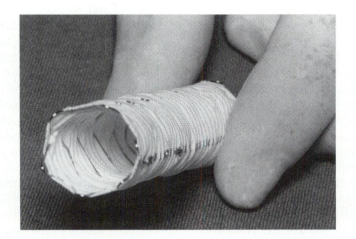

Figure 13–1. The Sydney endograft, a balloon-expandable Dacron prosthesis developed by White and Yu. (*Reproduced with permission: May J, White GH, Yu W, et al. Early experience with the Sydney and EVT prostheses for endoluminal treatment of abdominal aortic aneurysms. J Endovasc Surg. 1995;2(3):240–247.*)

"trombone technique."[11] This allows a second endograft to be deployed within and overlapping the first endograft.

Surgical Technique

The procedures were carried out in the operating room with the patient prepared and draped for open operation in the event of failed endoluminal repair. The femoral artery was exposed through a 5-cm vertical incision in the groin. On table, preprocedure angiography was carried out to identify the level of the renal arteries and the aortic bifurcation. These positions were marked on the image intensifier screen and the wheels of the machine locked to avoid errors of parallax. A longitudinally placed radio-opaque

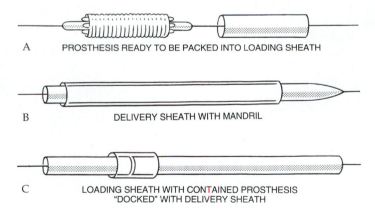

A   PROSTHESIS READY TO BE PACKED INTO LOADING SHEATH

B   DELIVERY SHEATH WITH MANDRIL

C   LOADING SHEATH WITH CONTAINED PROSTHESIS
     "DOCKED" WITH DELIVERY SHEATH

Figure 13–2. Preparation of the Sydney endograft for delivery: (**A**) Sydney prosthesis is mounted on a balloon catheter for packing into the loading sheath. (**B**) The appearance of the introducing sheath with mandrel. (**C**) Loading sheath and introducing sheath connected following withdrawal of mandrel. (*Reproduced with permission: May J, White GH, Yu W, et al. Early experience with the Sydney and EVT prostheses for endoluminal treatment of abdominal aortic aneurysms. J Endovasc Surg. 1995;2(3):240–247.*)

ruler was positioned beneath the patient as an additional point of reference. An introducing sheath with its mandrel was passed over a guide wire and through a femoral arteriotomy before being maneuvered into the aorta via the iliac arteries. When the sheath reached the level of the renal arteries, the mandrel was withdrawn and the endograft delivered via the sheath to a position immediately below the renal arteries. The introduction of the sheath, the delivery of the endograft, and its subsequent deployment were all performed under radiographic control. A postprocedure angiogram was performed to confirm exclusion of the aneurysmal sac from the circulation.

The procedure was performed entirely by the endoluminal route in 88 patients and by a combination of the endoluminal and extraluminal route in 25 patients. The techniques for the combined procedures have been described in detail in previous reports.[3,9,10] (Figs. 13–3A and B). The aim was to use an endoluminal tube graft wherever possible. Initially this resulted in type I aneurysms being treated by the endoluminal route and type II aneurysms being treated by a combination of the endoluminal and extraluminal route. With the development of a bifurcated version of the Sydney endograft and the availability of a bifurcated EVT device and bifurcated stentor device, the type II aneurysms are now more commonly managed by the endoluminal route alone.

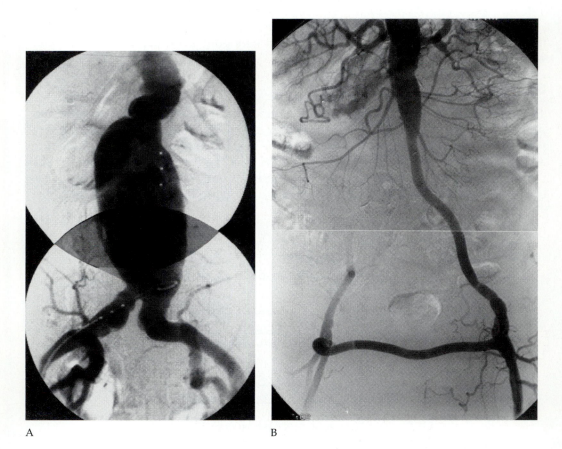

A   B

Figure 13–3. (A) Preoperative aortogram of patient with AAA and early aneurysmal disease in common iliac arteries. **(B)** Postoperative aortogram of patient in part A performed 2.5 years after endoluminal aortofemoral graft combined with femorofemoral crossover graft and occlusion of contralateral common iliac artery by detachable balloon. (*Reproduced with permission: May J, White GH, Waugh R, et al. Endoluminal repair of abdominal aortic aneurysms. Med J Aust. 1994;161:541–543.*)

TABLE 13–3. CAUSES OF FAILURE LEADING TO OPEN REPAIR

Access problems	2
Balloon related	
Malfunction	1
Aortic rupture	1
Stent related dislodgement	3
Graft thrombosis	1
Inability to deploy bifurcated graft	4
TOTAL	12

Follow-up

No patient has been lost to follow-up. This has involved clinical examination and contrast-enhanced CT within the first 10 days following operation, 6 months following operation, and annually thereafter. Any communication between the aneurysmal sac and the general circulation can be readily identified by extravasation of contrast. We believe it is less confusing to refer to this situation as an "endoleak"[12] rather than a "leak," which is in common usage. The latter term can be mistaken for an external rupture of the aneurysm rather than an internal communication in an intact aneurysm.

RESULTS

Endografts were able to be delivered and deployed successfully in the aortas of 101 patients. In the remaining 12 patients, endoluminal repair had to be abandoned in favor of open repair. The causes of failure in these 12 patients are listed in Table 13–3. There were six deaths within 30 days. Three were cardiac in nature, two primarily renal in nature, and one multisystem. All were procedure related. The outcome of the 113 patients undergoing endoluminal AAA repair is shown in Table 13–4, broken down according to the endoluminal method used. Of the 113 patients undergoing endoluminal AAA repair, 82 are currently alive and well with their AAA excluded from the circulation.

TABLE 13–4. OUTCOME OF ENDOLUMINAL AAA

System	Number of Procedures	Conversion		Endoleaks	Deaths	
		Primary	Secondary		Perioperative	Late
Modified Parodi	10	5	1	1	1	1
EVT tube	11	0	0	1	0	3
EVT bifurcated	4	2	0	0	1	0
Stentor bifurcated	14	0	1	0	1	0
Chuter	1	0	0	0	0	0
Sydney tube	41	1	4	5	2	2
Sydney aortoiliac	19	1	0	0	0	0
Sydney bifurcated	13	3	0	0	1	0

TABLE 13–5. LOCAL VASCULAR COMPLICATIONS

Femoral artery damage	4
Perforation of iliac artery	2
Dissection of iliac artery	2
Graft stenosis	2
Common iliac artery occlusion	4
Endoleak	
Spontaneous seal	1
Corrected endoluminally	2
Converted to open repair	2
Untreated	1
Renal arteries covered	2
Bleeding	
Return to OR	1
Hematoma	1
Wound complications	4
TOTAL	28

Complications

Complications have been classified according to the recommendations of the Ad Hoc Committee of the SVS and ISCVS on Uniform Reporting Standards for AAA. The local vascular complications are listed in Table 13–5. Of the six patients with endoleaks, two were corrected by secondary endoluminal repair (one of which subsequently developed a further endoleak and required conversion to open repair), two by conversion to open operation, and one by spontaneous seal. The remaining patient had an unrelated cerebrovascular accident 16 months after endoluminal repair and before the endoleak became apparent and no further intervention is planned.

The remote systemic complications are listed in Table 13–6.

CHANGES IN MORPHOLOGY OF AAA FOLLOWING ENDOLUMINAL REPAIR

The changes in morphology of AAAs that had been observed in follow-up CT have been reported by the authors previously.[13,14] Forty-seven patients in the study had AAA treated by the endoluminal method 12 months or longer ago. Endoleak was detected in 5 of these. The maximum diameter of the AAA increased in all 5 but was observed

TABLE 13–6. SYSTEMIC REMOTE COMPLICATIONS

Renal insufficiency	
Obstructive	2
Contrast media induced	5
Cardiac	
Congestive failure	2
Myocardial infarction	4
Cardiac arrhythmia	2
Stroke/TIA	3
TOTAL	18

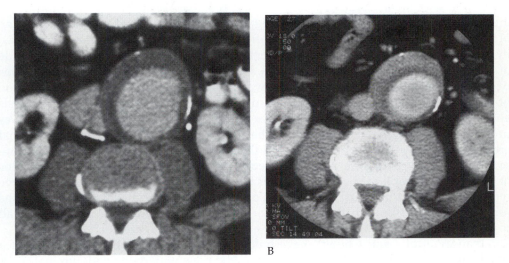

Figure 13–4. (A) Contrast-enhanced CT performed preoperatively in patient with 7.0-cm abdominal aortic aneurysm. **(B)** Contrast-enhanced CT performed 12 months following endoluminal repair of patient in part A. Diameter now measures 5.4 cm. (*Reproduced with permission: May J, White GH, Yu W, et al. A prospective study of changes in morphology and dimensions of abdominal aortic aneurysms following endoluminal repair: a preliminary report. J Endovasc Surg. 1995;2(4):343–347.*)

to decrease following secondary endoluminal repair. Forty-two patients had successful endoluminal repairs without evidence of endoleak. Following successful endoluminal repair the maximum transverse diameter of the AAA diminished progressively with time in all but three patients (Figs. 13–4A and B). This incremental diminution was 0.4 cm at 6 months, 0.8 cm at 12 months, and 1.1 cm at 18 months. Concurrent with this diminution in diameter of the aneurysmal sac, there was a paradoxical increase of 10% in the mean diameter of the proximal and distal neck of the aneurysm. Unlike the aneurysmal sac measurements, however, the increase in diameter of the aneurysmal necks was not progressive. Two of the three patients who demonstrated an increase in maximum transverse diameter in the aneurysmal sac at 6 months have subsequently seen a diminution in maximum transverse diameter at 12-month follow-up. The increase in diameter in the third patient was 2 mm over 12 months.

DISCUSSION

The two major disadvantages of endoluminal repair of AAA are that the long-term outcome is not known and the procedures themselves, by their nature, have some complications that are not seen with conventional operations. Damage to the iliac arteries, for example, would be rare with open AAA repair but a recognized hazard of passing an introducing sheath through these arteries as part of the endoluminal procedure. With regard to long-term outcome, it is reassuring that in medium-term follow-up with contrast-enhanced CT there has been shrinkage of AAA that had been isolated from the general circulation by endoluminal repair. Of more concern, however, is the authors' finding of expansion of the proximal and distal neck of AAA following endoluminal repair. The authors have hypothesised that this is due to deliberate oversizing of the endoprosthesis. Such oversizing is commonly practiced to avoid migration of the prosthesis when a noncompliant graft material is used. This concept is supported by the fact that the increase in neck diameter has not been progressive and the magnitude of the increase in diameter is the same as that by which the endoprosthesis was oversized. The alternative explanation, however, is that the natural history of expansion of the aneurysm is continuing unabated despite the insertion of the endoprosthesis and despite exclusion of the aneurysmal sac from the circulation. This process involves progressive aneurysmal degeneration in the aorta between the aneurysm and the renal arteries superiorly and the aneurysm and the aortic bifurcation inferiorly. If this were so, one might expect to see evidence of aneurysmal degeneration in autopsy specimens of patients with implanted endoprostheses who have died from other causes. We have reported three such patients[15,16] and have not observed aneurysmal degeneration in the neck of the aneurysms in these patients. The period of follow-up, however, in all patients was less than 2 years.

Ivancev et al.[17] and Chuter[18] have independently recorded distal migration of a proximal graft attachment device in patients who have undergone endoluminal AAA repair 1 or more years previously. This is important information and may have implications for the long-term outcome of endoluminal AAA repair. Both investigators were using endoprostheses that were anchored by modified Gianturco stents. With regard to the behavior of the aneurysmal neck following endoluminal repair, further relevant information has been reported by Baker et al.[19] They used ultrasound to determine the size of the aorta between the renal arteries and aortic grafts inserted at open repair of AAA in 95 patients at a median of 5 years previously. Forty (42%) had supragraft aortas greater than 3 cm diameter, 10 of which were greater than 4 cm and 2 greater than 5 cm. If this information were extrapolated to patients undergoing endoluminal AAA repair, one could anticipate a poor outcome in a proportion of patients. The only conclusion to be reached at this stage is that further careful and prolonged follow-up is mandatory for those centers using the endoluminal method.

REFERENCES

1. Parodi JC, Palmaz JC, Barone HD. Transfemoral intraluminal graft implantation for abdominal aortic aneurysms. *Ann Vasc Surg.* 1991;5:491–499.
2. May J, White GH, Yu W, et al. Results of endoluminal grafting of abdominal aortic aneurysms are dependent on aneurysm morphology. *Ann Vasc Surg.* 1996;10:254–261.
3. May J, White GH, Yu W, et al. Treatment of complex abdominal aortic aneurysms by a combination of endoluminal and extraluminal aorto-bifemoral grafts. *J Vasc Surg.* 1994;19:924–933.
4. Scott RA, Chuter TA. Clinical endovascular placement of bifurcated graft in abdominal aortic aneurysm without laparotomy. *Lancet.* 1994;343:413.
5. Yusuf SW, Baker DM, Chuter TAM, et al. Transfemoral endoluminal repair of abdominal aortic aneurysm with bifurcated graft. *Lancet.* 1994;344:650–651.
6. Moore WS, Vescera CL. Repair of abdominal aortic aneurysm by transfemoral endovascular graft replacement. *Ann Surg.* 1994;220:331–341.
7. Balm R, Eikelboom BC, May J, et al. Early experience with transfemoral endovascular aneurysm management (TEAM) in the treatment of aortic aneurysms. *Eur J Vasc Endovasc Surg.* 1996;11:214–220.
8. Chuter TAM, Wendt G, Hopkinson BR, et al. Transfemoral insertion of a bifurcated endovascular graft for aortic aneurysm repair: the first 22 patients. *J Cardiovasc Surg.* 1995;3:121–128.
9. May J, White GH, Yu W, et al. Endoluminal repair of complex abdominal aortic aneurysms. In: Yao J, Pearce WH, eds. *Arterial Surgery: Management of Challenging Problems.* Stamford, CT: Appleton & Lange; 1996;20:237–246.

10. May J, White GH. Specialised endovascular technique: combined surgical and endovascular approaches. In: White RA, Fogarty JJ, eds. *Peripheral Endovascular Interventions.* St. Louis, MO: Mosby Year Book; 1996;26:433–448.

11. Yu W, White GH, May J, Stephen MS. Endoluminal repair of abdominal aortic aneurysms using the trombone technique. *Asian J Surg.* 1996;19:37–40.

12. White GH, Yu W, May J. "Endoleak"—a proposed new terminology to describe incomplete aneurysm exclusion by an endoluminal graft. *J Endovasc Surg.* 1996;3:124–125.

13. May J, White GH, Yu W, et al. A prospective study of changes in morphology and dimensions of abdominal aortic aneurysms following endoluminal repair: a preliminary report. *J Endovasc Surg.* 1995;2(4):343–347.

14. May J, White GH, Yu W, et al. A prospective study of anatomic pathological changes in abdominal aortic aneurysms following endoluminal repair: is the aneurysmal process reversed? *Eur J Vasc Endovasc Surg.* 1996;11:1–7.

15. McGahan TJ, Berry GA, McGahan SL, et al. Results of autopsy 7 months after successful endoluminal treatment of an infrarenal abdominal aortic aneurysm. *J Endovasc Surg.* 1995;2:348–355.

16. May J, White G, Yu W, et al. Pathology of healing and changes in morphology of aortic aneurysms treated by endoluminal prostheses. In: Chuter TAM, Donayre CE, White RA, eds. *Endoluminal Vascular Prostheses* 2nd ed. Armonk, NY: Futura Publishing; 1996.

17. Ivancev K. Malmo experience with Ivancev prosthesis. Presented at Endovascular Aortic Aneurysm Surgery Symposium, April 1996, Nottingham, England.

18. Chuter TAM. Experience with Chuter bifurcated prosthesis. Presented at Endovascular Aortic Aneurysm Surgery Symposium, April 1996, Nottingham, England.

19. Baker DM, Hind R, Yusef W, et al. Do abdominal aortic aneurysms recur following repair? *Int Angiol.* 1995;(March):158.

14

Fate of Aortic Size Before and After Endovascular Technologies Tube Grafting

Augmented Data

Jon S. Matsumura, MD, and William H. Pearce, MD

The use of endovascular grafts for the treatment of abdominal aortic aneurysms (AAAs) offers an exciting alternative to the standard operative procedure. Although the conventional means of repair of AAAs has excellent long-term durability, the procedure is associated with significant morbidity and mortality.[1-4] Even though operative mortality has decreased, it is not known what percent of patients do not undergo surgery because of severe comorbid conditions. Endovascular repair of AAAs offers a less invasive method for the treatment of aortic aneurysm and will offer marginal operative candidates the possibility of definitive treatment. A number of reports of endovascular grafting for aneurysms have described technical success with varying periods of follow-up.[5-13] For this technology to replace the gold standard and be accepted by the medical community, endovascular grafting must protect patients from continued growth and rupture of their aneurysms.

In the past 5 years, many groups have reported their experience with endovascular grafting. Unfortunately, these series include many different grafts making comparison difficult. In the rush to embrace this technology, it is important to study each graft and delivery system in an objective and consistent fashion. In fact, endovascular grafts are being implanted outside of Food and Drug Administration (FDA)-approved protocols, sometimes with poor results.[14] We, along with 12 other centers in the United States, have participated in the Endovascular Technologies Inc. (EVT) trial using an FDA-approved protocol. Important features of this trial are the detailed record-keeping and long-term follow-up. In a recent study, EVT made available to our center the follow-up data for 34 patients who had undergone endovascular grafting and who had complete 1-year follow-up. These data were presented at the meeting of the Society for Vascular Surgery in Chicago, Illinois, in 1996.[15] Since that time an additional 13 patients have been added and also preoperative scans analyzed. This chapter presents these expanded data.

METHODS

Sixty-eight patients had endovascular graft placement beginning February 10, 1993, and continuing through January 24, 1995. These endovascular grafts were implanted in several institutions in phase I and phase II trials (see the acknowledgments for a list of participating centers and principal investigators). The phase I study design, device description, implantation technique, and short-term results have been described.[16] Using the demographic information and computed tomography (CT) scans supplied by EVT, complete data are available for 47 patients with both postimplantation and 1-year (between 11 to 13 months) CT scans. Eight patients have incomplete radiographic follow-up, 8 patients had immediate conversion to open procedure, 4 more patients were converted within the first year, and 1 patient died within the first year. The celiac aorta was picked as an internal control. The proximal neck was defined as the most cephalad image containing a complete hook set. The diameter of aneurysmal sac was the largest diameter of the aneurysm. Finally, the distal neck was defined as the most caudal image with a complete hook set. Comparable images were selected of these areas by matching calcification patterns in the aortic wall and bony landmarks of the adjacent spine. Radiographs were scanned on a VXR-8 (Vidar Systems Corporation, Herndon, VA) using 300 dpi on Adobe Photoshop (v3.0). The CT scans were cropped of all identifying data and coded. Using computerized planimetry (NIH Image, v1.57), the aortic image was enlarged, the perimeter traced, and measurements taken based on the accompanying calibrated scales. Area and perimeter were directly measured; major and minor transverse diameters were measured from best fit ellipses.

Preoperative angiograms were inspected for patency of the inferior mesenteric artery, lumbar arteries, and tortuosity of the infrarenal aorta. Attachment device fractures or hookbreaks were detected with radiographs and fluoroscopy. Postoperative CT scans were examined for evidence of perigraft flow as determined by contrast enhancement outside the lumen of the graft but within the aneurysm wall. After all parameters and measurements were completed, the codes were broken and subsequent analysis performed. The patients were placed in three groups based on perigraft leak: group I, no leak on any scan; group II, early leak that ceases before the 1-year scan; and group III, persistent leak. Selection of CT images, measurements, and interpretation of radiographs was performed by a single observer (JSM).

Paired two-tailed t tests were used to compare size changes. Pearson correlations were performed to assess relationship between aneurysm size change and covariates. A p value of <0.05 was selected for determination of statistical significance. Exploratory analyses are given with 95% confidence intervals in square brackets. Descriptive statistics are given to one standard deviation.

RESULTS

Forty-four of the 47 patients were male, and the mean age was 72 ± 8 years. The inferior mesenteric artery was patent before implantation in 38% of patients, and the mean number of patent infrarenal lumbar vessels was 4.5 ± 1.8. Nearly all of the infrarenal aortas were tortuous, presenting oblique cross-sections on standard imaging. In group I, there were 31 (66%) patients with no leaks; group II, 9 (19%) patients with early leaks; and group III, 7 (15%) patients with persistent leaks. Group II includes 7 patients with perigraft flow only on the postimplantation scan and none thereafter, 1

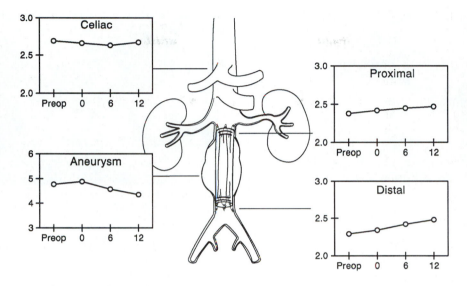

Figure 14–1. Aortic minor diameter size before and 1 year after implantation by anatomic location. Note the aneurysm graph has an expanded y axis.

patient with sealed leak following balloon dilation 2 months after implantation, and 1 with complete perigraft thrombosis 9 months after implantation. All grafts were patent.

The mean minor diameter preoperatively, at implantation, 6 months, and 1 year is depicted for all four areas of the aorta by leak group in Figure 14–1. Aneurysm minor diameter decreases from 4.88 ± 0.64 cm at implantation to 4.35 ± 0.86 cm at 1 year ($p < 0.0001$). In 36 patients the aneurysm size diminished and in 11 patients the aneurysm size increased over 1 year after endovascular grafting. The minor diameter of the celiac aorta (0.01 ± 0.19 cm (−0.07) [0.07, 0.09]) and proximal neck (0.05 ± 0.17 cm [−0.00, 0.09]) did not change significantly. However, the distal neck enlarged by 0.14 ± 0.27 cm [0.06, 0.22] at 1 year. Major diameter, perimeter, and area changes parallel the minor diameter changes. Figures 14–2 through 14–5 show the CT scans of a patient with dramatic aneurysmal shrinkage and distal neck enlargement.

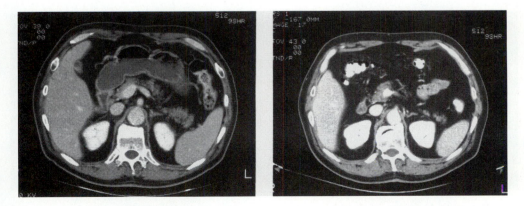

Figure 14–2. On the left is the aorta at the celiac artery immediately after implantation. On the right is the same area of aorta 1 year after implantation. There is no size change.

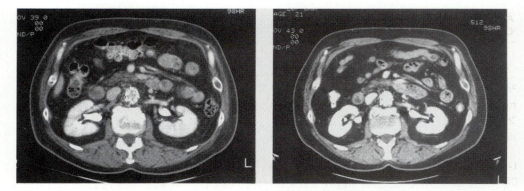

Figure 14–3. On the left is a proximal neck slice immediately after implantation. On the right is the same region 1 year after implantation. Size is essentially the same.

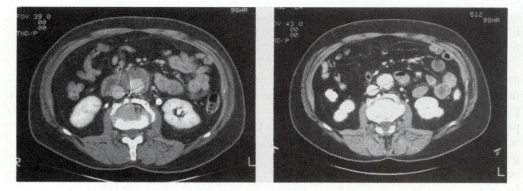

Figure 14–4. On the left is an aneurysm immediately after implantation; air is occasionally seen in the perigraft space. On the right is the same area of aneurysm 1 year after implantation. There is dramatic shrinkage.

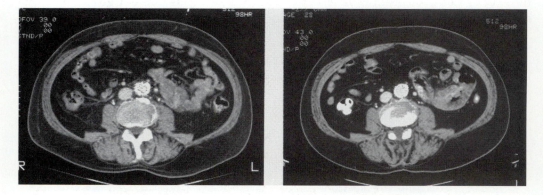

Figure 14–5. On the left is a distal neck slice immediately after implantation. On the right is the same area 1 year after implantation. There is slight enlargement.

TABLE 14–1. CHANGE IN AORTIC MINOR DIAMETER FROM PREOPERATIVE TO POSTIMPLANTATION SCAN AND FROM IMPLANTATION TO 1 YEAR

Mean Diameter (cm ± 1 SD)	Aneurysm	Celiac Artery	Proximal Neck	Distal Neck
Preoperative	4.77 ± 0.70	2.69 ± 0.31	2.38 ± 0.26	2.29 ± 0.29
Implantation	4.88 ± 0.64	2.66 ± 0.26	2.42 ± 0.29	2.34 ± 0.28
Change	0.11 ± 0.18	0.03 ± 0.17	0.04 ± 0.19	0.05 ± 0.25
95% confidence interval (CI) for change	[0.06, 0.16]	[−0.10, 0.04]	[−0.02, 0.10]	[−0.02, 0.12]
1 year	4.35 ± 0.86	2.67 ± 0.24	2.47 ± 0.28	2.48 ± 0.33
Change over 1 year	−0.53 ± 0.66	0.01 ± 0.19	0.05 ± 0.17	0.14 ± 0.27
95% CI for change	[−0.72, −0.34]	[−0.07, 0.09]	[−0.00, 0.09]	[0.06, 0.22]

Table 14–1 shows the size change and confidence intervals from preoperative to postimplantation scan, and from implantation to 1 year. The interval from preoperative CT to surgery was 76 ± 48 days (range: 1 to 252 days, median: 62 days). Aneurysm enlargement preoperatively of 0.11 cm is similar to that observed in untreated patients.[17] Proximal and distal neck do not change significantly from before to after the implantation procedure. Distal neck expansion occurs primarily in the 1 year after implantation.

Correlation of 1-year aneurysm size change with anatomic (inferior mesenteric artery patency, lumbar arteries, size of aneurysm), procedural (graft size and leak), and demographic (age) factors reveals two significant associations (Table 14–2). Younger patients are more likely to have greater shrinkage of their aneurysm. The mean age of patients with shrinkage was 72 ± 8 years, and the mean age of patients with expansion was 74 ± 8 years, indicating significant overlap in the individual ages of patients in these groups. This association was not detected with the previous report.[15] There continues to be a striking relationship between leak and aneurysm size (Fig. 14–6 and Table 14–3). In group I, the aneurysmal minor diameter decreased an average of 0.71 cm/year. In group II, minor diameter decreased by 0.47 cm/year, and in group III the aneurysms grew 0.19 cm/year. Twenty-seven of the 31 patients in group I had decreases in aneurysmal diameter and four had enlargement. Of these latter 4 group I patients, 1 had 0.05-cm growth with no further follow-up, and another had 0.15-cm growth followed by 0.03-cm shrinkage during the second year. The third had 0.06-cm shrinkage the first 6 months followed by 0.18-cm enlargement and a questionable perigraft leak on retrospective unblinded evaluation. The last patient had continuous 0.75-cm growth with no definite CT-detected leak. In group II, all aneurysms decreased in size, but in group

TABLE 14–2. PEARSON CORRELATIONS WITH ANEURYSM SIZE CHANGE (MINOR DIAMETER)

	N	Correlation	Unadjusted p Value
Size change	47	1.000	
Leak	47	0.473	0.001
Age	47	0.399	0.005
Graft size	47	0.140	0.349
Aneurysm size	44	−0.114	0.460
Inferior mesenteric patency	46	0.092	0.544
Lumbar arteries	46	0.007	0.961

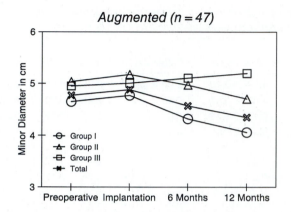

Figure 14–6. Aneurysm mean minor in relationship to leak group. The total cohort is represented with crosses. Group I (circles) and group II (triangles) have aneurysm shrinkage. Group III (squares) demonstrates aneurysm expansion.

III, all aneurysms enlarged. There were 12 (26%) patients with hookbreaks in the total cohort; 7 (23%) in group I, 4 (44%) in group II, and 1 (14%) in group III. There was no statistically significant relationship between hookbreaks and leak.

A closer look at the group III patients is revealing. Two patients with a small degree of enlargement (0.03 and 0.04 cm) in the first year have had further CT follow-up. Perigraft leaks are persistent and aneurysms have grown an additional 0.17 and 0.54 cm in the subsequent 12 and 18 months, respectively. Three others with leaks over 0.10 cm (0.23, 0.41, and 0.55 cm) have undergone secondary endovascular procedures including embolization of collaterals and repeat balloon dilation of the attachment systems in an attempt to close the leak, and follow-up after intervention is still pending. Further follow-up is not yet available on the last two patients with 0.01- and 0.09-cm growth.

Baseline characteristics of patients with complete and incomplete radiographic follow-up are listed in Table 14–4. There are no significant differences between the studied patients and those unavailable for 1-year follow-up.

TABLE 14–3. ANEURYSM MINOR DIAMETER AND OTHER FACTORS BY LEAK GROUP

Mean Diameter (cm ± 1 SD)	Total (n = 47)	Group I (n = 31)	Group II (n = 9)	Group III (n = 7)
Implantation	4.88 ± 0.66	4.77 ± 0.72	5.18 ± 0.27	5.01 ± 0.49
1 year	4.35 ± 0.86	4.06 ± 0.80	4.70 ± 0.62	5.20 ± 0.65
Change	−0.53 ± 0.66	−0.71 ± 0.64	−0.47 ± 0.56	0.19 ± 0.21
95% CI for change	[−0.72, −0.34]	[−0.94, −0.48]	[−0.84, −0.11]	[0.04, 0.35]
Shrinkage	36	27	9	0
Expansion	11	4	0	7
Hookbreaks	12 (26%)	7 (23%)	4 (44%)	1 (14%)
Lumbar arteries	4.5 ± 1.8	4.8 ± 1.9	3.7 ± 1.7	4.4 ± 1.4
IMA patent	18 (38%)	10 (32%)	3 (33%)	5 (71%)

TABLE 14–4. CHARACTERISTICS OF PATIENTS WITH COMPLETE DATA AND INCOMPLETE DATA

	Patients with Complete Discharge and 1-Year Measurement Data	Patients with Incomplete Data
Age (years)	72 ± 7.9	73 ± 7.2
Gender (male)	94%	89%
Aneurysm size (cm)	4.8 ± 0.7	5.2 ± 0.8
Graft size (cm)	2.4 ± 0.2	2.4 ± 0.2
Patent lumbar arteries (number)	4.5 ± 1.8	4.0 ± 1.9
Inferior mesenteric artery patent	39%	39%
Leak Group I	66%	61%
Group II	19%	17%
Group III	15%	22%

DISCUSSION

This study demonstrates that total endovascular exclusion of the aortic aneurysm results in significant reduction in aneurysm size. This finding is not surprising given the previous experience with the exclusion of aortic aneurysmal sacs and bypass procedures described by Shah et al.[18] While in the majority of patients the aneurysmal sac shrank after open exclusion and bypass, two patients who presented with continued enlargement of their aneurysmal sacs were found to have patent inferior mesenteric arteries (IMAs) and lumbar arteries. The aneurysmal sac continues to grow when any portion of it is left in continuity with arterial pressure. Failure of the endovascular graft to properly seal the aneurysmal sac from arterial pressure also results in continued expansion. The greatest degree of aneurysm shrinkage was found in group I in whom no leaks could be identified. In group II, persistent flow into the aneurysmal sac for varying times following the initial implantation probably accounts for the difference in shrinkage of the aneurysm found in this group as compared to group I. In group III, there was continued enlargement of the aneurysm (0.19 cm/year), which is comparable to that reported by Powell et al.[19] for untreated aneurysms. This observation is underscored by the recent report by Lumsden et al.[14] who described two patients who had undergone suboptimal endovascular grafting outside of their hospitals but who presented with rupture of their aneurysms.

Changes in the size of the aneurysm sac following endovascular grafting has been reported in several series. In the Eutrect experience with the EVT device, 9 patients were followed with helical CT, and in 7 of these patients the aneurysm volume decreased by 12 mL while in 2 patients the aneurysms enlarged.[10] May et al.[6] published 1-year CT follow-up on 30 patients, including 8 with the EVT graft, and found 26 patients with no leak had mean maximum aneurysm diameters of 5.18 cm preoperatively and 4.25 cm at 12 months. Four patients with endoleak had aneurysm enlargement from 6.46 to 7.75 cm.[6] In a report by Marin and colleagues[5] with a different type of an expandable device, six aneurysms shrunk while three enlarged. In their discussion and a CT study from their institution, these investigators associate persistent perigraft channels with continued aneurysmal enlargement.[5] Parodi and colleagues[7] have similarly described 3 patients with leaks past a few weeks, 1 of whom died of rupture and 2 died of other causes. In Parodi's series, 40 other patients with successful procedures without late leak had 10% to 20% reduction in aneurysm diameter after 17 months of follow-up.[7] Patients with persistent perigraft flow and aneurysm enlargement should undergo evaluation for additional therapeutic measures, including conversion to open repair. Also patients with definitive aneurysm enlargement should be suspected of having persistent perigraft flow even if it is not demonstrated by contrast-enhanced CT.

The etiology of perigraft leaks includes severely calcified aortic necks, graft size mismatch, and suboptimal stent placement. Many of these factors are correctable, and great effort has been and should continue to be directed at elimination of all causes of persistent leak. Hook placement can be avoided in heavily calcified areas or thrombus, graft dimensions must be carefully selected with consideration of the tortuosity of aneurysmal vessels, and deployment of attachment devices should be performed through the access that is most parallel to the line of flow of the necks, thus reducing sideways positioning of the hook crown. Devices have also been modified to reduce space between the graft and arterial wall, to encourage thrombosis of the perigraft space, and to reduce chance of metal fatigue. The management of perigraft leak postimplantation includes embolization of collateral pathways, balloon angioplasty of stents previously in place, and additional stent grafts.[16,20,21]

The association of young age with more rapid shrinkage of aneurysms is interesting. One may speculate that aneurysms in older patients are more calcified; however, shrinkage of calcified wall has been seen in collapsing aneurysms in this study. Although age correlates with aneurysm shrinkage in this larger study cohort, it does not discriminate adequately between patients who will or will not respond favorably.

With the EVT device and other endovascular grafting systems, attachment and stability of the graft within the arterial system are important considerations. The long-term outcomes of indwelling stents in the aorta in humans is not known. The EVT attachment system relies on a self-expanding stent with pinned hook devices to prevent migration and also relies on the arterial healing to augment this attachment. For this attachment system to function properly over long periods of time, it is important that the native aorta not continue to expand, allowing a perigraft leak to occur. In the short duration of this study (1 year), there does not appear to be any significant enlargement of the proximal aortic neck. The endovascular technique allows very precise placement of this device within a few millimeters of the renal vessels. It is probable that this device may successfully treat only the infrarenal portion of aneurysmal disease, and that nonexcluded segments of aorta are at continued risk for degeneration.[22-24] Since recurrent proximal aortic aneurysms occur in some instances more than a decade after open surgery, it will be important to follow these patients on a yearly basis.

The expansion of the distal neck is alarming, although the increment of enlargement is small over 1 year. The clinical significance of this enlargement is uncertain, but it does not appear to be statistically related to leak status or hook fractures. The expansion of the distal neck may be more related to the intrinsic biologic disease or other unknown factors. If continued expansion of the distal neck occurs, perigraft leaks may occur and become a clinical problem. In this case, bifurcation devices would become the preferred device configuration.

May et al.[25] from Sydney have also conducted detailed study of the proximal and distal aortic necks. In this recent report, 47 patients were studied with follow-up between 6 and 18 months after implantation of a variety of prostheses, including 10 patients with the EVT graft. Patients were grouped according to enlargement or shrinkage of the aneurysm and then further divided into length of follow-up, either 6, 12, or 18 months. Similar enlargement, ranging from 2.5 to 6.5 mm, of the proximal and distal neck was seen in the three groups with variable follow-up suggesting initial expansion and then plateau. Our study showed lesser degrees of dilation of the distal neck that seemed to occur primarily during the year following implantation and could not be associated with the procedure itself. These differences may be related to differences in the attachment system and its biologic effect on the aortic wall or may be due to differences in the methodology by which slices of CT scans were selected. Sporadic cases of late leak occurrence reinforce the widespread recommendations that continued close surveillance is a necessity following endovascular repair of aneurysms.

From a biologic point of view this study gives some insight into the pathophysiology of aneurysmal disease. The decrease in aneurysm size following exclusion supports the hypothesis that the process is pressure dependent. Other clinical studies with inflammatory aneurysms have demonstrated shrinkage of the aneurysm sac in most cases following open operative repair.[26] The mechanism by which the reduction of transmural wall pressure leads to decreases in inflammation is unknown. Clearly, the process of aortic enlargement and shrinkage is pressure dependent. The biomechanical changes that lead to these changes will initiate areas of research.

CONCLUSION

Endovascular grafting of abdominal aortic aneurysms is associated with reduction of aneurysm size 1 year following implantation. This shrinkage is related to permanent cessation of perigraft flow. There is no significant change of the aortic size at the levels of celiac or proximal neck, but the distal neck enlarges slightly. This 1-year follow-up supports the effectiveness of complete endovascular exclusion in selected patients. Longer follow-up, improved exclusion rates, and comparative trials are necessary before widespread use can be recommended.

Acknowledgments
We are grateful for the statistical analysis performed by Dorothy Dunlop, Institute for Health Services Research and Policy Studies, Northwestern University.
We are indebted to the participants and U.S. investigators, coinvestigators, and radiologists:

Emory University Hospital, Atlanta, GA
Primary investigator: Elliott Chaikof, MD
Coinvestigators: Alan Lumsden, MD, Thomas Dodson, MD,
Atef Salam, MD, Robert B. Smith, III, MD
Radiologists: Alan Zuckerman, MD, Stephen Kaufman, MD,
Louis Martin, MD

Henry Ford Hospital, Detroit, MI
Primary investigator: Calvin B. Ernst, MD
Coinvestigators: Daniel Reddy, MD, Joseph Elliott, MD,
Alexander Shepard, MD
Radiologist: P.C. Shetty, MD

Massachusetts General Hospital, Boston, MA
Primary investigator: David C. Brewster, MD
Coinvestigators: William M. Abbott, MD, Richard Cambria, MD
Radiologists: Stuart Geller, MD, John Kaufman, MD

Montefiore Medical Center, New York, NY
Primary investigator: Frank J. Veith, MD

Coinvestigator: Michael Marin, MD
Radiologist: Jacob Cynamon, MD

Miami Vascular Institute, Miami, FL
Primary investigator: Barry Katzen, MD, Orlando Puente, MD
Coinvestigators: Jose Alvarez, Jr., MD, Steven Kanter, MD
Radiologists: Barry Katzen, MD, James Benenati, MD,
Gerald Zemel, MD, Gary Becker, MD

Northwestern University Medical Center, Chicago, IL
Primary investigator: James S.T. Yao, MD
Coinvestigators: William H. Pearce, MD, Walter J. McCarthy, MD
Radiologists: Albert Nemcek, MD, Robert Vogelzang, MD

New York University Medical Center, New York, NY
Primary investigator: Thomas S. Riles, MD
Coinvestigators: Patrick Lamparello, MD, Mark A. Adelman, MD,
Gary Giangola, MD, Radiologist: Robert Rosen, MD

St. Thomas/Vanderbilt University Medical Center, Nashville, TN
Primary investigator: William H. Edwards, Sr., MD
Coinvestigators: William H. Edwards, Jr., MD, Thomas A. Naslund, MD

Stanford University Medical Center, Stanford, CA
Primary investigator: R. Scott Mitchell, MD
Coinvestigators: Christopher K. Zarins, MD, Edmund Harris, Jr., MD
Radiologist: Charles Semba, MD

University of Colorado, Denver, CO
Primary investigator: Robert B. Rutherford, MD
Coinvestigators: William C. Krupski, MD, Darrell Jones, PhD
Radiologists: David Kumpe, MD, Janette Durham, MD

University of California, Los Angeles, CA
Primary investigator: Wesley S. Moore, MD
Coinvestigators: Samuel S. Ahn, MD, J. Dennis Baker, MD,
William J. Quinones-Baldrich, MD, Hugh A. Gelabert, MD,
Herbert I. Machleder, MD, Richard W. Bock, MD, Rhoda Leichter, MD,
Radiologist: Antionette S. Gomes, MD

University of California, San Francisco, CA
Primary investigator: Jerry Goldstone, MD
Coinvestigator: Susan Wall, MD
Radiologist: Ernest Ring, MD

University of Texas Southwestern Medical Center, Dallas, TX
Primary investigator: G. Patrick Clagett, MD
Coinvestigators: Arun Chervu, MD, R. James Valentine, MD,
Stuart Myers, MD, Radiologists: George Miller, MD, Rebhi Awad, MD,
Margaret Hansen, MD, Helen Redman, MD, Jorge Lopez, MD

REFERENCES

1. Crawford ES, Saleh SA, Babb JW, et al. Infrarenal abdominal aortic aneurysm: factors influencing survival after operation performed over a 25-year period. *Ann Surg.* 1981;193(6):699–709.
2. Calcagno D, Hallett JW, Ballard DJ, et al. Late iliac artery aneurysms and occlusive disease after aortic tube grafts for abdominal aortic aneurysm repair: a 35-year experience. *Ann Surg.* 1991;214(6):733–736.
3. Glickman MH, Julian CC, Kimmins S, Evans WE. Aortic aneurysm: to tube or not to tube. *Surgery.* 1982;91(5):603–605.
4. Kazmers A, Jacobs L, Perkins A, et al. Abdominal aortic aneurysm repair in Veterans Affairs medical centers. *J Vasc Surg.* 1996;23:191–200.
5. Marin ML, Veith FJ, Cynamon J, et al. Initial experience with transluminally placed endovascular grafts for the treatment of complex vascular lesions. *Ann Surgery.* 1995;222(4):449–469.
6. May J, White GH, Yu W, et al. A prospective study of changes in morphology and dimensions of abdominal aortic aneurysms following endoluminal repair: a preliminary report. *J Endovasc Surg.* 1995;2(4):343–347.
7. Parodi JC. Endovascular repair of abdominal aortic aneurysms and other arterial lesions. *J Vasc Surg.* 1995;21:549–557.
8. Blum U, Langer M, Spillner G, et al. Abdominal aortic aneurysms: preliminary technical and clinical results with transfemoral placement of endovascular self-expanding stent-grafts. *Radiology.* 1996;198:25–31.
9. White GH, May J, McGahan T, et al. Historic control comparison of outcome for matched groups of patients undergoing endoluminal versus open repair of abdominal aortic aneurysms. *J Vasc Surg.* 1996;23:201–212.
10. Balm R, Kaatee R, Mali OR, Eikelboom BC. Vanishing aortic aneurysms following transfemoral endovascular aneurysm management with a tube graft: measurements with spiral CT angiography. Presented at ESVS '95, Scientific Program European Society for Vascular Surgery. P40–41A.
11. Chuter TAM, Wendt G, Hopkinson BR, et al. Transfemoral insertion of a bifurcated endovascular graft for aortic aneurysm repair: the first 22 patients. *Cardiovasc Surg.* 1995;3(2):121–128.
12. Moore WS, Vescera CL. Repair of abdominal aortic aneurysm by transfemoral endovascular graft placement. *Ann Surg.* 1994;220(3):331–341.
13. Edwards WH, Naslund TC, Edwards WH Sr, et al. Endovascular grafting of abdominal aortic aneurysms. *Ann Surg.* 1996;223(5):568–575.
14. Lumsden AB, Allen RC, Chaikof EL, et al. Delayed rupture of aortic aneurysms following endovascular stent grafting. *Am J Surg.* 1995;170:174–178.
15. Matsumura JS, Pearce WH, McCarthy WJ, Yao JST. Reduction in aortic aneurysm size, early results after endovascular graft placement. *J Vasc Surg.* 1996 (in press).
16. Moore WS, Rutherford RR. Transfemoral endovascular repair of abdominal aortic aneurysm: results of the North American EVT phase 1 trial. *J Vasc Surg.* 1996;23:543–553.
17. Ernst CB. Abdominal aortic aneurysm. *N Engl J Med.* 1993;328:1167–1171.
18. Shah DM, Chang BB, Paty PSK, et al. Treatment of abdominal aortic aneurysm by exclusion and bypass: an analysis of outcome. *J Vasc Surg.* 1991;13:15–22.
19. Powell JT, MacSweeney STR, Greenhalgh RM. The spontaneous course of small aortic aneurysm. In Yao JST, Pearce WHP, eds. *Aneurysms: New Findings and Treatments.* Norwalk, CT: Appleton & Lange; 1994:71–77.
20. Parodi JC. Endovascular repair of abdominal aortic aneurysms. In Whittemore A, ed. *Advances in Vascular Surgery.* St. Louis, MO: Mosby; 1993;1:85–106.
21. May J, White GH, Yu W, et al. Surgical management of complications following endoluminal grafting of abdominal aortic aneurysms. *Eur J Vasc Endovasc Surg.* 1995;10:51–59.
22. Plate G, Hollier LA, O'Brien P, et al. Recurrent aneurysms and late vascular complications following repair of abdominal aortic aneurysms. *Arch Surg.* 1985;120:590–594.
23. Coselli JS, LeMaire SA, Buket S, Berzin E. Subsequent proximal aortic operations in 123 patients with previous infrarenal abdominal aortic aneurysm surgery. *J Vasc Surg.* 1995;22:59–67.

24. Berman SS, Hunter GC, Smyth SH, et al. Application of computed tomography for surveillance of aortic grafts. *Surgery.* 1995;118:8–15.

25. May J, White GH, Yu W, et al. Prospective study of anatomic and pathological changes in abdominal aortic aneurysms following endoluminal repair: is the aneurysmal process reversed? *Eur J Vasc Endovasc Surg.* 1996;11:1–7.

26. Stella A, Gargiulo M, Faggioli GL, et al. Postoperative course of inflammatory abdominal aortic aneurysms. *Ann Vasc Surg.* 1993;7:229–238.

15

Stent-Graft

New Technique for Treatment of Aneurysms and Traumatic and Occlusive Arterial Lesions

Juan C. Parodi, MD, and Claudio J. Schonholz, MD

The diagnosis of abdominal aortic aneurysm (AAA) has been established with increasing frequency during the past two decades.[1] This observation probably is related to aging of the population, as well as to the extensive use of ultrasonography and computed tomography (CT) scanning for different pathologies.

Although AAA may occasionally cause distal embolization, rupture remains the most common and deadly complication. Elective replacement with a synthetic graft has proven to be the most appropriate method to prevent AAA rupture for nearly 40 years, and at respected medical centers, it has been associated with a postoperative mortality of less than 5%.[2]

Increasingly, vascular surgeons are encountering older patients with severe comorbid conditions. This can increase operative morbidity and may even elevate mortality of aortic surgery to a figure in excess of 60%.[3]

In patients with a prohibitive risk for surgery, other alternative forms of treatment such as axillofemoral bypass in conjunction with induced AAA thrombosis have been used. The procedure has now been abandoned despite preliminary reports of its initial success.[4]

In 1976, we began to develop a plan for endovascular treatment of AAA. Our current approach is predicated on the concept that stents may be used in place of sutures to secure the proximal and distal ends of a fabric graft extending the length of the AAA, thoracic aneurysm, or recanalized occluded artery. In arteriovenous fistulas (AVFs) and false aneurysms, a covered balloon or self-expandable stent has been used. A tubular Dacron or polytetrafluoroethylene (PTFE) graft, urethane fibers, or a segment of autologous deep vein has been used to cover stents.

ANIMAL STUDIES

To test the concept of intraluminal graft implantation, a canine aneurysmal model was used. A 6-cm segment of the infrarenal aorta was resected and replaced with a fusiform conduit made of crimped woven Dacron, measuring 8 cm in length.

Histologic studies demonstrated endothelium graft coverage of the experimental aneurysm neck, coupled with mural thrombus formation in the body of the aneurysm. Both of these changes were regularly encountered within a month after implantation of the aneurysmal graft. Six weeks later aneurysms were excluded using endoluminal graft deployment techniques. A noncrimped knitted Dacron tube of an appropriate diameter and length was attached to stents (Palmaz, Johnson & Johnson Interventional Systems). Two-thirds of each stent was covered by graft material, but one-third of the stent was left exposed to anchor the graft to the aortic wall. The graft was folded clockwise in two folds, mounted on a balloon catheter, placed over a guidewire, and loaded into a 14 French Teflon sheath. The right femoral artery was chosen for vascular access. Under fluoroscopy guidance the leading stent was advanced over the guide wire into the neck of the aneurysm, below the renal orifices and above the body of the aneurysm. Following the proper positioning of the device, the introducer sheath was withdrawn and balloon inflation used to secure the graft by deploying either one or two stents. In one group of dogs only a proximal stent was used, but in a second, larger group a distal stent was added to achieve total aneurysm exclusion. Angiography was then used to confirm correct stent-graft deployment and verify that the aneurysm was successfully excluded.

We operated on 43 dogs, in most cases to evaluate different models for experimental aneurysms or to test a variety of balloons and grafts. In our last group of dogs, we performed 6-month evaluations, obtaining color Doppler ultrasound (duplex) scans in some cases and complete pathologic studies in all animals. Using both optical and electronic microscopy, we found that both ends of stented grafts were covered by endothelium, and that the shaft of the graft was covered by a fibrin platelet barrier.

CLINICAL EXPERIENCE

Once we were satisfied that a Dacron graft could be delivered through a catheter and fixed firmly in place by balloon-expandable stents, we obtained permission from our institutional ethical committee to perform a pilot clinical study with a small group of patients who were fully informed regarding the nature of the procedure and subsequently were followed very carefully.

In September 1990, a patient with an AAA was treated and reported by us.[5] Since then, 128 patients with aneurysms, traumatic arterial lesions, and occlusive disease have been treated by our group (Table 15–1).

STENT-GRAFT DEVICE FOR ANEURYSMS

Details of the design of the stent-graft device have been described previously.[6] The balloon-expandable stent is a cylindrical tube with longitudinal slots that adopt a diamond shape when expanded. This design, initially described by Palmaz,[7,8] permits the stent to expand from a diameter of only 5 mm when collapsed to a diameter of more than 30 mm when expanded. The stent is 3.5 mm in length. The stent is made

TABLE 15–1. CLINICAL EXPERIENCE WITH STENT-GRAFT, SEPTEMBER 1990–JUNE 1996

		Number of Patients
Aneurysms: 103 patients		
Aortoaortic stent-graft	1 stent	8
	2 stents	42
Aortoiliac stent-graft		42
Aorto-bi-iliac stent-graft		8
Thoracic stent-graft		3
Vascular trauma		21
Occlusive disease		4

of annealed stainless steel, type 316L, because this alloy has been widely used in a variety of prosthetic applications.

Corrosion of implanted metal pieces usually occurs at sites of cracks and crevices on the metal surface. Therefore, the surface of metal stents must be uniform. The balloon-expandable stent is made as a single piece to avoid motion between parts. Micromotion between metal surfaces disrupts protective oxide films, allowing the area to corrode rapidly.

The knitted Dacron graft has a wall thickness of 0.2 mm and is manufactured using strong yarns with tensile and bursting strengths comparable to those of commercially available grafts. The compliance of the shaft of the graft (15%) is also similar to standard, knitted Dacron grafts. But the compliance of the segment overlapping the stent is 45% to adapt to needed expansion. Between these two segments, a transitional zone of intermediate compliance is interposed in an attempt to avoid abrupt changes in the diameter of the graft. The diameter and length of each graft is tailored to fit the individual patient, but the grafts we have employed most often are 18 to 20 mm in diameter and 8 to 12 cm in length (Figs. 15–1 and 15–2).

Because of its radiopacity, a thin gold wire is sutured to both ends of the graft. This permits the radiographic identification of both ends and the sides of the graft in order to correct torsion during implantation.

The balloon catheter we currently use (BALT Company, Paris, France) is constructed of nylon material and has some degree of compliance. This compliance allows us to use only two balloon sizes (25 and 30 mm in diameter). For aortoiliac grafting either a double balloon (25 and 12 mm in diameter) or two independent balloons are used.

The device is advanced under fluoroscopy guidance over a wire. We prefer a super stiff guide wire with a diameter of 0.038 inches. It facilitates the introduction of the device through tortuous iliac arteries, keeps the axis of our device parallel to that of the aorta, and by minimizing friction between the stent-graft and the aneurysmal wall prevents disruption of laminated thrombus that lines atherosclerotic aneurysms.

PROCEDURE

Under local or epidural anesthesia the patient is prepared and draped as for a standard AAA resection. In the three cases in which the thoracic aneurysm was treated, general anesthesia was utilized.

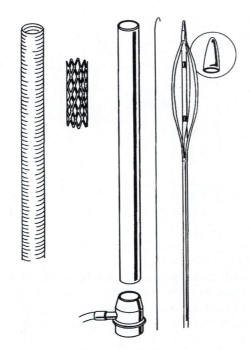

Figure 15–1. Stent-graft device: individual component (from left to right, graft, stent, sheath, wide wire, and balloon). (*Parodi JC. Endovascular repair of abdominal aortic aneurysms. Adv Vasc Surg. 1993;1:85–106.*)

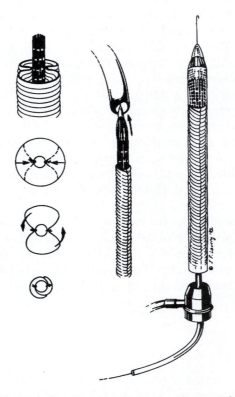

Figure 15–2. Stent-graft preparation: fixation of the graft to the stent, folding of the graft, and inclusion in the sheath. (*Parodi JC. Endovascular repair of abdominal aortic aneurysms. In Haimovici H, ed. Haimovici's Vascular Surgery. Blackwell Science; 1996:828–834.*)

A small incision is made over the chosen common femoral artery. Usually the straighter and wider artery is selected for access. A soft-tip guide wire is advanced in the aorta up to the level of the diaphragm. Over the wire a pigtail diagnostic catheter is placed inside the lumen of the aorta with the tip located proximally to the renal arteries. The first injection of 30 cc of contrast media is performed. The pigtail catheter has radiopaque marks engraved on its surface every 2 cm to facilitate lengths and diameters measurements using quantitative angiography.

With previously obtained images (angiogram and CT scan) and the new angiogram, target areas are defined. They could be the proximal neck of the aneurysm and distal cuff (if this latter exists) or the common iliac artery in the absence of the distal cuff.

The preloaded sheath containing the stent and graft mounted on a balloon is placed inside the lumen of the aneurysm under fluoroscopic guidance. Once in place, the sheath is removed and the cranial balloon is inflated with a diluted solution of ionic contrast media and saline. The balloon is kept inflated for 1 minute and then gently deflated (Fig. 15–3).

Before proceeding with balloon inflation, the main blood pressure is dropped using nitroglycerin solution. Pressure is kept at 70 mm Hg during balloon inflation. Lately we have used adenosine to stop the heart for few seconds and be able to precisely deploy the stent in cases of short necks. Temporary cardiac pacing was utilized.

The size of the balloon is selected beforehand according to the diameter of the neck of the aneurysm measured in the previous angiogram and CT scan. After securing the proximal stent, the second stent is placed. In some cases in which a double balloon device is used, the second balloon (either aortic or iliac) is positioned at the appropriate level and inflated, deploying the second stent. A final angiogram is performed. When an aortoiliac graft is placed, the procedure is completed by placing a femorofemoral graft and by the use of a detachable balloon or stent to occlude the contralateral common iliac artery. The occluding stent consists of an iliac stent covered by a Dacron tubular graft, which has a blind end created by a suture.

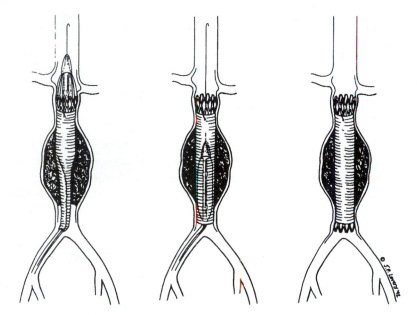

Figure 15–3. Stent-graft procedure. (*Parodi JC. Endovascular repair of abdominal aortic aneurysms. Adv Vasc Surg. 1993;1:85–106.*)

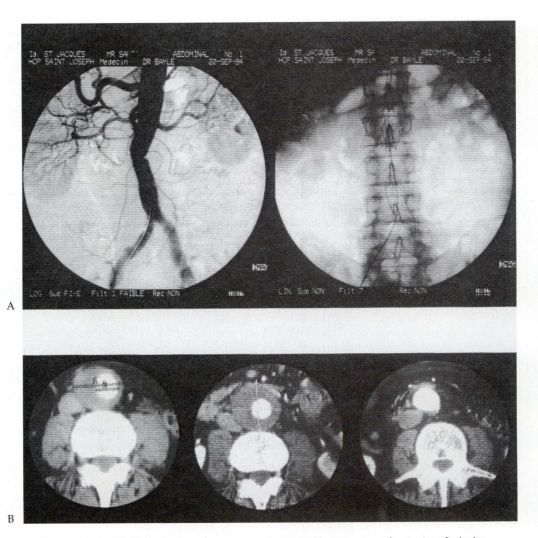

Figure 15–4. **(A)** Abdominal aortic aneurysm treated with an aortoaortic stent-graft device. **(B)** Angiography after treatment and 1-year follow-up CT scan show complete disappearance of the aneurysmal sac.

Time of the procedure varied according to the complexity of the case. When an aortoaortic procedure in a rather small aneurysm with nontortuous and wide lumen iliac arteries was performed, the procedure lasted 20 to 45 minutes (Fig. 15–4). When an aortoiliac graft plus a femorofemoral bypass and occlusion of the contralateral iliac were needed, the time spent in the operating room on occasion exceeded 3 hours.

STENT-GRAFT DEVICE FOR TRAUMA AND PROCEDURE

The goal of the technology is to obtain an occlusion of the tear of the arterial wall, which results in either a false aneurysm or an arteriovenous fistula from within the lumen by means of implanting a tubular metallic mesh (stent) covered by a Dacron fabric, a PTFE, a polycarbonate urethane polymer, or a vein (Fig. 15–5).

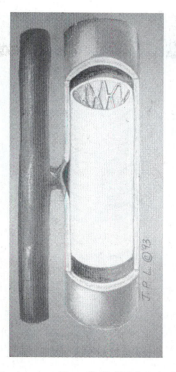

Figure 15–5. Covered stent for trauma. (*Parodi JC, Schönholz CJ. Traitment endovasculaire des traumatismes arteriels par Stent-graft. Impact Endovasculaire. 1996;1:30–34.*)

In those cases in which a Palmaz stent was used, the stent was mounted on an angioplasty balloon whose diameter matched that of the artery to be treated, having a final diameter in excess of 10% to 15% of the diameter of the artery in order to obtain a secure fixation.

Dacron, PTFE, or veins were attached to the stent with four 6/0 polypropylene sutures placed two in either end of the graft. These two sutures were placed 180 degrees apart from one another.

The device is compressed (crimping the stent and compressing and folding the graft; the balloon is undistended, folded, and compressed) in the introducer sheath. The sheath has a small diameter to facilitate its introduction and progression into the artery.

In two of our patients presenting a false aneurysm, infection was a concern. In one case, infection was a concern because the patient was suffering from AIDS and the second because the patient had an infected false aneurysm of the common femoral artery. In those two patients we decided to use an autologous vein. Autologous veins are known to be more resistant to infection when compared with synthetic material. In an additional young male (36 years old) a false aneurysm causing five consecutive cerebral infarctions developed after a post-traumatic carotid artery dissection. A vein-covered stent was placed near the base of the skull in the internal carotid artery with the purpose of creating a less thrombogenic surface and to cover the false aneurysm, which was the source of thrombus-generating cerebral infarction. Embolization subsided after the artery exclusions (Figs. 15–6A and B).

In one case we decided to use an iliac Johnson & Johnson stent covered with polycarbonate urethane fibers (Corvita Corporation, Miami, FL) to treat an AVF of the subclavian artery.

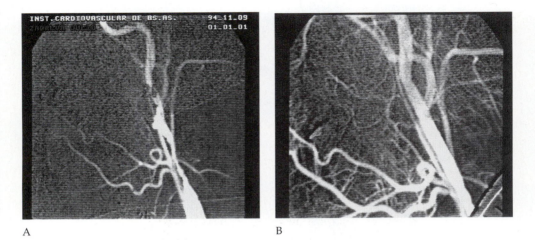

A   B

Figure 15–6. Internal carotid false aneurysm. (**A**) Diagnostic angiography and (**B**) post stent-vein treatment angiography.

The Corvita Endovascular Graft (CEG) is produced by coating a self-expanding metallic stent with biocompatible, elastomeric polycarbonate urethane (Corethane) fibers. It is manufactured in a variety of sizes to adapt to the injured vessel. A 9/10 French guiding catheter and 7/8 French pusher catheter were used over the wire for deployment (Fig. 15–7).

Between 1992 and March 1996, 21 patients with traumatic arterial lesions were treated with the stent-graft technique. Seventeen were males and 4 were females ages 15 to 63 years (mean, 36 years). Fifteen patients had post-traumatic AVFs and 6 false aneurysms.

The injured arteries were subclavian in 8 patients, axilar in 2 patients, aorta in 2 patients, common iliac in 2 patients, common carotid in 3 patients, superficial femoral artery (SFA) in 2 patients, common femoral in 1 patient, and internal carotid in 1 patient (Table 15–2).

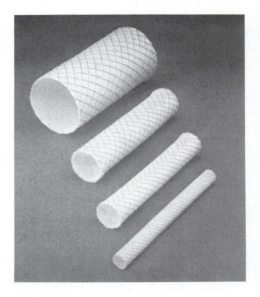

Figure 15–7. Corvita endovascular graft.

TABLE 15–2. VASCULAR TRAUMA TREATED WITH STENT-GRAFT

	Age	Sex	Arterial Injury	AVF-FA	Days	Device	Cause
1	20	M	Aortocava	AVF	2	Palmaz Dacron	Gunshot
2	15	F	Common iliac-cava	AVF	2	Palmaz Dacron	Iatrogenic laparoscopy
3	50	M	Axilar	AVF	1	Palmaz Dacron	Gunshot
4	23	M	Common carotid	FA	2	Palmaz vein	Gunshot
5	35	F	SFA	AVF	1	Palmaz Dacron	Gunshot
6	45	M	Subclavian	AVF	2	Palmaz PTFE	Gunshot
7	37	M	Internal	FA	4	Palmaz	Blunt
8	56	M	Common femoral	FA	10	Palmaz vein	Iatrogenic cardiac catheterization
9	24	M	Subclavian	AVF	3	Palmaz Dacron	Gunshot
10	56	M	Subclavian	AVF	3	Palmaz Dacron	Iatrogenic
11	22	M	Subclavian	AVF	2	Palmaz PTFE	Gunshot
12	30	M	Aortocava	AVF	3	Palmaz Dacron	Gunshot
13	56	F	Common carotid	FA	1	CEG	Iatrogenic
14	26	M	SFA	AVF	2	CEG	Gunshot
15	31	M	Axilar	FA	1	CEG	Gunshot
16	28	M	Subclavian	AVF	2	CEG	Gunshot
17	32	M	Common iliac	AVF	7	CEG	Gunshot
18	67	M	Subclavian	AVF	8	CEG + Palmaz PTFE	Iatrogenic
19	22	M	Common carotid	AVF	2	CEG	Stab wound injury
20	61	M	Subclavian	FA	2	Palmaz Dacron	Iatrogenic
21	52	F	Subclavian	FA	1	CEG	Iatrogenic

The causes of the lesions were gunshot wound in 12 patients, blunt trauma in 1 patient, stab wound injury in 1 patient, and iatrogenic (laparoscopic surgery, cardiac catheterization, and inadvertent arterial puncture during introduction of central vein catheters) in 7 patients.

All the procedures were similar in terms of the basic principles. Diagnosis was established by clinical findings, color duplex scanning, and arteriograms in every patient. Patients were treated under local anesthesia. The stent-graft was introduced from a remote site into the arterial tree either percutaneously or through a small cut down.

The arteries utilized as access sites were the common femoral in 17 cases, the superficial femoral artery in 1, common carotid artery in 1, and the axillary artery in two. Four different materials were used to cover stents: Dacron (8 cases), PTFE (1 case), polycarbonate urethane (9 cases) (Corvita Corporation), and autogenous vein (3 cases).

RESULTS

Aortic Aneurysm

All patients were followed by clinical examination, color duplex studies every 6 months, and CT scans once a year. Angiography was performed in some patients, and always performed in any patient in whom the color duplex or CT scans indicated or suggested any sign of leak, dilatation, or any change when compared with the study performed

TABLE 15–3. ASSOCIATED PATHOLOGIC CONDITIONS

Condition	Number of Patients
Severe chronic heart disease	53
Acute myocardial infarction	23
Severe pulmonary insufficiency	26
Renal insufficiency	5
Acute cerebral infarction	1
Two or more previous strokes	10
Hostile abdomen	2
Hepatic failure	2
Mild pulmonary insufficiency	12
Intermittent claudication	33
Disseminated intravascular coagulation (DIC)	1

immediately after the procedure. The average follow-up period was 34 months, with a range between 1 and 68 months.

"Early success" is defined as (1) graft covering the complete length of the aneurysm, and (2) watertight sealing of both ends of the graft firmly attached to intima of the artery without thrombus interposition.

"Late success" is defined as (1) persistence of initial success criteria, (2) absence of backflow from lumbar or inferior mesenteric artery after a 6-month period, and (3) absence of aneurysmal growth.

One hundred and three patients harboring aortic aneurysms were treated from September 1990 to March 1996. The average age was 73 years (range of 57 to 87 years); 10 patients were more than 80 years of age. Most patients had at least one associated morbid condition (Table 15–3). Fifty patients underwent aortic tube graft replacement, with 8 patients having only proximal stent, 42 aortoiliac stent-graft, 8 aorto-bi-iliac stent-graft, and 3 thoracic aneurysms.

Patients with successful procedures recovered very rapidly, had breakfast the next morning, and walked within 24 to 48 hours after the procedure. Typically they were discharged from the hospital after 3 or 4 days.

In our experience including all patients (intention to treat) we had the following results:

> Early failure in aortoaortic stent-graft procedures: 23%
> Early failure in aortoiliac stent-graft procedures: 24%
> Late failure in aortoaortic stent-graft procedures: 30%
> Late failure in aortoiliac stent-graft procedures: 5%

Early failures include (1) access problems that prevent proper deployment of the stent-graft, (2) major complications, (3) incomplete sealing, and (4) migration (one case).

Late failures had only one cause: perigraft leak usually from the distal end due to improper deployment of the stent-graft. The end of the graft was in direct contact with thrombus instead of being in contact with the intima of the neck of the AAA.

Arterial Trauma

Of 21 patients who sustained arterial injury, 20 patients had the false aneurysm or the AVF excluded successfully with the use of one or more stent-graft devices. The remaining patient had a subclavian AVF, and an additional procedure had to be done to occlude one additional AVF located in one of the branches of the subclavian artery. In this patient, a detachable balloon was placed in the scapular branch of the thoraco-cervical trunk.

All patients with long-standing AVF had significant stenosis at the site of injury. Stenosis had to be treated by inflating a shorter and stronger balloon. In many AVFs an association with a false aneurysm was clearly seen, but this finding did not change the strategy of the treatment.

When a high-flow AVF was treated with the CEG, the fistula remained open up to 24 hours, probably due to porosity of the graft. In only one patient, the fistula remained open for more than 7 days and the patient was treated with a PTFE Palmaz covered stent, obtaining a complete seal.

DISCUSSION

After 103 procedures for treating aneurysms and 25 for other conditions (AVFs, false aneurysms, and occlusive disease), it is possible to make some preliminary conclusions. First, the procedure is feasible and, when successfully applied, has the great attraction of simplicity. Second, the application of covered stents in trauma cases appears to be one of the main applications of this method because it transforms a somewhat complicated and potentially dangerous procedure into a simple and safe one. Also, associated stenosis can be treated with balloon angioplasty at the same time. In the near future stent-grafts could eventually be used in acute civilian or military injuries as a way to stop blood loss temporarily or definitively. In addition, this procedure can be combined with endovascular control of bleeding of secondary branches by using detachable balloons, coils, occluding stents, or the injection of fluids that become solid inside the body. The stent-graft is of particular appeal to apply to subclavian artery injuries, which often represent a real challenge even to the experienced surgeon. In the treatment of aortic aneurysms, however, there were more problems than those that initially could be predicted.[9] The procedure is simple in theory, but several details should be attended to before moving ahead with the widespread use of endovascular grafts. Measuring the diameter and length of the obstruction is crucial. We learned with great effort how to obtain reliable data. Enhanced CT scans, angiography with marked catheter, three-dimensional reconstruction using magnetic resonance (MR) or CT images, intraluminal measurements, and some geometric calculations helped us to obtain reasonably reliable data. Understanding that elongation occurs as dilatation of the aorta develops and in different planes allowed us to calculate more accurately the actual length of the artery. It appears that the final answer in regard to measurements will come from computer image processing using three-dimensional reconstruction of spiral CT or MR scans and probably a simulation program of insertion of a stent-graft device. In the meantime, we prefer to overestimate the length instead of underestimate it, because excess graft can be accommodated by the "accordian mechanism," accomplished by crimping the graft. If kinking results, it can be resolved by inserting an inner stent at that level.

Access problems accounted for several technical difficulties, including the presence of diffuse narrowing, stenotic, and tortuous iliac arteries. These abnormalities were responsible for difficulty in the entry of the rigid stent and the rather large diameter of the sheath. We overcame some of these problems by modifying the device and using different maneuvers during the procedure. Reducing the diameter of the sheath to 18 French was a remarkable advance toward the ideal device. Maneuvers such as the use of an extra-stiff wire, the "pull-down" maneuver, and sometimes implantation of a temporary conduit on the common iliac artery were also useful in overcoming some of the technical problems. The "pull-down" maneuver consists of dissecting free the common femoral and external iliac arteries, lifting the inguinal ligament up, and using blunt dissection to reach the iliac bifurcation from the groin (Fig. 15–8). Small branches should be divided between suture ligatures. When the arteries are free, by pulling the artery gently toward the feet of the patient, the tortuous artery becomes straighter, making the introduction of the sheath possible.

Changes in the shape or configuration of aneurysms are of interest. In the initial stages almost all aneurysms have a proximal neck and distal cuff of more than 3 cm; in the second stage, the distal cuff becomes shorter; and in the third stage, the distal cuff tends to disappear, while the proximal neck becomes shorter, but still longer than 2 cm. After this stage we found that elongation takes place, which creates tortuosity (Figs. 15–9A and B). Usually the distal curve opposes the proximal one. This results in a configuration in which if the convexity of the proximal neck is to the right, the distal cuff curves to the left, leaving the left iliac artery straight and the left with the tendency to produce a right angle.

Our findings indicate that in some patients a tubular graft is applicable when the distal aortic cuff is not present. An aorto-bi-iliac graft must be used as advocated by Chuter.[10] In addition, when the angle between the iliac arteries becomes larger than 90 degrees, an aortoiliac graft should be used with a femorofemoral bypass. We foresee that the three systems available will be applicable in patients harboring an AAA. Small and medium-size AAAs can benefit from an aortoaortic system, and large aneurysms can be treated with aorto-bi-iliac or aortoiliac systems with the addition of a femorofemoral bypass and exclusion of the contralateral common iliac artery.

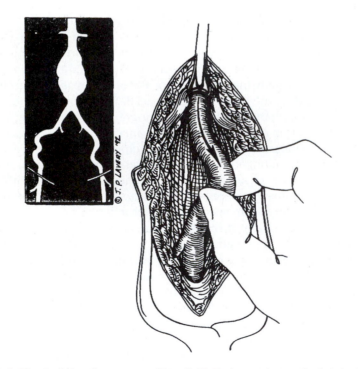

Figure 15–8. The "pull-down" maneuver. (*Parodi JC. Endovascular repair of abdominal aortic aneurysms. Adv. Vasc Surg. 1993;1:85–106.*)

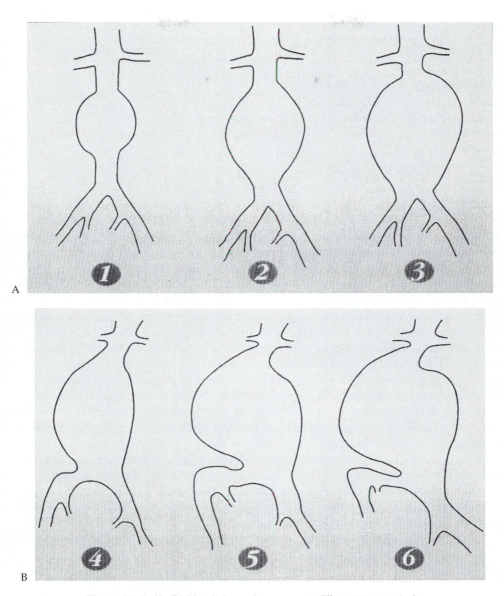

Figure 15–9. (A, B) Morphology of aneurysms: different stages, 1–6.

Because of their high radial force, balloon-expandable stents appear to be an ideal anchoring mechanism. We had one problem when the stent was incompletely deployed. Also, one patient had stent migration. It appears that intravascular ultrasound will be the ideal way to check the completeness of the stent deployment.

Microembolization is what we consider to be the main and more dreadful problem with this procedure. In this series, microembolization occurred five times, with death resulting in four patients. In the remaining case discrete microembolization of the right foot was successfully treated with intra-arterial administration of prostaglandin E1. The four cases died of massive microembolization, and these were technically difficult procedures in patients with large aneurysms. One patient was found to have visceral ischemia in the postmortem examination (Table 15–4).

TABLE 15–4. COMPLICATIONS

Complication	Number of Patients
Groin hematoma	2
Proximal leak (treated with a covered stent)	1
Injury to the external iliac artery (sutured)	1
Minimal distal microembolism treated by intra-arterial injection of prostaglandin	1
Migration	1
Massive microembolization	4
Distal leak	1

Reviewing our cases of embolization, it appears very clear that large and tortuous aneurysms pose an increased potential incidence of embolization. This is probably due to manipulation of the guide wire. On advancing the guide wire from the femoral artery into the aorta and then into the proximal neck, the operator will negotiate it inside a large and tortuous chamber coated with friable material. Sometimes it is very difficult to position the guide wire inside the proximal neck, because of the large cavity of the aneurysm and the relatively small orifice of the neck. Such maneuvers could eventually cause dislodgment of particles of the laminated thrombus. To eliminate this difficulty, it is advisable in all cases of large aneurysms with wide lumens to insert the guide wire percutaneously from the brachial artery. Occasionally, miscalculation of the length of the aneurysm created the need to change the device or to use complementary procedures such as implanting a third covered stent to increase the length of the device or to cover a leak. The more intraluminal manipulation we perform, the more the risk of dislodging particles from the aortic wall.

Microembolization can be minimized by the following maneuvers (1) In cases of large aneurysms with large lumens, the guide wire should be introduced from the brachial artery bringing it down to the femoral artery; and (2) care should be taken to measure precisely the length and diameters of the arteries and perform a simple well-planned procedure.

CONCLUSIONS

A word of caution is offered regarding definitive conclusions. We continue to find new abnormalities among the group of patients treated by us as long as 3 years after performing what we considered at the time a successful procedure. Hence, before this procedure can be offered to the community as an alternative treatment to eliminate AAAs, clear, unremarkable long-term experience should be available for presentation to the medical community. We are aware of the need to perform controlled trials with a large enough number of patients followed for a long period of time before introducing the endoluminal treatment in clinical practice. In the meantime, experience should be concentrated in a few centers with appropriate equipment and a skillful group of surgeons and interventional radiologists or cardiologists with experience in interventional vascular procedures.

Regarding other applications of the stent-graft combination, treatment of AVFs appears to be a simple and effective application. It can save time and prevent bleeding and peripheral nerve injuries. Treatment of false aneurysms in inaccessible places by the stent-graft technique also is promising, as is its use for vascular trauma. Arterial dissections, mostly aortic dissections, can probably be efficiently treated endoluminally by interrupting the flow through the intimal tear. Two of our cases showed how promising this approach could be.

The development of an "internal bypass" after balloon dilatation is an appealing idea in view of the failure of balloon dilatation in long stenosis or occlusions. In theory, isolating the inner surface of the treated artery eventually prevents any interaction between the damaged intima and the circulating elements and substances of the blood.

Our initial experience in treating thoracic aneurysms, one resulting from a type A dissection, an aneurysm of the descending thoracic aorta, and a thoracoabdominal aortic aneurysm with no compromise of the visceral arteries, indicates that the procedure is simpler than when treating AAA—and promising.

REFERENCES

1. Melton NJ, Bickerstaff LK, Hollier LH, et al. Changing incidence of abdominal aortic aneurysms: a population-based study. *Am J Epidemiol.* 1984;120:379–386.
2. Brown OW, Hollier LH, Pairolero PC, et al. Abdominal aortic aneurysm and coronary artery disease: a reassessment. *Arch Surg.* 1981;116:1484–1488.
3. McCombs RP, Roberts B. Acute renal failure after resection of abdominal aortic aneurysm. *Surg Gynecol Obstet.* 1979;148:175–179.
4. Karmody AL, Leather RP, Goldman M, et al. The current position of non resection treatment for abdominal aortic aneurysms. *Surgery.* 1983;94:591–597.
5. Parodi JC, Palmaz JC, Barone HD, et al. Transfemoral intraluminal graft implantation for abdominal aortic aneurysms. *Ann Vasc Surg.* 199;5:491–499.
6. Parodi JC, Barone HD. Transfemoral placement of aortic graft in aortic aneurysm: clinical experience in patients. In Yao JST, Pearce W, eds. *Aneurysms: New Findings and Treatments.* Norwalk, CT: Appleton & Lange; 1994:341–352.
7. Palmaz JC, Richter GM, Noeldge G, et al. Intraluminal stents in atherosclerotic iliac artery stenosis: preliminary report of multicenter study. *Radiology.* 1988;168:727–731.
8. Rees CR, Palmaz JC, Garcia O, et al. Angioplasty and stenting of completely occluded iliac arteries. *Radiology.* 1989;172:953–959.
9. Parodi JC. Endovascular repair of abdominal aortic aneurysms. *Adv Vasc Surg.* 1993;1:85–106.
10. Chuter T. Bifurcated endovascular graft insertion for abdominal aortic aneurysms. In: Greenhalgh RM, ed. *Vascular and Endovascular Surgical Techniques.* Philadelphia: WB Saunders; 1994:92.

V

Aorta and Its
Major Branches

16

Surgical Management of Acute
and Chronic Dissection of
Descending Thoracic Aorta

Edouard Kieffer, MD, and Quentin Desiron, MD

Whereas immediate surgical repair is widely accepted as the treatment of choice for dissection involving the ascending aorta,[1] management of chronic and especially acute dissection of the descending thoracic aorta remains controversial. In the latter situation most groups advocate surgery only if complications occur. As summarized by Miller[2,3] this conservative approach is based on three main assumptions: (1) early death can usually be avoided by medical therapy; (2) operative mortality is relatively high; and (3) long-term outcome is comparable after medical therapy and surgical treatment. However, these assumptions are based on results of historical series and do not take into account subgroups of patients at high risk for complications preventable by surgical treatment. Also recent progress now enables better perioperative management of patients who undergo emergency aortic repair. Finally early experience with endovascular treatment of ischemic complications of aortic dissection has been gratifying. The purpose of this chapter is to describe the therapeutic choices and our current surgical indications and techniques for acute and chronic dissection of the descending thoracic aorta.

CLASSIFICATION

Conventionally aortic dissections are classified as acute if they are seen within 14 days following the onset of symptoms and chronic if they are seen beyond 14 days.[4] The reason for this distinction is that the risk of life-threatening complications (especially rupture) is greatest in the first days following dissection.[5] De Bakey et al.[6] proposed an intermediate group of subacute dissection seen between 2 weeks and 2 months following symptoms but most authors consider this distinction to be unnecessary.

Classification of aortic dissection is important because clinical manifestations, prognosis, and therapeutic choices depend largely on the site and extent of dissection. Several classification systems have been made based on topographic features (Table

TABLE 16–1. CLASSIFICATION SYSTEMS OF AORTIC DISSECTION

Author [Reference]	Year	Institution	Involvement of Ascending Aorta	
			Present	*Absent*
De Bakey et al.[7]	1965	Baylor University	Types I and II	Type III
Daily et al.[8]	1970	Stanford University	Type A	Type B
Applebaum et al.[9]	1967	University of Alabama	Ascending	Descending
Meng et al.[10]	1981	Rush Medical College	Anterior	Posterior
Doroghazi et al.[11]	1984	Massachusetts General Hospital	Proximal	Distal

16–1).[7–11] The best known and probably most widely used system is the one described by DeBakey et al.[7] in 1965 which distinguished three types of aortic dissection: type I dissection involving the ascending aorta and a variable extent of the descending thoracic or thoracoabdominal aorta; type II dissection limited to the ascending aorta; and type III dissection involving the descending thoracic aorta without (type IIIa) or with (type IIIb) extension to the abdominal aorta.

Reul et al.[12] proposed more extensive subdivision of DeBakey type III dissection into four groups: type IIIa including dissections involving the upper half of the descending thoracic aorta, type IIIb including dissection involving the whole descending thoracic aorta, type IIIc including dissection involving the descending thoracic aorta and the abdominal aorta, and type IIId including retrograde dissection to the ascending aorta from an intimal tear in the descending thoracic aorta. Although these subgroups may be useful in selecting the aortic reconstruction technique, they add little to the previously mentioned two-subgroup breakdown of DeBakey's classification, that is, type IIIa including dissection limited to the descending thoracic aorta and type IIIb including dissection of the descending thoracic aorta with extension to the abdominal aorta.

In 1970 Daily et al.[8] proposed a simpler classification known as the Stanford classification system, which distinguishes type A dissections involving the ascending aorta and type B with no involvement of the ascending aorta. It should be emphasized that Stanford type B dissection can originate from and/or include the aortic arch. Type I and type II dissections of the DeBakey classification correspond to Stanford type A while type III of the DeBakey classification corresponds to Stanford type B. Other classification systems (Table 16–1) have been proposed using different terminology, but involvement of the ascending aorta is the main criteria of classification.

This chapter uses the conventional DeBakey classification system. We do not discuss the surgical management of dissections involving the aortic arch and dissecting aneurysms of the descending thoracic aorta developing after reconstruction of the ascending aorta in patients with type I dissection.

DESCRIPTION OF LESIONS

Aortic dissection is characterized by separation of the layers of aortic wall. Although dissection can result from an intramural hematoma with no connection to the aortic lumen, most dissections have an entry site due to localized intimal tear and one or more reentry sites allowing blood to circulate between the aortic lumen ("true lumen") and the dissected zone ("false lumen") (Fig. 16–1).[13] The most common entry site in type III dissection is the aortic isthmus. Location in the middle or lower part of the descending aorta is much less common, and location in the abdominal aorta is exceedingly rare.[14] Although it is usually transverse, the intimal tear can be round, straight, or curved. It does not generally involve the complete circumference of the aorta. At the level of the isthmus it is usually limited to the upper aspect of the aorta, within a few centimeters of the origin of the left subclavian artery.

Dissection can progress in retrograde and/or antegrade fashion. Progression usually takes place within seconds after the initial intimal tear but delayed progression is possible especially in patients with poorly controlled arterial hypertension. Retrograde progression of type III aortic dissection is rarely more than a few centimeters, stopping at the origin of the left subclavian artery. However, retrograde extension involving the posterior aspect of the aortic arch occurs in 10% to 15% of cases[1,15] and poses a significant surgical challenge especially since diagnosis using aortography (Fig. 16–2), computed tomography (CT) scanning or even transesophageal echocardiography may be difficult.

Antegrade progression usually follows a spiral path involving between one-half to two-thirds of the left lateral aspect of the descending thoracic aorta. It is rarely limited to the upper part of the descending thoracic aorta (Fig. 16–3). Dissection can stop at the diaphragm where the aortic orifice has a stiff, fibrous, consistency (type IIIa), but in most cases the whole abdominal aorta and even the iliac arteries are involved (type IIIb). Dissection of the thoracoabdominal aorta usually involves the left posterolateral aspect of the aorta with the visceral and right renal arteries branching from the true lumen and the left renal artery from the false lumen.[16] Exit (reentry) sites may correspond to the ostia of the disrupted collaterals (intercostal, lumbar, or visceral arteries) and/or occur at the distal end of dissection, that is, the aortic bifurcation, the

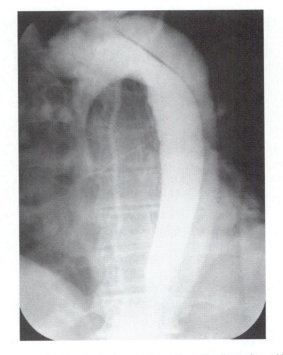

Figure 16–1. Aortogram showing typical acute type III aortic dissection with patency of both the true and false lumens. The initial (entry) intimal tear is located at the aortic isthmus.

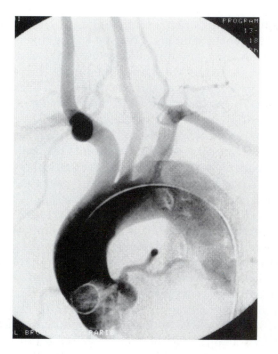

Figure 16–2. Aortogram showing acute type III aortic dissection with retrograde extension to the proximal transverse aortic arch.

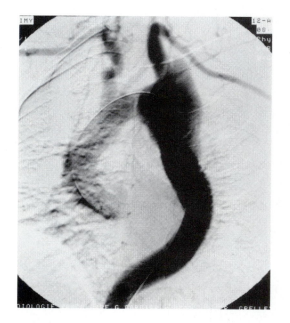

Figure 16–3. Aortogram showing limited acute type IIIa aortic dissection complicating pseudocoarctation of the distal transverse aortic arch.

iliac bifurcation, and even the femoral bifurcation. Flow rate in the false lumen is probably one of the main determinant factors for rupture, ischemic complications, and thrombosis.

NATURAL HISTORY

The natural history of dissection of the ascending and descending aorta is different. It is generally acknowledged that the risk of early death is much greater for type I and II dissections than for type III, which tends to have a more chronic course. To the contrary of proximal aortic dissections, type III dissection is not associated with a major risk of intrapericardial rupture, acute aortic insufficiency, and occlusion of the coronary arteries. Although the dismal early and late evolution of type III aortic dissection has been underlined in most reports, knowledge about the natural history of type III dissection is still incomplete. Most data come from early clinical and/or autopsy studies[17–21] and observations made after current medical treatment can hardly be considered as indicative of the natural course of the disease.

Surprisingly enough, and in contrast to abdominal aortic aneurysms, the rate of expansion of dissecting thoracic aortic aneurysm has been studied only recently. Dapunt et al.[22] reported on 17 patients with chronic type III aortic dissection studied by serial CT scanning with 3-D reconstruction. The mean increase in diameter was 0.59 cm/year while the probably more relevant increase in volume was 94.1 mL/year. Evaluation of the risk of rupture and appropriate surgical indications will probably benefit from such studies in the near future.

As a general rule the potential complications of acute as well as chronic dissection combine those of aneurysmal aortic disease to those of occlusive disease of the aortic branches.

Acute Dissection

The main risks of acute type III aortic dissections are rupture and ischemic complications. Both are usually lethal, accounting for mortality rates of up to 30% in the acute phase of dissection (Fig. 16–4)[19] unless successful emergency treatment is applied.

Rupture

Although the adventitia is the most resistant layer of the aorta, the incidence of rupture of the false lumen is high. Predisposing factors for rupture include poorly controlled hypertension, high flow rate within the false lumen, absence or small size of the reentry site(s), and increase in aortic diameter according to the law of Laplace.

The usual configuration of the entry site and false lumen explains why most ruptures complicating acute type III dissections occur in the left pleural cavity.[5,13] Due to associated rupture of the pleura, massive hemothorax ensues and death is usually prompt. This evolution is in distinct contrast with the more benign course of progressive and generally low-volume hemothorax due to transudation through the intact adventitia and pleura. Rupture can also occur into the mediastinum, the right pleural cavity,[5,23,24] the retroperitoneal space, or the peritoneal cavity. A few cases have been reported involving rupture into the pericardial cavity,[25] the esophagus,[5,26] the tracheobronchial tree, and the lung.[5]

Ischemic Complications

Ischemic complications are common in patients presenting acute type III dissection of the descending thoracic aorta with involvement of the abdominal aorta (type IIIb).[1,5,27–29]

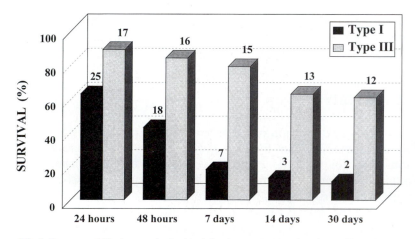

Figure 16–4. Compared 30-day survival rates following acute type I and type III aortic dissection showing the highly lethal nature of type I dissection as opposed to the more benign course of type III dissection. Numbers at the top of the bars refer to the actual number of patients in each group. (*Adapted from Lindsay J Jr, Hurst JW. Clinical features and prognosis in dissecting aneurysm of the aorta: a re-appraisal. Circulation. 1967;35:880–888.*)

In some cases ischemic manifestations may be the main clinical and prognostic features (Fig. 16–5). Any branch of the descending thoracic and abdominal aorta as well as the aorta itself can be affected and a variety of mechanisms can be involved.

Occurrence of high-grade stenosis or occlusion of the dissected aorta is rarely due to detachment of an intimal flap distal to an extensive intimal tear. If the tear is circumferential, intussusception of the intima can cause aortic obstruction.[30] In most cases, however, aortic obstruction is due to compression of the true lumen by the false lumen and is preferentially located at the thoracoabdominal junction.[31] An acute coarctation-like process can lead to severe hypertension with an enhanced risk of rupture and distal ischemia affecting the spinal cord, kidneys, digestive tract, and lower extremities. Spontaneous resolution can occur if a reentry site of sufficient size develops and flow is reestablished to the abdomen and lower extremities. If this does not occur, therapatic choices include surgical replacement of the descending thoracic aorta with reconstruction of the distal true lumen or creation of a reentry by fenestration of the intimal membrane separating the two lumens.

Narrowing of the abdominal branches of the aorta and the iliofemoral arteries is often due to compression of the true lumen by the false lumen at the origin of the vessel. However, other mechanisms can be observed.[1,27,32] Dissection can extend into the artery resulting in a reduction of the lumen. Dissection can disrupt the aortic intima at the origin of the artery and result in a waving intimal flap that blocks flow into the artery. Regardless of the mechanism, arterial stenosis can be complicated by extensive thrombosis with further reduction in the patency of the lumen.

Occurrence of ischemic symptoms due to occlusion of the aortic branches depends on the degree of obstruction, the duration of ischemia, the availability of sufficient collateral circulation, and the susceptibility of the organ system or extremity to ischemia. This multifactorial etiology probably explains the discrepancy between the incidence of aortic branch lesions reported in autopsy and clinical studies. In the autopsy series of Hirst et al.,[5] in which most patients died due to rupture, aortic dissection involving the abdominal aorta was associated with lesions of the visceral arteries in 27.7% of cases and lesions involving the arteries supplying the lower extremities in 26.1% of

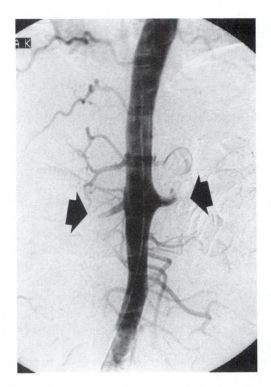

Figure 16–5. Aortogram showing bilateral renal artery occlusion (arrow) causing sudden anuria in a patient with a painless acute type III aortic dissection.

cases. In the clinical series of Cambria et al.[27] the corresponding incidences were only 8.7% and 11.7% respectively. Inasmuch as this diagnostic procedure does not examine the abdominal aorta and its branches, the increasing use of transesophageal echocardiography may be an explanation for the lower figures in recent clinical reports.[33] Likewise, CT scanning or magnetic resonance scanning (MRI) may be less sensitive for peripheral vascular lesions than aortography.

Clinical symptoms depend on the affected organ. Spinal cord ischemia can lead to paraplegia, paraparesis, and partial neurologic deficits such as Brown-Sequard's syndrome or isolated sphincter disturbances. These manifestations are uncommon but usually irreversible. Ischemia of the lower extremities is also uncommon. It is usually limited to a loss of one or both femoral pulses. Loss of pulse in the left upper extremity is also possible after retrograde extension of type III dissection or compression of the left subclavian artery by the aortic false lumen.[28] Ischemia involving the digestive tract may be associated with minor or no symptoms if only one of the main visceral arteries (celiac artery and superior mesenteric artery) is affected. However, because limited involvement is uncommon, intestinal infarction is a major life-threatening complication that warrants exploratory laparotomy before or after replacement of the proximal aorta in suspicious cases.[17] Renal ischemia can also be asymptomatic if the arterial lesion is unilateral and function of the contralateral kidney is normal. In patients with acute dissection, interpretation of hypertension and/or renal insufficiency can be confounded by a number of factors including the preexisting status of the kidneys and renal arteries[34] as well as the renal effects of hypotensive drugs administered to prevent aortic rupture.[9] Cardiopulmonary bypass used during reconstruction of the proximal aorta may also interfere with the visceral and/or renal circulation.

Chronic Dissection

Following initial medical management, most patients with acute type III aortic dissection survive long enough to reach the chronic phase of the disease. When used as the initial treatment of aortic dissection, surgery is usually palliative because complete removal of the dissected aorta is rarely possible. As a result careful surveillance is necessary in all patients to avoid the risk of late aortic rupture.

Fate of the False Lumen

Several cases of spontaneous cure of type III aortic dissection documented by CT scanning have been reported in the literature.[35-37] However, these cases are rare and have always involved patients with thrombosis of the false lumen and moderate aortic dilatation. In nearly 85% of cases the false lumen remains at least partially patent.[37] The risk of progressive dilatation of the false lumen (Fig. 16–6) leading to aneurysm formation has been estimated to be about 35%.[38] Aneurysm is usually limited to either the upper part of the descending thoracic aorta opposite the entry site or the infrarenal abdominal aorta. In most cases aneurysm involving the infrarenal abdominal aorta probably occurs in patients with preexisting degenerative lesions of the media. In other cases aortic dilatation progresses to extensive thoracoabdominal aneurysm. Aneurysm formation accounts for the risk of late rupture, which has been described as a major cause of late mortality following dissection of the descending thoracic aorta.[5,13,17–20,22] Complete thrombosis of the false lumen, once considered as a favorable prognostic

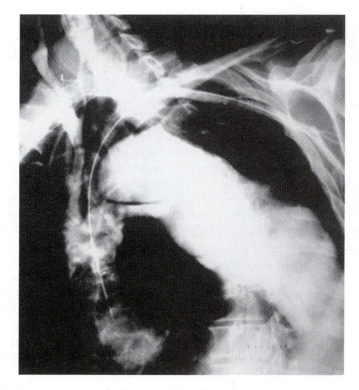

Figure 16–6. Aortogram showing huge dilatation of the false lumen and compression of the true lumen in a patient with chronic type III aortic dissection.

factor, does not protect against rupture since the diseased aorta may redissect[39] or follow the same evolution as degenerative aneurysm.[40]

Ischemic Complications

When initial ischemia has been transient or partial because of adequate collateral circulation, aortic branches involved in acute dissection can remain patent beyond proximal occlusive lesions. This can lead to chronic ischemia with intermittent claudication of the lower extremities, intestinal angina, renovascular hypertension, or ischemic renal insufficiency.[27-29] These ischemic complications are often but not always associated with aneurysm formation.

SURGICAL TECHNIQUES

A wide range of surgical techniques has been proposed for management of type III aortic dissection. Some are directed at the aortic lesion itself, some at the ischemic complications, and some at both lesions and complications. These methods can be used singly or in combination. In most cases only palliative repair is possible due to the extent of dissection and/or the high risks of complete aortic replacement during the acute phase.

Graft Replacement

The optimal goals of aortic replacement, especially in patients with acute type III aortic dissection, are to (1) remove the most threatening area; (2) close the entry site of the dissection; and (3) maintain or reestablish blood flow in the distal aorta and its branches.

The upper part of the descending thoracic aorta is the most frequently replaced segment in type III aortic dissection (Figs. 16–7 and 16–8). In such limited operations the risk of spinal cord ischemia is low provided that blood supply to the distal aorta is satisfactorily maintained intraoperatively.[1,41–43] In patients with extensive aneurysm involving the lower part of the descending thoracic aorta, total replacement of the descending thoracic aorta may be necessary. Construction of the lower anastomosis near the diaphragm can require thoracoabdominal incision. Though rarely used in patients with acute aortic dissection, replacement of the entire thoracoabdominal aorta using Crawford's inclusion graft technique[44] is often indicated in patients with chronic dissection since these lesions usually lead to formation of Crawford type I or II thoracoabdominal aneurysm (Fig. 16–9). Limited aortic replacement can also be indicated for lesions of the infrarenal aorta (rupture, expansion, or aneurysm)[45] but also during fenestration to reestablish circulation to the branches of the aorta (see later discussion). In rare cases replacement of the entire abdominal aorta is performed in combination with reimplantation of the visceral arteries directly or via an autogenous or prosthetic graft in order to treat visceral and/or renal ischemia.[46]

Replacement of the descending thoracic or thoracoabdominal aorta in patients with type III aortic dissection poses several technical problems. Preservation of the blood supply to the spinal cord and digestive tract is not a problem specific to management of aortic dissection. Extensive discussion of the indications and advantages of the various methods used for distal aortic perfusion is beyond the scope of this chapter. However, it should be underlined that replacement of a dissected descending thoracic or thoracoabdominal aorta is a delicate procedure in which clamping time is unpredictable and often longer than in operations for degenerative aneurysms. Svensson et al.[47] reported a high incidence (up to 24%) of spinal cord complications associated with

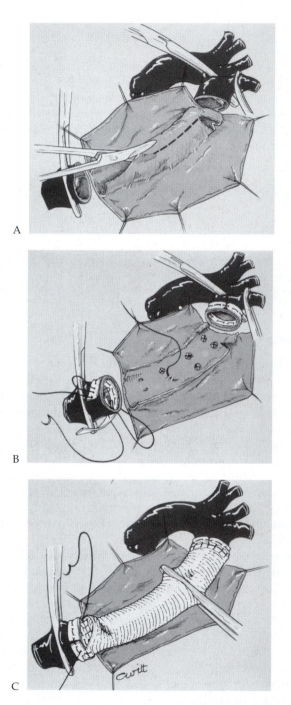

Figure 16–7. Conventional surgical technique for graft replacement of the upper part of the descending thoracic aorta in patients with acute type III aortic dissection: (**A**) resection of the intimal membrane and initial (entry) intimal tear; (**B**) reinforcement of both transected aortic ends with Teflon pledgets; and (**C**) graft anastomoses.

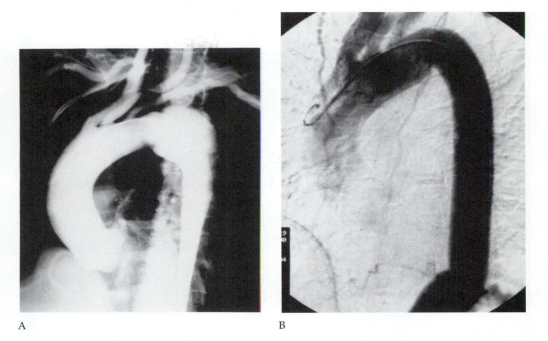

A   B

Figure 16–8. (A) Preoperative and **(B)** postoperative aortograms showing graft replacement of the upper part of the descending thoracic aorta in a patient with localized aneurysm at the entry site and compression of the distal true lumen complicating acute type III aortic dissection.

simple aortic cross-clamping during thoracoabdominal aortic replacement for extensive dissecting aneurysm. The efficacy of distal aortic perfusion in protecting the spinal cord, kidneys, and digestive tract has been well documented.[42,48] Distal perfusion also provides more effective decompression of the proximal aorta than pharmacologic manipulation during simple aortic cross-clamping. Decompression is important to avoid clamp injury and/or aortic rupture during clamping.

The choice of distal aortic perfusion technique depends on personal preference. Excellent clinical results have been obtained using a Gott shunt[43] or a left atriofemoral shunt with a centrifugal pump.[41,48] Despite the need for high-dose heparinization, our preference is partial cardiopulmonary bypass (femoral vein or pulmonary artery to femoral artery).[49–53] The main advantages of partial cardiopulmonary bypass are (1) to allow circulatory assistance before opening the chest and retrieval of blood in patients with intrapleural rupture,[50] (2) to ensure maximal oxygenation by compensating exclusion of the left lung, and (3) to be easily convertible to total cardiopulmonary bypass if necessary.[53]

Regardless of the method of distal aortic perfusion used, there is a small but certain risk of intraoperative visceral and spinal cord ischemia due to selective perfusion of the false lumen in the absence of a reentry site beyond the distal aortic clamp. This risk must be borne in mind from the beginning of the operation so that an alternative arterial perfusion site can be chosen in proper time. In some cases perfusion of the distal aorta must be preceded by fenestration of the infrarenal aorta or, more conveniently, by graft replacement of the aortic bifurcation in combination with proximal fenestration. The left limb of the bifurcated graft can be used for retrograde aortic perfusion.[54]

The poor quality of the aortic wall is a specific problem of surgical treatment of type III aortic dissection, in particular in patients presenting acute dissection or dissec-

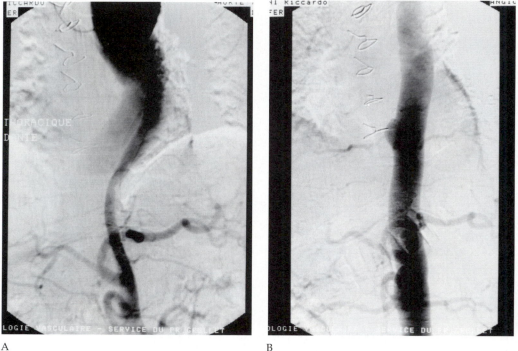

A   B

Figure 16–9. (A) Preoperative and **(B)** postoperative aortograms showing graft replacement of the thoracoabdominal aorta, including direct anastomoses of lower intercostal and visceral arteries to the aortic graft in a patient with chronic type III aortic dissecting aneurysm.

tion associated with preexisting conditions such as Marfan's syndrome. Aortoprosthetic anastomoses must be made after complete transection of the aorta[2,55] in order to enable proper placement of sutures including the aortic adventitia. Teflon pledgets are almost always used to reinforce the aortic edges (Fig. 16–7) and enable the anastomosis to withstand the shearing effect of each systolic thrust after clamp removal. Alternative suture reinforcement techniques recommended by other groups include application of gelatin resorcin formol (GRF)[56] or fibrin glue on the transsected edges of the aorta before suturing the graft and aortic banding with a Dacron tube graft in the immediate vicinity of both anastomoses.[57]

Construction of the proximal anastomosis in a healthy zone is important to successful repair and nearly always feasible. If dissection extends beyond the limit of resection, which is usually the case distally, two anastomoses techniques can be used depending on whether dissection is acute or chronic. In patients with acute dissection, dilatation of the aorta is moderate and the two lumens can be reassembled, thus maintaining or reestablishing satisfactory flow through the true lumen. In patients with chronic dissection and a patent false lumen the preferable technique consists of fenestration of the intimal membrane immediately below the future anastomosis followed by graft anastomosis to the two lumens in order to ensure that both remain patent (Fig. 16–10). In this regard it should be underlined that the false lumen often feeds one or more visceral or renal arteries and diverting flow into the true lumen would compromise supply to these arteries.

Another important precaution for successful outcome of surgical repair of aortic dissection is to avoid aortic injury during clamp placement. Although complete transection of the dissected aorta has been reported following clamp placement,[58] the most

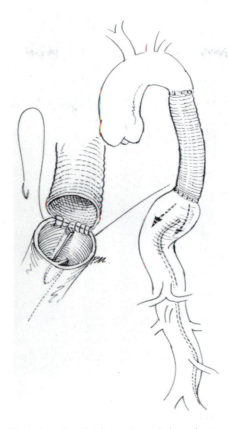

Figure 16–10. Preferred technique for distal anastomosis in patients with chronic type III aortic dissection. Following limited resection of the intimal aortic membrane below the future anastomosis, graft anastomosis is performed to the two distal aortic lumens.

frequent clamp-induced aortic lesion is an intimal tear, which can have serious consequences. In patients with acute dissection occurrence of an intimal tear distal to the distal anastomosis rules out any prospect of reassembly of the two lumens (Fig. 16–11). As in surgical repair of dissection involving the ascending aorta, distal aortic clamping can be easily avoided by using the "open" anastomosis technique. This is done by temporarily discontinuing distal aortic perfusion after construction of the proximal anastomosis and dividing the distal aorta beyond the distal aortic clamp before constructing the distal anastomosis. An intimal tear involving the aortic arch after clamp placement between the common carotid and left subclavian arteries can lead to dire complications. Retrograde dissection is nearly always rapidly fatal[12,43,52,59] unless deep hypothermia can be quickly instituted to achieve circulatory arrest and repair of the proximal aorta.[60] At best an intimal tear involving the aortic arch will lead only to formation of a juxta-anastomotic false aneurysm and require reoperation (Fig. 16–12). The use of ringed prosthetic grafts[61,62] has been fraught with technical difficulties[1] and has not eliminated anastomotic problems.

In view of these clamp-related complications, we and others[63,64] have advocated performing surgical correction of type III aortic dissection under elective deep hypothermic circulatory arrest. This technique provides a blood-free operative field and allows

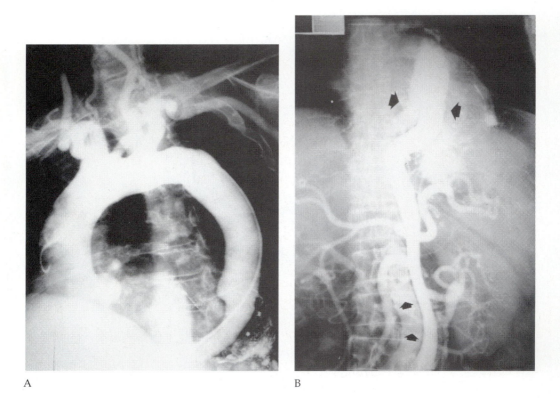

A   B

Figure 16–11. (A) Postoperative aortograms showing persistance of the false lumen in a patient with graft replacement of the upper part of the descending thoracic aorta. **(B)** Reentry sites in the distal aorta correspond to both spontaneous (*lower arrows*) and clamp-induced (*upper arrows*) communications between the true and false lumens.

precise aortic repair without clamping. Buffolo et al.[65] have taken advantage of the use of deep hypothermic circulatory arrest in type III aortic dissection by using median sternotomy to implant a distal "elephant trunk" into the descending thoracic aorta. Another important advantage of this technique is to allow better protection of the spinal cord during aortic clamping.[66] However, the etiology of spinal cord complications after surgery on the thoracoabdominal aorta is multifactorial and deep hypothermia is not a panacea. Before undertaking surgery for chronic type III aortic dissection we routinely perform selective preoperative arteriography of the intercostal and lumbar arteries to map spinal circulation so that we can preserve or reimplant critical arteries during surgery.[67]

Aortoplasty

In view of the high operative mortality associated with aortic replacement, various authors have proposed more conservative aortic repairs. A variety of techniques have been described but the common feature shared by all is suture of the intimal tear at the entry site. Reassembly of the two lumens is achieved in different ways. Several years ago Berger et al.[68] revived the old transverse suture technique that had been used previously by several authors.[11,42,69–71] Tanabe et al.[72] proposed injection of Ivalon into the false lumen to induce thrombosis. More recently Kawashima et al.[73] and Williams[74] described the so-called "tailored aortoplasty" technique designed to avoid graft replacement of the distal descending thoracic aorta and proximal abdominal aorta and thus

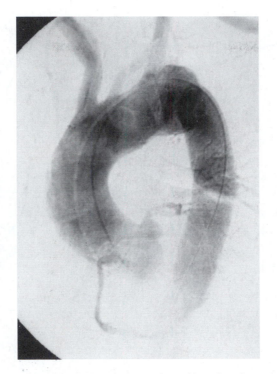

Figure 16–12. Late postoperative aortogram in a patient with graft replacement of the upper part of the descending thoracic aorta showing juxta-anastomotic false aneurysm due to clamp injury.

minimize spinal cord complications associated with extensive aortic replacement. In 1989 Fabiani et al.[75] reported one case of "glue aortoplasty" in which early postoperative aortogram was normal. Experience with these techniques is limited and long-term results have not been clearly documented.

Thromboexclusion

Thromboexclusion as described by Carpentier[76] in 1979 is based on a different principle from aortic replacement (Fig. 16–13). The first stage of the procedure consists of placing a prosthetic bypass graft between the ascending and abdominal aorta via median sternolaparotomy. The second stage consists of interrupting the aorta distal to the left subclavian artery. The true and false lumens are reassembled as a result of the reversed flow in the upper abdominal and descending thoracic aorta. The proximal part of the descending thoracic aorta including the site of entry and the most proximal portion of the dissected aorta are excluded by progressive thrombosis, theoretically with minimal risk for the blood supply to the spinal cord.

Although several authors have used this new technique with reasonably good clinical results,[77–80] its apparent simplicity has been deceptive. The special metal clamp used by Carpentier et al.[77] to achieve aortic interruption is the source of several difficulties. The first is placement. Exposure of the aorta distal to the left subclavian artery is often difficult and entails a low but certain risk of injury to the upper part of the false lumen.[78,79] Another problem is clamp migration, which can lead to compression of the left subclavian artery[77] or pulmonary artery. Clamp-induced aortic lesions can lead to fatal complications due to retrograde aortic dissection.[81] To avoid these complications some authors have proposed using sutures[82] or staples[80,83] in association with Dacron or Teflon pledgets instead of the clamp. Moreover, all authors agree that interruption

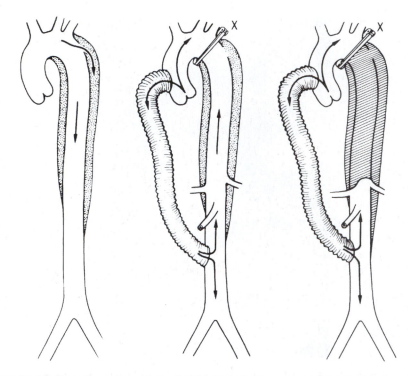

Figure 16–13. Thromboexclusion for acute type III aortic dissection as described by Carpentier et al.[77]

should be carried out on a flaccid aorta, which can be obtained either by proximal clamping, administration of hypotensive agents, or brief cardiac inflow occlusion by clamping of both venae cavae.[83] Some authors have also proposed interruption of the aorta between the left common carotid and subclavian arteries but this raises the need for either bypass from the ascending aorta-abdominal aorta bypass to the subclavian artery[80] or transposition of the subclavian artery into the common carotid artery.[82]

The main issues raised by the thromboexclusion technique involve its risk and efficacy. In comparison with aortic replacement thromboexclusion reduces but does not rule out the risk of aortic rupture[80] or spinal cord complications.[78–80] Moreover, there are no large series with sufficient follow-up to document the long-term fate of the aortic lesions left in place. To avoid late aneurysmal formation involving the descending thoracic aorta, Robicsek[84,85] and our group[82] tried a variant technique including complete interruption of the distal thoracic aorta either during the same procedure via the same anterior approach used for ascending aorta-abdominal aorta bypass or during a second procedure via left thoracotomy a few days later. However, we stopped using this technique several years ago because we found it to be as complicated and risky as aortic replacement.

Fenestration

Although fenestration is now only rarely mentioned in discussions of surgical techniques, it was the first surgical technique proposed for treatment of acute aortic dissection[86] and the first to achieve long-term survival.[87] The principle of fenestration is simple. It consists of creating a large reentry from the false lumen into the true lumen.

The dissected aorta is exposed, clamped, and opened. The intima is then resected with scissors up to the proximal clamp and the aortotomy is closed.

Based on analysis of the spontaneous course of aortic dissection it was initially speculated that equilibrating flow in the two lumens would be a simple and effective means of avoiding aortic rupture. This hypothesis proved to be wrong and we now know that the only way to prevent imminent rupture is aortic replacement. However, fenestration provides a cost-effective means of treating the ischemic complications of aortic dissection by reestablishing flow to the collateral and terminal branches of the abdominal aorta (Fig. 16–14).[29,31,79,88,89] It is for this purpose that fenestration still has a place in the surgeon's arsenal of techniques for management of aortic dissection.

Elefteriades et al.[90] recently described a simple technique for fenestration of the abdominal aorta. The infrarenal aorta is exposed by the retroperitoneal approach, clamped, and divided transversely in its midportion. The intimal membrane in the proximal segment is resected up to the proximal aortic clamp. The two lumens in the distal segment are reassembled using a circular suture and aortic continuity is reestablished by end-to-end anastomosis of the two aortic segments.

Like others[1,31] we prefer to perform fenestration via median laparotomy because it allows visual inspection of abdominal organs and bypass to any particular visceral or renal artery if the fenestration procedure fails to reestablish flow.[88] In this regard it

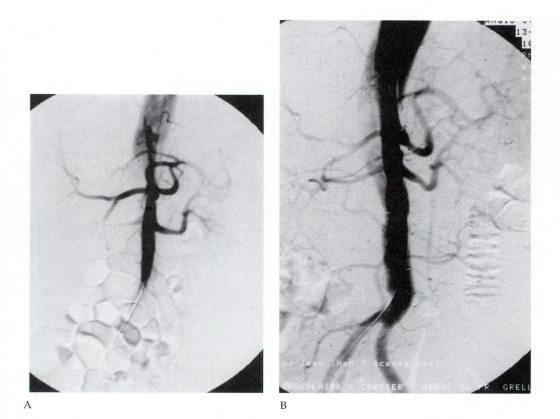

A   B

Figure 16–14. (A) Preoperative and **(B)** postoperative aortograms in a patient with acute type III aortic dissection with malperfusion of the renal and visceral arteries. Fenestration of the infrarenal abdominal aorta using a short interposition Dacron graft restored full patency of renal and visceral arteries with disappearance of all ischemic symptoms.

is important to underline that aortic fenestration cannot achieve effective revascularization in patients with extensive dissection, intimal flaps, or thrombosis of aortic branches.[1]

Additional problems associated with fenestration are that aorto-aortic anastomosis can be difficult and leaving the infrarenal abdominal aorta may lead to late aneurysm formation. For these reasons our preference goes to associated graft replacement of the infrarenal abdominal aorta.[45,88] A tube graft is usually sufficient (Fig. 16–14) and has the advantage of facilitating anastomosis to the distal true lumen. However, use of a bifurcated graft with distal anastomoses to the iliac or, more frequently, the femoral arteries may be indicated in patients presenting distal thrombotic occlusion or preexisting atherosclerotic lesions as well as in cases in which reassembly of the two lumens in the distal aortic segment is either unfeasible or unreliable.

Some authors have recommended clamping the supracoeliac aorta to allow resection of the intimal membrane at the level of the visceral arteries.[1] Our opinion is that this technique can be dangerous and is usually unnecessary since resection of infrarenal aortic intima is nearly always sufficient to reestablish satisfactory retrograde flow in the aortic branches (Fig. 16–14).

Isolated Revascularization of Aortic Branches

Isolated revascularization of the branches of the aorta is an alternative in case of contraindications to or failure of fenestration. Since the donor artery should ideally be located proximal to dissection, some authors have recommended long bypass either from the subclavian or axillary artery or from the ascending aorta. As a result isolated revascularization of aortic branches may become a complicated technique often with poor long-term patency rates. In most cases the revascularization procedure proceeds from a nondissected iliac artery (crossover femorofemoral bypass, iliorenal bypass, or iliosuperior mesenteric bypass) or another visceral artery (renomesenteric or mesentericorenal bypass, left splenorenal or renosplenic anastomosis, or right hepatorenal or renohepatic bypass).[91] A prosthetic graft used for fenestration of the infrarenal abdominal aorta can serve as the origin of a bypass, especially if fenestration fails to achieve revascularization.[31,88]

Endovascular Procedures

Like management of other types of vascular disease, treatment of aortic dissection has benefited from the introduction of endovascular techniques. Various endovascular procedures have been used for treatment of both the aortic lesions and ischemic complications. Two methods have been studied experimentally for endovascular treatment of aortic lesions, namely, stenting or stent-grafting[92–97] and placement of a balloon in the false lumen to close the entry and promote thrombosis.[98,99] Results of only one clinical trial involving stent-grafting in two patients with chronic type III aortic dissection have been reported.[100] One procedure was a technical failure and reoperation was required 3 months later.

Endovascular techniques have been much more successful for treatment of the ischemic complications of aortic dissection. Slonim et al.[101] reported results of stent placement and fenestration of the intima using a balloon catheter in a series of 22 patients with visceral and/or lower extremity ischemia. These two techniques were used separately in 16 and 3 patients, respectively, and in combination in 3 patients. One patient died of peritonitis due to irreversible intestinal ischemia 3 days after the procedure. Immediate clinical and anatomic results were good in all cases. During follow-up 3 patients required repeat endovascular treatment but no patient underwent conventional surgical treatment. In addition to the uncommonly high skills of the reporting radiology group, the main factors in achieving these excellent results were high-quality imaging facilities, catheterization of both arterial lumens, and intravascular ultrasonography. Careful preoperative workup is indeed necessary to identify the mechanism underlying ischemic complications and choose the most suitable technique, that is, fenestration of the intimal membrane if occlusion involves the aorta and stenting of the branch if occlusion involves the branch itself.

INDICATIONS

Acute Dissection

There is a general consensus that patients in whom type III acute aortic dissection is diagnosed or suspected should be given antihypertensive and negative inotropic treatment and kept under close clinical, hemodynamic and radiologic surveillance in an intensive care unit. The main goal of initial assessment is to determine whether the ascending aorta is intact since involvement of ascending aorta would be an indication for immediate surgery. However, there is little agreement concerning the role of surgery in the management of acute type III aortic dissection. Three approaches have been proposed:

1. For the reasons described at the beginning of this chapter most centers perform surgery only if there is demonstrable evidence of failure of medical therapy.[1,42,46,49,51,70,79,89,102–106] The main indications for surgery are rupture, expansion of the aorta, uncontrollable pain and/or hypertension, successive chest roentgenograms showing mediastinal enlargement, progressive hemothorax, and occurrence of ischemic complications involving the digestive tract, kidneys, or lower extremities. Using this approach most surgical procedures are performed under emergency conditions in unselected patients and postoperative mortality rates greater than 50% are still currently reported.[51,71,102,105] Limiting indications to surgery in such a selected group of poor-risk patients would also mean a higher incidence of rupture and reoperation in patients treated medically.

2. In contrast, the Stanford group[2,3,107] is recommending routine elective surgery in low-risk patients with type III acute aortic dissection. This attitude is based on recent reports showing a dramatic improvement in surgical results (see later discussion). The main advantage of this approach is that procedures are performed under much more favorable conditions. Late prognosis in survivors is probably better with fewer ruptures and operations.[3,107] However, many patients with type III dissection are elderly and present cardiovascular, cerebrovascular, pulmonary, and renal problems. Although these factors may not constitute absolute contraindications to surgery, they do worsen postoperative prognosis (Fig. 16–15).[3,108] Furthermore, this approach exposes some patients not at risk for aneurysm formation to unnecessary operative mortality and morbidity.

3. The third approach, which is the one advocated by our group, is intermediate between the conservative and surgical approach. It is intended to offer the best hope of avoiding uncontrollable late aortic complications while limiting the number of unnecessary early surgical procedures. This approach calls for surgery not

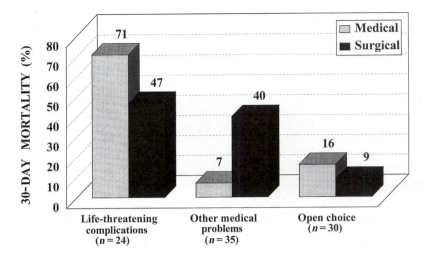

Figure 16–15. Compared 30-day mortality rates in three different groups of patients with acute type III aortic dissection receiving either medical or surgical treatment (see text). [*Adapted from Miller DC. The continuing dilemma concerning medical versus surgical management of patients with acute type B dissections. Sem Thorac Cardiovasc Surg. 1993;5:33–46 and from Glower DD, Fann JI, Speier RH, et al. Comparison of medical and surgical therapy for uncomplicated descending aortic dissection. Circulation. 1990;82(suppl IV):39–46.*]

only in patients presenting the previously mentioned compulsory indications but also in good-risk patients identified as being at risk for late rupture and aneurysm formation. Risk factors for rupture empirically accepted by most investigators include an aortic diameter greater than 5 cm, Marfan's disease or other connective tissue disorders, long-term corticosteroid therapy, and preexisting aortic abnormalities (coarctation or pseudocoarctation of the aortic isthmus, aberrant subclavian artery, and dystrophic aneurysm). Kato et al.[38] recently reported clinical data favoring indications for early surgery in selected low-risk patients with uncomplicated type III acute aortic dissection. They studied with CT scans 41 patients with type III aortic dissection who had been successfully treated medically during the acute phase. Aortic enlargement was defined as (1) maximum diameter of the dissected aorta ≥60 mm; (2) rapid enlargement of the dissected aorta >10 mm/ year; or (3) rupture of the dissected aorta. Multivariate analysis identified two strongly significant predictors of late aortic enlargement: a maximum aortic diameter of ≥40 mm during the acute phase and a patent primary entry site in the thoracic aorta. No aortic enlargement was observed in the other patients. Provided the operative risk is low, these authors advocate early surgery in this well-defined group of patients in order to avoid the added risks of rupture during medical therapy in the acute phase and a higher incidence of postoperative complications following surgery in the chronic phase.

Once the decision to operate has been made the next question is what type of procedure should be used. The choice depends on the surgical indication. In patients presenting aortic complications (rupture, expansion, and aneurysm) direct exposure and aortic replacement are mandatory. The extent of emergency graft replacement should be as limited as possible. In most cases of acute type III aortic dissections replacement can be limited to the upper part of the descending thoracic aorta or, more rarely, the infrarenal abdominal aorta.[45] Management of ischemic complications is more controversial. Most cardiovascular surgeons recommend replacement of the proximal aorta as a reliable method of reestablishing flow to the branches of the aorta.[28,109] With few exceptions vascular surgeons have questioned the reliability of this technique[27] and argue that more conservative procedures such as surgical fenestration of the abdominal aorta or current endovascular techniques achieve the same results more economically. For patients undergoing elective surgical correction for uncomplicated acute aortic dissection we feel that replacement of the proximal aorta with removal of the site of entry and reassembly of the two lumens is a more logical choice than thromboexclusion.

Regardless of whether or not surgery is performed during the acute phase of dissection, patients must be kept under strict long-term surveillance. The first goal of therapy is control of hypertension which is a statistically significant factor for aortic complications and late mortality.[3,6] Even in normotensive patients beta blockers should be administered because of their demonstrated protective effect against aortic dilatation. The second goal of postoperative surveillance is to allow CT scan or MRI surveillance every 6 months. The incidence of late aneurysm formation justifies the inconvenience and costs involved in long-term surveillance.

Chronic Dissection

Some patients with chronic type III aortic dissection develop chronic ischemic complications due to stenosis or occlusion of the aorta and/or renal, visceral, or iliac arteries. When such ischemic complications are not associated with aortic aneurysm or in poor surgical candidates, conservative techniques such as surgical bypass grafting or endovascular procedures can be used.[1,27,29,31,89,91,101] When dissection is associated with aortic aneurysm, aortic replacement is necessary and separate bypasses to the involved aortic branches can be performed from the aortic graft.[110]

The surgical indications for chronic dissecting aneurysm are the same as those for degenerative aneurysm of the descending thoracic or thoracoabdominal aorta.[1,6,47,51,107,109] Surgery is indicated in patients with complicated or symptomatic aneurysm, patients with evidence of progression on successive CT scans, and asymptomatic good-risk patients with aneurysms larger than 5 cm in diameter.

In patients with asymptomatic aneurysms careful workup is needed to evaluate the operative risk. In our group this workup includes echocardiography, coronary arteriography, Doppler ultrasonography of arteries to the brain, and respiratory function testing. Depending on the results of these investigations it may be necessary to perform other interventional or surgical procedures first (myocardial revascularization, carotid endarterectomy, or more rarely cardiac valvular replacement) or otherwise prepare the patient for aortic surgery (respiratory physiotherapy). Another important feature of the preoperative workup is spinal cord arteriography. Visualization of spinal cord vascularization greatly reduces the risk of postoperative spinal cord complications.[67] Conversely failure to visualize spinal cord vascularization may favor nonoperative management.

The extent of aortic replacement in patients with chronic type III aortic dissection is variable. A cautious and often feasible approach consists of replacement of only the aneurysmal zone (generally all or part of the descending thoracic aorta) and careful postoperative surveillance of the remaining dissected but nonaneurysmal aorta. However, extensive replacement is unavoidable in patients with thoracoabdominal aneurysm. Extensive aortic replacement is associated with a higher risk of spinal cord complications, which must be weighted against the possibly fatal consequences of aneurysm rupture.

CURRENT RESULTS

Early Results

Acute Dissection

Table 16–2 summarizes 30-day results of surgical management of acute type III aortic dissection in 10 series reported from 1990 to 1996 in the English literature.[43,89,102,103,105,106,109,111–113] Most patients in these series had graft replacement of the upper part of the descending thoracic aorta. Mortality rates ranged from 0%[106] to 69% (9/13).[105]

Interpretation of such conflicting data should obviously take into account important differences in referral patterns and indications for surgery from one institution to another. Schor et al.[106] acknowledged the fact that their outstanding surgical results (0 mortality) may well be explained by self-selection of the patients in a tertiary referral center. Although the same may apply to other studies reporting similarly good results,[109,111,112] the fact remains that substantial improvement in mortality rates following surgery for acute type III aortic dissection has occurred during the last 15 years, at least in selected patients operated on at selected medical centers.

On the other hand, the poor results reported in other series are obviously related to surgery being performed only in the most desperate situations. In the report by Neya et al.[105] 9 (69%) patients were operated on for aortic rupture and 7 (50%) patients were in hemorrhagic shock at the time of hospital admission. Adachi et al.[102] similarly reported a series of 39 patients in whom early surgery had been performed only for

TABLE 16–2. CURRENT 30-DAY RESULTS OF SURGICAL MANAGEMENT OF ACUTE TYPE III AORTIC DISSECTION

Author [Reference]	Period	Surgical Management	Number of Patients	Deaths	Paraplegia/ Paraparesis
Verdant et al.[43]	1974–1994	Aortic replacement	52	6	0
Neya et al.[105]	1979–1991	Aortic replacement	13	9	NA
Masuda et al.[111]	1979–1989	Aortic replacement	27	5	NA
Fradet et al.[103]	1980–1986	Aortic replacement			
		Initial	11	3	NA
		Secondary	6	5	NA
Grabitz et al.[89]	1981–1995	Aortic replacement	7	3	1
		Fenestration	7	1	0
		Extra-anatomic bypass	11	0	0
Svensson et al.[109]	1984–1989	Aortic replacement			
		Limited	17	1	NA
		Extensive	19	1	NA
Schor et al.[106]	1985–1995	Initial aortic replacement	17	0	0
		Secondary operations[a]	12	0	0
Adachi et al.[102]	1985–1989	Aortic replacement	10	6	NA
Coselli et al.[112,113]		Aortic replacement			
	1987–1995	Limited	28	4	2
	1986–1994	Extensive	16	1	2

NA, not available
[a] Includes three palliative procedures.

acute rupture. Of 10 patients operated on under emergency conditions due to massive bleeding, 6 (60%) died intra- or postoperatively. These series may reflect more closely the medical practice in the community setting.

In an attempt to compare medical and surgical therapy for uncomplicated type III aortic dissection Glower et al.[108] reported the combined experience of Stanford and Duke Universities. Miller[2] subsequently reanalyzed their data concerning acute type III aortic dissection (Fig. 16–15), clearly demonstrating the influence of surgical indications on postoperative results. Although mortality was high (47%) in patients operated on for life-threatening complications, it was still higher (71%) whenever those patients were treated medically. Patients without compelling indications for emergency surgery who had serious coexistent medical illnesses did obviously better following medical therapy. Finally low-risk patients without compelling indications for emergency surgery or serious coexistent medical illnesses had low, equivalent mortality rates following either medical or surgical therapy (16% versus 9%).

It has also been reported by Fradet et al.[103] that mortality following early surgery for acute type III aortic dissection is much higher when surgery is performed because of failure of medical therapy rather than as an initial therapy.

Ischemic complications involving the spinal cord, kidneys, digestive tract, or lower extremities have a significant influence on early mortality following graft replacement for acute type III aortic dissection. In the series of Fann et al.[28] operative mortality was 64% (7/11) in patients with vascular complications as opposed to 31% (9/29) in patients without vascular complications ($p < 0.002$). Mortality was 100% for patients with spinal cord ischemia, 67% for patients with renal ischemia, and 50% for patients with ischemia involving the lower extremities or compromised visceral perfusion. The fact that only renal ischemia showed independent predictive value for postoperative death at statistical analysis was probably due to the small number of patients.

The low rate of paraplegia/paraparesis in these series is probably explained by the usually limited extent of aortic replacement in the acute phase of dissection.

TABLE 16–3. CURRENT 30-DAY RESULTS OF AORTIC REPLACEMENT FOR CHRONIC TYPE III DISSECTING AORTIC ANEURYSM OF THE DESCENDING THORACIC/THORACOABDOMINAL AORTA

Author [Reference]	Period	Number of Patients	Extent of Replacement	Deaths	Paraplegia/ Paraparesis
Verdant et al.[43]	1974–1994	31	Thoracic	7	0
Kawashima et al.[73]	1977–1991	13	Thoracic	4	0
		15	Thoracoabdominal[a]	3	0
Grabitz et al.[89]	1981–1995	13	Thoracic	0	1
		24	Thoracoabdominal	7	5
Svennson et al.[109]	1984–1989	96	Thoracic	4	NA
		100	Thoracoabdominal	5	NA
Coselli et al.[112]	1987–1995	55	Thoracic	0	1
Coselli et al.[113]	1986–1994	77	Thoracoabdominal	4	2
Kitamura et al.[48, b]	1987–1993	15	Thoracic	0	0
		17	Thoracoabdominal	3	1
Kieffer[c]	1990–1994	31	Thoracic	2	2
		36	Thoracoabdominal	5	4

[a] These patients were managed by "tailored aortoplasty."
[b] Includes a few patients with acute dissections.
[c] Unpublished data.

TABLE 16–4. LATE ACTUARIAL SURVIVAL RATES (INCLUDING PERIOPERATIVE MORTALITY) FOLLOWING SURGICAL MANAGEMENT OF TYPE III AORTIC DISSECTION

Author [Reference]	Acute versus Chronic	Number of Patients	Survival (%)					
			1 Year	3 Years	5 Years	8 Years	10 Years	15 Years
Jex et al.[42]	Both	64	—	—	49	30	—	—
Svensson et al.[109]	Both	232	81	71	—	—	—	—
Kitamura et al.[48]	Both	65	—	—	70	—	70	—
Schor et al.[106]	Acute	17	93	—	68	—	—	—
Fann et al.[107]	Acute	46	56	—	48	—	29	11
	Chronic	34	78	—	59	—	45	27

Chronic Dissection

Table 16–3 summarizes late results of surgical management of chronic type III aortic dissection in seven series reported from 1990 to 1996 in the English literature,[43,48,73,89,109,112,113] to which we have added our own recent experience. Comparison to earlier series[6,8,12,52] demonstrates substantial improvement in mortality and paraplegia/paraparesis rates. Refinements in operative indications, surgical techniques, and perioperative care have obviously benefited those patients, the vast majority of whom are operated on electively. Despite many efforts in different directions, elimination of spinal cord complications has not been achieved and remains an important goal for future research.

Late Results

Detailed analysis of late results following surgery for acute type III aortic dissection have been reported by several groups.[6,42,105–107,109] Actuarial 5-year survival rates (including perioperative mortality) are in the 50% to 70% range (Table 16–4). Late deaths following surgical management of type III aortic dissection may be caused by cardiovascular disease, aortic complications, or unrelated causes. In these patients aneurysmal formation or redissection in untreated parts of the thoracic or abdominal aorta should be looked for by routine periodic surveillance of the entire aorta using CT scanning, MRI, or aortography. Elective reoperation should be offered to most good-risk patients in order to avoid late aortic rupture and reduce late mortality rates.

In most patients aortic dissection is nothing but an episode in the evolution of generalized aortic disease. Patients (and their physicians) should understand the lifelong nature of their disease in order to comply with the mandatory long-term aortic surveillance.

REFERENCES

1. Borst HG, Heinemann MK, Stone CD. *Surgical Treatment of Aortic Dissection.* New York: Churchill Livingstone; 1996.
2. Miller DC. Acute dissection of the descending thoracic aorta. *Chest Surg Clin North Am.* 1992;2:347–378.
3. Miller DC. The continuing dilemma concerning medical versus surgical management of patients with acute type B dissections. *Sem Thorac Cardiovasc Surg.* 1993;5:33–46.
4. DeSanctis RW, Doroghazi RM, Austen WG, Buckley MJ. Aortic dissection. *N Engl J Med.* 1987;317:1060–1067.

5. Hirst AE, Johns VJ, Kine SW. Dissecting aneurysm of the aorta: a reveiw of 505 cases. *Medicine.* 1958;37:217–279.

6. DeBakey ME, McCollum CH, Crawford ES, et al. Dissection and dissecting aneurysms of the aorta: twenty-year follow-up of five hundred twenty-seven patients treated surgically. *Surgery.* 1982;92:1118–1134.

7. DeBakey ME, Henly WS, Cooley DA, et al. Surgical management of dissecting aneurysms of the aorta. *J Thorac Cardiovasc Surg.* 1965;19:130–149.

8. Daily PO, Trueblood HW, Stinson EB, et al. Management of acute aortic dissections. *Ann Thorac Surg.* 1970;10:237–247.

9. Applebaum A, Karp RB, Kirklin JW. Ascending vs descending aortic dissections. *Am Surg.* 1976;183:296–300.

10. Meng RL, Najafl H, Javid H, et al. Acute ascending aortic dissection: surgical management. *Circulation.* 1981;64(suppl II):231.

11. Doroghazi RH, Slater EE, DeSanctis RW, et al. Long-term survival of patients with treated aortic dissections. *J Am Coll Cardiol.* 1984;3:1026–1034.

12. Reul GJ, Cooley DA, Hallman GL, et al. Dissecting aneurysm of the descending aorta: improved surgical results in 91 patients. *Arch Surg.* 1975;110:632–640.

13. Roberts WC. Aortic dissection: anatomy, consequences, and causes. *Am Heart J.* 1981;101:195–214.

14. Azodo MVU, Gutierrez OH, DeWeese JA. Abdominal aortic dissection with retrograde extension into the thoracic aorta. *Cardiovasc Intervent Radiol.* 1990;12:317–320.

15. Von Segesser LK, Killer I, Ziswiler M, et al. Dissection of the descending thoracic aorta extending into the ascending aorta: a therapeutic challenge. *J Thorac Cardiovasc Surg.* 1994;108:755–761.

16. Siegelman SS, Sprayregen S, Strasberg Z, et al. Aortic dissection and the left renal artery. *Radiology.* 1970;95:73–78.

17. Bickerstaff LK, Pairolero PC, Hollier LH, et al. Thoracic aortic aneurysms: a population-based study. *Surgery.* 1982;92:1103–1108.

18. Crawford ES, DeNatale RW. Thoracoabdominal aortic aneurysm: observations regarding the natural course of the disease. *J Vasc Surg.* 1986;3:578–582.

19. Lindsay J Jr, Hurst JW. Clinical features and prognosis in dissecting aneurysm of the aorta: a re-appraisal. *Circulation.* 1967;35:880–888.

20. Pressler V, McNamara JS. Thoracic aortic aneurysm: natural history and treatment. *J Thorac Cardiovasc Surg.* 1980;79:489–498.

21. Roberts CS, Roberts WC. Aortic dissection with the entrance tear in the descending thoracic aorta: analysis of 40 necropsy patients. *Ann Surg.* 1991;213:356–368.

22 Dapunt OE, Galla JD, Sadeghi AM, et al. The natural history of thoracic aortic aneuryms. *J Thorac Cardiovasc Surg.* 1994;107:1323–1333.

23. Faraci PA, Payne DD, Cleveland RJ. Type III aortic dissection with rupture into the right hemithorax. *J Cardiovasc Surg.* 1982;23:429–431.

24. Katagiri M, Takahashi M. Right hemothorax: an unusual presentation of ruptured aortic dissection. *J Cardiovasc Surg.* 1991;32:135–136.

25. Verdant A, Cossette R, Dontigny L, et al. Acute dissection of the descending thoracic aorta: repair in an unusual case. *Can J Surg.* 1984;27:390–391.

26. Roth JA, Parekh MA. Dissecting aneurysms perforating the esophagus. *N Engl J Med.* 1978;299:776.

27. Cambria RP, Brewster DC, Gertler J, et al. Vascular complications associated with spontaneous aortic dissection. *J Vasc Surg.* 1988;7:199–209.

28. Fann JI, Sarris GE, Mitchell RS, et al. Treatment of patients with aortic dissection presenting with peripheral vascular complications. *Ann Surg.* 1990;212:705–713.

29. Okita Y, Takamoto S, Ando M, et al. Surgical strategies in managing organ malperfusion as a complication of aortic dissection. *Eur J Cardiothorac Surg.* 1995;9:242–247.

30. Heinemann MK, Buehner B, Schaefers HJ, et al. Malperfusion of the thoracoabdominal vasculature in aortic dissection. *J Card Surg.* 1994;9:748–755.

31. Orend KH, Liewald F, Kirchdorfer B, Sunder-Plassmann L. Surgical management of descending aortic dissection. In: Weimann S, ed. *Thoracic and Thoracoabdominal Aortic Aneurysm.* Bologna: Monduzzi; 1994:103–108.

32. Walker PJ, Sarris GE, Miller DC. Peripheral vascular manifestations of acute aortic dissection. In: Rutherford RB, ed. *Vascular Surgery.* 4th ed. Philadelphia: WB Saunders; 1995:1087–1102.

33. Hughes JD, Bacha EA, Dodson TF, et al. Peripheral vascular complications of aortic dissection. *Am J Surg.* 1995;170:209–212.

34. Rackson ME, Lossef SV, Sos TA. Renal artery stenosis in patients with aortic dissection: increased prevalence. *Radiology.* 1990;117:555–558.

35. Albrechtsson U, Thorvinger B. Spontaneous resolution of a descending aortic dissection. *Acta Radiol.* 1989;30:305–306.

36. Hoshino T, Ohmae M, Sakai A. Spontaneous resolution of a dissection of the descending aorta after medical treatment with a β blocker and a calcium antagonist. *Br Heart J.* 1987;58:82–84.

37. Yamaguchi T, Naito H, Ohta M, et al. False lumens in type III aortic dissections: progress CT study. *Radiology.* 1985;157:757–760.

38. Kato M, Bai H, Sato K, et al. Determining surgical indications for acute type B dissection based on enlargement of aortic diameter during the chronic phase. *Circulation.* 1995; 92(suppl II):107–112.

39. Lui RC, Menkis AH, McKenzie FN. Aortic dissection without intimal rupture: diagnosis and management. *Ann Thorac Surg.* 1992;53:886–888.

40. Sanderson CJ, Rich S, Beere PA, et al. Clotted false lumen: reappraisal of indications for medical management of acute aortic dissection. *Thorax.* 1981;36:194–199.

41. Borst HG, Jurmann M, Bühner B, Laas J. Risk of replacement of descending aorta with a standardized left heart bypass technique. *J Thorac Cardiovasc Surg.* 1994;107:126–133.

42. Jex RK, Schaff HV, Piehler JM, et al. Early and late results following repair of dissections of the descending thoracic aorta. *J Vasc Surg.* 1986;3:226–237.

43. Verdant A, Cossette R, Pagé A, et al. Aneurysms of the descending thoracic aorta: three hundred sixty-six consecutive cases resected without paraplegia. *J Vasc Surg.* 1995;21:385–391.

44. Crawford ES. Thoracoabdominal and abdominal aortic aneurysms involving renal, superior mesenteric, and celiac arteries. *Ann Surg.* 1974;179:763–772.

45. Hunter JA, Dye WS, Javid H, et al. Abdominal aortic resection in thoracic dissection. *Arch Surg.* 1976;111:1258–1262.

46. Kasprzak PM, Raithel D. Surgical concepts for treatment of aortic dissections type B. In: Weimann S, ed. *Thoracic and Thoracoabdominal Aortic Aneurysm.* Bologna: Monduzzi; 1994:95–102.

47. Svensson LG, Crawford ES, Hess KR, et al. Experience with 1509 patients undergoing thoracoabdominal aortic operations. *J Vasc Surg.* 1993;17:357–370.

48. Kitamura M, Hashimoto A, Tagusari O, et al. Operation for type B aortic dissection: introduction of left heart bypass. *Ann Thorac Surg.* 1995;59:1200–1203.

49. Eisenmann B, Kretz JG, Kucharski K, Kieny R. Dissections de l'aorte thoracique descendante: traitement médical ou chirurgical? In: Kieffer E, ed. *Chirurgie de l'Aorte Thoracique Descendante et Thoraco-Abdominale.* Paris: Expansion Scientifique; 1986:227–235.

50. Faidutti B, Hahn C. Les dissections de l'aorte thoracique (27 observations). *J Chir.* 1969;98:503–520.

51. Glower DD, Speier RH, White WD, et al. Management and long-term outcome of aortic dissection. *Ann Surg.* 1991;214:31–41.

52. Miller DC, Stinson EB, Oyer PE, et al. Operative treatment of aortic dissections: experience with 125 patients over a sixteen-year period. *J Thorac Cardiovasc Surg.* 1979;78:365–382.

53. Pate JW, Richardson RL, Eastridge CE. Acute aortic dissections. *Am Surg.* 1976;42:395–404.

54. Coselli JS, Crawford ES. Femoral artery perfusion for cardiopulmonary bypass in patients with aortoiliac obstruction. *Ann Thorac Surg.* 1987;43:437–439.

55. Ergin MA, Galla JD, Lansman S, Griepp RB. Acute dissections of the aorta: current surgical treatment. *Surg Clin North Am.* 1985;65:721–741.

56. Chen YF, Chou SH, Chiu CC et al. Use of glutaraldehyde solution in the treatment of acute aortic dissections. *Ann Thorac Surg.* 1994;58:833–836.

57. Reul GJ Jr. New technique for surgical hemostasis of aorto-prosthetic anastomoses. *Cardiovasc Dis Bull Tex Heart Inst.* 1974;1:120–122.

58. Hume DM, Porter RR. Acute dissecting aortic aneurysms. *Surgery.* 1963;53:122–154.
59. Austen WG, DeSanctis RW. Surgical treatment of dissecting aneurysm of the thoracic aorta. *N Engl J Med.* 1965;272:1314–1318.
60. Graham JM, Stinnett DM. Operative management of acute aortic arch dissection using profound hypothermia and circulatory arrest. *Ann Thorac Surg.* 1987;44:192–198.
61. Krause AH, Chapman RD, Bigelow JC, et al. Early experience with the intraluminal graft prosthesis. *Am J Surg.* 1983;145:619–622.
62. Oz MC, Ashton R Jr, Singh MK, et al. Twelve-year experience with intraluminal sutureless ringer graft replacement of the descending thoracic and thoracoabdominal aorta. *J Vasc Surg.* 1990;11:331–338.
63. Kieffer E, Koskas F, Walden R, et al. Hypothermic circulatory arrest for thoracic aneurysmectomy through left-sided thoracotomy. *J Vasc Surg.* 1994;19:457–464.
64. Caramutti VM, Dantur JR, Favaloro MR, et al. Deep hypothermia and circulatory arrest as an elective technique in the treatment of type B dissecting aneuryms of the aorta. *J Card Surg.* 1989;4:206–215.
65. Buffolo E, Fonseca HP, Adrade JCS, et al. Surgical treatment of type B aortic dissection using the elephant trunk principle. *J Cardiovasc Surg.* 1992;33:59.
66. Kouchoukos NT, Daily BB, Rokkas CK, et al. Hypothermic bypass and circulatory arrest for operations on the descending thoracic and thoracoabdominal aorta. *Ann Thorac Surg.* 1995;60:67–77.
67. Kieffer E, Richard T, Chiras J, et al. Preoperative spinal cord arteriography in aneurysmal disease of the descending thoracic and thoracoabdominal aorta: preliminary results in 45 patients. *Ann Vasc Surg.* 1989;3:34–46.
68. Berger RL, Romero L, Chaudhry AG, et al. Graft replacement of the thoracic aorta with a sutureless technique. *Ann Thorac Surg.* 1983;35:231–239.
69. Parker FB Jr, Neville JF Jr, Hanson EL, et al. Management of acute aortic dissection. *Ann Thorac Surg.* 1975;19:436–442.
70. Ruberti U, Odero A, Arpesani A, et al. Acute aortic dissection: personal experience. *J Cardiovasc Surg.* 1988;29:70–79.
71. Viljanen T, Luosto R, Jarvinen A, Sariola H. Surgical treatment of aortic dissection in 60 patients. *Scand J Thorac Cardiovasc Surg.* 1986;20:193–201.
72. Tanabe T, Hashimoto M, Sakai K, et al. Surgical treatment of aortic dissection: application of Ivalon sponge to the dissected lumen. *Ann Thorac Surg.* 1986;41:169–175.
73. Kawashima Y, Shirakura R, Nakano S, et al. Long-term results of entry closure and aneurysmal wall plication with axillofemoral bypass: a new procedure for repair of DeBakey type 3 dissecting aneurysm. *Surgery.* 1993;113:59–64.
74. Williams GM. Treatment of chronic expanding dissecting aneurysms of the descending thoracic and upper abdominal aorta by extended aortotomy, removal of the dissected intima, and closure. *J Vasc Surg.* 1993;18:441–449.
75. Fabiani JN, Jebara VA, Carpentier A. Use of glue in treatment of type B aortic dissection. *Lancet.* 1989;2:1041.
76. Carpentier A. New approach to treatment of aortic dissections. *Lancet.* 1979;15:1291–1292.
77. Carpentier A, Deloche A, Fabiani JN, et al. New surgical approach to aortic dissection: flow reversal and thromboexclusion. *J Thorac Cardiovasc Surg.* 1981;81:659–668.
78. Carpentier A. Thromboexclusion: an alternative for type B dissection. *Sem Thorac Cardiovasc Surg.* 1991;3:242–244.
79. Elefteriades JA, Hartleroad J, Gusberg RJ, et al. Long-term experience with descending aortic dissection: the complication-specific approach. *Ann Thorac Surg.* 1992;53:11–21.
80. Odagiri S, Shimazu A, Shimokawaji M, et al. Use of a new stapling instrument for permanent occlusion of the aorta in the surgical procedure for thromboexclusion. *Ann Thorac Surg.* 1989;47:466–469.
81. Patra P, Petiot JM, Mainguene C, et al. Retrograde dissection of the aortic arch after exclusion-bypass of the descending thoracic aorta: a report of three cases. *Ann Vasc Surg.* 1989;3:341–344.
82. Kieffer E, Petitjean C, Richard T, et al. Exclusion-bypass for aneurysms of the descending thoracic and thoracoabdominal aorta. *Ann Vasc Surg.* 1986;1:182–195.

83. Ergin MA, O'Connor JV, Blanche C, et al. Use of stapling instruments in surgery for aneurysms of the aorta. *Ann Thorac Surg.* 1983;36:161–166.

84. Robicsek F, Allie DE. Long-range observations following two-stage occlusion of the descending thoracic aorta for type III dissection. *Ann Vasc Surg.* 1986;1:244–248.

85. Robicsek F. "Very long" aortic grafts. *Eur J Cardiothorac Surg.* 1992;6:536–541.

86. Gurin D, Bulmer JW, Derby R. Dissecting aneurysm of the aorta: diagnosis and operative relief of acute arterial obstruction due to this cause. *NY State Med J.* 1935;35:1200–1202.

87. DeBakey ME, Cooley DA, Creech O Jr. Surgical considerations of dissecting aneurysm of the aorta. *Ann Surg.* 1955;142:586–612.

88. Dinis da Gama A. The surgical management of aortic dissection: from uniformity to diversity, a continuous challenge. *J Cardiovasc Surg.* 1991;32:141–153.

89. Grabitz K, Sandmann W, Kniemeyer HW, Torsello G. Surgical management of complications in patients with acute and chronic dissection of the descending aorta. In: Weimann S, ed. *Thoracic and Thoracoabdominal Aortic Aneurysm.* Bologna: Monduzzi; 1994:227–234.

90. Elefteriades JA, Hammond GL, Gusberg RJ, et al. Fenestration revisited: a safe and effective procedure for descending aortic dissection. *Arch Surg.* 1990;125:786–790.

91. Andréassian B, Nussaume O, Kitzis M, et al. Dissection de l'aorte thoracique: chirurgie "ad hoc" des branches de l'aorte et de l'aorte à distance de l'entrée. In: Kieffer E, ed. *Chirurgie de l'Aorte Thoracique Descendante et Thoraco-Abdominale.* Paris: Expansion Scientifique; 1986:252–264.

92. Boudghene F, Sapoval M, Bigot JM, Michel JB. Endovascular graft placement in experimental dissection of the thoracic aorta. *JVIR.* 1995;6:501–507.

93. Charnsangavej C, Wallace S, Wright KC, et al. Endovascular stent for use in aortic dissection: an *in vitro* experiment. *Radiology.* 1985;157:323–325.

94. Kato N, Hirano T, Mizumoto T, et al. Experimental study for treatment of aortic dissection with expandable metallic stents. *JVIR.* 1994;5:417–423.

95. Marty-Ané C, Serres-Cousiné O, Laborde JC, et al. Use of endovascular stents for acute aortic dissection: an experimental study. *Ann Vasc Surg.* 1994;8:434–442.

96. Trent MS, Parsonnet V, Shoenfeld R, et al. A balloon-expandable intravascular stent for obliterating experimental aortic dissection. *J Vasc Surg.* 1990;11:707–717.

97. Yoshida H, Kakino T, Kajitani M, et al. Transcatheter placement of an intraluminal prosthesis for the thoracic aorta: a new approach to aortic dissection. *ASAIO.* 1991;37:272–273.

98. Akaba N, Ujue U, Umezarva K, et al. Management of acute aortic dissection with a cylinder-type balloon to close the entry. *J Vasc Surg.* 1986;3:890–894.

99. Carney WI, Rheinlander HF, Cleveland RJ, et al. Control of acute aortic dissection. *Surgery.* 1975;78:114–120.

100. Dake MD, Miller DC, Semba CP, et al. Transluminal placement of endovascular stent-grafts for the treatment of descending thoracic aortic aneurysms. *N Engl J Med.* 1994;331:1729–1734.

101. Slonim SM, Nyman Ulf, Semba CP, et al. Aortic dissection: percutaneous management of ischemic complications with endovascular stents and balloon fenestration. *J Vasc Surg.* 1996;23:214–253.

102. Adachi H, Kyo S, Takamoto S, et al. Early diagnosis and surgical intervention of acute aortic dissection by transesophageal color flow mapping. *Circulation.* 1990;82(suppl IV):19–23.

103. Fradet G, Jamieson WRE, Janusz MT, et al. Aortic dissection: a six year experience with 117 patients. *Am J Surg.* 1988;155:697–700.

104. Genoni M, von Segesser LK, Carrel T, et al. Aorten-dissektionen type B: operations, technick und resultate. *Helv Chir Acta.* 1994;60:1151–1157.

105. Neya K, Omoto R, Kyo S, et al. Outcome of Stanford type B acute aortic dissection. *Circulation.* 1992;86(suppl II):1–7.

106. Schor JS, Yerlioglu ME, Galla JD, et al. Selective management of acute type B aortic dissection: long-term follow-up. *Ann Thorac Surg.* 1996;61:1339–1341.

107. Fann JI, Smith JE, Miller DC, et al. Surgical management of aortic dissection during a 30-year period. *Circulation.* 1995;92(suppl II):113–121.

108. Glower DD, Fann JI, Speier RH, et al. Comparison of medical and surgical therapy for uncomplicated descending aortic dissection. *Circulation.* 1990;82(suppl IV):39–46.

109. Svensson LG, Crawford ES, Hess KR, et al. Dissection of the aorta and dissecting aortic aneurysms: improving early and long-term surgical results. *Circulation*. 1990;82(suppl IV):24–38.
110. Svensson LG, Crawford ES, Hess KR, et al. Thoracoabdominal aortic aneurysms associated with celiac, superior mesenteric, and renal artery occlusive disease: methods and analysis of results in 271 patients. *J Vasc Surg*. 1992;16:378–390.
111. Masuda Y, Yamada Z, Morooka N, et al. Prognosis of patients with medically treated aortic dissections. *Circulation*. 1991;84(suppl III):7–13.
112. Coselli JS, Plestis KA, La Francisca S, Cohen S. Results of contemporary surgical treatment of descending thoracic aortic aneurysms: experience in 198 patients. *Ann Vasc Surg*. 1996;10:131–137.
113. Coselli JS. Thoracoabdominal aortic aneurysms: experience with 372 patients. *J Card Surg*. 1994;9:638–647.

17

Mesenteric Ischemia

Current Surgical Techniques

*K. Wayne Johnston, MD, FRCS(C), and
Thomas F. Lindsay, MD, FRCS(C)*

The diagnosis of acute and chronic mesenteric ischemia is often difficult and management can be a major challenge. This paper reviews the early and long-term results of mesenteric arterial revascularization for acute and chronic ischemia. The data are based on the authors' recently published experience[1] and a review of the literature.

ACUTE MESENTERIC ISCHEMIA

Kach et al.[2] documented the etiology of acute mesenteric ischemia in 45 patients at laparotomy or autopsy: embolus, 35%; thrombosis, 27%; nonocclusive mesenteric ischemia, 9%; venous thrombosis, 11%; and undiagnosed, 18%. Clearly, the pathology observed in each hospital will vary based on the local referral pattern. For all causes, the mortality rates are very high as summarized by Taylor and Moneta[3]: embolus, 70%; thrombosis, 92%; and nonocclusive mesenteric ischemia, 92%.

Boley has been a proponent of early angiography and intra-arterial papaverine administration in an attempt to improve the results.[4] In patients who present with acute abdominal pain and the diagnosis of intestinal ischemia is suspected, in our experience, arteriography is useful and should be obtained if the study can be carried out expeditiously and if time permits. It will establish the diagnosis of nonocclusive mesenteric ischemia and allow treatment to be started immediately, identify the sites of embolic occlusion and ascertain if the embolus has broken up into smaller arteries. For patients with mesenteric thrombosis, this may help to decide which arteries are patent and suitable for a bypass. In each case, the risk of arteriography must be balanced against the chances that the delay required to obtain the procedure will represent a major increased metabolic risk to the patient or a greater risk of further bowel infarction.

Embolism

As in other sites, most emboli originate from pathology in the heart but occasionally an atherosclerotic or aneurysmal thoracic aorta may be the source. They usually lodge beyond the middle colic artery and consequently some perfusion to bowel remains. For this reason, the severity and location of the pain are variable.

Embolectomy is performed through a transverse or longitudinal arteriotomy in the superior mesenteric artery as it emerges from under the inferior edge of the pancreas at the base of the transverse mesocolon. To clear the small branches of fragments of embolic material, a small balloon catheter must be used and great care taken to avoid damage to the small arteries. A patch angioplasty may be necessary to close the artery. Following successful revascularization, Doppler signals should be recordable from the arteries at the junction of the bowel wall and the mesentery. Resection of necrotic segments of bowel is performed at the initial operation; however, evaluation of other segments is often very difficult and may have to be delayed until a "second look" is performed 24 hours later. Conservation treatment with catheter-directed fibrinolytic agents, catheter embolectomy, and anticoagulants may be considered for patients with small distal emboli and no peritoneal signs.[5]

Thrombosis

The overall mortality for all patients with mesenteric thrombosis is 92%.[3] In our series,[1] nine selected patients had mesenteric bypass grafts because of acute ischemia due to thrombosis. As in the series reported by Kaleya et al.,[4] prior symptoms of intestinal angina were common: six out of nine of our patients had a history of weight loss, five of nine food fear, and five of nine diarrhea. In eight cases, angiography demonstrated a >50% stenosis or occlusion in 75% of the celiac arteries, 88% of the superior mesenteric arteries, 38% of the inferior mesenteric arteries, and 13% of both internal iliacs because of abdominal aortic or iliac disease. Because of the emergency situation, a single bypass to the superior mesenteric artery was performed in seven of the nine patients. In addition to mesenteric revascularization, four patients required simultaneous bowel resection.

Both of the early deaths were due to bowel ischemia (mortality rate, 22%). Cumulative survival was 78% at 1 month, 65% at 1 year, and 52% at 5 years. Of the two late deaths, one was due to graft thrombosis and bowel infarction. McMillan et al.[6] reported similar results in nine patients with a mortality rate of 22% but with a 3-year patency rate of 92%.

There are few references in the literature to the results of the treatment of mesenteric thrombosis with bypass grafts; however, the results of our small series are encouraging and justify an aggressive approach to early diagnosis and revascularization in selected patients.

Nonocclusive Mesenteric Ischemia

Intestinal infarction can occur in the absence of arterial or venous occlusion because of prolonged vasoconstriction associated with hypoperfusion secondary to cardiac pathology, a septic process, or secondary to drug administration.[7] Arteriography demonstrates patent major arteries and tapered distal branches. Naturally, every effort is made to optimize the patient's hemodynamic status; however, intra-arterial papaverine administration (30 to 60 mg/h) may reduce vasospasm and be of benefit.[8] The timing of laparotomy for evaluation of the bowel is determined by the patient's status.

Mesenteric Venous Thrombosis

Although many cases are idiopathic in origin, mesenteric venous thrombosis may be secondary to hypercoagulable states, local inflammation, tumor invasion, or portal hypertension.[9] Most often, diagnosis is made intraoperatively by the detection of cyanotic edematous bowel and mesentery and segmental infarction with normal arterial pulsations. Infarcted bowel must be resected and heparin administered during the acute phase to prevent recurrent thrombosis. The duration of warfarin treatment depends on the etiology but certainly long-term treatment is justified if a hypercoagulable state is identified. Venous thrombectomy may have a role in the management of selected patients with extensive venous thrombosis, even though it is impossible to clear the small veins of thrombus, and recurrent thrombosis is likely.[10]

CHRONIC MESENTERIC ISCHEMIA

Delay in the diagnosis of chronic mesenteric ischemia averages 12 to 18 months[11–13] and often is made only after numerous investigations are negative. Although mesenteric atherosclerosis is common, the number of procedures performed even by large vascular centers are few. For example, our series of mesenteric bypass represented only 0.4% of our arterial procedures—data that are similar to that reported by others.[14]

Pathology

In an autopsy study, Reiner et al.[15] reported that mesenteric atherosclerosis was very common, occurring in 78% of the 88 older subjects studied. In the autopsies, they found severe stenosis (>50%) or occlusion of the celiac artery in 14%, superior mesenteric artery in 12%, and inferior mesenteric artery in 40%. Also, and of importance in predicting the results of surgical treatment, they observed that mesenteric vascular disease was frequent and that branch stenoses were present in most named arteries.

In general, patients who require intervention have extensive mesenteric arterial disease. For example, Cunningham et al.[16] reported involvement of both the celiac and superior mesenteric arteries in 98% and the inferior mesenteric in 50%. Also in their series, 25% of the patients had aortic occlusive or aneurysmal disease and 30% stenosis of one or both renals. Although most authors have stressed the importance of involvement of the celiac, superior mesenteric, and inferior mesenteric arteries, it should be recognized that significant collaterals to the bowel originate from the internal iliac arteries. In our series,[1] 56% of patients had severe bilateral reduction of internal iliac flow because of coexisting aortic disease or iliac involvement. This observation may be important in planning the operative procedure. While most patients have extensive disease with involvement of at least two arteries, if collaterals are inadequate, a severe lesion involving only the celiac or superior mesenteric arteries may cause significant symptoms or complications.

Diagnosis

All 21 patients in our series[1] complained of abdominal angina and as in other series had an average weight loss of 32 pounds.[14,17,18] An abdominal bruit was noted in only 24% of our cases, whereas others have reported an incidence of 70% to 85%.[11–13] Angiography confirmed extensive mesenteric artery occlusive disease with severe stenosis or occlusion in 100% of superior mesenteric arteries, 90% of celiac arteries, and 90% of inferior mesenteric arteries. Similar findings have been reported by others.[12,14,16,18,19]

Treatment Options

Percutaneous Transluminal Angioplasty

In general, percutaneous transluminal angioplasty (PTA) is not successful for lesions that involve the origin of renal arteries and it is generally assumed that PTA will have a similar limitation when applied to the celiac or superior mesenteric arteries. Matsumoto et al.[20] noted that PTA was technically successful in 70% of 19 patients and that 63% of the total number of patients were clinically improved for an average of 24 months. Rose et al.[21] compared the results of PTA and surgery in the same institution and observed better long-term results following surgery and concluded that PTA should be reserved for high-risk patients. Although the results of PTA are inferior to what can be achieved by surgery, in our limited experience, PTA has proven to have good early and intermediate results in treating selected high-risk patients with stenoses that do not involve the orifice of the superior mesenteric artery or lesions in one of the proximal branches. We have been reluctant to consider PTA for celiac stenosis because of the risk of rupture of the celiac artery, which is short and divides into the smaller caliber hepatic and splenic arteries. If the balloon inadvertently enters these smaller branches, which have a sharp angle to the celiac, with dilatation, rupture may occur. Following surgery, some patients will develop intimal hyperplasia in the region of the distal anastomosis or progressive atherosclerosis beyond the graft that may be amenable to PTA. The role of stents in treating mesenteric stenoses has not been defined.

Mesenteric Bypass

Bypass grafts have been constructed with the origin from virtually any artery in the abdomen. Frequently, grafts are taken in a retrograde direction from the abdominal aorta or an aortic bifurcation graft may be placed to provide a normal inflow site. Alternately a graft can be placed from the supraceliac aorta or lower thoracic aorta to provide prograde inflow to the mesenteric vessels.

Mortality Rate.   In our series of 21 cases, there were no in-hospital deaths but major complications occurred in 4.[1] A more representative mortality rate is 5% to 10% and death is often due to graft thrombosis and bowel necrosis.[12–16,18,19,22–24]

Postoperative Complications.   Systemic complications are frequent following major surgery in debilitated patients: 19% in our series and 10% in the report by McMillan et al.[6] Early graft thrombosis is of major concern and requires prompt detection and intervention to avoid a high mortality rate. Gewertz and Zarins[25] reported three patients who developed abdominal pain postoperatively when they began to eat, and arteriography showed patent grafts and severe diffuse vasospasm. They concluded that the clinical picture was due to a reperfusion syndrome. Following visceral revascularization, multisystem organ dysfunction was common in the report by Harward et al.[9] Pulmonary insufficiency, thrombocytopenia, and abnormal liver function were noted.

Long-Term Results.   Based on the results from our series, survival was 100% at 1 year, 93% at 2 years, 79% at 5 years, and 50% at 10 years. During follow-up, graft failure occurred in three patients (14%); two patients died, and one survived after reoperation. Results are reported by life table analysis in other studies as follows: McAfee et al.,[18] 5-year survival of 68%; and Kieny et al.,[19] 5-year survival of approximately 55%. When graft patency was assessed by duplex Doppler ultrasound, McMillan et al.[6] reported a 3-year graft patency of 89%.

Transaortic Endarterectomy

Cunningham et al.[16] noted that the perioperative mortality rate was higher in the transaortic endarterectomy group (7 of 48, 14.6%) by comparison to those having antegrade bypass (2 of 26, 7.7%); however, there were clear differences in the patient populations. For transortic endarterectomy, Cunningham et al. reported a 40% 10-year survival. Simple mesenteric artery endarterectomy is not a suitable procedure.

Management Decisions

Bypass Versus Transaortic Endarterectomy

Transaortic endarterectomy is preferred if the aortic plaque is localized to the visceral segment of the aorta and the renal arteries are involved along with the celiac and/or superior mesenteric artery. However, most cases can be revascularized using the bypass technique and the majority of vascular surgeons will be more adept with bypass techniques than direct thoracoabdominal surgery on the visceral aortic segment.

Prograde Bypass Versus Retrograde Bypass

Taylor and Moneta[3] summarized the literature and reported that the late success rate for prosthetic bypass grafts from the supraceliac aorta and infrarenal aorta were similar; specifically, 90% at 4.5 years for supraceliac grafts and 90% at 4.2 years for infrarenal grafts. In our series, there appeared to be a difference between retrograde and prograde grafts but it was not statistically significant: 3 of 16 retrograde bypass grafts thrombosed compared to 0 of 5 prograde bypasses. Several authors have argued in favor of a prograde bypass but without a comparative group.[9,19,26] McAfee et al.[18] could not confirm the superior results of a prograde bypass previously reported by Hollier et al.[13] from the same institution. McMillan et al.[6] reported 3-year patency rates of 95% and 93% from prograde and retrograde grafts, respectively. No series is large enough to determine the optimum approach, but in our experience, retrograde bypasses are more difficult because of their propensity to kinking and a prograde bypass is from the less diseased proximal aorta.

Single Bypass Versus Multiple Bypass

In general, complete intestinal revascularization is recommended. Based on analysis of the series from the Mayo Clinic, Hollier[13] suggested that recurrent symptoms after mesenteric artery bypass were related to incomplete revascularization. When only one artery was bypassed, 50% of patients had recurrent symptoms, whereas when two or three arteries were repaired, the recurrence rates fell to 29% and 11%, respectively. This observation was restated by McAfee et al.[18] after a reanalysis of the recent results from the Mayo Clinic and is further supported by Calderon et al.[12] However, Kieny et al.,[19] Gentile et al.,[23] and Cormier et al.[24] generally carried out only single artery bypass grafts and had a low rate of late recurrence. We performed a single graft to the superior mesenteric artery in only 3 of 21 cases. In the other cases, multiple bypasses were carried out to the superior mesenteric artery and celiac artery and/or the internal iliac arteries by concomitant aortic reconstruction. Although the difference did not reach statistical significance, of the patients who had only a single bypass graft, 2 of 5 died of bowel infarction, by comparison to 1 of 16 patients who had multiple grafts who survived reoperation because of graft occlusion. Since all series are relatively small and not randomized, it is unlikely that this issue will be resolved.

Type of Graft

Saphenous and prosthetic grafts were used equally in our series and seem to provide equal patency rates with 2 of 10 prosthetic grafts thrombosing during follow-up compared to 1 of 11 of the saphenous grafts. However, saphenous vein may be preferable for bypasses to small branch arteries or for retrograde bypasses since kinking is less likely to be a problem. McMillan et al.,[6] Calderon et al.,[12] and Cormier et al.[24] agree with this observation, but Hollier et al.[13] and Zelenock et al.[27] prefer saphenous vein.

Preoperative Intravenous Alimentation

Although it seems logical to consider hyperalimentation preoperatively in order to improve postoperative healing and increase the patient's strength and thereby reduce the chances of pulmonary complications and complications from delayed mobilization, there is no evidence to support this approach. In general, alimentation of catabolic patients increases body fat and extracellular water but not protein mass. Randomized trials of preoperative total parenteral nutrition have failed to demonstrate a reduction in mortality or complication rates in malnourished surgical patients.[28] Recent experience with the administration of human growth factor in burn patients and others with evidence of severe catabolism[29] suggests that this approach may increase protein mass and may have application to patients with severe mesenteric ischemia and weight loss; however, no reports using this approach in patients with mesenteric ischemia have been published. Continued oral intake in the form of food or an elemental diet may have limited benefit secondary to the inability of the bowel to absorb the nutrients. Conversely, the supply of nutrients may aid in preservation of the mucosa. Therefore it seems logical to allow the patients to eat as much as possible preoperatively, schedule surgical revascularization as soon as possible, and resume oral intake as soon as possible. Early postoperative enteral feeding has been shown to reduce the negative nitrogen balance following major vascular surgery.[30]

MESENTERIC REVASCULARIZATION AT TIME OF AORTIC SURGERY

Very few cases of concomitant mesenteric revascularization have been reported along with abdominal aortic aneurysm repair or an aortobifemoral bypass. For example, of the 666 cases reported in the Canadian Aneurysm Study,[31] superior mesenteric artery bypass was performed in only 2 cases. In our series, only 4 patients had concomitant surgery and Rheudasil et al.[14] reported 10 patients. The following criteria are suggested indications for considering concomitant mesenteric bypass: symptomatic intestinal ischemia, severe mesenteric artery disease, less severe mesenteric arterial disease but associated with an arterial reconstruction that is likely to reduce visceral blood flow such as inability to maintain normal pelvic blood flow, or clinically apparent bowel ischemia at the conclusion of the surgery.

CONCLUSION

Although rare, some patients with acute visceral ischemia can be saved by mesenteric revascularization. Chronic visceral ischemia can be treated successfully by arterial reconstruction with a relatively low operative risk and most patients receive long-lasting benefit. The number of cases reported in the literature does not permit definitive conclusions concerning operative management; however, based on the authors' experience, the following are suggested. The graft should originate from the supraceliac aorta or lower thoracic aorta, sites that are less prone to the development of atherosclerosis than the abdominal aorta. Grafts in the prograde direction are less likely to kink than retrograde grafts. The type of graft is not important but saphenous vein may be of benefit if the distal anastomosis is to a small visceral artery. Although priority must be given to revascularization of the superior mesenteric artery, complete mesenteric revascularization does not add significantly to the procedure and better long-term results may be obtained. More definitive conclusions on management will be obtained from multicenter trials or regional databases since revascularization for chronic mesenteric ischemia is an infrequent vascular reconstruction.

Acknowledgment
The authors acknowledge the secretarial assistance of Ms. P. Purdy.

REFERENCES

1. Johnston KW, Lindsay TF, Walker PM, Kalman PG. Mesenteric arterial bypass grafts—early and late results and suggested surgical approach for chronic and acute mesenteric ischemia. *Surgery.* 1995;118:1–7.
2. Kach K, Largiader F. Acute mesenteric infarcts—results of surgical therapy. *Helv Chir Acta.* 1989;56:23–27.
3. Taylor LM, Moneta GL. Intestinal ischemia. *Ann Vasc Surg.* 1991;5:403–406.
4. Kaleya RN, Sammartano RJ, Boley SJ. Aggressive approach to acute mesenteric ischemia. *Surg Clin North Am.* 1992;72:157–182.
5. Batellier J, Kieny R. Superior mesenteric artery embolism: eighty-two cases. *Ann Vasc Surg.* 1990;4:112–116.
6. McMillan WO, McCarthy NJ, Bresticker MR, et al. Mesenteric artery bypass: objective patency determination. *J Vasc Surg.* 1995;21:729–740.
7. Wilcox MG, Howard TJ, Plaskon LA, et al. Current theoretics of pathogenesis and treatment of nonocclusive mesenteric ischemia. *Dig Dis Sci.* 1995;40:706–716.
8. Schneider TA, Longo WF, Ure T, Vernavo AM III. Mesenteric ischemia. Acute arterial syndromes. *Dis Colon Rectum.* 1994;37:1163–1174.
9. Harward TR, Green D, Bergan JJ, et al. Mestenteric venous thrombosis. *J Vasc Surg.* 1989;9:328–333.
10. Ghaly M, Frawley JE. Superior mesenteric vein thrombosis. *Aust NZ J Surg.* 1986;56:277–279.
11. Rapp JH, Reilly LM, Qvarfordt PG, et al. Durability of endarterectomy and antegrade grafts in the treatment of chronic visceral ischemia. *J Vasc Surg.* 1986;3:799–806.
12. Calderon M, Reul GJ, Gregoric ID, et al. Long-term results of the surgical management of symptomatic chronic intestinal ischemia. *J Cardiovasc Surg.* 1992;33:723–728.
13. Hollier LH, Bernatz PE, Pairolero PC, et al. Surgical management of chronic intestinal ischemia. *Surgery.* 1981;90:940–946.
14. Rheudasil JM, Stewart MT, Schellack JV, et al. Surgical treatment of chronic mesenteric arterial insufficiency. *J Vasc Surg.* 1988;8:495–500.
15. Reiner L, Jimenez FA, Rodriguez FL. Atherosclerosis in the mesenteric circulation. Observations and correlations with aortic and coronary atherosclerosis. *Am Heart J.* 1963;66:200–209.
16. Cunningham CG, Reilly LM, Rapp JH, et al. Chronic visceral ischemia. *Ann Surg.* 1991;214:276–288.
17. Harward TRS, Brooks DL, Flynn TC, Seeger JM. Multiple organ dysfunction after mesenteric artery revascularization. *J Vasc Surg.* 1993;18:459–469.
18. McAfee MK, Cherry KJ Jr, Naessens JM, et al. Influence of complete revascularization on chronic mesenteric ischemia. *Am J Surg.* 1992;164:220–224.
19. Kieny R, Batellier J, Kretz J-G. Aortic reimplantation of the superior mesenteric artery for atherosclerotic lesions of the visceral arteries: sixty cases. *Ann Vasc Surg.* 1990;4:122–125.
20. Matsumoto A, Tegtmeyer CJ, Fitzcharles BK, et al. Percutaneous transluminal angioplasty of visceral arterial stenoses: results and long-term clinical follow-up. *J Vasc Interv Radiol.* 1995;6:165–174.
21. Rose SC, Quigley TM, Baker EJ. Revascularization for chronic mesenteric ischemia: comparison of operative arterial bypass grafting and percutaneous transluminal angioplasty. *J Vasc Interv Radiol.* 1995;6:339–349.
22. Stanton PE Jr, Hollier PA, Seidel TW, et al. Chronic intestinal ischemia: diagnosis and therapy. *J Vasc Surg.* 1986;4:338–344.

23. Gentile AT, Moneta GL, Taylor LM Jr, et al. Isolated bypass to the superior mesenteric artery for intestinal ischemia. *Arch Surg.* 1994;129:926–931.

24. Cormier JM, Fichelle JM, Vennin J, et al. Atherosclerotic occlusive disease of the superior mesenteric artery: late results of reconstruction surgery. *Ann Vasc Surg.* 1991;5:510–518.

25. Gewertz BL, Zarins CK. Postoperative vasospasm after antegrade mesenteric revascularization: a report of three cases. *J Vasc Surg.* 1991;14:382–385.

26. Beebe HG, MacFarlane S, Raker EJ. Supraceliac aortomesenteric bypass for intestinal ischemia. *J Vasc Surg.* 1987;5:749–754.

27. Zelenock GB, Graham LM, Whitehouse WM. Splanchnic arteriosclerotic disease and intestinal angina. *Arch Surg.* 1980;115:497–501.

28. The Veterans Affairs Total Parenteral Nutrition Cooperative Study Group. Perioperative total parenteral nutrition in surgical patients. *N Engl J Med.* 1991;325:525–532.

29. Wilmore DW. Catabolic illness. Strategies for enhancing recovery. *N Engl J Med.* 1991; 325(10):695–702.

30. Fletcher JP, Little JM. A comparison of parenteral nutrition and early postoperative enteral feeding on the nitrogen balance after major surgery. *Surgery.* 1986;100:21–24.

31. Johnston KW, Scobie TK. Multicenter prospective study of non-ruptured abdominal aortic aneurysms. I. Population and operative management. *J Vasc Surg.* 1988;7:69–81.

18

Surgical Management of Ischemic Nephropathy

Robert D. Riley, MD, Kimberley J. Hansen, MD, and Richard H. Dean, MD

The usefulness of renal revascularization in controlling hypertension secondary to renal artery occlusive disease is widely recognized. Although the criteria for patient selection are still controversial, there is no denying the durable benefit derived by many patients. Alternatively, severe occlusive disease may lead to inadequate effective renal plasma flow and diminished excretory function of the kidney. Traditionally, study of the sequelae of renovascular occlusive disease has centered on the pathophysiology and management of the resultant renovascular hypertension. More recent reports, however, have emphasized the potential for simultaneous retrieval of excretory function in some patients with combined hypertension and renal insufficiency.[1-3] These observations have renewed awareness of this functional consequence of renal ischemia and have led to the coining of the term *ischemic nephropathy.* By definition, ischemic nephropathy reflects the presence of anatomically severe occlusive disease of the extraparenchymal renal artery in a patient with excretory renal insufficiency. The severely azotemic patient with renovascular occlusive disease more clearly resembles the atherosclerotic patient with end-stage disease than does the nonazotemic patient. Although retrieval of function has immediate practical significance, the hazard of aggravating renal failure to a dialysis-dependent level or of placing the patient with dialysis dependence at a potentially higher operative risk by inappropriate surgery tempers enthusiasm for a nonselective approach to the management of these patients.

Morris and associates,[4] reporting in 1962 on eight azotemic patients with either severe bilateral renal artery occlusions or unilateral occlusive disease and an absent contralateral kidney, described a salutary effect of revascularization on both hypertension and renal function. Novick and colleagues[5] found a similar beneficial functional response to renal revascularization when bilateral lesions were corrected in azotemic patients. Nevertheless, little information in the literature accurately describes the incidence, prevalence, spectrum of clinical presentations, and natural history of ischemic nephropathy. Circumstantial evidence, however, suggests that it may be a more common cause of progressive renal failure in the atherosclerotic age group than was previously recognized. In a 1986 survey, 73% of patients with end-stage renal disease were in the atherosclerotic age group.[6] In a report by Mailloux and coworkers,[7] a presumed renovascular cause of end-stage renal disease (ESRD) increased in frequency from 6.7% for the period between 1978 and 1981 to 16.5% for the period between 1982 and 1985. The median age at the onset of ESRD for this group was the highest among all groups: the seventh decade of life. Each clinical characteristic is in concert with the demographic data on the authors' reported patient group with proven ischemic nephropathy.[8] In the authors' group, all patients had at least moderate hypertension, the mean age was 63 years old, and only 14% had diabetes mellitus. The authors believe these data argue that renovascular disease may be either the primary cause or a superimposed secondary accelerant of renal insufficiency in a larger proportion of patients with renal insufficiency than is commonly recognized. Using this premise as a guide, the authors currently screen all adult patients older than 50 years of age who have newly recognized renal insufficiency when hypertension of any level is a coexistent morbidity.

DIAGNOSTIC EVALUATION

Renal duplex sonography is the authors' preferred method for preliminary screening. Their experience with the use of renal duplex sonography as a screening technique was previously reported.[9] In this review, the authors found renal duplex sonography to have an overall accuracy rate of 96% for establishing the presence or absence of main renal artery occlusive disease. Because the term *ischemic nephropathy* implies the presence of global renal ischemia, the authors believe that renal duplex sonography, when performed by an experienced technician, is an adequate method for initially screening the patient with renal insufficiency. Through preliminary screening with renal duplex sonography, the authors limit the use of arteriography in patients with renal insufficiency to those with either positive findings on renal duplex sonography or severe hypertension.

The authors have continued to rely on standard cut-film arteriography in patients with renal insufficiency who have clinical or duplex sonographic evidence of renovascular disease. In the authors' experience, adequate assessment of the renal vasculature and the juxtarenal aorta requires multiple injections when intra-arterial digital subtraction angiography is employed. The use of a single midstream flush aortogram requires no more contrast material than that required for such multiple intra-arterial digital subtraction studies. In addition, standard arteriography provides information about cortical thickness and renal length, as well as improved clarity for interpretation of the renal artery anatomy. The fact that arteriography in patients with severe renal insufficiency, especially those with concomitant diabetes mellitus, can aggravate renal failure is widely recognized. Nevertheless, the authors believe that this risk is justified in such patients who have severe or accelerated hypertension or who have positive findings on renal duplex sonography. In these circumstances, the potential benefit derived from identification and correction of a functionally significant renovascular occlusive lesion exceeds the risk of arteriography.

Evaluation with renal vein renin (RVR) assays is useful less frequently in this patient population because the majority of patients have bilateral disease. Nevertheless, when a unilateral lesion is present, decisions regarding management should be based on both anatomic and functional assessments.

OVERALL EXPERIENCE WITH OPERATIVE MANAGEMENT

During the past two decades the introduction of new antihypertensive agents and percutaneous transluminal angioplasty (PTA) has changed many attitudes regarding the role of surgical intervention for renovascular disease (RVD).[10,11] New treatment alternatives combined with the increasingly older patient population seeking treatment for RVD have led many physicians to limit surgical intervention to patients demonstrating severe hypertension despite maximal medical therapy, patients demonstrating anatomic failures or disease patterns not amenable to PTA, or patients with RVD complicated by renal excretory insufficiency (i.e., ischemic nephropathy).[12] As a consequence of these changing attitudes and treatment strategies, the demography of the contemporary patient population has also changed.[13,14] Currently, patient populations are characterized by the predominance of atherosclerotic RVD complicated by site-specific atherosclerotic organ damage and renal insufficiency. Consequently, the contemporary results of surgical management of RVD differ significantly from earlier reported series.[15,16]

To examine the changes that have occurred in both the patient population presenting for operative management and the results of operation during the past two decades, we have reviewed our experience over a recent 54-month period.[17] During this period, we submitted 200 patients to operation for presumed renovascular hypertension, ischemic nephropathy, and renal artery aneurysms. Forty-three patients with nonatherosclerotic RVD included 12 men and 31 women, ranging in age from 5 to 66 years (mean age, 38 ± 17 years), who demonstrated either fibromuscular dysplasia (FMD) (39 patients: 34 medial fibroplasia, 4 intimal fibroplasia, 1 perimedial dysplasia), renal artery dissection (3 patients: 2 traumatic, 1 spontaneous), or transplant renal artery stenosis (1 patient). Of the remaining 157 patients with atherosclerotic RVD, there were 80 men and 77 women, with ages ranging from 37 to 80 years (mean age, 62 ± 9 years). Ninety (57%) of these patients were older than the age of 60, and 29 patients were in their eighth decade of life. Hypertension was present in 156 patients with atherosclerosis and ranged from 178/90 to 300/178 mm Hg (mean, 212/114 mm Hg). Hypertension had been recognized for 1 to 30 years (mean duration, 15 ± 7 years), and drug regimens used to control hypertension before surgery ranged from zero to six agents (mean, 2.8 ± 1.2 agents). Overall, 62% of patients had been hypertensive for more than 5 years, and 59% of patients required three or more antihypertensive medications. In addition to hypertension, 149 patients (95%) with atherosclerotic RVD demonstrated one or more risk factors for atherosclerosis, including cigarette use (128 patients), hyperlipidemia (35 patients), and diabetes mellitus (26 patients). Evidence of at least one of the following manifestations of organ-specific atherosclerotic damage was present in 147 patients with atherosclerotic RVD (94%): cardiac disease (75%), cerebrovascular disease (33%), and/or renal disease (60%). Only 8 patients were completely free of all organ-specific damage (Table 18–1).

Defined by a serum creatinine level of 1.3 mg/dL or greater after the removal of high-dose diuretics and angiotensin-converting enzyme inhibitors, 117 patients (75%) with atherosclerotic RVD had evidence of renal insufficiency (ischemic nephropathy). Seventy patients (45%) were considered to have severe insufficiency (serum creatinine >2.0 mg/dL), and 23 patients had extreme renal insufficiency (serum creatinine ≥3.0 mg/dL).

After operation five patients with atherosclerotic RVD died within 30 days of surgery. These were considered operative deaths, producing an overall operative mortality rate of 2.5% (0% for nonatherosclerotic RVD, 3.1% for atherosclerotic RVD). Operative deaths occurred in association with diffuse (two patients) and extreme (three patients) disease requiring either intermediate (three patients) or complex (two patients) repairs (Table 18–2). Definitions of severity of disease and complexity of operation are shown in Table 18–3. Operative deaths in two patients were a result of hemispheric cerebrovascular accidents apparent at the conclusion of the surgical procedure. Each

TABLE 18–1. PREVALENCE OF ASSOCIATED AORTOILIAC AND ORGAN-SPECIFIC ATHEROSCLEROSIS (*n* = 157 patients)

	No. of Patients	Clinical Manifestations	
Cardiac	117 (75%)	Angina	50
		MI	57
		LVH	92
		Strain pattern	35
		CABG/PTA	18
Cerebrovascular	52 (34%)	TIA	22
		CVA	28
		CEA	12
Renal	94 (61%)	Creatinine > 2.0 mg/dL	71
		Dialysis	11
		Nephrectomy	11
		Bypass/PTA	38
Aortoiliac	111 (72%)	Severe occlusive disease	86
		Aortic occlusion	17
		Aortic aneurysm	25
At least one manifestation present	147 (94%)		

MI, myocardial infarction; LVH, left ventricular hypertrophy; CABG, coronary artery bypass graft; PTA, percutaneous transluminal angioplasty; TIA, transient ischemic attack; CVA, cerebrovascular accident; CEA, carotid endarterectomy.

patient had a negative history and negative carotid duplex examination for significant extracranial carotid disease on the affected side. Two patients died after aspiration pneumonia and sepsis culminating in multisystem organ failure. One patient with hepatic cirrhosis died of postoperative bleeding after repair of a symptomatic renal artery aneurysm. There were no operative deaths among patients with nonatherosclerotic RVD, atherosclerotic patients with limited disease, or patients who had simple operative procedures. Two *ex vivo* reconstructions and two renal artery bypass grafts (1.4%) failed within 30 days of operation. In each case the kidney could not be salvaged at reoperation and a nephrectomy was required.

Patency of renovascular repairs was determined from 1 to 54 months after operation (mean, 16 months) in 158 patients (79%) with either angiography (32 patients), renal duplex sonography (RDS) (88 patients), or with both tests (38 patients). In addition to the failure of four repairs within 30 days of operation, follow-up angiography and RDS demonstrated two occlusions (both kidneys salvaged by reoperation) and two critical restenoses. The combined early and follow-up primary patency rate for 228 renal artery repairs studied with angiography or RDS was 97%. During this same time period, four

TABLE 18–2. OPERATIVE DEATHS

Age (yrs)	Disease		Complexity of Repair	Cause of Death
	Type	Extent		
64	As-RVD	Extreme	Intermediate	Pneumonia MSOF
66	As-RVD	Diffuse	Complex	Pneumonia MSOF
68	As-RVD	Diffuse	Complex	Postoperative bleeding
69	As-RVD	Extreme	Intermediate	CVA
70	As-RVD	Extreme	Intermediate	CVA

MSOF, multisystem organ failure; CVA, cerebrovascular accident.

TABLE 18–3. EXTENT OF ATHEROSCLEROSIS AND COMPLEXITY OF PROCEDURE DEFINITION AND PREVALENCE

Extent of Disease	No. of Patients (%)[a]	Procedure	No. of Patients (%)[b]
Limited disease Atherosclerosis of the renal artery(ies) and up to one extrarenal site	19 (12)	Simple Unilateral renal artery reconstruction Primary nephrectomy	63 (31)
Diffuse disease Atherosclerosis of the renal artery(ies) and two or more extrarenal sites	82 (52)	Intermediate Unilateral *in situ* branch repair Bilateral renal artery reconstruction Unilateral reconstruction with aortic repair	79 (40)
Extreme disease Diffuse atherosclerosis in combination with one or more of the following: (1) LVEF <30% (2) Clinical CHF (3) Serum creatinine >3.0 mg/d	56 (36)	Complex *Ex vivo* branch repair Bilateral reconstruction combined with aortic repair Reconstruction combined with suprarenal aortic or visceral artery repair	58 (29)

[a] Based on the 157 patients with atherosclerosis.
[b] Based on the entire 200 patients.

unoperated native renal arteries (6.6%) developed significant RVD contralateral to previous renovascular repairs.

HYPERTENSION RESPONSE

On the basis of criteria previously described, hypertension among the 195 survivors of surgery was considered cured in 41 patients (21%), improved in 137 (70%), and unchanged in 17 (9%) (Table 18–4). Overall, 91% of patients were considered to demonstrate a favorable hypertension response. Among the 43 patients with nonatherosclerotic RVD, hypertension was considered cured in 43%, improved in 49%, and unchanged in 8%. Among the 152 patients with atherosclerosis surviving operation, 15% were cured, 75% were improved, and 10% were unchanged. Among the patients with RVR assays, 98% of patients with lateralizing renin activity had a beneficial blood pressure response, whereas 87% of patients with nonlateralizing renin activity were improved. In this latter group 10 of 24 patients demonstrated severe bilateral RVD. Equivalent

TABLE 18–4. BLOOD PRESSURE RESPONSE TO OPERATION (n = 195 PATIENTS)

Response	All Patients		Nonatherosclerotic RVD Patients		Atherosclerotic RVD Patients	
	No.	%	No.	%	No.	%
Cured	41	21	19	44	22	15
Improved	137	70	21	49	116	76
Failed	17	9	3	7	14	9
Total	195		43		152	

blood pressure benefit was realized irrespective of patient age, duration of hypertension, complexity of repair, or extent of associated atherosclerotic disease.

EFFECT OF BLOOD PRESSURE RESPONSE ON LONG-TERM SURVIVAL

Since the logic for management of hypertension of any cause is to improve long-term cardiovascular morbidity and event-free survival, we reviewed the outcome of 71 patients who underwent operative management of renovascular hypertension (RVH) from 15 to 23 years previously.[18] Complete follow-up was available in 66 of the 68 patients who survived operation. Comparison of the initial blood pressure response to operation (1 to 6 months postoperatively) to the blood pressure status at the time of death or current date (up to 23 years later) shows that the effect of operative treatment is maintained over long-term follow-up (Fig. 18–1). In those patients who required repeat renovascular operation for recurrent RVH during follow-up, the majority of the operations were performed for the management of contralateral lesions that had progressed to functional significance (i.e., produced RVH).

Assessment of the effect of blood pressure response on late survival produced results that are not surprising. Although the subgroup of nonresponders is small, they experienced a significantly more rapid death rate during follow-up than did those patients who had a blood pressure response to operation (Fig. 18–2). This confirms the validity of the premise that inadequate management of RVH leaves the patient at higher risk of early death from cardiovascular events. The presence of angiographically diffuse atherosclerosis at the time of evaluation and operation was predictive of a more rapid rate of death during follow-up (Fig. 18–3). This difference in subsequent death rate was present, even though comparison between patients with diffuse atherosclerotic disease (ASD) and focal atherosclerotic (ASF) was undertaken only in patients experiencing a significant blood pressure response. In view of the suggestion by some physi-

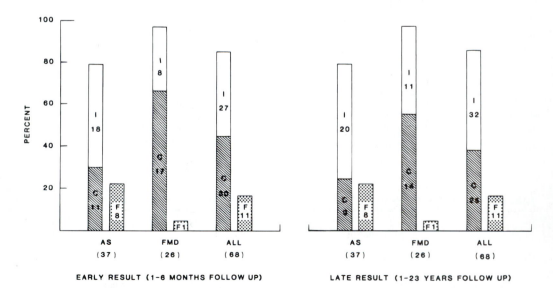

Figure 18–1. Bar graphs comparing initial benefit with late blood pressure response in the respective types of lesions. (*From Dean RH, Krueger TC, Whiteneck JM, et al. Operative management of renovascular hypertension. J Vasc Surg. 1984;1:234. Used by permission.*)

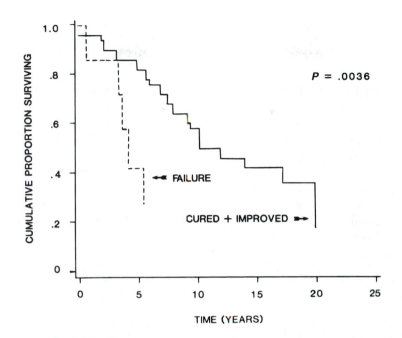

Figure 18–2. Kaplan-Meier life table analysis: survival by response to operation in 37 arteriosclerotic patients (deaths from cardiovascular causes). (*From Dean RH, Krueger, TC, Whiteneck, JM, et al. Operative management of renovascular hypertension. J Vasc Surg. 1984;1:234. Used by permission.*)

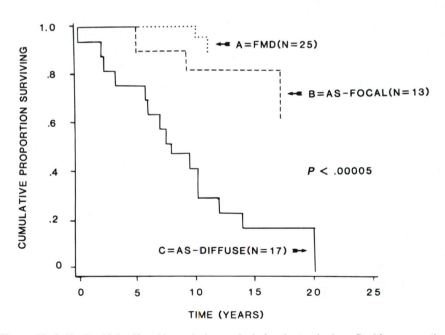

Figure 18–3. Kaplan-Meier life table analysis: survival of patients who benefited from operation by type and stage of disease (deaths from cardiovascular causes). FMD, fibromuscular dysplasia; AS-focal, focal atherosclerosis; AS-diffuse, diffuse atherosclerosis. (*From Dean RH, Krueger TC, Whiteneck JM, et al. Operative management of renovascular hypertension. J Vasc Surg. 1984;1:234. Used by permission.*)

cians that the presence of diffuse disease precludes a high rate of blood pressure response to operation, it is worthwhile to stress that there was no significant difference in frequency of response between the ASF (80%) and ASD (77%) groups in this study. In addition, although the presence of ASD was associated with a more rapid death rate, it does not preclude the probability of a longer survival in this subgroup when compared with a similar group of patients who either did not undergo operation or received no blood pressure benefit from such intervention. Furthermore, if one considers that ASD is only a later stage of ASF, it is not surprising that the end point of clinically significant disease, namely, death from cardiovascular events, arrives sooner when one begins follow-up or removes a risk factor, which causes its acceleration later in its natural history.

EXPERIENCE WITH ISCHEMIC NEPHROPATHY

To improve the understanding of ischemic nephropathy, the authors undertook a retrospective review of data collected during a 42-month period from 58 consecutive patients with ischemic nephropathy who had operative treatment at the authors' center (Bowman Gray School of Medicine at Wake Forest University).[8] The rate of decline in their renal function during the period before intervention and the impact of surgery on their outcome were examined. Patient ages ranged from 22 to 79 years (mean, 69 years). Based on serum creatinine values, immediate preoperative estimated glomerular filtration rates (EGFRs) ranged from 0 to 46 mL/min (mean, 23.85 ± 9.76 mL/min). Eight patients were dialysis dependent or anuric at the time of operation. Patients with at least three sequential measurements for calculations of EGFR changes during the 6 months before operation ($n = 32$) were used to describe the preoperative rate of decline in EGFR and the impact of operation on this decrease in the operative survivors. In addition, comparative analyses were performed of data from patients with unilateral versus bilateral lesions and patients classified as having improvement in EGFR versus no improvement after operation. Comparison of the immediate preoperative EGFR with the immediate postoperative EGFR for the entire group showed significant improvement in response to operation (Fig. 18–4).

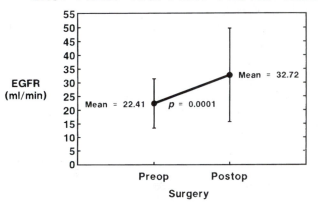

Figure 18–4. Comparison of the EGFR immediately before and at least 1 week after operation. The *p* value for differences is determined using the *t*-test for unpaired data. (*From Dean RH, Tribble RW, Hansen KJ, et al. Evolution of renal insufficiency in ischemic nephropathy. Ann Surg. 1991;213:446. Used by permission.*)

TABLE 18–5. ESTIMATED GLOMERULAR FILTRATION RATE RESPONSE VERSUS SITE OF OPERATION

| Operation | No. of Patients | Estimated Glomerular Filtration Rate (mL/min)[a] | | |
		Preoperative	*Postoperative*	*p Value[b]*
Unilateral	12	25.94 + 11.86	29.14 + 14.34	.1633
Bilateral	41	21.38 + 8.89	33.77 + 18.39	.0001

Note: Operative deaths and patients who were preoperatively dialysis dependent were excluded from the analysis.
[a] Values are mean ± SD.
[b] The *p* values are for the paired *t*-test.

The immediate impact of operation on the EGFR when results were examined according to the site of disease and operation is summarized in Table 18–5. In this evaluation, lesions (and procedures) to solitary kidneys and procedures consisting of unilateral revascularization with contralateral nephrectomy are recorded with the bilateral group. As noted in Table 18–5, when the groups were evaluated according to the site of operation, the bilateral group experienced a significant improvement in EGFR after operation ($p = 0.0001$). Although five patients (31%) in the unilateral group had an improvement in EGFR (a 20% or greater increase in EGFR) after operation (Table 18–6, no statistically significant benefit was seen when all patients with unilateral disease were collectively evaluated (see Table 18–5).

Figure 18–5 shows the rapid rate of change in EGFR for the entire group for the 6 months before operation and the beneficial impact of revascularization on this decline. Retrospective comparison of the rate of deterioration in EGFR before operation for the group who had improvement in EGFR by operation versus those receiving no benefit suggests that the rate of decline in GFR may have value in predicting the probability of retrieval of GFR by operation (Figs. 18–6 and 18–7). Unfortunately, the heterogenicity of individual slopes of change in EGFR prevent comment on a critical rate of decline that would predict retrieval of renal function by operation. Nevertheless, a rapidly deteriorating GFR should alert the physician to the potential presence of ischemic nephropathy and should argue for the likelihood of retrieval of function by operation when ischemic nephropathy is identified.

Renal revascularization had a beneficial impact on both the rate of decline in EGFR and EGFR itself when data for the entire group were analyzed collectively. Nevertheless, when data were analyzed with respect to the individual subgroups, the salutary effect of operation on the rate of deterioration of EGFR was seen only in the subset that experienced an immediate improvement in EGFR by operation.

TABLE 18–6. RENAL FUNCTION RESPONSE VERSUS SITE OF DISEASE IN PATIENTS WITH SEVERE RENAL INSUFFICIENCY ($n = 70$)

| Change in EGFR[a] | Unilateral | | Bilateral[b] | |
	No.	*%*	*No.*	*%*
Improved	5	31	29	54
No change	9	56	16	30
Worsened	2	13	9	16
Total	16		54	

[a] Significant change is ≥20% change in EGFR.
[b] Bilateral renal artery repair, unilateral repair of solitary kidney, or unilateral repair with contralateral nephrectomy.

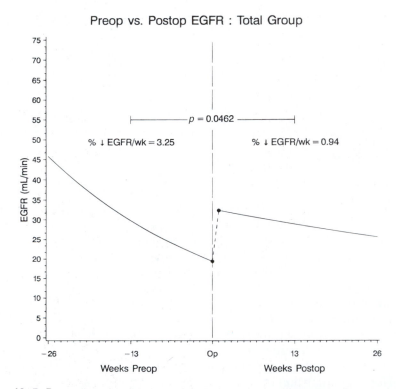

Figure 18–5. Percentage deterioration in EGFR per week for the entire group during the 6 months before (*n* = 50) and after (*n* = 32) operation. The immediate effect of operation on EGFR is also depicted. The *p* values for differences are determined using the *t*-test for unpaired data. Note the improvement in the slope of decline in EGFR after operation. (*From Dean RH, Tribble RW, Hansen KJ, et al. Evolution of renal insufficiency in ischemic nephropathy. Ann Surg. 1991;213:446. Used by permission.*)

This observation may have major clinical significance because the detrimental effect of renovascular occlusive disease may theoretically be from either of two causes. First, the lesion may limit renal perfusion to a degree that it affects excretory function. Second, it may be the source of microscopic atheroembolization that destroys functioning renal parenchyma. The authors' data suggest that correction of lesions causing reversible ischemia will provide both an immediate improvement in EGFR and a slowing of its rate of decline when compared with the preoperative rate of decline. Unfortunately, when the lesion was not producing significant reversible ischemia, as reflected by the absence of improvement in EGFR immediately after operation, no improvement in the rate of decline in EGFR was realized after operation. This argues that when atheroembolism is the only potentially active pathophysiologic consequence of the lesion, its correction may not lead to clinically important slowing of the rate of deterioration in renal function.

The authors' experience underscores the rapidity of the deterioration in renal function in patients with ischemic nephropathy and demonstrates the potential benefit of operation on both GFR and its rate of deterioration in this subset of patients. Nevertheless, the risk associated with operation is not inconsequential. Nevertheless, this risk and the rate of survival must be placed into context with the probability of survival without operation. In a study of the duration of survival following the institution of dialysis, Mailloux and coworkers[7] found that ESRD caused by uncorrected renovascular disease was associated with the most rapid

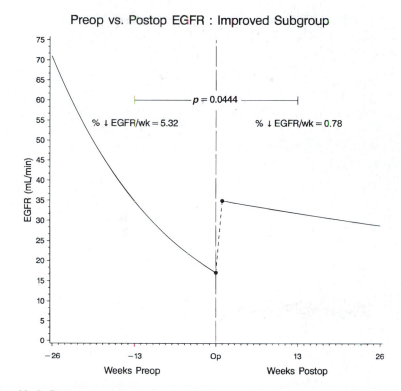

Figure 18–6. Percentage deterioration in EGFR per week during the 6 months before ($n =$ 23) and after ($n = 25$) operation in the group of patients who had at least a 20% improvement in EGFR following operation. The immediate effect of operation on EGFR in this group is also depicted. The p values for differences are determined using the t-test for unpaired data. Note the improvement in the slope of decline in EGFR after operation in this group. (*From Dean RH, Tribble RW, Hansen KJ, et al. Evolution of renal insufficiency in ischemic nephropathy. Ann Surg. 1991;213:446. Used by permission.*)

rate of death during follow-up. In their study, patients with renovascular disease had a median survival after the initiation of dialysis of only 27 months and a 5-year survival rate of only 12%. This equates with a death rate in excess of 20% per year. In this regard we have recently reported our experience with 20 patients who were dialysis dependent at the time of operation. There were no operative deaths in this group and 16 (80%) (Table 18–7) were rendered free of dialysis postoperatively.[19] Their life table survival curve is shown in Figure 18–8. Survival in those rendered dialysis independent was excellent. Those not freed from dialysis by operation had a death rate during follow-up similar to Mailloux's group not submitted to operation.

Not all patients with azotemia and even bilateral renal artery stenosis can be expected to benefit from revascularization. Preoperative indicators that influence the potential for functional retrieval in this group are the severity of the occlusive lesions and the type of hypertension. Functionally severe bilateral renal artery occlusions produce a particularly severe and difficult-to-control variety of hypertension. When such hypertension is present in combination with correctable bilateral stenosis or occlusions, revascularization should dramatically alleviate both the hypertension and the concomitant azotemia. In these patients, preoperative dependence on dialysis is not a negative factor for a successful outcome, even though some physicians do not believe that such revascularization can reverse long-standing dialysis dependence. This belief

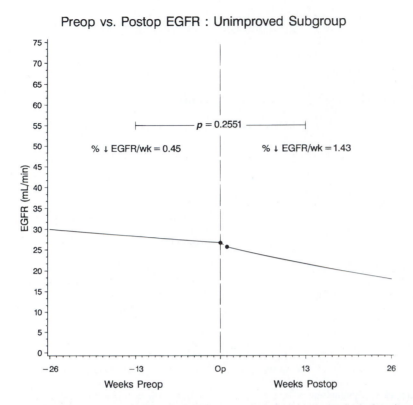

Figure 18–7. Percentage deterioration in EGFR per week during the 6 months before (*n* = 18) and after (*n* = 8) operation in the group of patients who had no significant immediate benefit in EGFR after operation. The *p* values for differences are determined using the *t*-test for unpaired data. Note the absence of improvement in the rate of deterioration of EGFR after operation in this group. (*From Dean RH, Tribble RW, Hansen KJ, et al. Evolution of renal insufficiency in ischemic nephropathy. Ann Surg. 1991;213:446. Used by permission.*)

has little practical significance because these patients have little to lose from revascularization. They have the greatest potential for retrieval of function with revascularization and only a minimal chance for prolonged survival without operation because of their dialysis-dependent renal failure combined with their severe, uncontrollable hypertension.

TABLE 18-7. IMMEDIATE AND LATE FUNCTION RESPONSE VERSUS SITE OF DISEASE

Dialysis Status	Unilateral (*n* = 4) No. of Patients (%)	Bilateral (*n* = 16) No. of Patients (%)	Total (*n* = 20) No. of Patients (%)
Immediate results[a]			
Dependent	3 (75)	1 (6)	4 (20)
Independent	1 (25)	15 (94)	16 (80)
Late results[b]			
Dependent	3 (75)	3 (19)	6 (30)
Independent	1 (25)	13 (81)	14 (70)

[a] *p* = 0.01, significant at the 0.05 alpha level after controlling for multiple comparisons.
[b] *p* = 0.06.

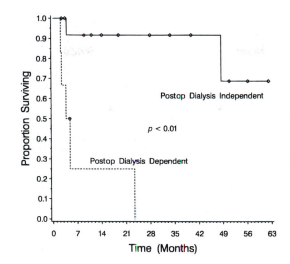

Figure 18–8. Product-limit estimate of patient survival according to dialysis status after operation ($n = 20$). (*From Hansen KJ, Thomason RB, Craven TE, et al. Surgical management of dialysis-dependent ischemic nephropathy. J Vasc Surg. 1995;21:197–211. Used by permission.*)

In contrast, the absence of hypertension in the patient with renovascular occlusions and azotemia should argue against the probability that revascularization will improve renal function. Such lesions are apparently not of physiologic significance because they are not producing an integral response to ischemia, namely, hypertension. Therefore, the physician should hesitate to consider revascularization in an azotemic normotensive patient because the risk of aggravating renal failure outweighs the probability that function will be improved by such intervention.

Consideration must also be given to the patient with chronic occlusive disease whose onset of oliguria or anuria is acute. This acute onset is usually the consequence of acute thrombosis in the stenotic artery to a solitary kidney or to the only kidney with previous significant residual function. Most of these patients will present with a history of hypertension, the severity of which was acutely accelerated, and the acute development of oliguric renal failure. Diagnostic evaluation of any patient presenting with such signs should include angiography. Although physicians were reticent in the past to perform angiography because of the nephrotoxic effect of the large amount of contrast material necessary for such an evaluation, the current use of "one-shot" aortography has greatly lessened the potential renal insult.

Although many physicians are tempted to react to the acute clinical presentation with immediate operation and attempted revascularization, a more carefully planned approach is superior. Because the acute event is usually at least 24 hours old and primarily represents a reduction in perfusion to below the critical level for maintaining urinary output, preoperative correction of metabolic derangements is essential to reduce the risk of surgical intervention. Thus, the patient may require several days of dialysis or the correction of other, more lethal cardiac derangements before renal revascularization can be attempted. The physician should remember that renal failure can be controlled by hemodialysis while hypertension and cardiac risk factors are decreased and that the amount of retrievable renal function is not dependent on the timing of intervention. In most of these patients, urine flow is almost instantaneous after completion of the revascularization, and the majority of patients will require no further dialysis in the immediate postoperative period.

REFERENCES

1. Scobie JE, Maher ER, Hamilton G, et al. Atherosclerotic renovascular disease causing renal impairment—a case for treatment. *Clin Nephrol.* 1989;31:119.
2. Bengtsson U, Bergentz S-E, Norback B. Surgical treatment of renal artery stenosis with impending uremia. *Clin Nephrol.* 1974;2:222.
3. Novick AC, Pohl MA, Schreiber M, et al. Revascularization for preservation of renal function in patients with atherosclerotic renovascular disease. *J Urol.* 1983;129:907.
4. Morris GC Jr, DeBakey ME, Cooley DA. Surgical treatment of renal failure of renovascular origin. *JAMA.* 1962;182:609.
5. Novick AC, Pohl MA, Schreiber M, et al. Revascularization for preservation of renal function in patients with atherosclerotic renovascular disease. *J Urol.* 1983;129:907.
6. *Annual Report.* Raleigh, NC: NC Kidney Council; 1986.
7. Mailloux LU, Bellucci AG, Mossey RT, et al. Predictors of survival in patients undergoing dialysis. *Am J Med.* 1988;84:855.
8. Dean RH, Tribble RW, Hansen KJ, et al. Evolution of renal insufficiency in ischemic nephropathy. *Ann Surg.* 1991;213:446.
9. Hansen KJ, Tribble RW, Reavis SW, et al. Renal duplex sonography: evaluation of clinical utility. *J Vasc Surg.* 1990;12:227.
10. Maxwell MH, Waks AU. Renovascular hypertension: current approaches to management. *Pract Cardiol.* 1987;13:128–137.
11. Cumberland DC. Percutaneous transluminal angioplasty: a review. *Clin Radiol.* 1983;34:25–36.
12. Vaughan ED, Case DB, Pickering TG, et al. Indication for intervention in patients with renovascular hypertension. *Am J Kidney Dis.* 1985;5:A136–A143.
13. Libertino JA, Flam TA, Zinman LN, et al. Changing concepts in surgical management of renovascular hypertension. *Arch Intern Med.* 1988;148:357–359.
14. Novick AC, Ziegelbaum M, Vidt DG, et al. Trends in surgical revascularization for renal artery disease. *JAMA.* 1987;257:498–501.
15. Stanley JC, Fry WJ. Surgical treatment of renovascular hypertension. *Arch Surg.* 1977;112:1291–1297.
16. Hansen KJ, Ditesheim JA, Metropol SH, et al. Management of renovascular hypertension in the elderly population. *J Vasc Surg.* 1989;10:266–273.
17. Hansen KJ, Starr SM, Sands RE, et al. Contemporary surgical management of renovascular disease, *J Vasc Surg.* 1992;16:319–331.
18. Dean RH, Krueger TC, Whiteneck JM, et al. Operative management of renovascular hypertension: results after 15-23 years follow-up. *J Vasc Surg.* 1984;1:234.
19. Hansen KJ, Thomason RB, Craven TE, et al. Surgical management of dialysis-dependent ischemic nephropathy. *J Vasc Surg.* 1995;21:197–211.

19

Results of Endovascular Stent-Grafting in Patients with Descending Thoracic Aortic Aneurysm

James I. Fann, MD, R. Scott Mitchell, MD,
Michael D. Dake, MD, and
D. Craig Miller, MD

With an annual incidence approximating 6 cases per 100,000 population, patients with thoracic aortic aneurysms are not infrequently encountered by vascular and cardiac surgeons.[1] The ascending aorta is affected most often (50% of all thoracic aortic aneurysms), with the descending thoracic aorta involved in less than one-half of cases (40%) and the aortic arch in a smaller fraction.[1,2] The vast majority of descending thoracic aortic aneurysms are the result of atherosclerosis, while medial degeneration is the most common etiology of ascending and arch aortic aneurysms.[2–4] Less frequent causes include infection, trauma, Marfan syndrome, and congenital aortic anomalies.

Atherosclerotic descending thoracic aortic aneurysms occur more frequently in men than women, with a mean age in the mid-60s at the time of diagnosis.[2–7] In this patient population, coexistent medical illnesses include coronary artery disease (29% of patients) and peripheral vascular disease; 13% to 29% of patients have an associated abdominal aortic aneurysm, 6% have cerebrovascular disease, and 4% suffer from peripheral arterial occlusive disease.[2–4,6–8] In addition, hypertension is present in more than one-half of cases, chronic obstructive pulmonary disease (COPD) in one-third, and congestive heart failure in 10%.[3,4,6,8]

Untreated, thoracic aortic aneurysms progressively enlarge and eventually rupture. Of those patients followed medically, 40% to 74% developed aneurysm rupture with a >90% fatality rate; up to one-third died from unrelated cardiovascular disease.[1,2,8] Of the patients who sustained a ruptured aneurysm, 68% occurred more than 1 month after the time of diagnosis. The average survival time was less than 3 years from the time of diagnosis.[2] For patients with thoracic aortic aneurysms not treated surgically, the actuarial survival estimates at 1 and 5 years were 60% and 20%, respectively.[1,2]

The conventional approach to management of patients with descending thoracic aortic aneurysms is open surgical aortic replacement with a tubular Dacron graft. An alternative method developed at Stanford University is endovascular stent-grafting; this technique is less invasive, potentially less expensive, and may be associated with lower morbidity than open surgical repair.[5,9–11] In this chapter, we review the results of the conventional approach and our initial experience with endovascular stent-grafting of descending thoracic aortic aneurysms.

CLINICAL EVALUATION

Because more than one-half of patients with descending thoracic aortic aneurysms are asymptomatic, the diagnosis is often suspected based on an abnormal chest radiograph or during evaluation for some other illness.[2,4,6,8] In patients with symptoms, back or chest pain is most common and is usually localized near the site of the aneurysm. Other signs and symptoms include compression or erosion of adjacent structures and are manifested as hoarseness from stretching or compression of the left recurrent laryngeal nerve, tracheal deviation and respiratory symptoms resulting from airway compression, hemoptysis from bronchial or pulmonary erosion, dysphagia from esophageal compression, neurologic deficits from spinal cord ischemia, and upper body venous distention due to superior vena cava syndrome.[5,6,8]

Evaluation prior to surgical repair includes assessment of the patient's cerebrovascular, cardiac, pulmonary, and renal status. Imaging of the descending thoracic aorta usually includes aortography and computed tomography (CT) or magnetic resonance imaging (MRI). In planning the surgical approach, aortography is useful in assessing adjacent aortic branches, including the intercostal arteries. CT (axial or spiral) or MRI provides valuable information regarding the pathoanatomic aspects of the aneurysm and other changes in contiguous structures. Coronary arteriography is obtained in those clinically suspected of having coronary artery disease.

CONVENTIONAL SURGICAL THERAPY

Because of the risk of rupture if untreated, therapeutic intervention is considered in all cases of descending thoracic aortic aneurysm. Operative repair is warranted in symptomatic patients; in those who are asymptomatic, an aneurysm diameter twice the diameter of a relatively normal contiguous segment of aorta (if such is present), an absolute size greater than 6 cm, or documented aneurysm enlargement over time are operative indications.[3,8] Smaller aneurysms are followed with serial CT or MRI scans every 6 to 12 months; surgical repair is recommended if progressive expansion occurs. Medical management is aimed at controlling associated diseases, such as hypertension and COPD.

Results with Conventional "Open" Surgical Procedures

The overall operative mortality rate for patients undergoing resection of descending thoracic aortic aneurysms averages 11%.[3,4,6,7,12–21] The operative mortality rate for patients who require emergency procedures is up to sevenfold higher than that for those individuals undergoing elective procedures. Emergency operation and congestive heart failure were independent risk factors for operative death in the earlier Stanford experience.[3] Factors that did not correlate significantly with hospital mortality included age, hypertension, chronic lung disease, previous myocardial infarction, angina, etiology of aneurysm, and aneurysm location.[3] The actuarial survival estimates for discharged patients were 70% to 79% at 5 years and 40% to 49% at 10 years.[3,4,6,12,20] Late deaths were due to cardiovascular and cerebrovascular events in 41% to 59% of cases and rupture of another aortic aneurysm in 20% to 25% of cases.[3,6]

Notwithstanding improved surgical techniques and intraoperative monitoring, major operative complications include paraplegia and renal insufficiency (due to hypoperfusion of the anterior spinal cord tracts and kidneys).[12,15] Emphasis has been properly placed on elective operation prior to rupture, preservation of spinal cord perfusion when feasible, expeditious operation, and prevention of hemorrhage and hypotension to improve the results. Although distal circulatory perfusion, including extracorporeal circulation (or temporary extravascular shunting in the past), is useful in providing cardiac decompression and reducing distal ischemic injury, it does not necessarily eliminate the risk of paraplegia (which averages 4%) or renal insufficiency (which averages 5%).[3,6,7,12-23]

Factors contributing to postoperative paraparesis or paraplegia include the degree of spinal cord ischemia during the aortic cross-clamp period (which is dependent on the extent of aneurysmal disease, available collateral channels, and cross-clamp time) and permanent exclusion of critical intercostal arteries with aortic graft replacement.[24-26] Important clinical determinants of postoperative renal failure include advanced age, atherosclerotic etiology, emergency operation, and preoperative renal dysfunction.[7,23]

ENDOVASCULAR STENT-GRAFTING

Evaluation of patients prior to endovascular stent-grafting of descending thoracic aortic pathology is similar to that for the conventional, open surgical approach; indeed, emergency conversion to an open procedure should the endovascular approach be unsuccessful is a real possibility in most patients. In addition, selection criteria have been developed and include the following: The proximal and distal aneurysm neck does not involve the origin of the left subclavian artery or the celiac axis; the aneurysm neck is of relatively small caliber (i.e., less than 4 cm); the aneurysm is fairly localized; the aneurysm is amenable to the placement of a stent-graft (e.g., patients with chronic dissection are usually excluded since the true lumen is small and distorted and the false lumen is large and eccentric); and there is adequate peripheral arterial or abdominal aortic access for the large (27 or 20 Fr outer diameter) delivery devices.[9] With greater experience, the strict requirement regarding the proximal neck has been modified such that involvement of the subclavian artery is no longer a contraindication since a left carotid-subclavian transposition (or bypass) can be performed beforehand to permit deployment of the endovascular stent-graft with the proximal fixation point in the distal arch.

Diagnostically, chest radiography is obtained followed by CT, preferably with spiral acquisition to provide a three-dimensional reconstruction of the descending thoracic aorta and arch.[9,27] Aortography is helpful to evaluate critical side branches, such as the intercostal, renal, and visceral arteries. The diameters and morphology of the femoral and iliac arteries are assessed to determine whether the delivery sheath can be passed safely, avoiding arterial injury or disruption. The relationship of the proximal aneurysm neck to the left subclavian artery and the distal neck to the celiac axis must be clearly defined. In addition, localization of patent intercostal arteries is important such that attempts can be made to preserve certain intercostal vessels at the time of stent-graft placement. It is possible, although not desirable, to use a segment of a noncovered stent body (attached proximally or distally to the stent-graft) to anchor the prosthesis within the neck of the aneurysm at the level of (or "covering") a patent intercostal or another branch artery, thus maintaining flow into the artery.

The advantage of the endovascular approach is that the thoracic aorta is not cross-clamped during stent-graft graft deployment; however, the risk of spinal cord ischemia and paraplegia is still present since critical intercostal vessels can be obliterated by the deployed stent-graft. In addition, reimplantation of intercostal arteries is not possible using the endovascular stent-graft approach, as is the case during an open procedure.

Stent-Graft Construction and Deployment

Unlike the balloon-expandable type of prosthesis used to treat abdominal aortic aneurysms, a self-expanding stent-graft is used in our approach because of the larger diameters of the descending thoracic aorta and because the largest affordable balloon catheter commercially available is only 2.5 cm in diameter.[9,28]

Each endovascular stent-graft prosthesis is custom fabricated and constructed of a stainless steel endoskeleton consisting of large-caliber Z-stents (Cook Inc., Bloomington, IN) covered with a Cooley Verisoft woven Dacron graft (Meadox Medicals, Inc., Oakland, NJ) (Fig. 19–1).[9] The graft crimps are ironed out to reduce the overall profile of the stent-graft. The diameter, length, taper or reverse taper, and curvature of the prosthesis (and the decision to cover all stent bodies with graft material) are based on the measurements obtained from the patient's spiral CT scan. The length of the stent-graft is calculated to allow for an additional 1.5 to 2 cm of stent-graft to serve as a friction anchor in the proximal and distal aneurysm necks.

The customized delivery sheath is made of Teflon and measures 27 or 20 Fr in external diameter. A plastic valve (Cook Urological, Inc., Bloomington, IN) is placed on the end of the delivery sheath to provide hemostasis during angiographic catheter manipulation and loading of the stent-graft. A tapered dilator is placed within the delivery sheath, and both sheath and dilator are advanced over a guide wire. After removal of the dilator and guide wire, a solid Teflon "pusher" rod is used to advance the compressed stent-graft (within the loading cartridge) into and up the delivery sheath.

Endovascular stent-grafting is performed in the operating room under general anesthesia usually with double-lumen endotracheal intubation.[9] Cardiopulmonary by-

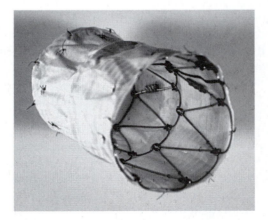

Figure 19–1. Endovascular stent-graft constructed of a stainless steel endoskeleton consisting of Z-shaped stent elements covered with a Cooley Verisoft woven Dacron graft.

pass standby is required in our opinion. The patient is placed in a 60-degree or full right lateral decubitus position depending on which fluoroscopic projection provides the best visualization of the descending thoracic aortic pathology. The femoral artery, iliac artery, infrarenal aorta, or a side limb graft (10-mm Dacron graft) attached to an abdominal aortic graft is used for access. Intraoperative aortography is performed with a portable radiographic image intensifier with digital road-mapping capability (Fig. 19–2). A transesophageal echocardiographic probe is placed for cardiac monitoring and for guidance in deploying the stent-graft.

The pigtail angiographic catheter is exchanged for a "super stiff" 0.035-inch guide wire, which is advanced into the aortic arch or descending thoracic aorta proximal to the aneurysm. The patient is heparinized (100 to 300 U/kg). A femoral or iliac arteriotomy, small aortotomy, or transverse incision in the side limb graft is made. Under fluoroscopic guidance, the large tapered dilator is passed over the guide wire and carefully advanced into the descending thoracic aorta; the delivery sheath is then advanced over the dilator. The dilator and guide wire are removed, leaving the delivery sheath in place. The stent-graft inside the loading cartridge is inserted into the mouth of the delivery sheath and advanced to the end of the sheath using the solid Teflon "pusher." The stent-graft and sheath are positioned using fluoroscopic guidance so that the proximal end of the stent-graft is located approximately 1 to 2 cm proximal to the aneurysm neck. Using intravenous esmolol and inhalational isofluorane, the mean arterial pressure is lowered to 50 to 60 mm Hg. The stent-graft is deployed by firmly holding the "pusher" in position and retracting the delivery sheath. After deployment of the stent-graft, the blood pressure is allowed to rise, the "pusher" is removed, and a guide wire reinserted under fluoroscopic guidance. A pigtail catheter is passed over the guide wire into the ascending aorta or arch, and a completion aortogram is performed (Fig. 19–3). Finally, the delivery sheath is removed and the arteriotomy or distal aortotomy repaired. Protamine sulfate is given for heparin neutralization. Follow-up radiologic evaluations are obtained based on protocol (Fig. 19–4).

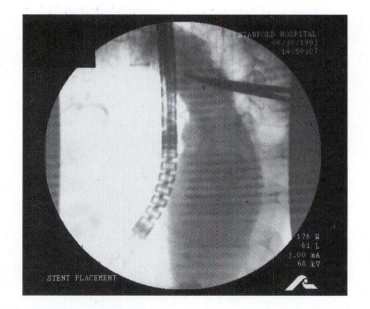

Figure 19–2. Intraoperative angiogram of descending thoracic aortic aneurysm. The transesophageal echocardiographic probe is present, and the level of the proximal neck is marked by an externally placed metallic clamp.

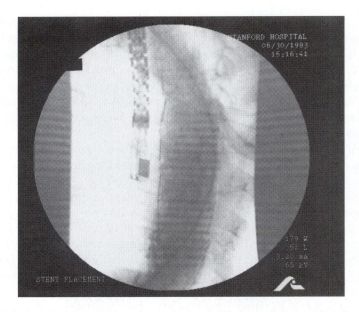

Figure 19–3. Completion angiogram demonstrating deployment of stent-graft and exclusion of flow into aneurysm.

Special Considerations

For patients with a proximal descending thoracic aortic aneurysm extending to the origin of the left subclavian artery, a left carotid-subclavian transposition (or bypass) is necessary prior to the endovascular stent-graft procedure in order to establish an adequate proximal neck (or "landing zone") without jeopardizing subclavian artery flow by the deployed stent-graft.[9] After the subclavian to carotid anastomosis is per-

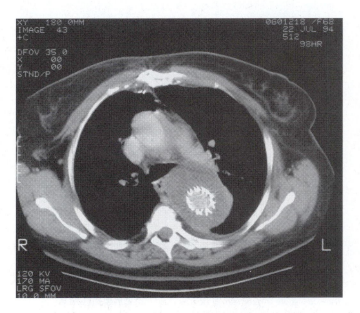

Figure 19–4. Axial CT with contrast demonstrating stent-graft situated within descending thoracic aorta with exclusion of flow into the aneurysm sac.

formed with the patient in the supine position, the patient is repositioned, prepped, and redraped for the stent-graft procedure.

Patients with large or symptomatic abdominal aortic and thoracic aortic aneurysms (not thoracoabdominal aortic aneurysms) have been successfully treated with a conventional open abdominal aortic aneurysm repair coupled with placement of a descending thoracic aortic stent-graft. Thoracic aortic stent-graft placement is facilitated by sewing a side limb (10-mm Dacron graft) onto the abdominal aortic graft; alternatively, if a bifurcation graft is necessary, one limb of this graft may be used. The side limb is used for delivery sheath access, and the stent-graft is deployed in the above manner. At the conclusion of the procedure, the auxiliary side limb is oversewn.

In patients with multiple thoracic aortic aneurysms (involving the ascending aorta or arch as well as the descending thoracic aorta), it is possible to replace the ascending aorta and arch using the "elephant trunk" technique initially; this is followed at a later date, if necessary, with stent-grafting of the descending thoracic component of the aneurysm. The proximal end of the stent-graft is deployed inside the distal opening of the elephant trunk graft.[10,29]

Occasionally, there may be residual blood flow into the aneurysm sac after initial stent-graft deployment as seen on completion angiography. In this situation, it is necessary to place an additional stent-graft "extension" segment (either distal or proximal to the first stent-graft) in order to exclude all flow into the aneurysm.

Current Results with Stent-Grafting

In our early experience from Stanford published in 1994, Dake et al.[9] reported 13 patients who underwent successful stent-graft placement for descending thoracic aortic pathology. Average follow-up was only 12 months. After stent-grafting, complete thrombosis of the aneurysm was achieved in 12 patients, and partial thrombosis in one patient. In this pilot series, there were no instances of death, paraplegia, stroke, or distal embolization. These preliminary results demonstrated that endovascular stent-grafting was feasible in highly selected patients.[9]

Our present experience with endovascular stent-grafting of the descending thoracic aorta includes 81 patients (61 men and 20 women) with descending thoracic aortic disease (Table 19–1). Seventy-six patients underwent stent-graft placement at Stanford University, and 5 patients underwent the stent-graft procedures at outside institutions by one of the authors (MDD). The results presented herein (except for the actuarial estimate of survival) include the entire series of 81 patients. It is important to note that approximately one-half of these patients were judged by cardiovascular surgeons not to be open operative candidates due to multiple risk factors.[11] The predominant pathology was atherosclerotic or degenerative aneurysmal disease, occurring in 67 patients (Table 19–2). The institutional review board-sanctioned imaging protocol for preprocedure evaluation, intraoperative deployment, and postprocedure follow-up is summa-

TABLE 19–1. PATIENT CHARACTERISTICS

Number of patients	81
Men : women	3 : 1
Mean age (range)	66 years (35–88 years)
True : false aneurysms	2 : 1
Diameter of aneurysms (range)	6.2 cm (5–11)
Mean follow-up (range)	13.2 months (1–45 months)

TABLE 19–2. ETIOLOGY OF DESCENDING THORACIC AORTIC PATHOLOGY

	No.
Atherosclerotic/degenerative	67
Dissection	5
Traumatic aneurysm	7
Pseudoaneurysm	4
Mycotic aneurysm (healed)	2

TABLE 19–3. IMAGING PROTOCOL (INSTITUTIONAL REVIEW BOARD APPROVED)

Timing	Radiographic Procedure		
	CXR	CT	Angiography
Preprocedure	X	X	X
Intraoperative			X
Predischarge	X	X	X
Two months postprocedure	X		
Six months postprocedure	X	X	X
One year postprocedure	X	X	X
Two years postprocedure (and annually thereafter)	X	X	

CXR, chest radiography; CT, spiral computed tomography.

TABLE 19-4. SITES OF ACCESS FOR ENDOVASCULAR STENT-GRAFTING

Site	No.
Femoral	52
Old AFB graft limb	9
Iliac	3
Transverse aortic arch	1
Abdominal aorta	25
For access (only)	7
Concomitant AAA repair	18
Surgical aortic tube graft	8
Surgical AFB graft	9
Endovascular AAA stent-graft	1

AFB, aortobifemoral bypass graft limb; AAA, abdominal aortic aneurysm.

rized in Table 19–3. All patients underwent CT with spiral reconstruction and angiography prior to consideration for stent-grafting. Fifty-two patients were approached using a femoral arteriotomy, 3 through an iliac arteriotomy, and 25 via the abdominal aorta (Table 19–4). In those who required the abdominal aortic approach, 7 patients were accessed via a small aortotomy (inadequate distal access), and 18 patients underwent concomitant abdominal aortic aneurysm repair. The mean diameter of the diseased descending thoracic aorta was 6.2 cm (range of 5 to 11 cm); the mean diameter of the stent-graft was 3.5 cm (range of 2.4 to 4.5 cm), and the average length of the stent-graft was 10.2 cm (range of 5 to 22 cm).

Patient follow-up (100% complete) averaged only 13.2 months, since a large fraction of patients underwent stent-grafting in 1995 and 1996. There were 7 early or procedure-related deaths (early mortality rate of 9 ± 3% [±70% confidence limit]) (Tables 19–5 and 19-6). The paraplegia rate was 4 ± 2%, and the stroke rate was 5 ± 3%. No patient to date has required conversion to an open surgical approach. In 4 patients (5 ± 3%), thrombosis of the aneurysm was incomplete after stent-graft deployment: Three subsequently died, 2 of whom sustained sudden, unexpected late deaths (categorized as possible treatment failures), and 1 developed fatal aneurysm rupture into the esophagus (Table 19–7). With regard to cerebrovascular accidents, angiographic manipulation and stent-graft instrumentation at the level of the aortic arch were associated with 3 presumably embolic strokes (Table 19–8). Another patient sustained an intracerebral hemorrhage during an otherwise uneventful stent-graft deployment; this patient was heparinized during the procedure, but there was no identifiable period of hypertension in the intraoperative or postprocedure period. Paraplegia occurred in 3 patients, 2 of whom had complicated intraoperative and postprocedure courses; in 1 patient, stent-grafting was uncomplicated, but the entire descending thoracic aorta had to be excluded (Table 19–9).

For the 76 patients who underwent endovascular stent-grafting at Stanford University, the actuarial survival estimates were 87 ± 4% at 1 year, 81 ± 6% at 2 years, and 81 ± 6% at nearly 4 years (Fig. 19–5). Given the high-risk nature of this specific patient cohort, these results are satisfactory. This survival curve compares with a 5-year actuarial survival estimate of 70% to 79% in patients who underwent open surgical repair in the past.[3,4,6,12,20] A total of 5 patients died late. Two deaths were sudden, and 1 was due to aneurysm rupture; thus, these 3 deaths can be categorized as 1 definite and 2 possible treatment failures (Tables 19–10 and 19–11). Five patients developed late recanalization or filling of the aneurysm sac over time; 3 of these were successfully treated with secondary radiologic embolization procedures, 1 underwent open surgical repair (with exclusion of the descending thoracic aorta), and 1 continues to be followed expectantly.

Limitations and Unknowns

There are a number of real and potential limitations inherent in this technique of endovascular stent-grafting. The current delivery system is very large, which requires adequate arterial and aortic access. From the technical standpoint, the deployment process is relatively imprecise, and the position of the stent-graft cannot be adjusted after deployment.

A major question involves the unknown stability of stent-graft fixation and the ultimate fate of the aneurysm. After deployment, the stent-graft is held in place simply by friction fixation to the proximal and distal necks of the aneurysm; thus, stent-graft migration is a possibility, especially if one neck dilates over time.[9] It is also possible that the aneurysm may continue to expand despite being thrombosed outside the

TABLE 19–5. EARLY DEATHS OR COMPLICATIONS OF ENDOVASCULAR STENT-GRAFTING

	No.
Early or procedure-related deaths	7 (9 ± 3%)
Incomplete thrombosis	4 (5 ± 3%)
Stroke	4 (5 ± 3%)
Paraplegia	3 (4 ± 2%)
Myocardial infarction	1
Proximal dissection	1
Ruptured iliac artery	1
Open surgical conversion	0
Stent-graft infection	0
Distal embolization	0

Data presented as mean ± 70% confidence limit.

TABLE 19–6. CLINICAL DATA REGARDING EARLY OR PROCEDURE-RELATED DEATHS

Time of Death (Postprocedure)	Clinical Data
27 days	83-year-old man with an atherosclerotic descending thoracic aortic aneurysm who developed aspiration pneumonia and respiratory failure.
31 days	66-year-old man with an atherosclerotic descending thoracic aortic aneurysm who underwent complex redo suprarenal aneurysm resection followed by stent-grafting; complicated by coagulopathy, hypotension, paraplegia, and renal failure.
18 hours	79-year-old man with an atherosclerotic descending thoracic aortic aneurysm who sustained avulsion of previous aortoiliac anastomosis during delivery sheath introduction.
42 days	75-year-old woman with a contained rupture of a distal arch and descending thoracic aortic aneurysm who underwent a left subclavian-carotid bypass followed by stent-grafting; complicated by multiple cerebellar infarcts, pneumonia, and sepsis.
36 hours	69-year-old woman with a symptomatic penetrating atherosclerotic ulcer of the mid-descending thoracic aorta; complicated by massive left cerebral hemorrhage.
19 days	72-year-old woman with an atherosclerotic descending thoracic aortic aneurysm; complicated by respiratory failure and sepsis.
2 hours	29-year-old man who sustained multiple trauma with traumatic aortic tear, liver failure, coagulopathy, and multiple organ failure.

TABLE 19–7. OUTCOME OF PATIENTS WITH INCOMPLETE ANEURYSM THROMBOSIS AFTER ENDOVASCULAR STENT-GRAFTING

Patient No.	Aortic Pathology	Follow-up
4	Chronic traumatic false aneurysm	Alive and well at 35 months
8	Subacute type B dissection superimposed on saccular atherosclerotic aneurysm	Sudden death at 13 months
27	Fusiform atherosclerotic aneurysm	Fatal aortoesophageal fistula at 4 months
63	Atherosclerotic aneurysm	Multiple cerebellar infarcts, died after 42 days

TABLE 19–8. CLINICAL DATA REGARDING PATIENTS WITH EARLY STROKE

Patient No.	Clinical Data
63	Stroke and death: 75-year-old woman with distal arch and descending thoracic aortic aneurysm who underwent a left subclavian-carotid bypass followed by stent-grafting; developed multiple cerebellar infarcts.
64	Stroke and death: 69-year-old woman with penetrating atherosclerotic ulcer of the descending thoracic aorta; developed massive left cerebral hemorrhage.
67	Stroke: 66-year-old woman who underwent arch aneurysm repair with profound hypothermic circulatory arrest followed by descending thoracic aortic stent-grafting accessed via the aortic arch; developed left occipital infarct, resolving.
70	Stroke: 72-year-old woman with distal arch aneurysm who underwent stent-grafting; developed left hemiparesis with mild residual deficit.

TABLE 19–9. CLINICAL DATA REGARDING PATIENTS WITH PARAPLEGIA

Patient No.	Clinical Data
15	66-year-old woman with atherosclerotic descending thoracic aortic aneurysm whose intraoperative course was complicated by aortic obstruction with hypotension; developed paraplegia and renal failure.
23	66-year-old man with an atherosclerotic descending thoracic aortic aneurysm who underwent complex redo suprarenal aneurysm resection followed by stent-grafting; hospital course complicated by coagulopathy, hypotension, paraplegia, renal failure, and death.
50	78-year-old man with descending thoracic aortic intramural hematoma who underwent uncomplicated stent-grafting of entire descending thoracic aorta.

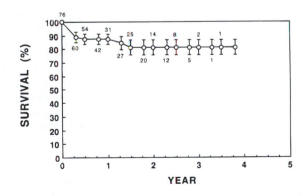

Figure 19–5. Actuarial survival of the 76 patients in the Stanford University experience.

TABLE 19–10. LATE COMPLICATIONS OR DEATHS AFTER ENDOVASCULAR STENT-GRAFTING

	No.
Late deaths	5
Sudden, unexplained	2
Aneurysm rupture	1
Stroke	1
Congestive heart failure multisystem organ failure	1
Late recanalization or aneurysm filling	5
Interventional radiology treatment	3
Reoperation	1
Observation	1
Stent-graft infection	0
Distal embolization	0
Stent-graft migration	0

prosthetic stent-graft. Although we have not observed stent-graft migration to date, there was one case of aneurysm rupture; also, 2 patients died suddenly and unexpectedly, which in the absence of an autopsy should be considered to be possibly related to progressive aneurysm expansion and rupture. In addition, late aneurysm filling or recanalization of a tract around the stent-graft has been observed in 5 patients.

Other limitations include anatomic constraints, such as the need for adequate proximal and distal aortic necks, the confounding presence of critical aortic branches in the diseased aorta, and the fact that only relatively straight segments of aorta can be managed in this manner. Placement of the stent-graft close to the distal arch appears to be associated with a higher incidence of strokes, presumably due to catheter manipulation in the ascending aorta or arch. Finally, the long-term efficacy and clinical outcome of endovascular stent-grafting of descending thoracic aortic aneurysms remains totally unknown. Only 5- to 10-year follow-up of a larger number of patients with serial imaging studies will answer this key question.

TABLE 19–11. CLINICAL DATA REGARDING LATE DEATHS

Patient No.	Time of Death (Postprocedure)	Clinical Data
8	409 days	66-year-old man who underwent stent-grafting of descending thoracic aortic dissection with incomplete thrombosis of aneurysm; died suddenly (no postmortem).
27	109 days	79-year-old man who underwent stent-grafting of descending thoracic aortic aneurysm; sustained fatal aortoesophageal fistula.
34	463 days	88-year-old man who underwent stent-grafting of descending thoracic aortic aneurysm; sustained late fatal stroke.
55	61 days	69-year-old man who underwent stent-grafting of descending thoracic aortic aneurysm with complete thrombosis of aneurysm; died suddenly (no postmortem).
66	31 days	81-year-old man who underwent stent-grafting of descending thoracic aortic aneurysm with complete thrombosis of aneurysm; discharged and later developed cardiopulmonary failure and multiple organ failure.

CONCLUSION

Endovascular stent-grafting of the descending thoracic aortic aneurysms is a reasonable alternative approach to open surgical repair for high-risk patients and those considered to be inoperable by conventional techniques. Patients who are most likely to benefit include the very elderly, those with markedly compromised cardiac, pulmonary, or renal status, and individuals who have undergone previous complex operations on the descending thoracic aorta. In addition, endovascular stent-grafting is a useful adjunct for patients with abdominal and descending thoracic aortic aneurysms that need to be treated concomitantly. The abdominal aneurysm is repaired in a conventional fashion and stent-grafting is simultaneously employed for the thoracic component. The current results suggest that this minimally invasive approach may be associated with less early morbidity compared to open thoracotomy and repair. The promise of truly long-term efficacy of this technique awaits 5- to 10-year follow-up investigations.

REFERENCES

1. Bickerstaff LK, Pairolero PC, Hollier LH, et al. Thoracic aortic aneurysms: a population-based study. *Surgery*. 1982;92:1103–1108.
2. Pressler V, McNamara JJ. Thoracic aortic aneurysm: natural history and treatment. *J Thorac Cardiovasc Surg*. 1980;79:489–498.
3. Moreno-Cabral CE, Miller DC, Mitchell RS, et al. Degenerative and atherosclerotic aneurysms of the thoracic aorta. *J Thorac Cardiovasc Surg*. 1984;88:1020–1032.
4. Pressler V, McNamara JJ. Aneurysm of the thoracic aorta. *J Thorac Cardiovasc Surg*. 1985;89:50–54.
5. Fann JI, Miller DC. Descending thoracic aortic aneurysms. In: Baue AE, Geha AS, Hammond GL, et al., eds. *Glenn's Thoracic and Cardiovascular Surgery*. 6th ed. Norwalk, CT: Appleton and Lange; 1995:2255–2272.
6. DeBakey ME, McCollum CH, Graham JM. Surgical treatment of aneurysms of the descending thoracic aorta. *J Cardiovasc Surg*. 1978;19:571–576.
7. Livesay JJ, Cooley DA, Ventemiglia RA, et al. Surgical experience in descending thoracic aneurysmectomy with and without adjuncts to avoid ischemia. *Ann Thorac Surg*. 1985;39:37–46.
8. McNamara JJ, Pressler VM. Natural history of arteriosclerotic thoracic aortic aneurysms. *Ann Thorac Surg*. 1978;26:468–473.
9. Dake MD, Miller DC, Semba CP, et al. Transluminal placement of endovascular stent-grafts for the treatment of descending thoracic aortic aneurysms. *N Engl J Med*. 1994;331:1729–1734.
10. Fann JI, Dake MD, Semba CP, et al. Endovascular stent-grafting after arch aneurysm repair using the "elephant trunk." *Ann Thorac Surg*. 1995;60:1102–1105.
11. Mitchell RS, Dake MD, Semba CP, et al. Endovascular stent-graft repair of thoracic aortic aneurysms. *J Thorac Cardiovasc Surg*. 1996;111:1054–1062.
12. Hamerlijnck RP, Rutsaert RR, DeGeest R, et al. Surgical correction of descending thoracic aortic aneurysms under simple aortic cross-clamping. *J Vasc Surg*. 1989;9:568–573.
13. Borst HG, Jurmann M, Buhner B, Laas J. Risk of replacement of descending aorta with a standardized left heart bypass technique. *J Thorac Cardiovasc Surg*. 1994;107:126–133.
14. Verdant A. Descending thoracic aortic aneurysms: surgical treatment with the Gott shunt. *Can J Surg*. 1992;35:493–496.
15. Najafi H, Javid H, Hunter J, et al. Descending aortic aneurysmectomy without adjuncts to avoid ischemia. *Ann Thorac Surg*. 1980;30:326–335.
16. Crawford ES, Walker HSJ, Saleh SA, Normann NA. Graft replacement of aneurysm in descending thoracic aorta: results without bypass or shunting. *Surgery*. 1981;89:73–85.

17. Cooley DA, Baldwin RT. Technique of open distal anastomosis for repair of descending thoracic aortic aneurysms. *Ann Thorac Surg.* 1992;54:932–936.
18. von Segesser LK, Killer I, Jenni R, et al. Improved distal circulatory support for repair of descending thoracic aortic aneurysms. *Ann Thorac Surg.* 1993;56:1373–1380.
19. Lawrence GH, Hessel EA, Sauvage LR, Krause AH. Results of the use of the TDMAC-heparin shunt in the surgery of aneurysms of the descending thoracic aorta. *J Thorac Cardiovasc Surg.* 1977;73:393–398.
20. Hilgenberg AD, Rainer WG, Sadler TR. Aneurysm of the descending thoracic aorta. *J Thorac Cardiovasc Surg.* 1981;81:818–824.
21. Najafi H. 1993 Update: descending aortic aneurysmectomy without adjuncts to avoid ischemia. *Ann Thorac Surg.* 1993;55:1042–1045.
22. Cartier R, Orszulak TA, Pairolero PC, Schaff HV. Circulatory support during crossclamping of the descending thoracic aorta. *J Thorac Cardiovasc Surg.* 1990;99:1038–1047.
23. Schepens MA, Defauw JJ, Hamerlijnck RP, Vermeulen FE. Risk assessment of acute renal failure after thoracoabdominal aortic aneurysm surgery. *Ann Surg.* 1994;219:400–407.
24. Svensson LG, Patel V, Robinson MF, et al. Influence of preservation or perfusion of intraoperatively identified spinal cord blood supply on spinal motor evoked potentials and paraplegia after aortic surgery. *J Vasc Surg.* 1991;13:355–365.
25. Laschinger JC, Izumoto H, Kouchoukos NT. Evolving concepts in prevention of spinal cord injury during operations on the descending thoracic and thoracoabdominal aorta. *Ann Thorac Surg.* 1987;44:667–674.
26. Laschinger JC, Cunningham JN, Nathan IM, et al. Experimental and clinical assessment of the adequacy of partial bypass in maintenance of spinal cord blood flow during operations on the thoracic aorta. *Ann Thorac Surg.* 1983;36:417–426.
27. Rubin GD, Walker PJ, Dake MD, et al. Three-dimensional spiral computed tomographic angiography: an alternative imaging modality for the abdominal aorta and its branches. *J Vasc Surg.* 1993;18:656–665.
28. Parodi JC, Palmaz JC, Barone HD. Transfemoral intraluminal graft implantation for abdominal aortic aneurysms. *Ann Vasc Surg.* 1991;5:491–499.
29. Borst HG, Laas J. Surgical treatment of thoracic aortic aneurysms. In: Karp RB, Laks H, Wechsler AS, eds. *Advances in Cardiac Surgery.* St. Louis, MO: Mosby Year Book; 1993:4:47–87.

VI

The Ischemic Extremity

20

Infection Control in Lower Extremity Revascularization

Douglas A. Coe, MD, and Jonathan B. Towne, MD

Despite advances in vascular surgical techniques and development of improved antimicrobial agents, wound complications after infrainguinal revascularization remain a formidable problem. Although the exact incidence of lower extremity graft infection is low, ranging between 1% to 5%, morbidity in terms of subsequent amputation and mortality are significant. In prosthetic reconstructions, the risk of infection exists for the life of the graft, with late infections possible years after implantation. Principles of treatment of wound and graft infection have emerged and depend largely on the graft material, timing of infection vis-à-vis the initial operation, the microbiology of the infectious process, and the clinical status of the patient. A basic knowledge of risk factors, etiology, bacteriology, presentation, and treatment options is required to minimize morbidity and mortality in these difficult patients.

INCIDENCE

The exact incidence of infrainguinal bypass graft infection is unknown, but has been reported to be between 1.5% and 12% for prosthetic grafts and 0% to 1.7% for autogenous grafts if all time periods are considered.[1,2] Several important risk factors predispose to subsequent graft infection. Wound healing complications such as skin or subcutaneous tissue necrosis, cellulitis, hematoma, or lymphatic leak significantly increase the risk of subsequent graft infection. Local wound complications occur in up to 44% of infrainguinal bypass procedures,[3] and up to one-third of graft infections have preceding wound problems. In their study assessing risk factors for primary graft infections, Edwards et al.[4] identified postoperative wound infection as the primary predisposing factor in 33% of subsequent graft infections. Likewise, Cherry and coworkers[5] reviewed 39 cases of infrainguinal graft infections and found that postoperative wound infection occurred in 28% of cases. The presence of a groin incision greatly increases the risk of both wound and graft infection. In a study of 2,411 consecutive prosthetic arterial reconstructions, 3.5% of 489 femoroperipheral reconstructions developed graft infection, and of note was that graft infection occurred only when a groin incision had been used.[6] Other risk factors for infectious complications include emergency bypass procedures and the need for early reoperation for graft thrombosis or bleeding. In a review of their arterial graft infections, Hoffert et al. found that 50% of conduit infections had required early reoperation for postoperative hematoma formation, and in Kent's series, infectious complications were associated with emergent operations in 13% of cases.[1,3]

Multiple factors predispose to wound infections and relate to specific patient characteristics and to the occurrence of other early postoperative complications. In a review of 126 consecutive patients who underwent *in situ* vein bypass, Reifsnyder et al.[7] found that early graft revision (<4 days) and the presence of a lymph leak significantly increased the risk for postoperative wound infection. However, factors such as age, race, diabetes, duration of operation, and presence of gangrene or ulceration did not significantly influence the incidence of infectious complications in that series. Wengrovitz and coworkers[8] retrospectively studied 163 subcutaneous saphenous vein bypasses and found on regression analysis that chronic steroid use, ipsilateral ulceration, and pedal bypasses predicted an increased incidence of wound infection. They also identified female gender, diabetes, use of continuous incisions, and procedures for limb salvage as factors associated with wound complications in their group of patients. Furthermore, a prospective evaluation of wound complications in 79 infrainguinal incisions identified postoperative complications in 44% of incisions, 25% of which were wound infections. The only predictors of wound complications in this group included age, obesity, and presence of venous stasis.[3]

The natural history of graft infection depends partly on the timing of presentation, which has a widely variable interval between implantation and recognition of the infection. Multiple studies have indicated that wound and graft infections tend to occur early. In Lorentzen's study, 85% of graft infections occurred in the first 30 days.[6] Likewise, Liekweg et al.[9] reported that 85% of groin wound infections in their series presented within 5 weeks of the initial operation. However, graft infection may not become clinically evident for months to years after placement.[6,10] Early graft infections are usually easily identified due to associated wound complications and signs of systemic inflammation. Graft infections that present in a delayed fashion, however, usually do not present with signs of sepsis and are associated with more nonspecific symptoms.

Morbidity and mortality associated with graft infection depend not only on the timing of presentation, but also on microbiology, graft location, and method of treatment. Unrecognized or inadequately treated infringuinal graft infection has a mortality rate ranging between 0% and 22% and results in amputation in between 8% to 53% of cases, with one series reporting an amputation rate of 79%.[10-12]

PATHOPHYSIOLOGY

The primary cause of infectious wound or graft complications involves contamination at the time of surgery. Contamination can occur when the graft contacts the skin and from breaks in surgical technique. Emergent operations increase the risk for infectious complications potentially because of lack of attention to sterile technique and possibly due to immunologic status of the stressed patient. Early reoperation also increases the risk of infection secondary to increased exposure of the graft to potential contamination and from any retained thrombus or debris that can serve as potent culture media. In addition, factors such as prolonged operative times and extended preoperative hospitalization are thought to contribute to risk of wound and graft infection. Levy et al.[13] prospectively obtained skin flora cultures on the day of admission, day of surgery, and 5 days postoperatively in patients undergoing lower extremity revascularization.

They demonstrated that patients enter the hospital colonized with slime-producing coagulase-negative staphylococci and that strains shift from predominantly susceptible to predominantly resistant species.

Colonization of native artery can be a source of graft contamination. Macbeth and colleagues[14] cultured arterial specimens and surrounding tissue (as controls) from patients undergoing clean, elective prosthetic arterial reconstructions. Forty-three percent of arterial segments were culture positive with *Staphylococcus epidermidis* as the most common isolate while all controls were sterile. Correlation of culture data to subsequent suture line disruption in infected grafts at their institution revealed that positive arterial cultures were associated with disruption in 57% of cases, whereas there were no anastomotic disruptions in patients with negative arterial cultures.[14] Durham and associates[15] corroborated these data with a 43% culture positive rate and noted that graft infections occurred only in culture positive arteries. In addition, they found that positive arterial cultures had no predictive value regarding graft infection at initial operations, but that positive arterial cultures were associated with eventual graft infection in 28% of patients undergoing subsequent vascular reconstructions.

Another potential source of graft infection is from hematogenous or lymphatic seeding from remote sites of infection or colonization. Experiments in dogs have demonstrated intravenous infusion of 10^7 colony-forming units of *S. aureus* will produce clinical graft infection in nearly 100% of animals in the early postoperative period.[16] The lymphatic system has also been implicated in the pathogenesis of graft infection originating from a distal septic focus such as an infected ischemic foot ulcer by both hematogenous spread and from direct seeding of the graft. Experimentally, transection of lymphatics at the graft site in the presence of a distal infection leads to significantly more graft infections compared to lymphatic ligation and excision.[17] They concluded that lymphatic bacterial transport contributed to graft infection both from direct graft seeding and from transmission of bacteria to the blood leading to hematogenous seeding of the graft. The propensity for a graft to become infected decreases with time due to development of a pseudointimal layer and incorporation within surrounding tissues, but the graft can remain at significant risk for up to a year after implantation. Even years after implantation, the graft can be seeded by bacteremia thought to be due to an incomplete pseudointimal lining. To what extent this mechanism contributes to the pathogenesis of graft infection in humans is unknown, but bacteremia has been associated with such procedures as central venous or bladder catheterization, gastrointestinal endoscopy, dental or genitourinary instrumentation, and in patients harboring remote infections such as pneumonia, endocarditis, and distal foot infections.

The potential for graft infection is also influenced by the patient's immunocompetence and immune factors associated with the graft itself. The sequence of events involved with vascular graft infection is initiated by adhesion of bacteria to the graft surface. Subsequent colonization and biofilm production leads to activation of the host's immune response, producing an inflammatory reaction involving perigraft tissues and the graft–artery anastomosis.[18] Prosthetic materials initiate an inflammatory response characterized by an acidic, ischemic environment that is inhibitory to normal host defenses and antibiotic activity, further promoting bacterial replication. Autogenous grafts, however, develop rich microvascular connections and are thereby much more resistant to bacterial growth and subsequent infection. Patients with impaired immunocompetence such as those with malnutrition, malignancy, chemotherapy, chronic steroid use, and chronic renal failure are potentially at increased risk of infectious complications due to inadequate host defense.

The degree to which the previous sequence of events occurs also depends in large part on the bacterial species and the characteristics of the graft material. The virulence of coagulase-positive staphylococci is enhanced by release of exotoxin and an extracellular mucin, which protects the organism against antibiotics, antibodies, and phagocytes.[19] In addition, bacterial adhesion to graft materials is related to physical characteristics of the graft. Bacterial adherence to Dacron has been shown to be 10 to 100 times greater than to polytetrafluoroethylene (PTFE).[20] This interaction is particularly important in less virulent strains responsible for delayed infection. Organisms such as *S. epidermidis* reside in the interstices of the graft and produce an extracellular glycocalyx biofilm, which provides an excellent protective environment for persistent growth.

The site of contamination and subsequent infection usually starts at one point along the course of the graft and can involve either the body of the graft or the anastomotic region. If the process is able to decompress through a sinus tract to the skin, the infection can remain localized. If, however, external drainage does not occur, infected fluid will track along the course of the graft in the potential space between the conduit and perigraft tissues to involve the entire conduit. If anastomotic involvement ensues, destruction of the involved artery will occur, leading to disruption of the anastomosis with pseudoaneurysm formation.

MICROBIOLOGY

The bacteriology of graft infections has changed over the years and is influenced by multiple factors. Most infections are due to bacteria, but other microorganisms have been recovered including fungi, and in aortic grafts, mycobacteria and mycoplasma.[21,22] In the past, *S. aureus* was the predominant pathogen and was isolated in up to 50% of cases. More recently, graft infections due to *S. epidermidis* and gram-negative bacteria have increased in frequency. Specimen acquisition and culture technique has a significant impact on the species recovered. Sampling error can occur when lower numbers of bacteria are present despite gross clinical signs of infection. In particular, delayed infections due to *S. epidermidis* and other coagulase-negative staphylococci are frequently associated with negative culture results.[23]

The timing of graft infection has significant implications as to the bacteriology involved in the process. Early infections, those that present within 4 months of surgery, are associated with particularly virulent strains of bacteria, with *S. aureus* being the most prevalent. These bacteria produce exotoxin and enzymes that enhance its virulence and induce an intense local and systemic inflammatory response. Although less common, gram-negative organisms such as *Proteus, Klebsiella,* and *Enterobacter* can also be responsible for early graft infections. *Pseudomonas*, an aerobic gram-negative rod, is a particularly aggressive pathogen and is frequently associated with anastomotic breakdown with bleeding.

Delayed graft infections (those presenting months to years after implantation) are usually associated with less virulent bacteria. *Staphylococcus epidermidis* and other coagulase-negative organisms have limited ability for tissue invasion and generally require the presence of a foreign body for prolonged survival.[24] Colonization by coagulase-negative staphylococci is confined to a perigraft biofilm, which contains a relatively low concentration of organisms. However, with time, the biofilm is recognized by the host's defenses, producing an inflammatory response with tissue-damaging effects. The process is insidious with few signs of systemic inflammation (fever, leukocytosis), but is capable of anastomotic disruption with pseudoaneurysm formation or development of cutaneous fistulas.

Acquisition of bacteria from graft and wound infections is necessary to guide subsequent antibiotic therapy. Studies often demonstrate a significant incidence of negative cultures despite convincing evidence of infection.[4,5,25–27] This can be due to absence of tissue invasion, presence of a surface biofilm, low numbers of organisms, and concomitant antibiotic use. Virulent strains of bacteria (coagulase-positive staphylococci, gram-negatives) are easily recovered due to invasion of the bloodstream and more advanced tissue invasion. However, coagulase-negative staphylococci do not infiltrate tissues to the same extent and often will be missed on routine swab culture; more sensitive techniques are required for their isolation. One such method involves submersion of a portion of several different regions of the graft and surrounding tissue in broth media with disruption of the graft using either mechanical grinding or ultrasonication. This disperses the organisms in the media for increased bacterial growth despite negative Gram stain and routine culture results.[23] In addition, there should be communication between the surgeon and the microbiology laboratory regarding the clinical situation and potential suspected pathogens.

PRESENTATION

The way in which graft infection presents can range from having deceptively subtle signs and symptoms to massive infection with life-threatening systemic sepsis or hemorrhage. Peripheral infections are generally easier to diagnose than their intracavitary counterparts, but prompt diagnosis and treatment is necessary if subsequent morbidity and mortality are to be avoided.

Classification schemes of infection after infrainguinal bypass have been proposed by several authors. Szilagyi first graded wounds based on depth of involvement: grade I applied when only the dermis was involved; grade II infections extended to the subcutaneous tissues but did not invade the graft; and grade III infections directly involved the graft.[10] A modification of this classification defined grade III infections as those that affected the body of the graft but neither of the anastomoses; grade IV included infections that directly involved an anastomosis but was not associated with bacteremia or hemorrhage; and grade V described infected anastomoses associated with sepsis or bleeding at the time of presentation.[28]

Wound healing complications such as hematoma, lymphocele, or tissue necrosis usually precede deeper involvement. Timing of infection determines to a large extent how the process will present. Early graft infections will usually present in conjunction with wound infection and are associated with signs of systemic sepsis including fever, leukocytosis, and bacteremia. The initial presenting sign of graft infection in up to a quarter of patients is anastomotic disruption with potential exsanguinating hemorrhage.[4] Groin wounds are most commonly involved, and the majority of patients presenting with graft infection at the groin present with overt signs of wound sepsis with abscess formation, cellulitis, sinus tract development, or graft exposure.[29] Less commonly, deeper infection may be heralded by distal petichiae from septic microembolization, graft thrombosis, or a pulsatile mass over an anastomotic site. These infections tend to occur within the first weeks of surgery and are generally associated with coagulase-positive staphylococci or virulent gram-negative organisms.

The diagnosis of delayed graft infection is more difficult due to the less virulent nature of the causative organisms and the presence of a perigraft biofilm. Involvement can occur anywhere along the graft but most commonly occurs at femoral anastomoses. Systemic signs are usually absent though the patient may complain of malaise, localized pain and tenderness. Commonly there is inflammation of perigraft tissues with erythema of the overlying skin, a palpable perigraft inflammatory mass, or a cutaneous sinus tract. Many of the superficial signs are temporarily improved with systemic antibiotics, only to return with cessation of therapy.

In addition to careful attention of incisions and bypass routes, thorough examination of the distal extremity must be performed seeking signs of ischemia, distal embolization of microemboli, and sources of infection such as infected foot lesions. Furthermore, other sources of systemic infection such as pneumonia, upper urinary tract infection, and endocarditis should be sought as a potential source for hematogenous seeding of the graft.

Laboratory studies in patients with suspected infrainguinal graft infections are nonspecific and frequently of little assistance in confirming the diagnosis. Leukocytosis with a left shift is common in patients presenting with early wound and graft infection, but may be normal in delayed infections. Likewise, the erythrocyte sedimentation rate (ESR) is elevated but is a nonspecific finding. Blood cultures should be obtained but can be negative in a significant number of documented infections. Urinalysis should be performed, and culture data should be obtained from other sites, such as foot and surgical wound drainage, to rule out other sources of infection.

DIAGNOSIS

Radiologic Studies

The prompt diagnosis of infrainguinal graft infection is mandatory if morbidity and mortality are to be minimized. Both anatomic and functional imaging techniques, when used in a complementary fashion, are highly accurate for identifying the presence and extent of infection and for planning management strategy.

Ultrasonography

Duplex ultrasonography has great utility in the evaluation of patients with suspected graft infection, and is considered by some to be the initial diagnostic modality of choice.[30] Duplex imaging is particularly useful in the evaluation of pulsatile masses, and can differentiate perigraft fluid collections and hematomas from pseudoaneurysms with a high degree of accuracy[31] (Figs. 20–1, 20–2, and 20–3). If an abnormal fluid collection is identified, aspiration under ultrasound guidance can be performed. Graft incorporation can be determined, and vessel patency is easily confirmed using color-flow and spectral analysis.

The advantages of this modality include its widespread availability, and that it does not involve radiation exposure or the use of intravenous contrast. It is noninvasive and easily portable, which makes it useful in the initial evaluation of critically ill patients. Also, visualization in multiple planes can provide important information not readily available with other techniques. However, scan quality is extremely technician dependent and intra- and interexaminer studies may not be consistent. Furthermore, ultrasound is unable to differentiate infected from sterile fluid collections and tissue plane resolution is inferior to that of other imaging modalities. For these reasons, it has been suggested that ultrasound should be relegated to cases where other imaging techniques are not available, or to patients too ill to be transported to the radiology department.[32]

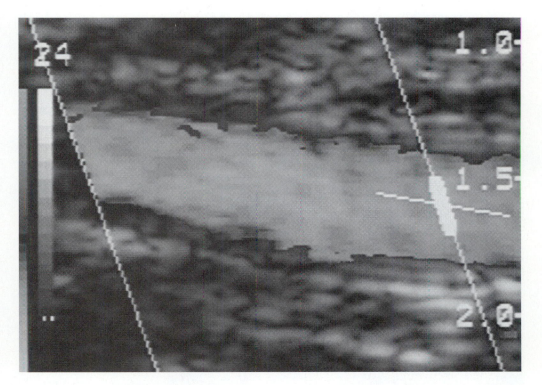

Figure 20–1. Normal color-flow image of postoperative graft.

Computed Tomography

Although computed tomography (CT) scanning is more commonly used in the evaluation of suspected intra-abdominal graft infection, it has utility in diagnosing peripheral graft infections as well. As with ultrasonography, CT can identify abnormal fluid collections and the presence of anastomotic pseudoaneurysms (Fig. 20–4). CT-guided needle aspiration can be performed if an abnormal fluid collection is identified. In addition, the entire length of the conduit can be examined, and vessel patency can be determined. However, CT is superior to ultrasound in defining various characteristics of the inflammatory process. Loss of normal tissue planes and presence of air around the graft, indicative of soft tissue inflammation, are among the CT criteria for graft infection[33] and are more clearly visualized by CT when compared to ultrasound. Unlike ultrasonography, CT is not technician dependent and has higher consistency with sequential scans.

Magnetic Resonance Imaging

Magnetic resonance imaging (MRI) is a relatively new modality for assessment of patients with possible graft infection. Most studies evaluating the efficacy of MRI in diagnosing graft infection have been with caviteric prostheses where it has a reported overall accuracy of 88% to 94%.[34,35] Criteria for graft infection are similar to those of CT scan and include identification of abnormal perigraft fluid collections and loss of normal tissue planes around the graft. However, MRI has several advantages over CT scanning. First, MRI has the ability to reconstruct images in multiple planes, thereby providing better visualization of the extent of the infectious process.[36] Second, intrave-

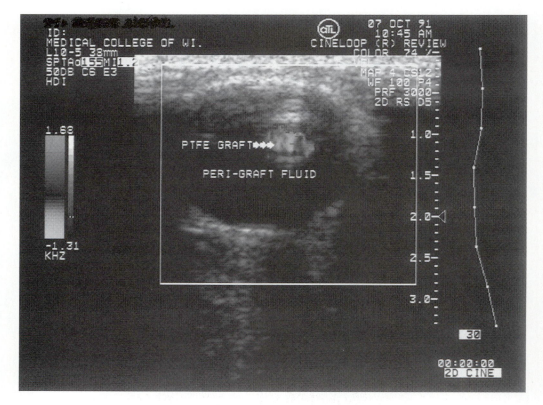

Figure 20–2. Cross-section of PTFE graft showing perigraft fluid.

nous contrast is not required to determine vessel patency due to a black "flow void" created by flowing blood on the MR image.[36] Finally, MRI is thought by some to be more sensitive in revealing small fluid collections and soft tissue changes due to better resolution between tissue and fluid densities.[34,35]

Disadvantages of MRI include its inability to differentiate infected from sterile fluid collections, and the inability to differentiate perigraft gas from calcium.[35] At the present time, image acquisition times are relatively long, and MR-guided aspiration is cumbersome. Furthermore, the technology is costly and not universally available, and there exists a population of patients who are unable to tolerate the procedure.

Functional Imaging

Radionuclide scans using indium-111-labeled leukocytes and polyclonal immunoglobulin G (IgG) have an adjunctive role in the diagnosis of vascular graft infection. They cannot be performed in the early postoperative period due to nonspecific uptake of the signal by healing tissues. A study by Sedwitz et al.[37] reported a sensitivity of 100% but a specificity of 50% and an accuracy of 53% for detecting wound complications. A negative scan was very reliable in ruling out an infectious process in this series. LaMuraglia and colleagues[38] studied 25 patients suspected of having graft infection using indium-111-labeled human IgG and reported a sensitivity of 93%, a specificity of 100%, with an accuracy of 96%.[38] IgG scans are generally preferred over leukocyte scans because of the abscence of red cell and platelet labeling, and lack of exposure of the staff to blood products. Currently, functional imaging is best utilized in conjunction with anatomic imaging to better determine the location and extent of infection.

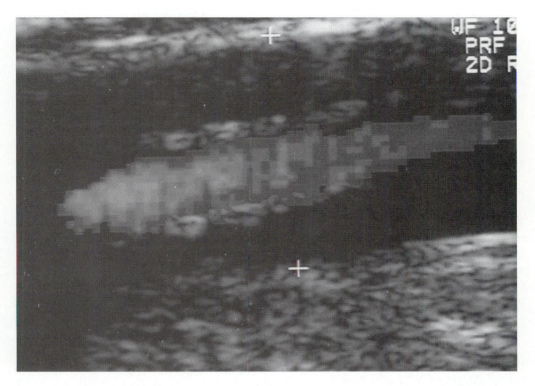

Figure 20–3. Longitudinal view of infected graft in Figure 20–2 demonstrating perigraft fluid.

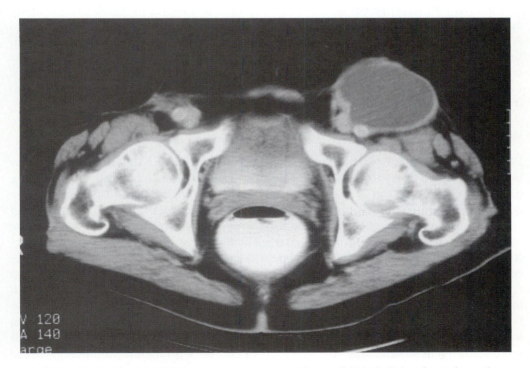

Figure 20–4. CT scan showing perigraft fluid surrounding graft in both limbs of aortofemoral grafts at inguinal ligament.

Contrast Angiography

Angiography provides little diagnostic information when evaluating a patient for graft infection, but is vital for planning therapeutic strategies. Angiograms will demonstrate vessel occlusion and pseudoaneurysms, but these are also well demonstrated using duplex ultrasound and CT scanning. The utility of angiography comes in assessing the proximal and distal vascular tree for subsequent arterial reconstruction.

MANAGEMENT

General Principles

The basic goals of therapy in patients with lower extremity graft infection are the irradication of infection and maintenance of adequate distal perfusion. Management in these patients must be highly individualized and is dependent on factors such as the severity of the patient's clinical presentation (anastomotic hemorrhage, hemodynamic instability, signs of systemic sepsis), the extent and microbiology of the infection, the type of graft, patient comorbidity, and status of the patient's native vasculature. All surgical options should be considered, but the axiom "life over limb" must always be observed when formulating the therapeutic plan.

Initial treatment involves a thorough history and physical examination to determine the acuity of the patient's illness. Patients who present in shock due to sepsis or hypovolemia from hemorrhage require expeditious evaluation and initiation of treatment. Aggressive resuscitation efforts with blood and fluid volume in an intensive care setting are imperative in these critically ill patients. Broad-spectrum antibiotics are started early in the patient's initial hospital course, and development of a surgical strategy can proceed during the initial resuscitative period.

For patients who present with less acute symptomatology, time exists to thoroughly evaluate and optimize the patient's comorbid conditions in preparation for surgery. Again, a broad-spectrum antibiotic should be started, and then tailored based on sensitivity results from wound or aspiration culture. Imaging studies should be performed concomitantly to determine the nature, extent, and location of the infectious process. Finally, frank discussions with the patient regarding potential surgical options, morbidity, and mortality should also take place.

Wound Infection

Wound infection after infrainguinal arterial reconstruction is common and can occur in up to 44% of procedures.[3] Risk factors and classification of wound infection are discussed previously and impact on subsequent treatment. Class I and II infections are considered "minor" and generally respond to operative debridement, local wound care, and intravenous antibiotics.[28] Class III wounds with graft exposure are of more concern and are associated with more conduit complications. Prime management objectives of these wounds are early surgical debridement, drainage of any clinically significant fluid collections, and conformation of autogenous tissue coverage.[39] Ouriel and colleagues[2] managed wounds in 16 patients with exposed autogenous vein grafts with local wound care and delayed autogenous tissue coverage until adequate granulation had developed. They reported hemorrhage or thrombosis in 56% of cases managed in this manner. Alternatively, Reifsnyder and colleagues[7] described their experience with wound complication management with early operative debridement, autogenous tissue coverage when indicated, three times daily dressing changes, and parenteral antibiotics in 55 wound infections, 13 of which were graft-threatening. This management protocol resulted in no deaths, no limb loss, and universal graft salvage. There must be a high index of suspicion of graft involvement in any wound infection, and early surgical inspection to rule out graft involvement is required if overt conduit infection is to be avoided.

Prosthetic Graft Infection

Treatment options for prosthetic graft infection include total graft excision, excision with *in situ* revascularization, excision with extra-anatomic reconstruction, and graft preservation techniques using aggressive debridement, autogenous tissue coverage, and local wound care. Graft excision is generally required if any of the following conditions exist: (1) signs of systemic sepsis; (2) anastomotic disruption with hemorrhage; (3) presence of gram-negative organisms on culture; (4) involvement of the entire graft; and (5) associated graft thrombosis. Removal of the entire graft in these situations is essential if the infection is to be cleared. Attempts at graft preservation in this setting almost always result in recurrence or progression of the infection with the risk of systemic toxicity and delayed exsanguinating hemorrhage.

It is uncommon to remove the infected prosthesis without the need to revascularize. If the conduit was previously occluded or the original procedure was performed for claudication, collateral development may have occurred to a sufficient degree to prevent limb-threatening ischemia and immediate revascularization may not be required. Generally, if ankle Doppler signals are absent at the time of surgery, critical ischemia with its associated increase in morbidity and limb loss can be anticipated if revascularization is not performed.

If the indications for graft excision do not include anastomotic bleeding or overwhelming systemic toxicity, and distal revascularization is required, staged surgical therapy can be done by first performing the revascularization followed by graft excision several days later. Morbidity and mortality can be reduced and lower extremity ischemia is avoided using this technique. However, if the patient presents with hemorrhage or septic shock, control of bleeding and graft excision are the initial priorities and staged operations are not recommended. The conduit of choice for arterial reconstruction is autogenous vein or endarterectomized iliac or superficial femoral artery. Autogenous tissue is frequently unavailable in these patients, in which case prosthetic reconstruction using PTFE through remote, noninfected tissue planes should be performed.

Early graft infections are usually associated with more severe complications such as anastomotic bleeding or sepsis, complex wound infections, and particularly virulent bacterial pathogens (gram-negative aerobes, coagulase-positive staphylococci) and therefore almost always require excision. Principles of graft removal include excision of the entire graft, wide debridement and irrigation of the surrounding tissues, closure of arteriotomies and arterial stumps with monofilament suture, and aggressive antibiotic therapy. In addition, patients with questionable limb viability should be started on systemic heparin anticoagulation.

Graft infections that occur months to years after implantation are generally indolent, less extensive, and present with vague signs and symptoms. The infecting organisms are most commonly mucin-producing strains of *S. epidermidis,* although other coagulase-negative staphylococci can be isolated using appropriate techniques. In these cases, if the infection is localized and pseudoaneurysm or graft thrombosis has not occurred, graft preservation may be attempted. This therapy entails (1) repeated, aggressive surgical debridement; (2) autogenous tissue coverage; (3) local wound care with dressing changes; and (4) long-term intravenous antibiotics. Several studies have reported successful graft preservation in more than 90% of cases with significantly better limb salvage using this strategy and recommend this treatment in selected PTFE graft infections.[5,11,40]

Another method of treating prosthetic graft infection is excision with *in situ* replacement using autogenous or PTFE conduits. As with graft preservation treatment, the patient cannot be septic or present with hemorrhage. Essential components of *in situ* graft replacement include perioperative vancomycin, exclusion of virulent gram-negative bacteria on culture, wide debridement and irrigation of perigraft tissue and anastomotic sites, and rotational muscle flap coverage.[41] Towne et al.[42] reported results of this treatment in 20 patients with prosthetic graft infection including both aortic and infrainguinal conduits. Coagulase-negative staphylococci were isolated in 17 (85%) cases. In this series, all wounds healed, all grafts remained patent, there was no limb loss, and all replacement grafts remained well incorporated.[42] *In situ* replacement of biofilm graft infections is effective for treating localized graft healing problems, but because of the indolent nature of this type of infection, subsequent infection of previously uninvolved graft segments can occur.

Autogenous Graft Infection

The incidence of confirmed lower extremity autogenous graft infection is exceedingly low and often goes unreported in large series.[43-47] Autogenous grafts are much more resistant to infection, but irreversible graft damage can ensue particularly if gram-negative pathogens are involved.[2] Management objectives are the same as those with prosthetic graft infections: complete resolution of the infectious process and preservation of distal perfusion.

As with prosthetic graft infections, graft excision is usually required if the infection manifests as systemic toxicity, graft thrombosis, anastomotic disruption with bleeding or pseudoaneurysm formation, or if gram-negative bacteria are involved. In these situations, reconstruction using either *in situ* replacement or extra-anatomic bypass can be utilized. However, if the infection is localized and anastomoses are intact in a patent conduit, graft preservation procedures as described previously can be attempted with favorable results.[48]

REFERENCES

1. Hoffert PW, Gensler S, Haimovici H. Infection complicating arterial grafts. *Arch Surg.* 1965;90:427–435.
2. Ouriel K, Geary KJ, Green RM, DeWeese JA. Fate of the exposed saphenous vein graft. *Am J Surg.* 1990;160:148–150.
3. Kent KC, Bartek S, Kuntz KM, et al. Prospective study of wound complications in continuous infrainguinal incisions after lower limb arterial reconstruction: incidence, risk factors, and cost. *Surgery.* 1996;119:378–383.
4. Edwards WH Jr, Martin RS III, Jenkins JM, Edwards WH Sr. Primary graft infections. *J Vasc Surg.* 1987;6:235–239.
5. Cherry KJ Jr, Roland CF, Pairolero PC, et al. Infected femorodistal bypass: is graft removal mandatory? *J Vasc Surg.* 1992;15:295–305.
6. Lorentzen JE, Nielsen OM, Arendrup H, et al. Vascular graft infection: an analysis of sixty-two graft infections in 2411 consecutively implanted synthetic vascular grafts. *Surgery.* 1985;98:81–86.
7. Reifsnyder T, Bandyk D, Seabrook G, et al. Wound complications of the *in situ* vein bypass technique. *J Vasc Surg.* 1992;15:843–850.

8. Wengrovitz M, Atnip RG, Gifford RRM, et al. Wound complications of autogenous subcutaneous infrainguinal arterial bypass surgery: predisposing factors. *J Vasc Surg.* 1990;11:156–163.

9. Liekweg WG Jr, Greenfield LJ. Vascular prosthetic infections: collected experience and results of treatment. *Surgery.* 1977;81:335–342.

10. Szilagyi DE, Smith RF, Elliot JP, Vrandecic MP. Infection in arterial reconstruction with synthetic grafts. *Ann Surg.* 1972;176:321–333.

11. Calligaro KD, Westcott CJ, Buckley RM, et al. Infrainguinal anastomotic arterial graft infections treated by selective graft preservation. *Ann Surg.* 1992;216:74–79.

12. Kikta MJ, Goodson SF, Bishara RA, et al. Mortality and limb loss with infected infrainguinal bypass. *J Vasc Surg.* 1987;5:566–571.

13. Levy MF, Schmitt DD, Edmiston CE, et al. Sequential analysis of staphylococcal colonization of body surfaces of patients undergoing vascular surgery. *J Clin Microbiol.* 1990;28:664–669.

14. Macbeth GA, Rubin JR, McIntyre KE Jr, et al. The relevance of arterial wall microbiology to the treatment of prosthetic graft infections: graft infection vs. arterial infection. *J Vasc Surg.* 1984;1:750–756.

15. Durham JR, Malone JM, Bernhard VM. The impact of multiple operations on the importance of arterial wall cultures. *J Vasc Surg.* 1987;5:160–169.

16. Moore WS. Experimental studies relating to sepsis in prosthetic vascular grafting. In: Duma RJ, ed. *Infections of Prosthetic Heart Valves and Vascular Grafts.* Baltimore: University Park Press; 1977:267–285.

17. Rubin JR, Malone JM, Goldstone J. The role of the lymphatic system in acute arterial prosthetic graft infections. *J Vasc Surg.* 1985;2:92–98.

18. Bandyk DF, Bergamini TM. Infection in prosthetic vascular grafts. In: Rutherford RB, ed. *Vascular Surgery.* 4th ed. Philadelphia: WB Saunders; 1995:588–603.

19. Dougherty SH, Simmons RL. Infections in bionic man: the pathophysiology of infections in prosthetic devices—part II. *Curr Prob Surg.* 1982;19:269–318.

20. Schmitt DD, Bandyk DF, Pequet AJ, Towne JB. Bacterial adherence to vascular prostheses: a determinant of graft infectivity. *J Vasc Surg.* 1986;3:732–740.

21. Doscher W, Krishnasastry KV, Deckoff SL. Fungal graft infections: case report and review of the literature. *J Vasc Surg.* 1987;6:398–402.

22. Dale BAS, McCormick JStC. Mycoplasma hominis wound infection following aortobifemoral bypass. *Eur J Vasc Surg.* 1991;5:213–214.

23. Bergamini TM, Bandyk DF, Govostis D, et al. Identification of *Staphylococcus epidermidis* vascular graft infections: a comparison of culture techniques. *J Vasc Surg.* 1989;9:665–670.

24. Geary KJ, Tomkiewicz ZM, Harrison HN, et al. Differential effects of a gram-negative and a gram-positive infection on autogenous and prosthetic grafts. *J Vasc Surg.* 1990;11:339–347.

25. Bandyk DF, Bergamini TM, Kinney EV, et al. *In situ* replacement of vascular prostheses infected by bacterial biofilms. *J Vasc Surg.* 1991;13:575–583.

26. Yeager RA, Porter JM. Arterial and prosthetic graft infection. *Ann Vasc Surg.* 1992;6:485–491.

27. Mertens RA, O'Hara PJ, Hertzer NR, et al. Surgical management of infrainguinal arterial prosthetic graft infections: review of a thirty-five-year experience. *J Vasc Surg.* 1995;21: 782–791.

28. Samson RH, Veith FJ, Janko GS, et al. A modified classification and approach to the management of infections involving peripheral arterial prosthetic grafts. *J Vasc Surg.* 1988;8:147–153.

29. Goldstone J, Moore WS. Infection in vascular prostheses: clinical manifestations and surgical management. *Am J Surg.* 1974;128:225–233.

30. O'Brien T, Collin J. Prosthetic vascular graft infection. *Br J Surg.* 1992;79:1262–1267.

31. Polak JE, Donaldson MC, Whittemore AD, et al. Pulsatile masses surrounding vascular prostheses: real-time US color flow imaging. *Radiology.* 1989;170:363–366.

32. Merrell SW, Lawrence PF. Diagnosis of graft infection: anatomic and functional techniques. *Semin Vasc Surg.* 1990;3:89–100.

33. Haaga JR, Baldwin N, Reich NE, et al. CT detection of infected synthetic grafts: preliminary report of a new sign. *AJR.* 1978;131:317–320.

34. Auffermann W, Olofsson PA, Rabahie GN, et al. Incorporation versus infection of retroperitoneal aortic grafts: MR imaging features. *Radiology.* 1989;172:359–362.

35. Olofsson PA, Auffermann W, Higgins CB, et al. Diagnosis of prosthetic aortic graft infection by magnetic resonance imaging. *J Vasc Surg.* 1988;8:99–105.
36. Justich E, Amparo EG, Hricak H, Higgins CB. Infected aortoiliofemoral grafts: magnetic resonance imaging. *Radiology.* 1985;154:133–136.
37. Sedwitz MM, Davies RJ, Pretorius HT, Vasquez TE. Indium 111-labeled white blood cell scans after vascular prosthetic reconstruction. *J Vasc Surg.* 1987;6:476–481.
38. LaMuraglia GM, Fischman AJ, Strauss HW, et al. Utility of the indium 111-labeled human immunoglobulin G scan for the detection of focal vascular graft infection. *J Vasc Surg.* 1989;10:20–28.
39. Gordon IL, Pousti TJ, Stemmer EA, et al. Inguinal wound fluid collections after vascular surgery: management by early reoperation. *South Med J.* 1995;88:433–436.
40. Perler BA, Vander Kolk CA, Dufresne CR, Williams GM. Can infected prosthetic grafts be salvaged with rotational muscle flaps? *Surgery.* 1991;110:30–34.
41. Krupski WC. Infected vascular graft. In: Cameron JL, ed. *Current Surgical Therapy.* 5th ed. St. Louis, MO: Mosby; 1995:690–701.
42. Towne JB, Seabrook GR, Bandyk D, et al. *In situ* replacement of arterial prosthesis infected by bacterial biofilms: long-term follow-up. *J Vasc Surg.* 1994;19:226–235.
43. Bergamini TM, Towne JB, Bandyk DF, et al. Experience with *in situ* saphenous vein bypass during 1981 to 1989: determinant factors of long-term patency. *J Vasc Surg.* 1991;13:137–149.
44. Taylor LM, Edwards JM, Porter JM. Present status of reversed vein bypass grafting: five-year results of a modern series. *J Vasc Surg.* 1990;11:193–206.
45. Leather RP, Shah DM, Chang BB, Kaufman JL. Resurrection of the *in situ* saphenous vein bypass: 1000 cases later. *Ann Surg.* 1988;208:435–442.
46. Donaldson MC, Mannick JA, Whittemore AD. Femoral-distal bypass with *in situ* greater saphenous vein: long-term results using the Mills valvulotome. *Ann Surg.* 1991;213:457–465.
47. Veith FJ, Gupta SK, Ascer E, et al. Six-year prospective multicenter randomized comparison of autologous saphenous vein and expanded polytetrafluoroethylene grafts in the infrainguinal arterial reconstructions. *J Vasc Surg.* 1986;3:104–114.
48. Calligaro KD, Veith FJ, Schwartz ML, et al. Management of infected lower extremity and autologous vein grafts by selective graft preservation. *Am J Surg.* 1992;164:291–294.

21

Endovascular Technique in *In Situ* Vein Graft

David Rosenthal, MD, and Giancarlo Piano, MD

The first successful femoropopliteal *in situ* saphenous vein bypass was reported by Karl Victor Hall of Oslo, Norway, in 1962.[1] Since this initial report, surgeons have attempted to simplify the two principal technical components of the operation: (1) rendering the saphenous vein valves incompetent and (2) occluding the venous side branches. Unfortunately, to accomplish this, an incision must be made in the length of the leg over the course of the saphenous vein, which can be fraught with hazard, especially in the diabetic patient where wound complications can be devastating.

In an attempt to make the *in situ* vein bypass technique less invasive, we developed an operative approach that would allow the surgeon to render the vein valves incompetent and occlude venous side branches from within the saphenous vein—an "endovascular" technique in *in situ* vein graft.

CLINICAL STUDIES

In an effort to determine if endovascular occlusion of venous side branches could be performed, an electronically steerable nitinol catheter was developed to occlude venous side branches with embolization coils. Between June 1990 and December 1993, 97 patients underwent 99 endovascular *in situ* femorodistal popliteal or tibial bypasses in a multicenter study.[2,3]

At operation, standard incisions were made over the proximal femoral artery/vein and over the saphenous vein at the site of the distal anastomosis. The saphenous vein was mobilized for enough length to permit each anastomosis and posterior ligation. After heparinization the saphenous vein was divided from the common femoral vein, and the most proximal valve in the vein was excised with scissors. Initially in this study, an angioscope was inserted into the proximal portion of the saphenous vein, either directly or through a transsected large proximal side branch, and the angioscope passed down the saphenous vein to identify venous side branches, which were located and marked on the skin. By turning off the overhead operating room lights the angioscope light transilluminated through the skin and side branches was identified. Retro-

271

grade "stripper" valvulotomes were inserted through the distal portion of the divided saphenous vein and advanced proximally. The angioscope identified the location of each competent valve while irrigation with a 5% dextrose/heparin (1,000 IU/L)–papaverine (30 mg/L) solution from the angioscope maintained the valve leaflets in a closed position for valvulotomy.

After completion of valvulotomy, the angioscope was removed and reinserted through the distal saphenous vein. The nitinol alloy catheter (CRI, Catheter Research, Inc., Indianapolis, IN) was then inserted into the proximal saphenous vein. Venous side branches were entered with the articulating CRI catheter under angioscopic surveillance. Fluoroscopy surveillance verified placement of the CRI catheter in a venous side branch and confirmed coil placement after ejection in 46 operations, whereas fluoroscopic surveillance only was used in 53 operations. Side branch occlusion was performed with 2-mm × 4-cm, 3-mm × 6-cm, and 4-mm × 6-cm platinum coils (Target Therapeutics, San Jose, CA). The length of the occlusion coils before embolization (4 to 6 cm) is unrelated to the final coil configuration in the side branch because the coil "balls up" after deployment (Fig. 21–1). Tiny (1- to 2-mm) tributaries were left patent, and intraoperative arteriography verified venous side branch occlusion and saphenous vein bypass patency.

All patients were given 325 mg aspirin after operation and were evaluated clinically in the immediate postoperative period (30 days); midterm follow-up extended to 24 months. Graft patency was evaluated by color-flow duplex ultrasonography or Doppler ultrasonography. Bypass occlusion was confirmed by duplex or arteriographic evaluation and all bypasses were evaluated every 3 months.

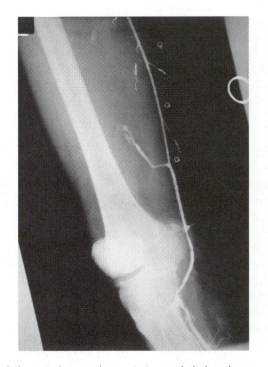

Figure 21–1. Completion arteriogram demonstrates occluded saphenous side branches and patent *in situ* bypass. (*Reproduced with permission: Rosenthal D, Dickson G, Rodriguez FJ, et al. Infrainguinal endovascular in situ saphenous vein bypass: ongoing results. J Vasc Surg. 1994;20:390.*)

RESULTS

Sixty-eight femorodistal popliteal and 31 femorocrural *in situ* bypasses were performed in 97 patients utilizing the endovascular occlusion technique. Nine complications related to the various types of valvulotomes occurred early in the series when we were less experienced with these devices. Three valvulotome heads (two Olympus, one Leather) "detached," and venotomies were necessary to retrieve them; one of these resulted in a graft failure. Six other saphenous vein perforations required vein patch angioplasty in five cases and a primary repair in one case. The perforations occurred when the valvulotome caught at a side branch orifice and "sheared" the vein.

In 99 *in situ* operations, endovascular occlusion of 342 saphenous vein side branches (average 4.6 side branches per case) was performed. Of the 342 side branches cannulated, 288 (84%) were totally occluded, and 54 (16%) were partially occluded with 411 platinum occlusion coils at the time of "completion" arteriograms. Side branches initially occluded remained occluded and 51 of the 54 partially occluded side branches thrombosed during follow-up by color-flow ultrasonography. In general, venous side branches at or above the knee, because they were larger, were the ones more easily cannulated and occluded.

Wound complications after the endovascular bypasses occurred in 5% (5 of 99) of patients. These were minor (hematoma in two, seroma in two, and skin edge slough in one), but prolonged the hospital stay in these patients.

After operation, the mean hospital length of stay (LOS) was 4.1 days (range 1 to 16 days). Five "missed" arteriovenous fistulas (AVFs) were identified by completion arteriography at the end of operation; these were ligated uneventfully.

The 24-month bypass graft patency rate was 77% (Fig. 21–2).[2,3] During midterm follow-up, 12 graft failures occurred. Five were perioperative failures, attributed to technical error in four cases and an "inadequate" vein in the fifth. In one patient the valvulotome head detached, and at venotomy to retrieve the head, a 3 cm intimal injury was noted. Three other technical failures were in early cases in which the CRI catheter and angioscope were "aggressively used" in a small vein (2.5 mm) and failure was thought to be due to intimal injury. The last patient had a 2.0-mm "sclerotic vein below the knee," which thrombosed 4 days after operation. The other 7 graft failures occurred during the first 3 months; these diabetic patients had gangrene (Rutherford Grade II, category 5).[4] These patients had poor arterio-

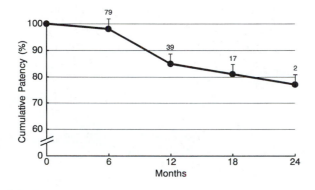

Figure 21–2. Cumulative 24-month patency of endovascular *in situ* vein bypass. Numbers at intervals indicate grafts at risk. (*Reproduced with permission: Rosenthal D, Dickson C, Rodriguez FJ, et al. Infrainguinal endovascular in situ saphenous vein bypass: ongoing results. J Vasc Surg. 1994;20:390.*)

graphic runoff and failures were thought to be due to the severe distal disease present and not a mechanical injury to the vein graft.

COMMENTS

Infrainguinal *in situ* saphenous vein bypass remains among the most challenging operations facing the vascular surgeon today. These patients often have complicated medical and surgical problems, and the increasing awareness of rising health care costs in the United States today has made "minimally invasive" operations most attractive.

Gupta and Veith[5] demonstrated the inadequacy of Diagnosis Related Group (DRG) reimbursement for limb salvage arterial reconstructions. Their study evaluated the cost of 209 patients in 10 hospital centers from various geographic and practice patterns who underwent *in situ* saphenous vein bypasses for limb salvage. The net reimbursement to the hospital for each *in situ* patient was a loss of $5,616, or a total study loss of $1,173,744. The basic cause of this problem was the protracted hospital LOS. In their report the mean LOS for these *in situ* patients was 18.8 days (Gupta, personal communication, May 1993). This information is corroborated by data from the Health Care Finance Administration, Office of Payment Policy, on the CPT codes 35583 and 35585 (femoropopliteal and tibial *in situ* vein bypasses), in which the average hospital LOS for 15,299 cases was 12.8 days. This, in large part, was due to the morbidity associated with an incision in the leg, the length of which can be fraught with hazard, especially in the diabetic patient where wound complications can be devasting.

Wound complications after femoropopliteal-tibial bypass with saphenous vein are common and have been reported in up to one-third of cases and are usually due to ischemia of the posterior "flap" along the thigh incision, which may cause cellulitis, lymphangitis, edema, and fat necrosis.[6–8] In our study, wound complications occurred in only five (5%) patients, as the femoropopliteal bypasses, whenever possible, were performed through two incisions, while anterior tibial grafts required a third incision for anastomosis. Thus, by obviating the need for an incision the length of the leg, the potential for wound complications and hospital LOS were greatly reduced.

CURRENT TECHNIQUE

The endovascular bypass procedure has been simplified since our initial studies and we have continued to refine the instrumentation and technique of operation. Today,

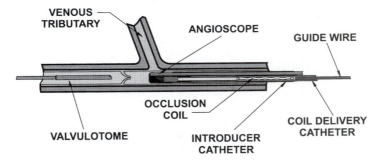

Figure 21–3. Retrograde valvulotome and side branch occlusion system.

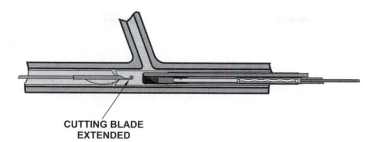

**CUTTING BLADE
EXTENDED**

Figure 21–4. Under angioscopic surveillance, the valvulotome is extended and the valve cusp engaged.

we perform endovascular *in situ* bypass using a prototype valvulotome and side branch occlusion system (Baxter, Vascular, Irvine, CA) that is elegant in its simplicity and user friendly. The component parts are a retrograde valvulotome, which houses an irrigating catheter (for heparin–papaverine–saline flush) introduced from the distal saphenous vein (Fig. 21–3). The side branch occlusion system is introduced from the proximal saphenous vein and is made up of a movable angioscope, an introducer catheter, within which is the coil delivery catheter, which contains a preloaded occlusion coil and a guide wire.

During valvulotomy, the angioscope is placed in the "extended position," which allows us to visualize the vein lumen in a 360-degree, circumferential fashion. The valvulotome cutting blades are kept in the retracted position to minimize any potential for intimal trauma. When a set of valve cusps is identified, the cutting blade is extended and the valve cusps engaged (Fig. 21–4). With general traction on the valvulotome, valvulotomy of one valve cusp under direct angioscopic surveillance is performed. The valvulotome is rotated 180 degrees, the contralateral cusp is engaged, and valvulotomy again performed.

Most major side branches are located at the site of the vein valves; therefore, side branch occlusion can be immediately performed after valvulotomy. During side branch occlusion, the angioscope is placed into the "retracted position," which better allows the operator to visualize the side branch orifice. The coil delivery catheter, which contains the occlusion coil and guide wire is then guided into the side branch (Fig. 21–5). The guide wire is advanced and a coil deployed out of the delivery catheter, into the venous side branch, and the side branch is embolized (Fig. 21–6). With this new system, valvulotomy and side branch occlusion may be easily and safely performed with one pass down the saphenous vein through two incisions.

The limitations of the endovascular bypass are, first and foremost, the size and quality of the saphenous vein. In veins less than 3 mm in diameter, it may be too difficult to maneuver the catheter into venous side branches without causing intimal

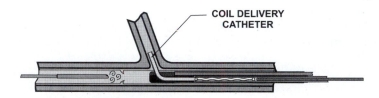

**COIL DELIVERY
CATHETER**

Figure 21–5. The coil delivery catheter containing an occlusion coil and guide wire is guided into the side branch.

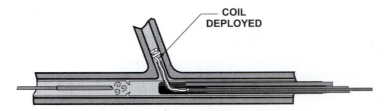

Figure 21–6. The coil is deployed and the side branch embolized.

injury. In general, venous side branches at or above the knee, because they are larger, are most easily cannulated and occluded, but endovascular occlusion of all saphenous vein side branches may not be possible in each vein graft. The technique, however, continues to evolve and as refinement and catheter design continue and operator experience increases, it is hoped these limitations will be solved. Indeed, with the latest generation valvulotome and side branch occlusion system, we have performed 12 endovascular infrainguinal *in situ* bypasses for limb salvage in recent months. In 9 of these 12 patients, the operations were performed through two incisions; 3 patients required extra incisions to ligate perforator veins. The mean hospital LOS was 3.8 days, and there was one wound complication: a full thickness skin slough in a patient who inadvertently left his popliteal incision staples in place for 21 days. One retained AVF was identified, and one graft has failed.

If the endovascular bypass long-term patency rates remain similar to classic *in situ* bypass patency rates, the benefits we will see of decreased hospital LOS, reduced wound-related complications, shortened recuperation, and, therefore, increased health care savings gives the endovascular *in situ* vein graft concept strong consideration as a possible future operation for infrainguinal revascularization.

REFERENCES

1. Hall KV. The great saphenous vein used *in-situ* as an arterial shunt after extirpation of the vein valves. *Surgery.* 1962;51:492–495.
2. Rosenthal D, Herring MB, O'Donovan T, et al. Endovascular infrainguinal *in situ* saphenous vein bypass: a multicenter preliminary report. *J Vasc Surg.* 1992;16:453–458.
3. Rosenthal D, Dickson C, Rodriguez FJ, et al. Infrainguinal endovascular in situ saphenous vein bypass: ongoing results. *J Vasc Surg.* 1994;20:389–395.
4. Rutherford RB, Flanigan DP, Gupta SK, et al. Suggested standards for reports dealing with lower extremity ischemia. *J Vasc Surg.* 1986;4:80–94.
5. Gupta SK, Veith FJ. Inadequacy of Diagnosis Related Group (DRG) reconstructions. *J Vasc Surg.* 1990;11:348–357.
6. Schwartz ME, Harrington EB, Schanzer H. Wound complications after *in situ.* bypass. *J Vasc Surg.* 1988;7:802–807.
7. Utley JR, Thomason ME, Wallace JD, et al. Preoperative correlates of impaired wound healing after saphenous vein excision. *J Thorac Cardiovasc Surg.* 1989;98:147–149.
8. Wengrovitz M, Atnip RG, Gifford RM, et al. Wound complications of autogenous subcutaneous infrainguinal arterial bypass surgery: predisposing factors and management. *J Vasc Surg.* 1990;11:156–163.

22

Current Status of Thrombolytic Therapy in Occlusion of Native Arteries and Bypass Grafts

Kenneth Ouriel, MD

Peripheral arterial occlusion is associated with pain with ambulation when mild, and with pain at rest and threatened tissue loss when severe. The process may occur in the setting of underlying atherosclerotic disease and a preexisting native arterial or bypass graft stenosis; alternatively, an embolus or hypercoagulable state may result in occlusion of a previously normal arterial segment or graft. Operative intervention has long been the standard therapy for peripheral arterial occlusion. Thrombolytic therapy has gained widespread acceptance during the last two decades, with the potential to restore arterial flow through a less invasive technique than open surgical intervention.

PATIENT CHARACTERISTICS

Ischemic symptoms from peripheral arterial occlusion are traditionally grouped into two categories: nonthreatening ischemia (claudication alone) and limb-threatening ischemia (rest pain, ischemic ulceration, or gangrene). The severity of symptoms following the occlusion of a peripheral artery or bypass graft is dependent on the adequacy of collateral circulation around the process.[1] Limb-threatening symptoms are rare in the absence of multilevel arterial occlusion. Thus, the solitary superficial femoral occlusion at the adductor canal is usually associated with claudication alone, whereas obstruction of the superficial femoral and popliteal vessels is commonly associated with rest pain progressing to tissue loss. Cardiac emboli to the periphery constitute a special case. These emboli tend to lodge at the common femoral arterial bifurcation, obstructing flow to both the superficial femoral artery and the profunda femoris artery. In the absence of prior occlusive disease, collaterals are virtually absent and the leg becomes acutely ischemic with pain, pallor, paresthesia, and coolness below the level of the groin.

Lower limb ischemia has been categorized into acute and chronic varieties. Acute limb ischemia is defined by patient presentation with symptoms with a well-defined onset, generally within 14 days. Chronic ischemic symptoms are more insidious in onset and it is frequently impossible for the patient to identify the point of onset with precision.

The results of therapy for peripheral arterial occlusion are dependent on the severity of ischemia. The randomized study of Veith et al.[2] documented decreased graft patency in patients with claudication compared to those with limb-threatening ischemia. Similarly, Jivegaard et al.[3] observed a correlation between the severity of ischemia and the perioperative mortality rate associated with surgical revascularization. With these considerations in mind, Rutherford et al.[4] published a grading scheme for acute limb ischemia. This scheme was an attempt to standardize the severity and, in this manner, allow the rational comparison of data from different studies. The criteria were adopted by the Society of Vascular Surgery and the North American Chapter of the International Society for Cardiovascular Surgery and have been dubbed with the colloquialism "SVS/ISCVS criteria." Limbs may be subcategorized into one of these gradations of ischemia using the SVS/ISCVS criteria. The least ischemic category comprises those limbs without limb-threatening symptoms, generally with claudication alone. The middle category includes limbs that are threatened but where therapeutic intervention can still salvage the extremity. The final category identifies those limbs with irreversible ischemia where therapeutic interventions can be predicted to be futile. As such, studies evaluating novel operative or thrombolytic treatment modalities have generally included patients with SVS/ISCVS Category II ischemia; threatened, but not irreversibly so.

TREATMENT OF PERIPHERAL ARTERIAL OCCLUSION

The primary therapeutic objective in the setting of peripheral arterial occlusion is the restoration of blood flow through recanalization of the occluded native artery or bypass graft (thrombectomy or thrombolysis) or through placement of a new bypass graft around the occlusive process. Surgical intervention in the setting of acute limb ischemia consisted of balloon catheter thromboembolectomy following the introduction of the device by Fogarty et al.[5] in 1963. Although balloon catheter thromboembolectomy remains appropriate for embolic problems, many have advocated placement of a new bypass graft conduit for all other etiologies. At present, surgical methods remain the standard form of therapy with which all newer modalities must be compared. Open surgical techniques are safe and efficacious in the setting of chronic peripheral arterial occlusion. Surgical intervention in the setting of acute occlusion has been associated with a high rate of amputation and patient demise, presumably as a result of the fragile medical status of this patient subgroup (Table 22–1). Blaisdell et al.[6] were among the first to identify the high rate of morbidity and mortality associated with surgical intervention for acute limb ischemia. They suggested that immediate operative intervention be delayed, treating the patient with high-dose heparin therapy until stabilization could be achieved. Although this therapeutic strategy never became fully accepted,

TABLE 22–1. HISTORICAL RESULTS OF OPERATION FOR LIMB ISCHEMIA, TABULATED IN HOSPITAL OR AT 1 MONTH FOLLOWING THE PROCEDURE

Author	Year	Etiology	Amputation (%)	Death (%)
Blaisdell et al.[6]	1978	Embolism, thrombosis	30	25
Jivegaard et al.[3]	1986	Embolism, thrombosis	19	26
Yeager et al.[7]	1992	Graft thrombosis	30	15

later studies by such investigators as Jivegaard et al.[3] and Yeager et al.[7] confirmed the high mortality associated with surgical intervention.

Thrombolytic dissolution of the occluding fibrin–platelet thrombus has been employed as an alternative to surgery. Plasminogen activators such as streptokinase, urokinase, and recombinant tissue plasminogen activator have been administered directly into the thrombus through a catheter-directed approach. Thrombolytic agents provided two potential advantages over standard surgical methods. First, the obstructing thrombus or thromboembolus could be ameliorated using techniques less invasive than open operation. Second, patency of the original conduit or native artery could be restored, obviating the need to harvest a new graft.

Despite these advantages of thrombolytic techniques, successful thrombolysis must be followed by an endovascular or open surgical approach to unmasked stenotic lesions, lesions thought to be the causative etiology of the occlusive event (Table 22–2). Thrombolytic techniques should not be considered to be replacement modalities for open surgical repair; this is possible and appropriate in a minority of cases. For example, successful thrombolysis of an occluded vein graft is likely to uncover a stenotic lesion responsible for the failure of the conduit.[8] This lesion must then be addressed with a directed surgical technique such as patch angioplasty or an endovascular modality such as balloon angioplasty. Only in rare cases of embolic events or prosthetic graft occlusion will thrombolysis be sufficient as the sole intervention.

The evaluation of novel treatment modalities must include the careful evaluation of long-term follow-up data. Primary outcome measures such as limb salvage and patient mortality must be assessed and compared with the results of standard therapy. Benefits such as limitations in the frequency and magnitude of required interventions and decreases in the economic burden of treatment are relevant secondary end points that become important once equivalence in the primary outcome measures has been proven.

In the United States, patients with peripheral arterial occlusion are generally admitted under the direct care of a vascular surgeon as the primary decision maker. Patients with acute and severe limb ischemia are usually sent directly to the hospital emergency department and vascular surgical consultation is immediately requested. Patients with more chronic symptoms or symptoms of a lesser order of severity are sent to the vascular surgical outpatient office. In each case, the vascular surgeon assumes responsibility as the primary caregiver. Nevertheless, the appropriate treatment of these patients is always multidepartmental, involving the interventionalist in a direct role and occasionally cardiologists, hematologists, and vascular medicine specialists in consultation. Following admission, diagnostic arteriography is performed by the interventionalist.

TABLE 22–2. SECONDARY TREATMENT MODALITIES UTILIZED FOLLOWING SUCCESSFUL THROMBOLYSIS

Clinical Scenario Following Thrombolysis	Therapeutic Alternatives
Complete dissolution of arterial embolus	Long-term anticoagulation
Open graft without a residual lesion	Long-term anticoagulation
Solitary lesion in saphenous vein graft	Surgical patch angioplasty; balloon dilatation
Multiple lesions in saphenous vein graft	Replacement of some or all of the graft
Atherosclerotic stenosis of native artery, short	Surgical endarterectomy; balloon dilatation; bypass grafting
Atherosclerotic stenosis of native artery, long	Bypass grafting

The interventionalist reviews the diagnostic arteriogram and confers with the vascular surgeon with respect to the most appropriate management of the patient: immediate surgery, thrombolysis, or an endovascular intervention such as balloon angioplasty, stenting, or atherectomy. If a thrombolytic strategy is elected, interplay between the interventionalist and vascular surgeon is continuous and ongoing. Decisions regarding the termination of thrombolytic infusion or the performance of subsequent surgical or endovascular interventions are usually made by the vascular surgeon, albeit with considerable input from the interventional team.

CLINICAL TRIALS OF THROMBOLYSIS FOR PERIPHERAL ARTERIAL OCCLUSION

Thrombolysis for peripheral arterial occlusion was not attempted until the mid-1950s, despite the discovery of streptokinase more than two decades previously by Tillett and Garner.[9] Purity of the agents was a problem, forcing Tillett to limit use to extravascular disease processes; specifically, the dissolution of loculated hemothoraces.[10] Despite Tillett's initial experience with the intravascular administration of varying doses of streptokinase in 11 volunteer subjects,[11] Cliffton and Grossi[12] were the first to report the use of thrombolytic agents for intravascular thrombus using a combination of streptokinase and plasminogen to generate plasmin. Cliffton and Grossi assumed that the exogenous plasmin was the substance responsible for dissolution of the thrombus. Later studies, however, would reveal that excess streptokinase in the preparation was the active agent, converting endogenous fibrin-bound plasminogen to plasmin.[13]

Anecdotal experiences predominated in the three decades that followed the initial clinical reports, using both systemic[14–18] and intra-arterial[19–21] thrombolytic routes of administration to address peripheral arterial thrombosis. Dotter et al.[22] popularized the use of catheter-directed streptokinase thrombolysis, reporting success rates well above those observed with systemic administration with what they termed "selective, low-dose therapy."

These anecdotal experiences were followed by retrospective, sometimes consecutive series of thrombolytic techniques. Investigators such as Hess et al.,[20] McNamara and Fischer,[23] and Graor et al.[21] reported their individual experience with large numbers of patients treated with remarkable results. Urokinase became the agent of choice for peripheral arterial occlusion,[1] with thrombolytic success rates of greater than 80% and patient mortality rates of less than 10%.

Prior to the 1990s, however, no randomized comparison existed of thrombolysis with standard surgical intervention. The need for a prospective comparison became clear with the publication of several reports with poorer thrombolytic success rates than originally reported.[24–26] A randomized trial of recombinant tissue plasminogen activator (rt-PA) versus surgical thrombectomy appeared in the European literature,[27] but its small size of 20 patients precluded meaningful conclusions.

A randomized trial of intra-arterial urokinase versus surgical intervention was reported by the Rochester group in 1994.[28] This adequately powered study enrolled 114 patients with severe, limb-threatening acute limb ischemia. Decreased in-hospital cardiopulmonary complications and a corresponding improvement in patient survival were realized in the urokinase group (Table 22–3). There was no difference in the rate of amputation, with limb salvage in approximately 20% of the patients. The data must be viewed with caution, however, because the study population comprised a subgroup

TABLE 22–3. RESULTS OF THE ROCHESTER TRIAL OF UROKINASE VERSUS OPERATION IN THE INITIAL TREATMENT OF PATIENTS WITH LIMB-THREATENING PERIPHERAL ARTERIAL OCCLUSION[a]

	Amputation Rate		Mortality Rate	
	30 Days (%)	*12 Months (%)*	*30 Days (%)*	*12 Months (%)*
Urokinase (57)	9	18	12	16
Operation (57)	14	18	18	58
	n.s.[b]	n.s.	n.s.	$p = 0.01$

[a] From Ouriel et al.[28]
[b] Not significant.

with very recent onset (mean less than 24 hours duration) and very severe ischemia (mean ankle–brachial index 0.04).

Shortly after the publication of the Rochester trial, the Surgery or Thrombolysis for Ischemia of the Lower Extremity (STILE) trial appeared.[29] The STILE trial was a multicenter randomized comparison of rt-PA, urokinase, and operation in patients with nonembolic lower extremity ischemia of less than 6 months duration. As such, the study included both acute and chronic peripheral arterial occlusions. The trial documented a death or amputation rate of 38% in patients who presented within 2 weeks of the onset of symptoms, compared with 10% in patients presenting after 2 weeks. There was no mortality differences noted (Table 22–4).

The STILE trial utilized a composite index of adverse clinical outcomes as the primary study end point. This outcome measure included the objective and clinically relevant outcomes of death and amputation but added additional measures such as renal failure and wound complications—events less tightly linked to the thrombolytic procedure. In addition, "ongoing ischemia" was added to the list of adverse events triggering the major end point, a measure that is subjective and difficult to assess. In fact, a benefit in the composite index was detected by the safety committee of the STILE trial and forced the premature termination of the study despite a lack of differences in limb salvage or mortality.

The Thrombolysis or Peripheral Arterial Surgery (TOPAS) study was the most recently completed thrombolytic trial, comparing recombinant urokinase (r-UK) with operative intervention in the treatment of peripheral arterial occlusions less than or equal to 14 days in duration.[30] The TOPAS trial was originally designed to mimic the Rochester study. As such, the sample sizes were chosen based on event rates observed in the Rochester study. The results of the initial phase of the TOPAS trial suggested that the amputation rate and mortality associated with thrombolytic therapy were equal to that of immediate operation (Table 22–5). The 4,000 IU/min r-UK dose was chosen as the "best dose." In a comparison of the clinical results in the 4,000 IU/min group

TABLE 22–4. RESULTS AT 1 MONTH OF THE STILE TRIAL OF THROMBOLYSIS OR OPERATION IN NONEMBOLIC LOWER LIMB ISCHEMIA

		Thrombolysis (%)	Operation (%)
Native artery	Death	4.1	7.1
	Major amputation	4.1	2.0
Bypass graft	Death	3.8	0
	Major amputation	7.7	15.2

TABLE 22–5. RESULTS OF THE TOPAS PHASE I TRIAL OF THROMBOLYSIS (4000 IU/MIN RECOMBINANT UROKINASE) VERSUS OPERATION FOR ACUTE LOWER LIMB ISCHEMIA (1 YEAR FOLLOW-UP DATA)

	Recombinant Urokinase (%)	Operation (%)
Survival	86.1	84.3
Amputation-free survival	74.6	65.4

and the surgical group, the 1-year mortality rate (14% versus 16%) and the amputation-free survival rate (75% versus 65%) did not differ significantly.

It is interesting to note that the presentation and publication of the Rochester data correlated with a slowing of overall patient acquisition in the TOPAS trial, concurrent with inclusion of less severely ill patients in the study (evidenced by a decreased mortality rate in the operative group as the study progressed). As the TOPAS trial progressed, it became evident that the patients enrolled differed substantially from those entered into the Rochester trial. The mortality and amputation rates were significantly lower in TOPAS, such that there was little chance of achieving differences in the primary end point. Moreover, publication of the Rochester data created investigator bias toward thrombolysis for acutely ischemic extremities. The investigators were unwilling to randomize those patients who would benefit the most from thrombolysis—the medically fragile subpopulation with recent onset of severely ischemic symptoms. These factors likely accounted for the equivalent mortality rates in the TOPAS thrombolytic and operative treatment arms.

Once the end points of death and amputation were found to be equivalent, the secondary end points gained increased importance in the comparative study. The most important secondary end point in the TOPAS trial was the quantification of the severity of the interventions during 6-month follow-up. Interventions were ranked on the basis of long deliberation by a committee of vascular practitioners, ranging from lowest severity (medical or thrombolytic intervention alone) to open surgical procedures, amputation, and death. Although no differences were detected with regard to amputation or death, significant benefit in lowering the requirement for open surgical interventions was observed in the thrombolytic group. The fact that the need for invasive interventions was lower in the thrombolytic group over the duration of follow-up attests to the durability of thrombolytic interventions in the TOPAS trial.

The secondary benefit of lowering the magnitude of invasive interventions is a factor that is likely to be of great importance to patients and their families. It is appropriate to rely on secondary end points only when the primary end points are equivalent between treatment groups. A preliminary overview of the TOPAS data suggested that the primary end point of amputation-free survival was equivalent in the r-UK and surgical groups. It was apparent that the results were better in graft occlusions than native arterial occlusions, with trends toward lower mortality and amputation rates when the occlusive process involved a bypass graft.

FACTORS AFFECTING THE RESULTS OF CLINICAL TRIALS

The results of clinical trials of thrombolysis versus operation are dependent on two factors: (1) the skill of the clinical management team in interventional and surgical techniques; (2) the patient selection criteria defining the composition of the study population. Although the STILE trial has been criticized on the basis of poor thrombolytic technical results with failure to cannulate the thrombus successfully in a significant percentage of patients, it is likely that differences in selection criteria are the most significant factor accounting for differences in study results.

Medically fragile patients with recent onset of severe ischemia comprise the subpopulation most likely to benefit from thrombolytic interventions. The perioperative mortality rate is excessive in this subgroup,[6,28] presumably due to the inability of these patients to tolerate well open surgical interventions without adequate preparation. Exclusion of this subgroup from the study population would bias the results against thrombolysis, as was probably observed in the TOPAS trial. In a similar manner, inclusion of patients with chronic ischemia is likely to bias the results against thrombolysis. This phenomenon was observed in the STILE trial; thrombolytic benefits were observed only after subgroup analyses were performed with *post hoc* stratification into acute and chronic subgroups.

Given the data generated by the three adequately powered comparisons of thrombolysis and operation, it is unlikely that new comparative trials will be possible. Investigator sentiment is such that preconceived notions regarding the most appropriate form of therapy render patient acquisition difficult. Subsequent trials are likely to be directed at an evaluation of newer thrombolytic agents and strategies rather than comparisons with operation. Thus, the data currently available may represent the only opportunity to compare critically thrombolysis and operation for peripheral arterial occlusion.

COMPARISON OF THROMBOLYTIC RESULTS IN NATIVE ARTERIES VERSUS BYPASS GRAFTS

Several studies have analyzed thrombolytic results with regard to the nature of the occluded conduit, native artery or bypass graft. Braithwaite and colleagues[31] assessed the results of catheter-directed thrombolysis in 201 patients entered into the British Thrombolysis Study Group database. Clinical results were similar in the 123 native arterial and 78 bypass graft occlusions. Berkowitz and associates[32] retrospectively analyzed the results of thrombolytic treatment of bypass graft occlusions and found no differences in outcome with regard to whether the graft was saphenous vein, other autogenous vein, or prosthetic material.

The results of the prospective trials do not corroborate those of the nonrandomized series. A multivariate analysis of the data from the Rochester trial revealed an increased rate of complete clot dissolution in prosthetic bypass grafts versus native arteries, with a 1.2-fold increment in the odds ratio.[33] The STILE data documented a 1-month mortality rate of 4% in both the native artery and bypass graft subgroups, with a major amputation rate of 4% in the native artery patients versus 8% in the bypass graft patients.[29] At first glance one would surmise that limb salvage was better in native arteries versus bypass graft, until the data are addressed in concert with the results of operation. The corresponding rate of amputation following operative therapy was 2% in the native artery subgroup versus 15% in the bypass graft subgroup. These data imply an incremental benefit of thrombolytic therapy over operation with respect to limb salvage in patients with bypass graft occlusion, a benefit that was not observed in native arterial occlusions. An initial review of the TOPAS data would confirm this impression, with improved clinical results in occluded bypass grafts compared with native arteries.

OVERALL STRATEGY IN THE TREATMENT OF PERIPHERAL ARTERIAL OCCLUSIVE DISEASE

The severity of symptoms is the most important clinical parameter with which to formulate clinical strategies. Patients with non–lifestyle-limiting claudication may be best managed without arteriographic investigation, managing symptoms conservatively with exercise, cessation of smoking, and occasionally the oral pharmacologic agent pentoxifylline. Severe claudication that has a negative impact on the ability of the patient to conduct activities of daily living may be appropriately treated with balloon dilatation or operative bypass. The role of thrombolysis in this clinical setting has been limited to the dissolution of native artery clot prior to angioplasty.

Patients with threatened limbs in the form of rest pain or tissue loss carry a high risk of limb loss without intervention. These patients should undergo arteriography with consideration of endovascular intervention for focal lesions and bypass grafting for more diffuse disease. Patients with acute occlusions may be best treated with catheter-directed thrombolytic therapy, addressing unmasked lesions with an operative or endovascular approach. Recent data suggest that bypass graft occlusions may be associated with a better thrombolytic response than native arterial occlusions. In all cases, however, the appropriate therapy must be tailored to the clinical presentation, the anatomic distribution of disease, and the experience of the clinical team.

REFERENCES

1. McNamara TO, Bomberger RA, Merchant RF. Intra-arterial urokinase as the initial therapy for acutely ischemic lower limbs. *Circulation.* 1991;83(suppl I):I-106–I-119.
2. Veith FJ, Gupta SK, Ascer E, et al. Six-year prospective multicenter randomized comparison of autologous saphenous vein and expanded polytetrafluoroethylene grafts in infrainguinal arterial reconstructions. *J Vasc Surg.* 1992;3:104–114.
3. Jivegaard L, Holm J, Schersten T. Acute limb ischemia due to arterial embolism or thrombosis: influence of limb ischemia versus pre-existing cardiac disease on postoperative mortality rate. *J Cardiovasc Surg.* 1988;29:32–36.
4. Rutherford RB, Flanigan DP, Gupta SK, et al. Suggested standards for reports dealing with lower extremity ischemia. *J Vasc Surg.* 1986;4:80–94.
5. Fogarty TJ, Cranley JJ, Drause RJ, et al. A method for extraction of arterial emboli and thrombi. *Surg Gynecol Obstet.* 1963;116:241.
6. Blaisdell FW, Steele M, Allen RE. Management of acute lower extremity arterial ischemia due to embolism and thrombosis. *Surgery.* 1978;84:822–834.
7. Yeager RA, Moneta GL, Taylor LM Jr, et al. Surgical management of severe acute lower extremity ischemia. *J Vasc Surg.* 1992;15:385–393.
8. Ouriel K, Shortell CK, Green RM, DeWeese JA. Differential mechanisms of late failure of autogenous and prosthetic bypass conduits. *J Cardiovasc Surg.* 1995;3:469–473.
9. Tillett WS, Garner RL. The fibrinolytic activity of hemolytic streptococci. *J Exp Med.* 1933;58:485–502.
10. Tillett WS, Sherry S. The effect in patients of streptococcal fibrinolysin (streptokinase) and streptococcal deoxyribonuclease on fibrinous, purulent, and sanguinous pleural exudations. *J Clin Invest.* 1949;28:173.
11. Tillett WS, Johnson AJ, McCarty WR. The intravenous infusion of the streptococcal fibrinolytic principle (streptokinase) into patients. *J Clin Invest.* 1955;34:169–185.
12. Cliffton EE, Grossi CE. Investigations of intravenous plasmin (fibrinolysin) in humans; physiologic and clinical effects. *Circulation.* 1956;14:919.
13. Alkjaersig N, Fletcher AP, Sherry S. The mechanism of clot dissolution by plasmin. *J Clin Invest.* 1959;38:1086.
14. Marder VJ. The use of thrombolytic agents: choice of patient, drug administration, laboratory monitoring. *Ann Intern Med.* 1979;90:802–812.
15. Sherry S, Fletcher AP, Alkjaersig N. Developments in fibrinolytic therapy for thromboembolic disease. *Ann Intern Med.* 1959;50:560.

16. Camiolo SM, Thorsen S, Astrup T. Fibrinogenolysis and fibrinolysis with tissue plasminogen activator, urokinase, streptokinase-activated human globulin, and plasmin. *Proc Soc Exp Biol Med.* 1971;138:277–280.

17. Sharma GVRK, Cella G, Parisi AF, Sasahara AA. Thrombolytic therapy. *N Engl J Med.* 1982;306:1268–1276.

18. Martin M. Thrombolytic therapy in arterial thromboembolism. *Prog Cardiovasc Dis.* 1979; 21:351–374.

19. McNicol GP, Douglas AS. Treatment of peripheral vascular occlusion by streptokinase perfusion. *Scand J Clin Lab Invest.* 1964;16(suppl 78):23–29.

20. Hess H, Ingrisch H, Mietaschk A, Rath H. Local low-dose thrombolytic therapy of peripheral arterial occlusions. *N Engl J Med.* 1982;307:1627–1630.

21. Graor RA, Risius B, Young JR, et al. Low-dose streptokinase for selective thrombolysis: systemic effects and complications. *Radiology.* 1984;152:35–39.

22. Dotter CT, Rosch J, Seaman AJ. Selective clot lysis with low-dose streptokinase. *Radiology.* 1974;111:31–37.

23. McNamara TO, Fischer JR. Thrombolysis of peripheral arterial and graft occlusions: improved results using high-dose urokinase. *Am J Roentgenol.* 1985;144:769–775.

24. Sicard GA, Schier JJ, Totty WG, et al. Thrombolytic therapy for acute arterial occlusion. *J Vasc Surg.* 1985;2:65–78.

25. Ricotta J. Intra-arterial thrombolysis. A surgical view. *Circulation.* 1991;83:I120–I121.

26. Ricotta JJ, Green RM, DeWeese JA. Use and limitations of thrombolytic therapy in the treatment of peripheral arterial ischemia: results of a multi-institutional questionnaire. *J Vasc Surg.* 1987;6:45–50.

27. Nilsson L, Albrechtsson U, Jonung T, et al. Surgical treatment versus thrombolysis in acute arterial occlusion: a randomised controlled study. *Eur J Vasc Surg.* 1992;6:189–193.

28. Ouriel K, Shortell CK, DeWeese JA, et al. A comparison of thrombolytic therapy with operative revascularization in the treatment of acute peripheral arterial ischemia. *J Vasc Surg.* 1994;19:1021–1030.

29. The STILE Investigators. Results of a prospective randomized trial evaluating surgery versus thrombolysis for ischemia of the lower extremity. The STILLE trial. *Ann Surg.* 1994;220:251–268.

30. Ouriel K, Veith FJ, Sasahara AA. Thrombolysis or peripheral arterial surgery: phase I results. *J Vasc Surg.* 1996;23:64–75.

31. Braithwaite BD, Petrik PV, Ritchie AWS, Earnshaw JJ. Computerized angiographic analysis of the outcome of peripheral thrombolysis. *Am J Surg.* 1995;170:131–135.

32. Berkowitz HD, Kee JC. Occluded infrainguinal grafts: when to choose lytic therapy versus a new bypass graft. *Am J Surg.* 1995;170:136–139.

33. Ouriel K, Shortell CK, Azodo MVU, et al. Predictors of success in catheter-directed thrombolytic therapy of acute peripheral arterial occlusion. *Radiology.* 1994;193:561–566.

23

CT Angiography in Evaluation of Thoracic Outlet Syndrome

William S. Rilling, MD, Albert A. Nemcek, Jr., MD, Robert L. Vogelzang, MD, and Jon S. Matsumura, MD

Thoracic outlet syndrome (TOS) is a general term used to describe a variety of disorders caused by compression of the subclavian artery, subclavian vein, and/or the brachial plexus. These structures are subject to compression in well-defined anatomic regions as they pass from the chest (or neck) to the arm. The specific regions include, from medial to lateral, the interscalene triangle, the costoclavicular space, and the retropectoral or quadrilateral space. Although the clinical presentation can be extremely variable, the majority of patients with TOS have well-defined congenital or acquired abnormalities in one or more of these regions.[1-3] Radiologic evaluation can be helpful in defining the nature and location of these abnormalities, to allow for precise and timely surgical treatment.

A conventional radiologic workup in patients with TOS initially includes plain radiography of the chest and cervical spine. These studies reveal relevant osseous abnormalities such as cervical ribs, clavicular callus or tumor, abnormally long transverse processes of the seventh cervical vertebral body, and some first rib anomalies. However, many osseous abnormalities such as first rib or clavicular exostoses or subtle post-traumatic changes of the first rib are not easily identified on plain films. Many patients subsequently undergo conventional angiography or venography depending on their presenting symptoms. Arteriography is performed to include provocative positioning of the upper extremity and defines the location of impingement as well as associated vascular complications including poststenotic dilatation or aneurysm, local intimal injury, thrombosis, and distal embolization. Duplex scanning and color-flow Doppler imaging can also be helpful in evaluating dynamic vascular compression in these patients.[4]

More recently, cross-sectional imaging techniques have been used in the evaluation of TOS. Conventional axial computed tomography (CT) can be helpful especially in patients without osseous abnormalities on plain radiographs.[5] Magnetic resonance imaging (MRI) and specialized techniques such as magnetic resonance angiography have also been used to demonstrate vascular compression.[6] MRI can also be used for detailed imaging of the brachial plexus[7] and may demonstrate fibrous bands that cause neural compression and are not visualized with other imaging methods.[8]

With the recent advent and subsequent widespread use of helical CT scanners, CT angiography (CTA) has emerged as a powerful tool in vascular imaging. CTA has proven valuable in many thoracic, abdominal, and peripheral applications. For example, in many centers CTA has virtually replaced preoperative angiography in the evaluation of abdominal aortic aneurysms and potential renal donors.[9,10] CTA is also well suited for evaluating the thoracic outlet. With current techniques, detailed angiographic images of this region can be produced. The surrounding osseous structures, which are frequently the key to the pathogenesis of this disorder, are imaged in exquisite detail and can be evaluated with multiplanar and three-dimensional reconstructions. Finally, the surrounding soft tissue elements, particularly the scalene and subclavius muscles, are also well demonstrated with helical CT and CTA.

TECHNIQUE

Because CTA is a relatively recent development, techniques for optimal performance of CTA continue to be developed. This section describes the technique that has evolved at our institution during the past 2 years. In patients with suspected arterial or neural compression, 20 ga or larger peripheral venous access is established in the asymptomatic upper extremity. Iodinated contrast (300 mg I/cc) is injected at a rate of 3 cc per second for a total of 80 cc, with a 25-second delay from the start of injection to image acquisition. Scans are performed with 3.2-mm collimation from just above the aortic arch to the level of the C6 vertebral body with a 1:1 pitch; axial scans are reconstructed with overlapping slices every 1.5 mm. The region of interest can then be covered with approximately 60 to 70 slices, which requires a breath hold of about 20 to 25 seconds. We have found that, with appropriate breathing instruction, most patients can perform this easily. The scan is performed with the symptomatic extremity in both the arm down (neutral) position and with the arm held in abduction and external rotation.

The protocol is altered slightly in patients with venous compression or symptoms of venous thrombosis. The peripheral IV is placed in the symptomatic extremity. A dilute contrast mixture (30 cc of the iodinated contrast listed earlier diluted to 170 cc with normal saline) is injected at the same rate and volume as for evaluation of the arteries, with a decrease in the scan delay to 5 seconds and all other scan parameters unchanged. This dilute contrast mixture provides excellent visualization of the veins without the artifacts associated with injection of full-strength contrast in the ipsilateral venous system.

Once the scan is performed, the data must be processed for optimal display and interpretation. First, the source axial images are reviewed for other abnormalities (e.g., Pancoast tumor) that could be related to the patient's symptoms. Axial views of the C7 transverse processes are reviewed to document their position relative to the scalene musculature. Impingement of the C7 transverse processes into the interscalene space can be associated with neural compression.[5] Multiplanar reconstructions (MPR) are then performed in the sagittal and curved coronal planes, the latter following the course of the vessels of interest. Sagittal reconstructions demonstrate the interscalene triangle and costoclavicular space and any associated compression of the artery or vein. Curved coronal reconstructions simulate the traditional arteriographic and venographic appearances and show associated vascular abnormalities such as aneurysms or stenoses.

Three-dimensional shaded surface displays are also performed. These reconstructions can be displayed on a data station and manipulated to show the vessels and adjacent osseous structures in various orientations. This allows for optimal conceptualization and visualization of any osseous abnormalities such as cervical rib, bifid first rib, postoperative and post-traumatic changes, and the relationship of these abnormalities to the artery or vein. Maximum intensity projection (MIP) angiograms, which have proven valuable for other CTA applications, are technically difficult to optimize in the thoracic outlet due to the numerous osseous structures immediately adjacent to the vessels. We have not yet found MIP reconstructions helpful for evaluation of TOS and do not perform them routinely.

ADVANTAGES

CTA has many advantages in the evaluation of TOS. First, the various reconstructions, especially sagittal and coronal MPRs, allow for optimal visualization of the anatomy of this complex region. In sagittal reformations, the subclavian artery is visualized as an ovoid contrast-enhanced structure situated between the anterior and middle scalene muscles in the interscalene triangle and between the first rib and clavicle in the costoclavicular space. The subclavian vein is also visualized as an ovoid contrast-enhanced structure anterior to the scalene muscle and anterior and slightly inferior to the subclavian artery in the costoclavicular space. With abduction, the head of the clavicle moves posteriorly and slightly cephalad, narrowing the costoclavicular space. We have had the opportunity to evaluate several normal subjects with this technique, and have noted that the subclavian vein is compressed to some degree in all. The vein is compressed between the clavicle with the attached subclavius muscle or tendon and the anterior scalene muscle (Fig. 23–1). The anterior and middle scalene muscles, interscalene space, and subclavius muscle are all visualized well with this technique. In many cases, the width of the scalene insertions and the base of the interscalene triangle can be measured and compared to reported normal values in cadaver studies.[1,11] Musculotendinous vascular compression can also be seen, including venous compression by a hypertrophied subclavius muscle and tendon as seen in Paget–Schroetter syndrome (Fig. 23–2).

CTA clearly demonstrates the congenital osseous anomalies and acquired bony abnormalities that are so prevalent in this patient population. Although many osseous abnormalities such as cervical ribs are clearly demonstrated on plain radiographs, CTA shows these abnormalities as well as their direct relationship to the artery, vein, or brachial plexus. CTA also simultaneously shows vascular complications such as stenosis, occlusion, or aneurysm (Figs. 23–3 and 23–4). In addition, subtle abnormalities such as hypertrophied scalene tubercles of the first rib or other exostoses narrowing the costoclavicular space can be seen (Fig. 23–5). In a recent series of patients with TOS studied with conventional axial CT,[5] 75% of patients with normal plain films had an abnormal finding on their CT. As described earlier, the most frequent finding in these patients was abnormal impingement of the C7 transverse process into the interscalene triangle.

To date, we have performed CTA on 18 consecutive patients who presented to our institution with suspected TOS. Of these 18 patients, 9 presented with symptoms of arterial compression, 5 with symptoms of venous compression, and 4 with suspected neural compression. Seven of these patients have currently undergone surgery. Osseous impingement mechanisms were correctly identified by CTA in all 7 patients, including 5 with cervical ribs, 1 with clavicular callus, and 1 with an anomalous first rib. We

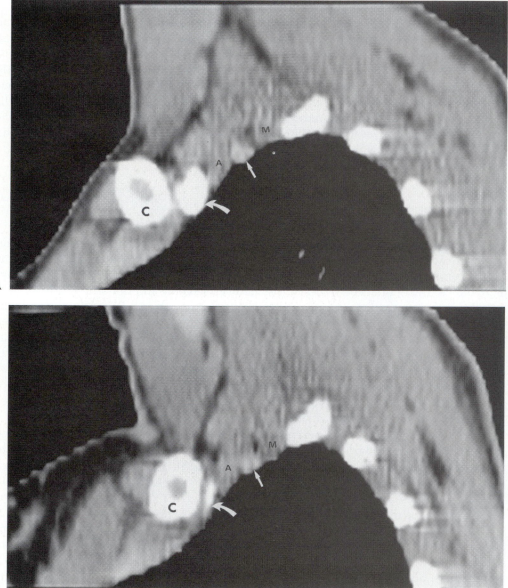

Figure 23–1. Sagittal reconstructions of spiral CT scan of the interscalene triangle in a normal volunteer. Dilute contrast has been injected in an ipsilateral arm vein. Arm in (**A**) neutral position and in (**B**) abduction. C, clavicle; A, anterior scalene muscle; M, middle scalene muscle; straight arrow, subclavian artery; curved arrow, subclavian vein. Note narrowing of subclavian vein in **B** as it is compressed between the clavicle and anterior scalene muscle.

have also found excellent correlation between conventional arteriography and venography and the CTA studies. Arteriographic/venographic correlation was obtained for 13 extremities in 11 patients. CTA correctly identified subclavian aneurysm or poststenotic dilatation (3 patients), arterial occlusion or compression with provocative positioning (4 patients), and venous thrombosis or stenosis (5 patients). One patient had a medial subclavian venous web that was not identified on the CTA. Two patients with normal arteriograms in this series had no evidence of arterial compression on the CTA studies.

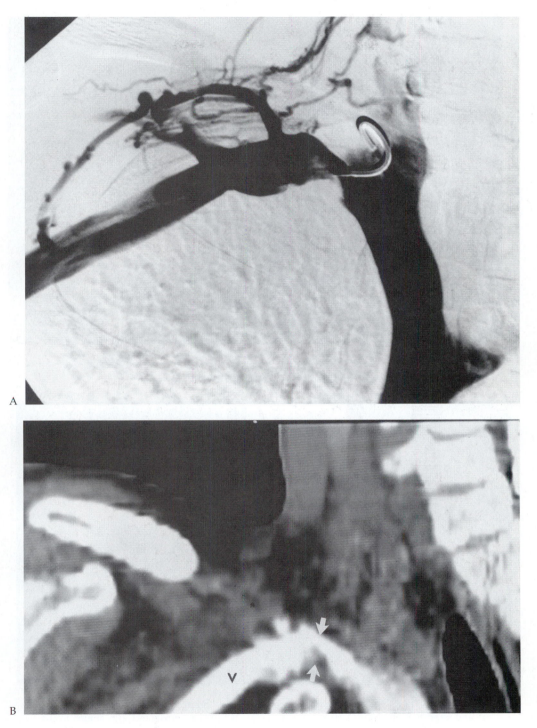

Figure 23–2. Radiographic studies on a 32-year-old woman with Paget–Schroetter syndrome, following urokinase thrombolysis of subclavian vein thrombosis. (**A**) Digital subtraction venogram shows marked stenosis of the medial subclavian vein. (**B**) Corresponding curved coronal reconstruction of spiral CT shows subclavian vein (v) with medial stenosis (*arrows*) (*continued*).

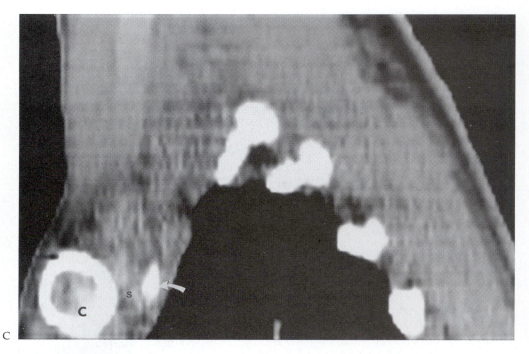

Figure 23–2. (*Continued*). (**C**) Sagittal CT reconstruction shows marked narrowing of the subclavian vein (*curved arrow*) due to large subclavius muscle (s). C, clavicle.

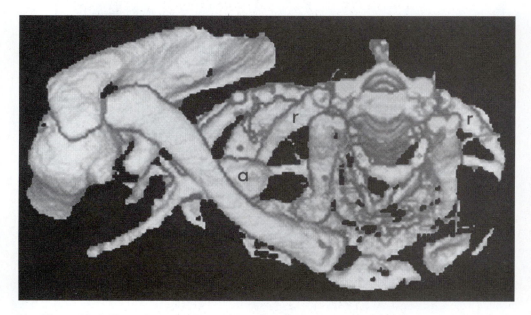

Figure 23–3. Three-dimensional shaded surface display in patient with bilateral cervical ribs (r) and large right subclavian artery aneurysm (a). The patient presented with emboli to the right hand.

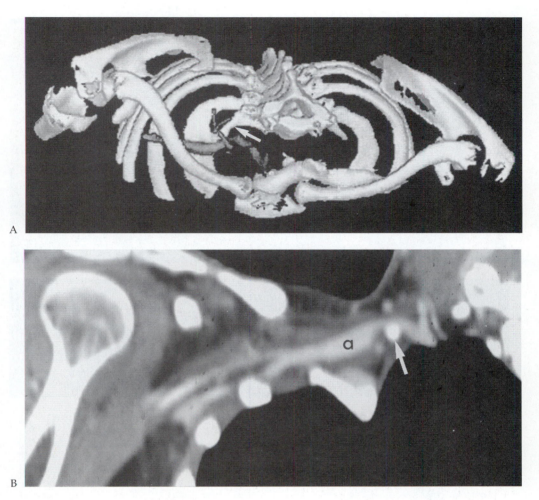

Figure 23–4. (A) Three-dimensional shaded surface display in patient with bilateral cervical ribs and right-sided symptoms of thoracic outlet syndrome. Note that the right cervical rib (*arrow*) is the larger of the two and articulates with the first rib causing deviation of subclavian artery (*shaded dark gray*). (**B**) Curved coronal reconstruction shows superior deviation of the subclavian artery (a) by the cervical rib (*arrow*). Note the poststenotic dilatation of the subclavian artery.

Due to its minimally invasive nature, CTA may be helpful in the evaluation of patients with confusing clinical presentation. The clinical manifestations of TOS are quite variable, and in many patients the diagnosis is uncertain. Patients with neural compression can be especially difficult to diagnose. CTA in these patients is a useful modality to evaluate the thoracic outlet for vascular compression and other abnormalities that could cause neural compression (Fig. 23–6). Many patients in this population have anomalous fibromuscular bands causing compression. Although these bands are not directly visualized, secondary signs can be seen such as a prominent scalene tubercle or hook-like extensions of the C7 transverse processes. In these patients with a questionable clinical diagnosis of TOS, a normal CTA study can obviate the need for conventional angiography.

The precise localization of osseous or muscular impingement, superb anatomic definition, and simultaneous imaging of vascular complications are all valuable in surgical planning for TOS. Clearly, optimal surgical approach varies depending on the location of

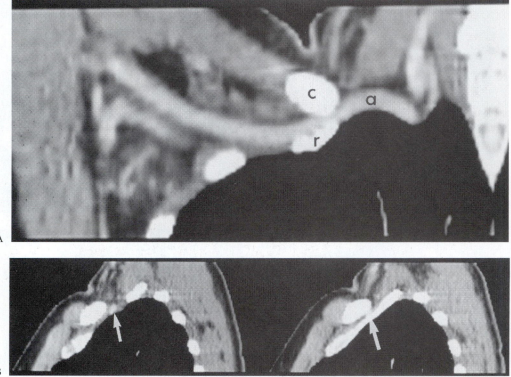

Figure 23–5. (A) Curved coronal spiral CT reconstruction in a young female volleyball player with right arm symptoms demonstrates compression of the right subclavian artery (a) in the costoclavicular space with the arm abducted. Note the unusual contour of the superior surface of the first rib (r). c, clavicle. **(B)** Sagittal reconstructions in the same patient, with subclavian artery designated by arrows. The image on the left is just medial to the costoclavicular space, and on the right at the costoclavicular space, both with the arm abducted. Note the narrowed costoclavicular space and resultant subclavian artery compression.

impingement, presence of congenital or acquired anatomic abnormalities, and the need for vascular repair and/or reconstruction. CTA can thus facilitate the planning of surgical approach and targets for resection. In addition, CTA can be helpful in postoperative follow-up, especially in patients with recurrent or persistent symptoms. Long-term postsurgical outcome is strongly influenced by the extent of first rib resection.[12] CTA with reformatted images demonstrates the extent of first rib resection as well as residual impingement in the costoclavicular space. In addition, reformations can easily detect cases in which there has been inadvertent resection of the second rather than the first rib, a situation that can be responsible for persistent symptoms. Patency and appearance of bypass grafts can simultaneously be evaluated with this technique (Fig. 23–7).

LIMITATIONS

Despite its excellent depiction of thoracic outlet anatomy and the many other advantages described earlier, CTA has some limitations in the evaluation of TOS. First, CTA cannot replace conventional angiography/venography. Subtle intraluminal abnormalities such as intimal irregularities and venous webs are more clearly defined by conventional

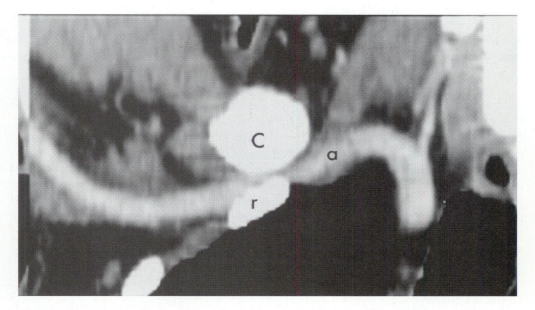

Figure 23–6. Curved coronal reconstruction in a patient presenting with symptoms of neural compression and history of clavicular fracture. A large amount of clavicular callus (c) is present, which markedly narrows the costoclavicular space and compresses the subclavian artery (a). r, first rib.

angiography, and may not be detected by CTA at all. Also, patients with suspected distal emboli require conventional angiography for confirmation.

A subgroup of patients with TOS, particularly throwing athletes, have axillary artery and/or branch vessel compression.[2,3,13,14] Although the axillary artery is well visualized with CTA, neither we nor others have had the opportunity to evaluate any patients with axillary artery compression with this technique, and its use in this regard must be regarded as speculative at this time. These patients can develop branch vessel aneurysm with distal embolization.[15] Branch vessels are inconsistently visualized and suboptimally evaluated with current CTA; however, we have noted anecdotally that the posterior circumflex humeral artery is usually well demonstrated on the three-dimensional reconstructions.

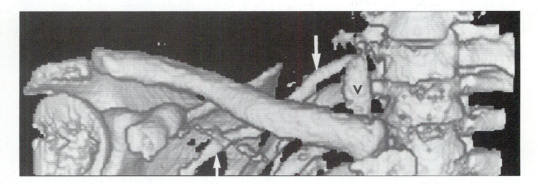

Figure 23–7. Professional baseball catcher with history of subclavian vein thrombosis, status—postaxillary vein to jugular vein bypass performed due to persistent symptoms after first rib resection. Three-dimensional shaded surface display shows patent bypass graft (*arrows*) to internal jugular vein (v). The right first rib is absent.

The majority of scalene muscle anomalies are not clearly demonstrated with CTA. While scalene and subclavius muscular hypertrophy and associated vascular compression are well demonstrated (Fig. 23–2), subtle scalene anomalies such as the presence of a scalenus minimus muscle are difficult to visualize.

Congenital fibromuscular bands and scalene muscle anomalies, which are not well seen with CTA, are common in both TOS patients and the general population.[16] Due to their prevalence, the significance of these anomalies is uncertain. However, they may represent the anatomic substrate on which chronic repetitive trauma, muscular hypertrophy, or injury act to cause symptoms.[17,18]

A final limitation of CTA is its inconsistent direct visualization of the brachial plexus. In many patients, especially those with sufficient perivascular and perimuscular fat, the brachial plexus fibers are clearly visible. However, this is not the case in all patients and MRI probably provides more consistent and detailed images of the brachial plexus. Obliteration of the normal perivascular fat posterior to the subclavian artery may be a secondary sign of brachial plexus impingement that can be seen with CTA.

CONCLUSION

Thoracic outlet syndrome is a heterogeneous and complex disorder in which the diagnosis and optimal treatment rely on identifying the location and etiology of neurovascular compression. CTA elegantly demonstrates the anatomy of the thoracic outlet and can identify both osseous and musculotendinous mechanisms of impingement. Vascular complications such as thrombosis, stenosis, and aneurysm are simultaneously identified. In our own series, osseous impingement mechanisms were correctly identified with CTA and there was good correlation with standard arteriography and venography. Further investigation is needed to determine the utility of this modality in evaluating the quadrilateral space, branch vessel complications, and scalene muscle anomalies.

REFERENCES

1. Makhoul RG, Machleder HI. Developmental anomalies at the thoracic outlet: an analysis of 200 consecutive cases. *J Vasc Surg*. 1992;16:534–542.
2. Pearce WH, Tropen BI, Baxter BT, Yao JST. Arterial complications in the thoracic outlet. *Semin Vasc Surg*. 1990;3:236–241.
3. Durham JR, Yao JST, Pearce WH, et al. Arterial injuries in the thoracic outlet syndrome. *J Vasc Surg*. 1995;21:57–70.
4. Longley DG, Yedlicka JW, Molina EJ, et al. Thoracic outlet syndrome: evaluation of the subclavian vessels by color duplex sonography. *AJR*. 1992;158:623–670.
5. Bilbey JH, Muller NL, Connell DG, et al. Thoracic outlet syndrome: evaluation with CT. *Radiology*. 1989;171:381–384.
6. Ohkawa Y, Isoda H, Hasegawa S, et al. MR angiography of thoracic outlet syndrome. *JCAT*. 1992;16:475–477.
7. Collins JD, Disher AC, Miller TQ. The anatomy of the brachial plexus as displayed by magnetic resonance imaging: technique and application. *J Nat Med Assoc*. 1995;87:489–498.
8. Panegyres PK, Moore N, Gibson R, et al. Thoracic outlet syndromes and magnetic resonance imaging. *Brain*. 1995;118:819–821.
9. Zeman RK, Silverman PM, Berman PM, et al. Abdominal aortic aneurysm: findings on three dimensional display of helical CT data. *AJR*. 1995;164:917–922.
10. Rubin GD, Alfrey EJ, Dake MD, et al. Assessment of living renal donors with spiral CT. *Radiology*. 1995;195:457–462.

11. Telford ED, Mottershad S. Pressure at the cervico-brachial junction (an operative and anatomical study). *J Bone Joint Surg.* 1948;30B:249–263.
12. Mingol A, Feldhaus RJ, Farina C, et al. Long term outcome after transaxillary approach for thoracic outlet syndrome. *Surgery.* 1995;118:840–844.
13. Kee ST, Dake MD, Wolfe-Johnson B, et al. Ischemia of the throwing hand in major league baseball pitchers: embolic occlusion from aneurysms of axillary artery branches. *J Vasc Interv Radiol.* 1996;6:979–982.
14. McCarthy WJ, Yao JST, Shafer MF, et al. Upper extremity arterial injury in athletes. *J Vasc Surg.* 1989;9:317–327.
15. Nijhuis HHAM, Muller-Wiefel HM. Occlusion of the brachial artery by thrombus dislodged from a traumatic aneurysm of the anterior circumflex humeral artery. *J Vasc Surg.* 1991;13:408–411.
16. Juvonen T, Satta J, Laitala P, et al. Anomalies at the thoracic outlet are frequent in the general population. *Am J Surg.* 1995;170:33–36.
17. Machleder HI. Thoracic outlet syndromes: new concepts from a century of discovery. *Cardiovasc Surg.* 1994;2:137–145.
18. Sanders RJ, Ratzin-Jackson CG, Banchero N, Pearce WH. Scalene muscle abnormalities in traumatic thoracic outlet syndrome. *Am J Surg.* 1990;159:231–236.

24

Measuring Functional Outcomes for Patients with Intermittent Claudication

Joseph Feinglass, MD, PhD, and Walter J. McCarthy, MD

The last two decades have witnessed a substantial increase in rates of interventional revascularization procedures for lower extremity peripheral arterial disease (PAD).[1] This increase in hospitalization for lower extremity bypass graft surgery and lower extremity angioplasty mirrors a similarly rapid increase in coronary revascularization procedures for older Americans.[2] In both cases, in addition to expected benefits in prolonging life or preventing amputation, surgeons, interventional radiologists, and cardiologists have embraced new, often complementary, endovascular and surgical techniques as methods to improve patients' quality of life.

Traditionally, lower extremity revascularization procedures were reserved for patients with rest pain, skin ulcers, or gangrene.[3] However, treatment of disabling intermittent claudication may account for a significant portion of the recent overall increase in lower extremity procedures. This may also be one reason why investigators reviewing the per capita doubling of peripheral bypass procedures in Maryland from 1979 to 1989 found no concomitant decrease in the lower extremity amputation rate.[4,5]

PAD patient outcomes traditionally reported in the vascular surgery literature have focused on clinical end points such as perioperative mortality and complications, arterial patency, limb salvage, restenosis, and graft failure rates. However, few studies have explicitly measured the relationship between hemodynamic improvement and patients' own perceptions of the impact of treatment on symptoms or disability. It was therefore of interest to determine methods of measuring self-reported functional outcomes, particularly for patients with less advanced vascular disease who were making decisions about discretionary revascularization procedures for intermittent claudication.

Led by investigators from Northwestern University Medical School, a team of participating Chicago-area vascular surgery offices and clinics is conducting a multicenter prospective outcomes study of medical, surgical, and endovascular management of claudication. This research was designed to take advantage of recent advances in the reliabilty and validity of patient self-reported health status surveys, while at the same time monitoring changes in patients' lower extremity hemodynamics using noninvasive Doppler blood pressure measurements. This chapter describes how the Chicago Area Intermittent Claudication Research Study is addressing the challenge of measuring self-reported functional status and community walking ability for patients with claudication.

EPIDEMIOLOGY OF INTERMITTENT CLAUDICATION

Estimates of the prevalence of intermittent claudication derived from population studies vary by geographic setting and time interval, and have been sensitive to questionnaire documentation of exertional calf pain.[6] Data derived from noninvasive Doppler lower extremity studies in older cardiovascular health population cohorts indicate an approximate 1.5% to 2% prevalence of symptomatic intermittent claudication (one-third female) among older Americans, increasing somewhat in the seventh decade of life.[7-9] However, these studies indicate that individuals with classic claudication symptoms represent only a small portion (<20%) of all subjects with clinically documented, often asymptomatic lower extremity PAD as indicated by an abnormal ankle-brachial index (ABI). An abnormal ABI is a marker for atherosclerosis in other vascular beds and is independently associated with at least a fourfold increased risk of mortality over 5 years and an even higher rate of nonfatal cardiovascular events.[10-12]

The vascular surgery literature maintains a general consensus that while some patients with claudication will experience improvement, 10% to 20% are likely to experience significant disease progression within 5 years of the onset of symptoms, with an approximate 5% amputation rate.[13] A total of 6% of the 1969 patients enrolled in the placebo arm of the 14-country ketanserin study underwent revascularization procedures for worsening leg ischemia within 1 year of follow-up; other referral center studies suggest up to 25% of patients with claudication undergo revascularization within 5 years of referral.[13,14]

MEDICAL MANAGEMENT AND EXERCISE THERAPY

Given studies indicating up to a ninefold relative risk of developing intermittent claudication for smokers and that continued smoking is a major risk factor for the subsequent development of rest pain, graft failure, and amputation, smoking cessation is probably the most critical health intervention for patients with claudication.[14-17] Medical management of vascular disease should also focus on controlling frequently coexisting cardiovascular risk factors such as hyperlipidemia, hypertension, and diabetes.[18] There is also a general consensus that physical training improves participants' pain-free walking performance. One meta-analysis of 21 published studies found a mean increase in distance to the onset of claudication pain of 179% (and a 122% improvement in distance to maximal claudication pain) after an exercise program.[19] Controversy remains about whether exercise benefits are related to collateral circulation, improved muscle metabolism, or other adaptations.[20] The duration of walking distance gains beyond active exercise program participation is less well known, as is the relationship between pain-free treadmill walking distances and patients' community walking ability. The only FDA-approved drug for claudication is pentoxyfilline, but reviews of randomized controlled trials conclude that existing data are inadequate to refute or support efficacy claims for clinically meaningful improvement.[21]

SURGICAL AND ENDOVASCULAR MANAGEMENT

Given perceived limitations on pharmacologic and exercise therapy, relief from disabling intermittent claudication has increasingly been sought through surgical and
endovascular revascularization.[22] A recent meta-analysis of pooled data from 17 studies
with several hundred patients with femoropopliteal disease suggests an approximate
overall 73% 5-year patency rate for saphenous vein bypass (49% for polytetrafluoroethylene grafts) and 45% 5-year patency for lower extremity angioplasty. However, results
were significantly better when only patients with claudication and stenotic lesions were
analyzed separately from those with critical ischemia.[23]

Few studies to date have actually gone further to document the relationship between
improved arterial blood flow and functional status. In one small study, investigators reported no significant correlation between a 0.37 mean improvement in resting ABI and
a mean 58% improvement in community walking distance scores for 14 surgical bypass
patients at 12 weeks after surgery for claudication.[24] In virtually the only randomized trial
to compare reconstructive surgery (with and without subsequent physical training) to
training alone for 75 patients with claudication, the physical training group, with no improvement in ABI after about 1 year, experienced 24% of the gain in mean symptom-free
walking distance of the bypass surgery and training group and 37% of the surgery alone
group. However, depending on whether patients limited by comorbidities or treatment
compliance were censored in the results, 75% to 95% of surgically treated patients, compared to 10% to 20% of the physical training alone group, had unrestricted maximal walking distances greater than 600 meters at follow-up.[25]

THE CHICAGO AREA INTERMITTENT CLAUDICATION
RESEARCH STUDY

For patients with intermittent claudication, and particularly for those who seek specialty
referral for their condition, it can be hypothesized that patient satisfaction with medical
care is related to at least three domains:

1. inversely to symptom significance, including patient perceptions of the severity
   of claudication and other leg pain;
2. positively related to community walking ability over time;
3. positively related to the quality of physician–patient communication about
   treatment decisions. While it may be hard for patients to judge the quality
   of care they have received, better understanding by clinicians of clinical and
   psychosocial predictors of patients' long-term functional outcomes, often at the
   center of patients' concerns when referred to a vascular specialist, has the potential to improve patients' ultimate satisfaction with care for their condition.[26]

In 1991, a group of Chicago-area vascular surgeons began to conduct a coordinated,
multicenter research program designed to better understand functional outcomes for
vascular disease patients. The principal focus of this effort was to further the rigor of
clinicians' functional assessments of intermittent claudication, to describe patient self-
reported outcomes over time, and to examine differences in medical, surgical, and
endovascular treatment effects.

FUNCTIONAL STATUS ASSESSMENT

One aim of initial pilot research was to test explicitly the extent to which there is a readily
measurable, clinically meaningful correlation between limb perfusion (or severity of

lower extremity vascular disease) and physical functioning. This relationship is often obscured by the confounding effects of comorbid conditions and sociodemographic factors. Despite this complexity, the perceived relationship between limb perfusion and functioning often influences recommendations for bypass surgery or angioplasty.

Both generic and condition-specific functional status survey measures are required to determine the range of patient characteristics that affect functional outcomes over time. Generic survey items are designed to measure a broad scale of functioning with a relatively wide spread, or range, of possible responses. Describing patients with claudication along a broad continuum allows for comparison to normal, healthy respondents of the same age, and to other patients with or without different chronic diseases. Generic survey items are usually arranged from basic "floor" items, such as those related to difficulty in performing activities of daily living such as bathing, dressing and toileting, to broad "ceiling" items, such as difficulty engaging in vigorous activities such as running, lifting heavy objects, or strenuous sports.

Standardized scores computed across multiple items provide a functional status scale. A valid, reliable, and responsive functional status scale provides a unidimensional range of "easy" to "difficult" items, is capable of reproducing item hierarchy in different patient groups and practice settings, and unites multiple attributes into a single index, which allows calibration across a continuum of functioning.[27] To be useful to clinicians, the "clinimetric" units produced by this scale should have a clear and meaningful interpretion and be approximately as reliable as physical measurements derived from laboratory tests or physical examination. Condition-specific functioning measures, such as those designed to measure walking capability or distance to claudication pain onset, add more precise measurement of specific disabilities along the overall continuum of functioning.

A few studies have attempted to measure functioning for patients with PAD. One study of patients with more severely ischemic lower extremity disease who had undergone aortobifemoral bypass found functional deficits as severe as those for patients with congestive heart failure or recent myocardial infarction.[28] This study employed the physical functioning scale from the Medical Outcomes Study, now used in the 36-item SF36 Health Survey (SF36).[29] The SF36 has been administered to a population sample of the general U.S. adult population and has been used to profile health status for a variety of specific chronic conditions. It calculates scales representing eight discrete dimensions of health: physical functioning, physical and emotional role functioning, bodily pain, general health perceptions, vitality, fatigue, social functioning, and mental health. All scores are standardized with a "ceiling" of 100 (best) and a "floor" of 0 (worst). The physical functioning (PF) score is based on 10 items rating the degree of difficulty experienced when performing moderate and vigorous activities, carrying groceries, climbing stairs, and walking various distances. Approximately 50% of people with PF scores in the 50 to 59 range reported being able to walk one block without limitation due to health as opposed to 90% of those with scores in the 70 to 79 range. The mean PF score for the general U.S. population is 84.2 (SD = 23.3); the mean for the general U.S. male population older than age 65 is 65.8, for females older than 65 it is 61.9. The Cronbach, a reliability coefficient measuring internal consistency, is 0.93.[29]

Regensteiner and colleagues[30] have also developed the condition-specific PAD Walking Impairment Questionnaire (WIQ), an 11-item survey designed specifically to analyze community walking function for patients with peripheral arterial disease. The walking distance score measures the degree of difficulty in walking, without stopping to rest, for several distances up to five blocks. It is scored from a 0 (inability to walk) to 1 (unrestricted walking ability) range. The WIQ summary score for distance was found to be highly correlated with peak treadmill walking time, moderately correlated with treadmill time to onset of claudication pain, and to have test–retest reliability and sensitivity to changes related to exercise rehabilitation and surgical treatment.[30] To control for potential differences in physical capacity, separate speed and distance summary scores are computed. In a separate study by Northwestern investigators, calibrating "ceiling" effects in a population of young, healthy college students, the WIQ speed and distance scores were indeed found to be uncorrelated.[31]

DIFFERENCES IN FUNCTIONAL STATUS AFTER TREATMENT: PILOT RESEARCH

To test the responsiveness of measures of functional status to differences in treatment, Northwestern investigators at two private, one academic, and one Department of Veterans Affairs vascular surgery clinics identified patients with prior visits for claudication from medical and blood flow laboratory records. A survey was then mailed to several hundred patients without signs of rest pain, gangrene, skin ulcers, or prior lower extremity revascularization procedures at the time of an index office visit between 1 and 5 years previous to the survey. A total of 187 patients returned completed questionnaires (54%).[32]

Along with the SF36 and WIQ instruments, patients completed a 16-item chronic disease checklist. In addition to medical history questions, patients were specifically asked to rate the degree to which symptoms of chronic conditions (e.g., hip or knee arthritis pain, sciatica or back pain, deafness or blindness) other than peripheral vascular disease interfered with their ability to walk. The highest Likert scale measure of comorbidity walking impairment on any symptom was used to weight four hierarchical walking difficulty levels ("very much," "much," "some," "none or slight"). These levels of comorbidity walking impairment were found to be monotonically correlated with SF36 PF scores for claudication patients in subsequent analyses. Patients also responded to a series of 30 items about smoking and exercise habits, severity, duration, and tolerance of leg symptoms, sociodemographic characteristics, and satisfaction with treatment.

Table 24–1 presents an overall comparison of characteristics of patients who ultimately had bypass surgery ($n = 41$, including 13 patients who underwent both angioplasty and bypass procedures), angioplasty alone ($n = 39$), or continued noninvasive management ($n = 107$) over the 1 to 5 years of study follow-up. Patients who had undergone interventional management had significantly higher functioning levels on all measures as compared to noninvasively managed respondents.[32]

Multiple regression analysis was used to test the significance of differences in SF36 PF after controlling for treatment group differences in sociodemographic characteristics, follow-up time, location of stenoses, initial ABI at index office or clinic visit, duration of claudication symptoms, smoking, and the severity of comorbid conditions. Table 24–2 presents the multiple regression model results. Statistically significant predictors of higher SF36 PF included initial ABI (coefficient = 47.8, $p < 0.001$), bypass surgery (coefficient = 9.7, $p = 0.03$), moderate comorbidity walking impairment (coefficient = -18.6, $p < 0.001$), and severe comorbidity walking impairment (coefficient = -38.1, $p < 0.001$).

To determine the likelihood that observed differences between treatment groups were an artifact of placebo effects or selection of patients for procedures, an identical model was estimated including three ABI/treatment group interaction variables. These

TABLE 24–1. DEMOGRAPHIC, DISEASE SEVERITY, AND SELF-REPORTED FUNCTIONAL OUTCOME MEASURES FOR PATIENTS WITH INTERMITTENT CLAUDICATION UNDERGOING PERIPHERAL BYPASS SURGERY, ANGIOPLASTY, OR NONINVASIVE MANAGEMENT AFTER 1 TO 5 YEARS FROM INDEX OFFICE VISIT

	(N = 187)		
	Bypass Surgery (N = 41)	*Angioplasty (N = 39)*	*Noninvasive Management (N = 107)*
Demographics			
Mean age (years)	64.0 ± 9.6[b]	63.3 ± 8.7[b]	69.0 ± 10.0
Male (%)	75.6	79.5[a]	58.9
High school graduate (%)	80.5[a]	66.7	63.6
Married (%)	56.1	43.6	43.9
Nonwhite race (%)	20.0	5.0[a]	20.6
Current smoker (%)	36.6	15.4	23.8
Disease Severity and Impairment			
Mean ABI	0.52 ± .15	0.59 ± .14	0.56 ± 0.16
Aortoiliac disease (%)	46.3[a]	46.2[a]	23.4
Duration of symptoms (years)	5.8 ± 4.9	4.5 ± 2.3	6.2 ± 6.4
Mean follow-up time (months)	34.4 ± 15.8	30.9 ± 16.0	32.4 ± 18.3
History of cardiovascular disease (%)	51.2	61.5	43.9
Comorbidity walking impairment:			
None/slight (%)	31.7[a]	30.8[a]	15.8
Some (%)	24.4	28.2	26.2
Much/very much (%)	43.9	41.0	57.9
Functional Outcome Measures			
SF36 physical functioning (mean)	65.2 ± 29.9[b]	61.8 ± 26.0[a]	52.2 ± 25.7
WIQ walking distance (mean)	0.68 ± .35[c]	0.59 ± .35[b]	0.43 ± 0.33
Leg symptoms improved since initial visit (%)	78.0[c]	74.3[c]	28.0
Would choose the same treatment again (%)	78.0[c]	71.8[c]	25.2
Satisfaction with treatment	3.8 ± 1.5[b]	3.7 ± 1.5[b]	3.1 ± 1.1

Note: Bypass surgery includes 13 patients who underwent bypass surgery and angioplasty, as well as 28 patients who underwent bypass surgery alone. ABI, ankle-brachial index at index visit. Satisfaction with treatment was measured on a scale of 1 (very dissatisfied) to 5 (very satisfied). Statistical tests compare bypass and angioplasty groups to noninvasive management.
[a] Significantly different from noninvasively managed patients, $p < 0.05$.
[b] Significantly different from noninvasively managed patients, $p < 0.01$.
[c] Significantly different from noninvasively managed patients, $p < 0.001$.
Adapted with permission from: Reifler D, Feinglass J, Slavensky R, et al. Functional outcomes for patients with intermittent claudication: bypass surgery versus angioplasty versus noninvasive management. *J Vasc Med Biol*. 1994;5:203–211, Table 2.

interaction variables test the significance of *initial* ABI (as recorded at the time of the index visit) in predicting *subsequent* functioning, 1 to 5 years later at the time of the survey. If the higher functioning of the revascularized patients was indeed a product of improved peripheral blood flow, pretreatment ABI should not be significantly related to functioning for the bypass and angioplasty patients, but would remain highly significant as a predictor of functioning for the noninvasively managed patients.

The main effect of bypass surgery remained significant ($p = 0.04$) in the full model, whereas the interaction of bypass surgery and initial ABI was not significant. These results indicate the lack of significance for bypass patients of initial ABI as a predictor of subsequent functioning. The interaction of noninvasive management and initial ABI

**TABLE 24–2. MULTIPLE REGRESSION MODEL OF SF36 PHYSICAL FUNCTIONING
SCORE FOR PATIENTS WITH INTERMITTENT CLAUDICATION
AFTER 1 TO 5 YEARS FROM INDEX OFFICE VISIT**

	$N = 187$; $R^2 = 0.42$		
	Coefficient	Standard Error	P Value
Age	.287	0.190	0.13
Male sex	−6.32	3.70	0.09
High school graduate	1.53	3.65	0.68
Married	6.24	3.38	0.07
Current smoker	4.16	4.07	0.31
Initial ABI	47.8	12.2	<0.001
Aortoiliac disease	0.071	3.77	0.99
Duration of symptoms (years)	0.055	0.311	0.86
Follow-up time (months)	0.062	0.096	0.52
Moderate comorbidity walking impairment	−18.6	4.75	<0.001
Severe comorbidity walking impairment	−38.1	4.35	<0.001
Angioplasty	5.04	4.48	0.26
Bypass surgery	9.73	3.37	0.03
Constant	29.4	18.8	0.11

Adapted with permission from: Reifler D, Feinglass J, Slavensky R, et al. Functional outcomes for patients with intermittent claudication: bypass surgery versus angioplasty versus noninvasive management. *J Vasc Med Biol.* 1994;5:203–211.

remained highly significant ($p < 0.001$), indicating the continued negative effects of abnormal lower extremity blood flow for those patients. These results are consistent with a hypothesis that higher levels of functioning for bypass patients were indeed related to improved blood flow. The third interaction variable, testing the significance of baseline ABI for patients who underwent angioplasty alone, was also significant ($p = 0.02$). This finding would be consistent with a less significant effect of angioplasty on intial ABI (or a high postangioplasty restenosis rate).

THE INTERMITTENT CLAUDICATION PROSPECTIVE OUTCOMES STUDY

In the summer of 1993, investigators from Northwestern University Medical School were awarded a 3-year grant from the Agency for Health Care Policy and Research (AHCPR) for a prospective outcomes study of intermittent claudication. Patients in the study were enrolled during 1993 to 1995 at visits to 1 of 16 academic, community, or Veterans Administration (VA) vascular surgery offices or clinics. Figure 24–1 presents a list of these participating Chicago-area vascular surgeons and clinical sites.

Patients with a complaint of claudication were enrolled if they were without previous leg revascularization procedures and had no signs of progressive disease such as ischemic rest pain, skin ulcers, or gangrene. Diagnosis was confirmed by an abnormal resting ABI (≤ 0.94) at the time of the index visit, as per epidemiologic criteria.[33] Ankle systolic pressure was computed from blood flow laboratory reports as the lowest leg mean of the dorsalis pedis and posterior tibial arteries.

The study design calls for three subsequent home health visits by project visiting nurses at approximately 6-month intervals. Project home health nurses perform Doppler lower extremity exams with portable equipment, collect follow-up patient questionnaires, and verify patient reports about any lower extremity revascularization proce-

OFFICES	PHYSICIANS
Section of Vascular Surgery, Cook County Hospital *Chicago*	Richard Keen, M.D.
Cardiovascular & Vascular Surgical Associates *Edward Hospital* *Naperville*	Dean M. Govostis, M.D.
Department of Cardiovascular and Thoracic Surgery *Evanston/Glenbrook Hospitals* *Evanston*	John F. Golan, M.D. Joseph R. Schneider, M.D.
Department of Vascular And Interventional Radiology *Illinois Masonic Medical Center* *Chicago*	Manuel Madayag, M.D.
Section of Peripheral Vascular Surgery *Loyola University Medical Center* *Maywood*	William H. Baker, M.D. Howard P. Greisler, M.D. Fred N. Littooy, M.D.
Hines Veterans Administration Hospital *Hines*	Fred N. Littooy, M.D.
Vascular Surgery *La Grange Memorial Hospital* *La Grange*	David A. Loiterman, M.D.
Lutheran General Hospital *Des Plaines* *Northwest Community Hospital* *Arlington Heights* *Resurrection Medical Center* *Chicago*	Sidney P. Haid, M.D. Thomas W. Kornmesser, M.D. Thomas A. Painter, M.D.
Division of Vascular Surgery *Division of Interventional Radiology* *Northwestern Memorial Hospital* *Chicago*	Walter J. McCarthy, M.D. William H. Pearce, M.D. James S. T. Yao, M.D. Robert Vogelzang, M.D.
Lakeside Veterans Administration Medical Center *Chicago*	William H. Pearce, M.D.
St. Francis Hospital *Evanston*	Kevin Halstuk, M.D.
Vascular Surgery *South Suburban Hospital* *Hazel Crest*	Mulji Pauwaa, M.D.
Department of Vascular Surgery *University of Chicago Hospitals* *Chicago*	Hisham S. Bassiouny, M.D. Bruce L. Gewertz, M.D. James F. McKinsey, M.D. Giancarlo Piano, M.D.
Division of Vascular Surgery *Department of Surgery, University of Illinois-Chicago Hospitals* *Chicago*	Henrik Baraniewski, M.D. Darwin Eton, M.D. James J. Schuler, M.D.
Westside Veterans Administration Medical Center *Chicago*	Henrik Baraniewski, M.D.

Figure 24–1. Chicago area intermittent claudication study list of participating clinical study sites.

dures (or other hospitalizations) subsequent to the enrollment visit. The home visit protocol has been described in detail elsewhere.[34]

Initial cross-sectional data on 555 enrolled patients have recently been analyzed.[35] Because of a focus on ABI measurement, data from approximately 50 other enrolled patients with noncompressible arteries but diagnostic waveforms were excluded. Enrolled patients are from throughout the greater Chicago metropolitan area, with more than 100 separate postal zip codes stretching from the Wisconsin border to western Illinois and northern Indiana. Table 24–3 presents chronic disease-related impairment data at enrollment.

The mean SF36 PF score for all 555 study patients was 45.8 (SD = 22.5), about equal to the lower 25th percentile of the U.S. population age 65 and older.[29] The mean WIQ score for all patients was 0.32 (SD = 0.27). The mean age was just under 69; 10.3% were age 80 or older. Three-quarters of study patients reported graduating high school and almost 20% reported working full or part time. Almost 60% were married; 27.6% reported living alone. A total of 110 (19.8%) female and 91 (16.4%) African-American

TABLE 24–3. CHRONIC DISEASE COMORBIDITIES AT ENROLLMENT IN THE PROSPECTIVE OUTCOME STUDY OF INTERMITTENT CLAUDICATION

	N = 555			
	Mean/ Frequency	*SD/Percent*	*Mean (SD) PF Score*[a]	*Mean (SD) WIQ Score*[b]
Hypertension	381	(68.6%)	45.1 (22.7)	0.31 (0.26)
Myocardial infarction	189	(34.0%)	42.8 (21.6)	0.30 (0.24)
Angina	174	(31.4%)	42.5 (21.8)	0.25 (0.24)
Congestive heart failure	76	(13.7%)	39.3 (21.3)	0.28 (0.25)
Diabetes	182	(32.8%)	44.6 (22.8)	0.28 (0.25)
Arm or leg paralysis/ cerebrovascular disease	115	(20.7%)	37.2 (20.1)	0.27 (0.25)
Cancer (except skin cancer)	80	(14.4%)	44.7 (25.1)	0.28 (0.25)
Allergies	117	(21.1%)	45.3 (27.1)	0.34 (0.26)
Knee arthritis	169	(30.5%)	41.0 (23.1)	0.27 (0.26)
Other arthritis	254	(45.8%)	43.9 (22.4)	0.31 (0.25)
Back pain	183	(33.0%)	41.2 (22.4)	0.27 (0.25)
Lung disease	88	(15.9%)	39.3 (22.5)	0.26 (0.26)
Skin disease	97	(17.5%)	43.5 (20.3)	0.31 (0.26)
Impaired hearing	137	(24.7%)	45.7 (27.1)	0.34 (0.27)
Impaired vision	115	(20.7%)	42.8 (20.9)	0.32 (0.29)
Comorbidity walking impairment:				
None/slight	246	(44.4%)	49.8 (23.5)	0.36 (0.27)
Mild	120	(21.6%)	48.0 (21.3)	0.35 (0.25)
Moderate	100	(18.0%)	45.1 (19.8)	0.31 (0.26)
Severe	89	(16.0%)	34.3 (20.7)	0.23 (0.24)

[a] SF36 Health Survey physical functioning score 0 (worst)–100 (best).
[b] PAD Walking Impairment Questionnaire 0 (worst)–1 (unrestricted).
Adapted with permission from: Feinglass J, McCarthy WJ, Slavensky R, et al. The effect of lower extremity blood pressure on physical functioning for patients with intermittent claudication. *J Vasc Surg.* 1996;24:503–510, Table 2.

patients were included. About one-third reported engaging in "regular physical exercise" of various types. The mean lowest leg ABI was 0.59 (SD = 0.16) with a range of 0.12 to 0.94; only 8 patients had ABIs above 0.90. Patients reported an average of about 5 years of claudication symptoms. Patients with a longer duration of symptoms had significantly lower PF ($p = 0.02$) and WIQ ($p = 0.03$) scores.

In answer to specific questions about leg symptom significance, more than 40% of all patients described their PAD symptoms as "severe" or "very severe." These patients had 10-point lower PF scores than the sample mean ($p < 0.001$). Patients reporting severe leg symptoms had a mean WIQ distance score of only 0.20 (SD = 0.20), compared to the rest of the cohort with a mean WIQ distance score of 0.41 (SD = 0.27; $p < 0.001$). A total of 93 patients (16.8%) reported being unable to walk even one block without stopping to rest, and 60 patients (11%) reported they either "could not do" or "had much difficulty" walking 50 feet. A total of 140 patients (25.2%) reported being "limited a lot" in walking one block on the SF36.

Patients from VA vascular clinics had significantly lower PF scores and a much higher prevalence of walking impairment due to comorbid conditions. Table 24–3 presents prevalences of major comorbid conditions and patient ratings of the overall severity of comorbid symptoms with respect to walking impairment. Two-thirds of the sample were hypertensive, one-third diabetic, and one-third reported clinically evident coronary artery disease. One-fourth of the 125 female patients reported taking estrogen; another one-fourth had tried estrogen replacement but stopped. Self-reported aspirin or coumadin use was about 60%, the current reported prevalence of smoking was 30% to 35%, 25% reported taking lipid-lowering agents, and 20% reported taking pentoxfylline.

LOWER EXTREMITY BLOOD FLOW AND PHYSICAL FUNCTIONING

Stepwise multiple regression analysis was used to explore the cross-sectional relationship of lower extremity blood flow, as measured by the ABI, and patients' SF36 PF and WIQ scores. The analysis was controlled for sociodemographic characteristics, clinic site, comorbid conditions and smoking, and duration of leg symptoms. Exercise habits and employment characteristics were excluded because they are confounded with the dependent functioning variables.

Table 24–4 presents the results of the stepwise regression analysis of SF36 PF scores. A total of nine candidate variables were significant at the $p < 0.05$ level. ABI was indeed a significant predictor ($p = 0.004$) of PF score. Other positively associated variables included male sex and a completed high school education; negatively associated variables included enrollment at a VA clinic, severe comorbidity walking impairment (as opposed to no or mild comorbidity walking impairment), and a history of arm or leg paralysis, cerebrovascular disease, congestive heart failure, coronary disease, knee arthritis, or chronic back pain. The model of WIQ scores provided virtually the same results, with a history of diabetes also a significant negative predictor ($p = 0.04$). ABI was even more significant ($p < 0.0001$) in the WIQ model; the coefficient of 0.33 on ABI indicates that a 10.3% increase in WIQ walking distance is associated with a 0.3 increase in ABI.

When interpreting these cross-sectional results, keep in mind that findings represent mean effects across the whole patient sample. Obviously patients with an initially

TABLE 24–4. STEPWISE MULTIPLE REGRESSION MODEL OF SF36 PHYSICAL FUNCTIONING SCORE
PROSPECTIVE OUTCOMES STUDY OF INTERMITTENT CLAUDICATION BASELINE ENROLLMENT DATE

	$N = 555;\ R^2 = 14.5$		
	Coefficient	Standard Error	P Value
Lowest leg ABI	18.8	5.7	.001
Male sex	5.1	2.6	.047
High school graduate	4.8	2.1	.025
Severe comorbidity walking impairment	−10.1	2.5	<.001
Paralysis/CVD	−8.0	2.3	<.001
COPD	−5.0	2.5	.045
CHF/CAD	−4.2	1.8	.022
Knee arthritis/back pain	−3.7	1.8	.040
VA clinic patient	−5.5	2.1	.008
Constant	37.7	4.2	<.001

Key: CVD, history of cerebrovascular disease; COPD, history of chronic obstructive pulmonary disease; CHF/CAD, history of congestive heart failure/coronary artery disease (myocardial infarction or angina).
Adapted with permission from: Feinglass J, McCarthy WJ, Slavensky R, et al. The effect of lower extremity blood pressure on physical functioning for patients with intermittent claudication. *J Vasc Surg.* 1996;24:503–510, Table 4.

high ABI or functioning level would have an attenuated relationship between these variables. Conversely, the predicted effects of ABI on functioning for the subset of patients with low ABI, low functioning, and few significant comorbidities would be much stronger than the mean effects. The results thus mirror current clinical judgment about the best candidiates for interventional management of PAD.

FUTURE RESEARCH AIMS

When 18-month follow-up is completed, longitudinal data and survival analyses will be used to determine the prognostic significance of lower extremity bypass surgery and percutaneous transluminal angioplasty on longer term PAD and functional end points. About 120 to 140 patients are expected to undergo lower extremity revascularization procedures; attrition due to death, incapacitation due to illness, and other causes are expected to account for about 15% to 20% of the original sample. Special emphasis will be placed on estimating the effects of modifiable risk factors, in particular smoking, exercise, and specific cardiovascular medications, on the incidence of four classes of outcomes: all cause mortality, cardiovascular (CV) disease events, progression of PAD, and change in functional status. All analyses will be controlled by baseline sociodemographic characteristics, severity of comorbid conditions, leg symptom duration, and lower extremity hemodynamics. Mail and telephone follow-up, review of medical records, and acquisition of death certificates will be used to document clinical end points of death, acute CV events requiring hospitalization, and PAD progression as measured by lower extremity rest pain, skin ulcers, gangrene, graft failure, restenosis, or foot amputation.

Power estimates based on a cumulative 15% event rate (a rate less than or equal to that expected for each outcome class) with 0.8 power ($\alpha < .05$) provide detectable odds ratios of 1.35 or greater with a 400-patient sample.[36] The prognostic significance of LE revascularization for functional outcomes will also be tested with linear regression models. The sample needed to detect a 10-point difference in repeated PF score between two self-selected groups, with 0.8 power and a $p < 0.05$ (two-sided test), with intertemporal correlation of 0.6, is only 69 patients per treatment group (i.e., bypass or angioplasty); even greater precision is afforded by the repeated measures design.

Outcomes based on patient self-reported health status are becoming increasingly important indicators of the quality and appropriateness of medical care. Private and government third-party insurers as well as individual patient "consumers" will increasingly use such outcomes to evaluate their association with providers. Increasing competition and the growth of integrated delivery systems will undoubtedly require vascular surgeons to undertake more rigorous functional assessment of patients and to document long-term results. The Chicago Area Intermittent Claudication Research Study, together with similar efforts across the United States, will hopefully provide important benchmarks for future efforts in multispecialty vascular disease management.

REFERENCES

1. Stanley JC, Barnes RW, Ernst CB, et al. Vascular surgery in the United States: workforce issues. *J Vasc Surg*. 1996;23:172–181.
2. Boutwell RC, Mitchell JB. Diffusion of the new technologies in the treatment of the Medicare population: implications for patient access and program expenditures. *Int J Tech Assessment Health Care*. 1993;9:62–75.

3. Coffman JD. Intermittent claudication—be conservative. *N Engl J Med.* 1991;325:577–578.

4. Tunis SR, Bass EB, Steinberg EP. The use of angioplasty, bypass surgery, and amputation in the management of peripheral vascular disease. *N Engl J Med.* 1991;325:556–562.

5. Becker GJ, Ferguson JG, Bakal CW, et al. Angioplasty, bypass surgery, and amputation for lower extremity peripheral artery disease in Maryland: a closer look. *Radiology.* 1993;186:635–638.

6. McDermott MM, McCarthy W. Intermittent claudication: the natural history. *Surg Clin North Am.* 1995;75:581–591.

7. Kannel WB, McGee DL. Update on some epidemiologic features of intermittent claudication: the Framingham study. *J Am Geriatr Soc.* 1985;33:13–18.

8. Vogt MT, Wolfson S, Kuller LH. Lower extremity arterial disease and the aging process: a review. *J Clin Epidemiol.* 1992;45:529–542.

9. Newman AB, Siscovick DS, Manolio TA, et al. Ankle-arm index as a marker of atherosclerosis in the cardiovascular health study. *Circulation.* 1993;88:837–845.

10. Criqui MH, Langer RD, Fronek A, et al. Mortality over a period of 10 years in patients with peripheral arterial disease. *N Engl J Med.* 1992;326:381–386.

11. Violi F, Criqui M, Longini A, Castiglioni C. Relation between risk factors and cardiovascular complications in patients with peripheral vascular disease: results from the A.D.E.P. study. *Atherosclerosis.* 1996;120:25–35.

12. Simonsick EM, Guralnik JM, Hennekens CH, et al. Intermittent claudication and subsequent cardiovascular disease in the elderly. *J Gerontol.* 1995;50A:M17–M22.

13. McDaniel MD, Cronenwett JL. Basic data related to the natural history of intermittent claudication. *Ann Vasc Surg.* 1989;33:273–277.

14. Dormandy JA, Murray GD. The fate of the claudicant—a prospective study of the 1969 claudicants. *Eur J Vasc Surg.* 1991;131–133.

15. Jonason T, Ringqvist L. Factors of prognostic importance for subsequent rest pain in patients with intermittent claudication. *Acta Med Scand.* 1985;218:27–33.

16. Jelnes R, Gaardsting O, Hougaard Jensen K, et al. Fate in intermittent claudication: outcome and risk factors. *Br Med J.* 1986;293:1137–1140.

17. Cronenwett JL, Warner KG, Zelenock GB, et al. Intermittent claudication: current results of nonoperative management. *Arch Surg.* 1984;119:430–436.

18. Wilt TJ. Current strategies in the diagnosis and management of lower extremity peripheral vascular disease. *J Gen Int Med.* 1992;7:87–101.

19. Gardner AW, Poehlman ET. Exercise rehabilitation programs for the treatment of claudication pain. *JAMA.* 1995;274:975–980.

20. Ernst E, Fialka V. A review of clinical effectiveness of exercise therapy for intermittent claudication. *Arch Intern Med.* 1993;153:2357–2360.

21. Radack K, Wyderski RJ. Conservative management of intermittent claudication. *Ann Intern Med.* 1990;113:135–146.

22. Isner JM, Rosenfield K. Redefining the treatment of peripheral artery disease: role of percutaneous revascularization. *Circulation.* 1993;88:1534–1557.

23. Hunink MGM, Wong JB, Donaldson MC, et al. Patency results of percutaneous and surgical revascularization for femoropopliteal arterial disease. *Med Decis Making.* 1994;14:71–81.

24. Regensteiner JG, Hargarten ME, Rutherfort RB, Hiatt WR. Functional benefits of peripheral vascular bypass surgery for patients with intermittent claudication. *Angiology.* 1993;44:1–10.

25. Lundgren F, Dahllof AG, Lundholm K, et al. Intermittent claudication-surgical reconstruction or physical training? A prospective randomized trial of treatment efficiency. *Ann Surg.* 1989;209:346–355.

26. Fowler FJ, Bin L. Comparing survey measures of quality of medical care. In Warnecke R, ed., *Health Survey Research Methods: Conference Proceedings.* Hyattsville, MD: U.S. Department of Health and Human Services, Public Health Service, Centers for Disease Control and Prevention, National Center for Health Statistics; 1996;9–14.

27. Haley SM, McHorney CA, Ware JE. Evaluation of the MOS SF-36 physical functioning scale (PF10): I. unidimensionality and reproducibility of the Rasch item scale. *J Clin Epidemiol.* 1994;47:671–684.

28. Schneider JR, McHorney CA, Malenka DJ, et al. Functional health and well-being in patients with severe atherosclerotic peripheral vascular occlusive disease. *Ann Vasc Surg.* 1993;7:419–428.

29. Ware JE, Snow KK, Kosinski M, Gandek B. *SF-36 Health Survey: Manual & Interpretation Guide.* Boston: The Health Institute, New England Medical Center; 1993.

30. Regensteiner JG, Steiner JF, Panzer RJ, Hiatt WR. Evaluation of walking impairment by questionnaire in patients with peripheral artery disease. *J Vasc Med Biol.* 1990;2:142–152.

31. Feinglass J, Yarnold PR, Martin GJ, McCarthy WJ. Prevalence of walking impairment in young, healthy adults. *Percept Motor Skills.* 1993;77:417–418.

32. Reifler D, Feinglass J, Slavensky R, et al. Functional outcomes for patients with intermittent claudication: bypass surgery versus angioplasty versus noninvasive management. *J Vasc Med Biol.* 1995;5:203–211.

33. Hiatt WR, Marshall JA, Baxter J, et al. The effect of diagnostic criteria on the prevalence of peripheral arterial disease: the San Luis Valley diabetes study. *Circulation.* 1995;91:1472–1479.

34. Feinglass J, McCarthy WJ, Slavensky R, et al. The effect of lower extremity blood pressure on physical functioning for patients with intermittent claudication. *J Vasc Surg.* 1996;24:503–510.

35. Feinglass J, Slavensky R, Tang L. The intermittent claudication research study: vascular outcomes research using home health nurses. *J Vasc Nursing.* 1996;14:8–11.

36. Rubenstein LV, Gail MH, Santner TJ. Planning duration of a comparative clinical trial with loss to follow-up and a period of continued observation. *J Chron Dis.* 1981;34:469–479.

VII

Vascular
Emergencies

25

Endovascular Stent-Grafts for Treatment of Traumatic Pseudoaneurysms and Arteriovenous Fistulas

Michael L. Marin, MD, Frank J. Veith, MD, and Takao Ohki, MD

An increase in civilian trauma during the past decade is clearly linked to an overall rise in handgun-associated injuries. Penetrating trauma to the vascular system from any high-velocity missile may be complicated by arterial occlusions, pseudoaneurysms, and arteriovenous fistulas (AVFs). During the past 30 years, the optimal management of these vascular lesions has been refined by both military and civilian trauma experiences.[1–6] Arterial injuries that demonstrate a pulse deficit in association with severe limb or organ ischemia, expanding arterial hematomas, or active hemorrhage from an injured vessel clearly mandate urgent surgical exploration and arterial repair. The direct surgical repair of these vascular injuries may be complicated by several factors, including inaccessibility of the vascular lesion when trauma occurs to a vessel within a central body cavity. In addition, false aneurysms and AVFs may markedly distort local anatomy and induce significant venous hypertension, further increasing the challenge of a standard surgical repair often at a cost of considerable blood loss. Alternative treatments using catheter-directed techniques may reduce procedural risks and improve outcome in those patients who are stable after a vascular injury. One such therapy employs endovascular stent-grafts to repair the injured vessels directly from the luminal surface.[7–11] These devices permit minimally invasive arterial repairs to be performed from readily accessible sites in the vasculature that are remote from the area of arterial trauma. This chapter reviews a clinical experience with the placement of stent-grafts for the treatment of arterial pseudo-aneurysms and AVFs at the Montefiore Medical Center in New York.

TECHNIQUES AND DEVICES

Transluminally placed stent-grafts for treating traumatic arterial lesions were initially conceptualized by Dotter[12] in 1969, and one of the first clinical applications of this

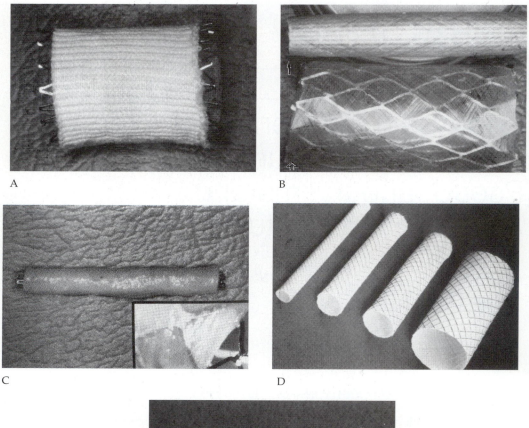

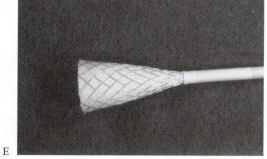

Figure 25–1. Endovascular covered stents. (**A**) Dacron graft material may be used to cover the balloon expandable stents. These devices have been used by Parodi[7] to treat traumatic lesions. (**B**) Polyurethane can be fabricated directly onto a stent. This material has "elastic" properties, permitting a closed stent (*thin arrow*) to remain well covered following deployment (*thick arrow*). (**C**) Autogenous vein can be used to cover stents, creating biological stent-grafts. The collapsed stent-graft assumes a small profile, which effectively covers the struts of the stent following deployment (*inset*). (**D**) Corvita endovascular stent-graft for arterial trauma. This polyurethane-covered stent structurally resembles the Wallstent. (**E**) Delivery catheter system for the Corvita stent-graft. A central "pusher" catheter ejects the self-expanding device out of the distal end of the sheath.

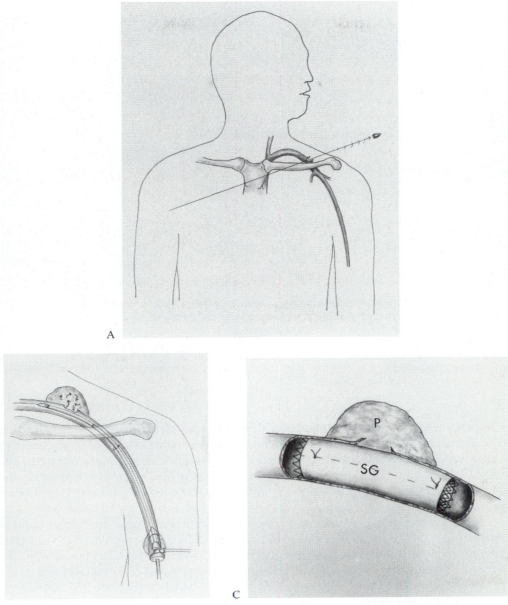

A

B

C

Figure 25–2. Schematic drawing of stent-graft repair of an arterial injury. (**A**) A bullet wound partially disrupts the wall of the vessel. (**B**) The stent-graft device is delivered to the site of injury via a remote arteriotomy. (**C**) Once deployed, the stent-graft covers the hole in the vessel. SG, stent-graft; P, pseudoaneurysm. (*Reprinted with permission: Marin ML, Veith FJ, Panetta TF, et al. Transluminally placed endovascular stented graft repair for arterial trauma. J Vasc Surg. 1994;20:466–473.*)

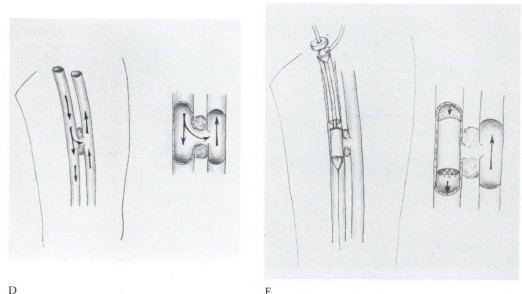

D   E

Figure 25–2. (**D**) When an arteriovenous fistula forms following a vascular injury, the same principles apply for stent-graft repair. In this example, the stent-graft device is inserted in the superficial femoral artery at a site remote form the arterial injury. (**E**) Following deployment, the stent-graft occludes the AVF. (*Reprinted with permission: Marin ML, Veith FJ, Panetta TF, et al. Transluminally placed endovascular stented graft repair for arterial trauma. J Vasc Surg. 1994;20:466–473.*)

technology was performed by Volodos et al.[13] using a Dacron graft and a self-expanding stent to treat a thoracic aortic pseudoaneurysm. Experimental and clinical experiences to date have demonstrated success with several different devices for treating traumatic arterial lesions (Fig. 25–1).[7,8,14] The ideal composition of the external covering on the stent and the best mechanism for stent deployment have not as yet been identified in the treatment of traumatic lesions.

At the Montefiore Medical Center, we have predominantly used the Palmaz balloon expandable stent in conjunction with a thin-walled polytetrafluoroethylene (PTFE) graft covering to perform arterial repairs of pseudoaneurysms and AVFs (Fig. 25–2). The stents varied between 2 to 3 cm in length and were fixed inside 6-mm Gore-tex grafts (W.L. Gore and Associates, Flagstaff, AZ) by 2 "U" stitches (Fig. 25–3A). The stent-graft was then mounted onto a balloon angioplasty catheter, which had a tapered dilator tip firmly attached to the end of the balloon catheter (Fig. 25–3B). The entire device was contained within a 12 French delivery system for over-the-wire insertion either percutaneously or through an arterial cut-down.

We recently participated in a Food and Drug Administration (FDA) phase I trial of the Corvita stent-graft device for arterial trauma (Corvita Corporation, Miami, FL). This device is fabricated from a self-expanding stent of braided wire similar in construction to the Wallstent (Schneider Corporation, Minneapolis, MN). The stent is covered with polyurethane fibers (Fig. 25–1D). The stent-graft may be cut to the desired length in the operating room using wire-cutting shears and then loaded into a specially designed delivery sheath (Fig. 25–1E). This sheath has a central "pusher" catheter that is responsible for discharging the graft at the desired location.

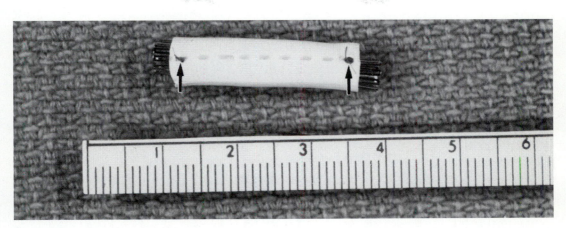

A

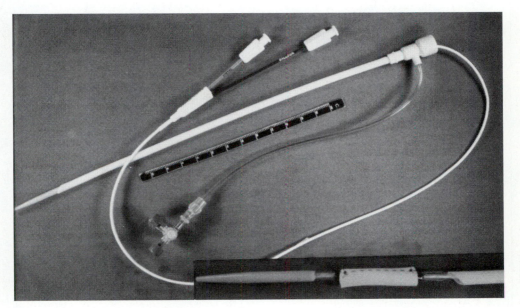

B

Figure 25–3. (A) An endovascular stent-graft. A segment of PTFE is attached to a stainless steel slotted balloon expandable (Palmaz) stent using two 5-0 prolene "U" stitches (*arrows*). (*Reprinted with permission: Marin ML, Veith FJ, Panetta TF, et al. Transluminally placed endovascular stent-graft repair for arterial trauma. J Vasc Surg. 1994;20:466–473.*) (**B**) The stent-graft is mounted on an angioplasty balloon and placed into a sheath prior to insertion. Note the presence of a dilator tip at the end of the balloon catheter, which provides a smooth taper within the catheter (*inset*).

TABLE 25–1. STENT-GRAFTS FOR ARTERIAL TRAUMA

Sex/ Age	Mechanism of Injury	Vessel(s) Involved	Pseudo-aneurysm	Arterio-venous Fistula	Anes-thesia	Associated Injuries	Injury to Repair Time Interval	Stent-Graft Length (cm)	Access	Hospital Stay (days)	Patency (months)	Complications
M/22	Bullet	LSFA	Yes	No	Local	Soft tissue right thigh; left deep venous thrombosis	12 h	3	LSFA arteriotomy	6	2[a]	Distal emboli (treated with catheter suction thrombectomy)
F/85	Surgical trauma	RCIA	Yes	Yes	Local	None	8 years	5[b]	LCFA percutaneous	4	5	Wound hematoma
M/49	Catheterization	RCIA	Yes	Yes	Epidural	None	18 months	5	Right femoral	5	5	—
M/68	Iliac graft disruption	LCIA	Yes	No	Epidural	None	1 month	9	Left femoral	5	6	—
M/66	Aortic graft disruption	Aorta	Yes	No	Epidural	None	1 week	10	Left femoral	5	11	—
M/76	Aortic disruption	Aorta	Yes	No	Epidural	None	3 days	7	Left femoral	7	13	—
M/18	Bullet	RASA	Yes	No	Local	None	6 h	3	Right brachial artery	3	14	—
M/22	Bullet	RASA	Yes	No	Local	Hemothorax	3 h	3	Right brachial artery	6	14	—
M/18	Bullet	RSA	Yes	Yes	Local	Hemothorax	48 h	3	Right brachial artery	4	23	—
F/78	Catheterization	RSA	Yes	No	Local	Hemothorax	24 h	3	Right brachial arteriotomy	8 weeks[c]	30	—
M/78	Catheterization	LCIA	Yes	No	Epidural	None	4 months	2	LCFA arteriotomy	2	30	—
M/35	Bullet	RASA	Yes	No	Local	Brachial plexus	3 weeks	3	Right brachial arteriotomy	4	31	—
M/24	Knife	LASA	Yes	No	General	Pneumothorax; hemothorax	4 h	3	Left brachial arteriotomy	7	35	Stent compression
M/28	Bullet	RSFA	Yes	No	Local	Left open femur fracture	12 h	3	RSFA arteriotomy	9	38	—
M/20	Bullet	LSFA LSFV	Yes	Yes	General	Soft tissue buttock	36 h	3	LSFA percutaneous	5	40	—

[a]Died 2 months postprocedure (homicide). [b]Corvita stent-graft. [c]Hospitalized for multiple medical problems.

Abbreviations: LSFV, left superficial femoral vein; LSFA, left superficial femoral artery; RSFA, right superficial femoral artery; RSA, right subclavian artery; LCIA, left common iliac artery; RCIA, right common iliac artery; RASA, right axillary subclavian artery; LASA, left axillary subclavian artery; LCFA, left common femoral artery.

RESULTS

As shown in Table 25–1, 15 patients received 15 stent-grafts to treat traumatic arterial lesions. The age of the patients receiving these grafts ranged between 18 and 85 years. Thirteen patients were male. Seven injuries occurred as a result of gunshot wounds (Fig. 25–4); 1 as a result of a knife wound; there were 3 iatrogenic needle catheterization injuries; 1 arterial trauma sustained at the time of gynecological surgery; and 3 that occurred as a result of arterial graft disruptions (Figs. 25–5 and 25–6). All injuries were associated with an adjacent pseudoaneurysm. In four instances the arterial injury formed a fistula to an injured adjacent vein. Associated injuries were present in 7 patients with arterial trauma and in 1 with an iatrogenic arterial injury (Table 25–1). One patient who had an axillary pseudoaneurysm repaired with a stent-graft required a vein patch of a small brachial artery at the catheter insertion site at the conclusion of the procedure. Stent-graft patency was 100% with no early or late graft occlusions. One patient with a left axillary-subclavian stent-graft developed a compression of the stent at 12 months, which was treated with balloon angioplasty. This problem recurred 3 months later and no intervention was done. This compressed device has not thrombosed with follow-up over 2 years. Mean follow-up for all stent-grafts was 24 months with a range of 5 to 40 months.

DISCUSSION

The prompt diagnosis and treatment of penetrating vascular trauma are essential to avoid the delayed sequelae that may occur when significant injuries to arteries are not diagnosed.[15–18] Traumatic AVFs and pseudoaneurysms involving nonessential vessels, such as the branches of the hypogastric or deep femoral arteries, can be effectively treated by catheter-directed arterial embolization.[19,20] Long-term follow-up of coil-treated lesions has been favorable. Small, anatomically favorable groin pseudoaneurysms secondary to catheterization injuries may be effectively treated with ultrasound-guided compression. Other injuries to vital arteries have traditionally required direct surgical repair of the damaged vessel employing either lateral repairs or prosthetic vascular conduits to restore critical arterial flow and avoid delayed complications.

Endovascular methods are rapidly evolving to treat a variety of vascular problems, including arterial trauma.[7–9,20] Endovascular therapy using balloon angioplasty of large vessels such as the iliac arteries appears to be a safe and effective alternative to surgery for some forms of stenotic and occlusive vascular disease.[21] This form of therapy may be successfully extended to more complex lesions by the use of intra-arterial stents.[22] The blending of intravascular stent and prosthetic graft technologies has resulted in the evolution of new devices (stented grafts) with a wide range of potential applications in the vascular system. Early feasibility studies of these devices have shown them to be technically capable of excluding experimentally created arterial aneurysms with the potential for treating other lesions.[23–25] Clinical experiences with stented grafts for trauma have been reported by several investigators.[7–9]

This chapter has reviewed the preliminary experience at the Montefiore Medical Center with stented grafts for the treatment of traumatic arterial lesions. Follow-up of these patients extends to 40 months. In this series, device insertion was accomplished with uniform technical success, and a satisfactory repair of the arterial lesion has been maintained in all cases with preservation of the arterial flow through the injured critical segment. Distal embolization occurred in one patient and this was managed by catheter-based suction thrombectomy of a small plaque embolism in the superficial femoral artery.

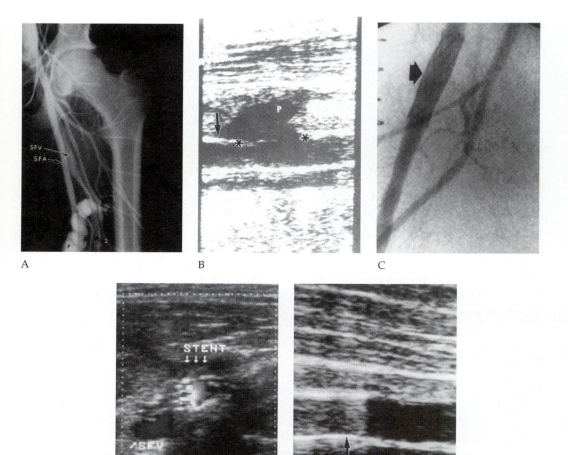

A   B   C

D,A   D,B

Figure 25–4. (A) Femoral arteriogram after gunshot wound to left thigh. An AVF associated with a large pseudoaneurysm is seen between the left superficial femoral artery (SFA) and the superficial femoral vein (SFV). Selective catheterization of the deep femoral artery (1) and the SFA branch (2) showed that these vessels were not injured. p, pseudoaneurysm. **(B)** Duplex ultrasonographic image of SFA depicted in part A. Loss of the intimal stripe (*arrow*) and associated pseudoaneurysm (p) is seen. Arterial defect measures approximately 13 mm (distance between asterisks). **(C)** Completion arteriogram demonstrates patency of the SFA, proper positioning of the stent-graft (*arrow*), and no evidence of the AVF or extravasation. Metal clips were placed in the skin before the procedure to facilitate fluoroscopic localization of the AVF and proper placement of the stent-graft. **(D)** Transverse and longitudinal duplex ultrasonographic images of stent-graft repair of SFA after 3 months. *A,* transverse image of artery and vein at level of stent can be identified with evidence of normal flow in arteries. *B,* longitudinal duplex ultrasonogram identifies stent-graft within artery (*arrow*). Minimal changes in peak systolic velocities are appreciated between the native SFA and that portion of the vessel that is covered by the stent-graft. (*Reprinted with permission: Marin ML, Veith FJ, Panetta TF, et al. Percutaneous transfemoral insertion of a stented graft to repair a traumatic femoral arteriovenous fistula. J Vasc Surg. 1993;18:299–302.*)

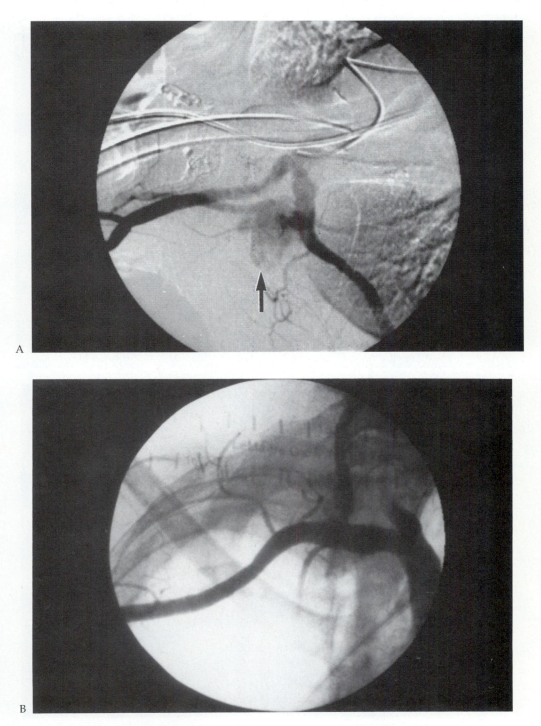

Figure 25–5. (A) This arteriogram shows a large pseudoaneurysm of the subclavian artery (*arrow*) just distal to the right vertebral artery that occurred after an attempted subclavian vein catheter insertion. **(B)** Following stent-graft placement through the right brachial artery, the pseudoaneurysm was excluded. Vertebral artery flow was maintained. (*Reprinted with permission: Marin ML, Veith FJ, Panetta TF, et al. Transluminally placed endovascular stented graft repair for arterial trauma. J Vasc Surg. 1994;20:466–473.*)

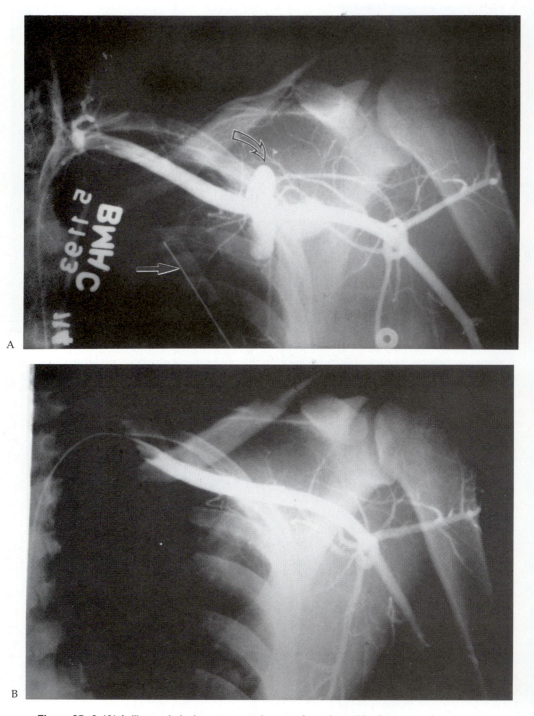

Figure 25–6. (A) Axillary-subclavian artery arteriogram of a patient with a large pseudoaneurysm (*curved arrow*) after a stab wound to the chest resulting in a hemopneumothorax (*straight arrow*, chest tube). **(B)** Following transluminal insertion of the stent-graft device, the pseudoaneurysm was repaired and flow was restored. (*Reprinted with permission: Marin ML, Veith FJ, Panetta TF, et al. Transluminally placed endovascular stented graft repair for arterial trauma. J Vasc Surg. 1994;20:466–473.*)

Endovascular stent-grafts inserted from a remote site in the arterial tree have several advantages over conventional repairs. When compared with standard operative repair of similar lesions, stent-grafts appear to be associated with less blood loss and a reduced requirement for anesthesia and dissection in the traumatized field. These advantages are particularly important in those patients with large, central vessel injuries or truncal AVFs with venous hypertension. Standard surgical repair of such lesions is notoriously difficult and is associated with significant blood loss. Stent-graft repair of these central or truncal artery false aneurysms avoids the need for extensive operations through major body cavities. These advantages are also important in patients who are critically ill from coexisting traumatic injuries or underlying major medical comorbidities. In the presence of these dire circumstances, the use of stent-grafts already appears justified to treat some traumatic lesions of major, critical arteries.

At present, controversy exists regarding the best conduit for the management of extremity arterial trauma distal to the subclavian and common femoral vessels, and this concern would be expected to extend to the use of prosthetic stent-grafts. Autogenous vein, which has excellent early and late patency rates, is preferred by most surgeons.[26] Autogenous veins have also been used to fashion stent-grafts for the treatment of arterial trauma in infected fields as well as to repair arterial injuries located in the carotid circulation where mural thrombus would present the greatest risk for embolization. Alternatively, others have achieved satisfactory results with conventional surgery using prosthetic grafts for extremity arterial wounds.[27] While long autogenous grafts for arteriosclerotic ischemia have been associated with better patency rates than arterial reconstructions performed with prosthetics, short (≤3-cm) prosthetic graft segments are likely to function satisfactorily in the axillary and superficial femoral arteries. However, this premise remains to be proven by longer patient follow-up. Even if late failure of stent-grafts in these locations occurs, percutaneous transluminal angioplasty or a subsequent elective vein graft bypass could then be performed in a field free of traumatized tissue and contamination and when the status of the venous circulation in a traumatized limb is known. Obviously, if the function of prosthetic stent-grafts in the superficial femoral and axillary arteries is poor, an autogenous vein-covered stent device could be considered as an alternative.

One theoretical problem with stent-graft repairs involves the potential for stimulating intimal hyperplasia at the stent-graft arterial junction. Although any form of traumatic injury to an artery may induce hyperplastic activity in the cells that compose the arterial wall, the Palmaz intra-arterial stent has been shown to cause a relatively limited intimal hyperplastic response in experimental studies as well as in the treatment of stenotic or occluded iliac arteries in patients.[22] In the latter setting, prolonged patency has been the rule.

Despite the potential disadvantages of using a thrombogenic stent-graft device that could stimulate intimal hyperplasia to treat a traumatic lesion of the axillary or femoral arteries, the advantages of minimally invasive deployment, decreased blood loss, and the ability to insert stent-grafts under local anesthesia through remote sites make this endovascular technique for repair of penetrating vascular injuries a potentially important tool that may be considered for more widespread use. This is already true for multiple trauma and critically ill patients with central artery injuries. Long-term follow-up of these repairs will be necessary to fully evaluate the safety and efficacy of these devices in extremity arteries and in other less critical circumstances.

CONCLUSION

Intravascular stents have become important tools for the management of vascular lesions; however, stents in combination with vascular grafts have only recently been applied clinically. This chapter describes an experience with stent-grafts for the treatment of penetrating arterial trauma. The use of stent-grafts appears to be associated with decreased blood loss, a less invasive insertion procedure, reduced requirements for anesthesia, and a limited need for an extensive dissection in a traumatized field. These advantages are especially important in patients with central AVFs or false aneurysms, particularly those who are critically ill from other coexisting injuries or medical comorbidities. In these circumstances, the use of stent-grafts already appears justified for the treatment of traumatic arterial lesions. Although the early results are encouraging, documentation of long-term effectiveness must be obtained before these devices can be recommended for widespread or generalized use in the treatment of major arterial injuries.

REFERENCES

1. Drapanas T, Hewitt RL, Weichert RF, Smith AD. Civilian vascular injuries: a critical appraisal of three decades of management. *Ann Surg.* 1970;172:351–360.
2. Burnett HF, Parnell CL, Williams GD, Campbell GS. Peripheral arterial injuries: a reassessment. *Ann Surg.* 1976;183:701–709.
3. Perry MO, Thal ER, Shires GT. Management of arterial injuries. *Ann Surg.* 1971;173:403–408.
4. Feliciano DV, Bitondo CG, Mattox KL, et al. Civilian trauma in the 1980s. A 1-year experience with 456 vascular and cardiac injuries. *Ann Surg.* 1984;199:717–724.
5. Jahnke EJ, Jr, Seeley SF. Acute vascular injuries in the Korean war: an analysis of 77 consecutive cases. *Ann Surg.* 1953;138:158–177.
6. Rich NM, Spencer FC. *Vascular Trauma.* Philadelphia: WB Saunders; 1978.
7. Parodi JC. Endovascular repair of abdominal aortic aneurysms and other arterial lesions. *J Vasc Surg.* 1995;21:549–557.
8. Marin ML, Veith FJ, Panetta TF, et al. Transluminally placed endovascular stented graft repair for arterial trauma. *J Vasc Surg.* 1994;20:466–473.
9. Becker GJ, Benenati JF, Zemel G, et al. Percutaneous placement of a balloon-expandable intraluminal graft for life-threatening subclavian arterial hemorrhage. *J Vasc Interv Radiol.* 1991;2:225–229.
10. May J, White G, Waugh R, et al. Transluminal placement of a prosthetic graft-stent device for treatment of subclavian artery aneurysm. *J Vasc Surg.* 1993;18:1056–1059.
11. Schmitter SP, Marx M, Bernstein R, et al. Angioplasty-induced subclavian artery dissection in a patient with internal mammary artery graft: treatment with endovascular stent and stent-graft. *AJR.* 1995;165:449–451.
12. Dotter CT. Transluminally-placed coilspring endarterial tube grafts. Long-term patency in canine popliteal artery. *Invest Radiol.* 1969;4:329–332.
13. Volodos NL, Karpovich IP, Troyan VI, et al. Clinical experience of the use of self-fixing synthetic prostheses for remote endoprosthetics of the thoracic and the abdominal aorta and iliac arteries through the femoral artery and as intraoperative endoprosthesis for aorta reconstruction. *Vasa Suppl.* 1991;33:93–95.
14. Rivera FJ, Palmaz JC, Encarnacion CE, et al. Aneurysm and pseudoaneurysm balloon expandable stent/graft bypass: clinical experience. *J Vasc Interv Radiol.* 1994;5:19. Abstract.
15. Feliciano DV, Cruse PA, Burch JM, Bitondo CG. Delayed diagnosis of arterial injuries. *Am J Surg.* 1987;154:579–584.
16. Richardson JD, Vitale GC, Flint LM, Jr. Penetrating arterial trauma: analysis of missed vascular injuries. *Arch Surg.* 1987;122:678–683.
17. Ben-Menachem Y. Vascular injuries of the extremities: hazards of unnecessary delays in diagnosis. *Orthopedics.* 1986;9:333–338.
18. Escobar GA, Escobar SC, Marquez L, et al. Vascular trauma: late sequelae and treatment. *J Cardiovasc Surg.* 1980;21:35–40.

19. Rosch J, Dotter CT, Brown MJ. Selective arterial embolization. A new method for control of acute gastrointestinal bleeding. *Radiology.* 1972;102:303–306.
20. Panetta TF, Sclafani SJA, Goldstein AS, Phillips TF. Percutaneous transcatheter embolization for arterial trauma. *J Vasc Surg.* 1985;2:54–64.
21. Johnston KW, Rae M, Hogg-Johnston SA, et al. 5-Year results of a prospective study of percutaneous transluminal angioplasty. *Ann Surg.* 1987;206:403–413.
22. Palmaz JC, Laborde JC, Rivera FJ, et al. Stenting of the iliac arteries with the Palmaz stent: experience from a multicenter trial. *Cardiovasc Interv Radiol.* 1992;15:291–297.
23. Mirich D, Wright KC, Wallace S, et al. Percutaneously placed endovascular grafts for aortic aneurysms: feasibility study. *Radiology.* 1989;170:1033–1037.
24. Laborde JC, Parodi JC, Clem MF, et al. Intraluminal bypass of abdominal aortic aneurysm: feasibility study. *Radiology.* 1992;184:185–190.
25. Balko A, Piasecki GJ, Shah DM, et al. Transfemoral placement of intraluminal polyurethane prosthesis for abdominal aortic aneurysm. *J Surg Res.* 1986;40:305–309.
26. Keen RR, Meyer JP, Durham JR, et al. Autogenous vein graft repair of injured extremity arteries: early and late results with 134 consecutive patients. *J Vasc Surg.* 1991;13:664–668.
27. Feliciano DV, Mattox KL, Graham JM, Bitondo CG. Five-year experience with PTFE grafts in vascular wounds. *J Trauma.* 1985;25:71–82.

26

Use of Transesophageal Echocardiography in Diagnosis of Aortic Dissection

Stephen P. Wiet, MD, and David D. McPherson, MD

Transesophageal echocardiography (TEE) allows excellent imaging of the heart due to the close relationship of the esophagus to the heart and lack of lung interference. In addition, the thoracic aorta (particularly the proximal ascending aorta and descending thoracic aorta from the arch to the diaphragm) is in close proximity to the esophagus, allowing detailed visualization of its structure and function. Initially, TEE was performed with monoplane probes, which provided transverse imaging sections radiating from the probe. The addition of biplane TEE with longitudinal interrogation planes radiating from the probe has allowed for better evaluation of the ascending thoracic aorta and aortic arch, giving more complete visualization of the thoracic aorta. Figure 26–1 illustrates the relationship of the aorta to the esophagus from the aortic valve to the diaphragm. The imaging planes have been superimposed, demonstrating both horizontal and vertical imaging planes. Multiplane TEE is the newest development that permits interrogation in multiple planes and in varying degrees from longitudinal to transverse, further enhancing the ability of TEE to visualize the entire thoracic aorta. Therefore, it is not surprising that diseases of the thoracic aorta, including dissections, aneurysms, and atherosclerosis, represent expanding indications for TEE.

This chapter describes the procedure, its utility for diagnosing aortic dissection, and comparison to other imaging techniques such as computed tomography (CT), aortography, and vascular magnetic resonance imaging (MRI).

PROCEDURE

Prior to each procedure, informed consent is obtained. If indicated, intravenous antibiotic prophylaxis for bacterial endocarditis is given. Lidocaine viscous and cetacaine spray preparations are used as oropharyngeal anesthesia. Glycopyrolate may be given to decrease secretions. Intravenous midazolam (Versed) is given as a short-acting anxiolytic in incremental doses. The patient is oriented into the left lateral position and

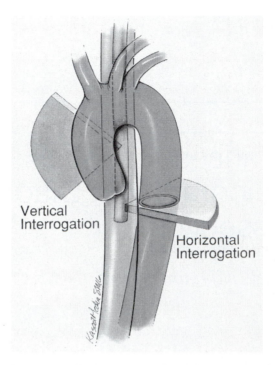

Figure 26–1. This figure illustrates the relationship between the esophagus and the thoracic aorta. Note that the esophagus is in proximity to the descending thoracic aorta from the arch to the diaphragm. The imaging fans, transverse to the right and longitudinal to the left, are radiating from the probe. (*Reprinted with permission: Wiet SP, McPherson DD. Role of transesophageal echocardiography in diagnosing diseases of the thoracic aorta. In: Yao JST, Pearce WH, eds. Aneurysms: New Findings and Treatments. Norwalk, CT: Appleton and Lange: 1994.*)

the tip of the probe is advanced into the esophagus. Images of the aorta, including ascending arch and descending thoracic aorta, are recorded up to the gastroesophageal junction, which is the level of the diaphragm. In addition, a cardiac transesophageal examination is performed. While imaging, Doppler (for flow information) and contrast studies (if shunts are suspected) are performed. Images are recorded on videotape. At the conclusion of the study, the probe is withdrawn and the patient observed for 1 to 2 hours prior to discharge to home or ward.

Dimensions of TEE probes for adult imaging range in maximum diameter of the distal imaging end from 11 to 13 mm. Pediatric imaging probes are approximately 6 to 8 mm in maximal diameter and can be used in children weighing more than 10 kg. Because TEE is essentially a modified gastroscopy in which the majority of images are taken at the mid and distal esophageal level, absolute contraindications to TEE include esophageal disease (cancer, stricture, esophageal varices), and relative contraindications include infectious disease of the esophagus and cancer of the stomach (especially the fundus) and severe cervical arthritis. Relative contraindications would require gastroenterologic passage of the probe. In uncooperative patients, patients on ventilators, or those undergoing operative procedures, an anesthesiologist generally is responsible for sedation and passes the probe. With experience, TEE is a relatively benign procedure and can be performed in critically ill patients with little if any risk of complication, including dissection extension.

UTILITY FOR EVALUATION OF AORTIC DISSECTION

Patients with suspected thoracic aorta dissection require immediate diagnostic evaluation so that urgent therapeutic interventions can be performed.[1-4] Detailed information concerning the dissection, the location of the entry site, the formation of thrombus in the false lumen, and evidence of pericardial effusion or aortic regurgitation are required to select the best management plan and to assess the patient's prognosis.[1-3]

Figure 26–2 identifies the three types of aortic dissections according to the DeBakey classification: Type I originates in the ascending aorta and extends into and beyond the arch and descending thoracic aorta; Type II originates in and is confined to the ascending aorta; and Type III originates in the descending aorta and either stops above the diaphragm (IIIa) or extends below the diaphragm (IIIb). Although there are variations of this classification, such as Type III dissections that extend back into the ascending aorta, for identification of the site and origin of dissection, and treatment approach planning, this classification has stood the test of time.

Figures 26–3, 26–4, and 26–5 schematically illustrate TEE imaging sections obtained from patients in our laboratory with a complex Type I aortic dissection. Figure 26–3 illustrates the proximal ascending aorta with the dissection flap. Figure 26–4 demonstrates the dissection flap and the true and false lumen in the descending thoracic aorta with the interluminal communication between the true and false lumen well illustrated by color Doppler. Figure 26–5 demonstrates the dissection flap and thrombus in the false lumen in both transverse and longitudual imaging planes. Therefore, visualizing the presence of a pericardial effusion, aortic insufficiency, extent of the dissection and dissection flap, differentiation of true from false lumen, identification of thrombus in the false lumen, and identification of interluminal communication is easily accom-

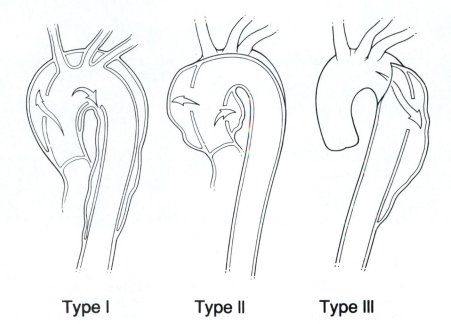

Type I   Type II   Type III

Figure 26–2. This figure illustrates the DeBakey classifications of aortic dissections. Type I involves the entire aorta; Type II the ascending aorta; and Type III the descending aorta.

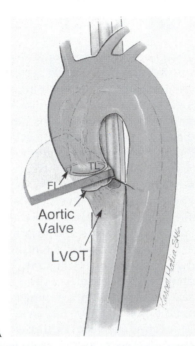

A

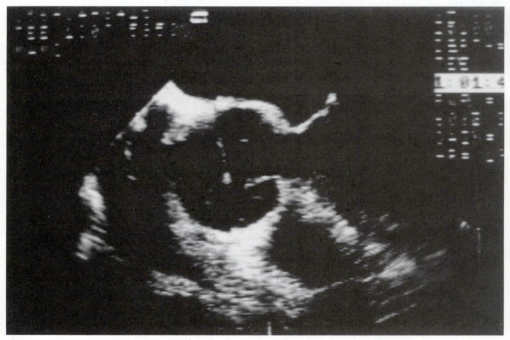

B

Figure 26–3. (A) Schematic of and [**B; C**, (see color insert)] TEE of the left ventricular outflow tract (LVOT) and ascending aorta in a patient with a Type I dissection. The dissection flap (B) separates the true from the false lumen, and in C (see color insert) color-flow Doppler enhances the demarcation between the true and false lumen. (*Reprinted with permission: Wiet SP, McPherson DD. Role of transesophageal echocardiography in diagnosing diseases of the thoracic aorta. In: Yao JST, Pearce WH, eds. Aneurysms: New Findings and Treatments. Norwalk, CT: Appleton and Lange: 1994.*)

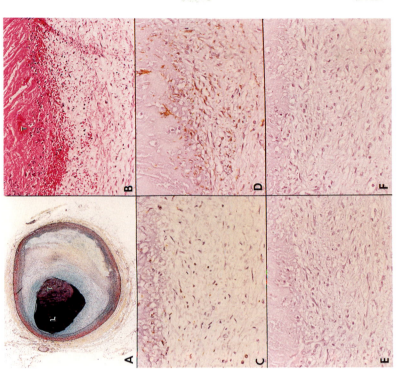

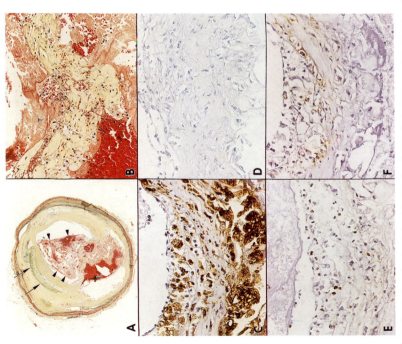

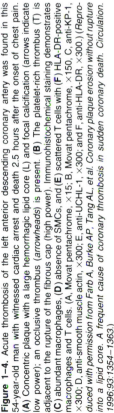

Figure 1–4. Acute thrombosis of the left anterior descending coronary artery was found in this 54-year-old man with witnessed cardiac arrest and death 2.5 hours after the onset of chest pain. (**A**) Concentric plaque with a large hemorrhagic lipid core (L) and focal calcification (arrows indicate low power); an occlusive thrombus (*arrowheads*) is present. (**B**) The platelet-rich thrombus (T) is adjacent to the rupture of the fibrous cap (high power). Immunohistochemical staining demonstrates (**C**) abundant macrophages, (**D**) absence of SMCs, and (**E**) scattered T cells with (**F**) HLA-DR-positive macrophages and T cells. (A, Movat pentachrome, ×15; B, Movat pentachrome, ×150, C, anti-KP-1, ×300; D, anti-smooth muscle actin, ×300; E, anti-UCHL-1, ×300; and F, anti-HLA-DR, ×300.) (*Reproduced with permission from Farb A, Burke AP, Tang AL, et al. Coronary plaque erosion without rupture into a lipid core. A frequent cause of coronary thrombosis in sudden coronary death. Circulation. 1996;93:1354–1363.*)

Figure 1–5. This 33-year-old woman had sudden collapse and witnessed cardiac arrest shortly after eating. Acute thrombosis of the left anterior descending coronary artery was found at autopsy, and the thrombosed segment is shown at low power in **A**. An eccentric plaque containing a nonocclusive thrombus (T) is present, and the remainder of the lumen (L) is filled with dark-gray barium gelatin. The eroded plaque surface is seen at high power in **B**, and numerous spindle-shaped cells are present in the plaque. The thrombus (T) consists predominantly of platelets, and the luminal plaque surface is cellular and rich in proteoglycans (green color by Movat staining in **A**). (**C**) Occasional macrophages are present in the plaque and thrombus. (**D**) Actin immunohistochemical staining identifies the cells at the luminal surface in contact with the thrombus as SMCs. Stains for T cells in **E** and HLA-DR in **F** are negative. (A: Movat pentachrome, ×15; B: hematoxylin-eosin, ×150; C: anti-KP-1, ×300; D: anti-smooth muscle actin, ×300; E: anti-UCHL-1, ×300; and F: anti-HLA-DR, ×300.) (*From same source as Figure 1–4.*)

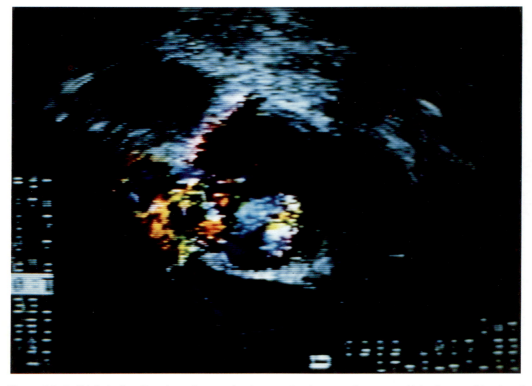

Figure 26–3. (C) Colorflow Doppler enhances the demarcation between the true and false lumen. (*Reprinted with permission: Wiet SP, McPherson DD. Role of transesophageal echocardiography in diagnosing diseases of the thoracic aorta. In: Yao JST, Pearce WH, eds. Aneurysms: New Findings and Treatments. Norwalk, CT: Appleton & Lange, 1994.*)

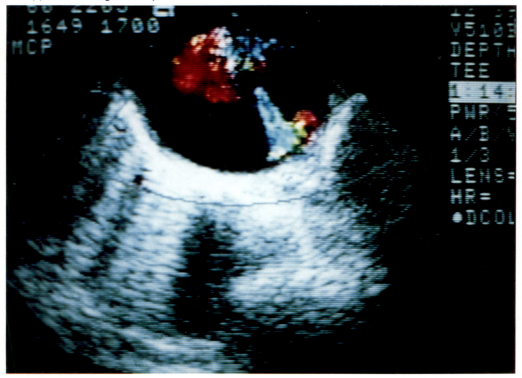

Figure 26–4. (B) TEE of the interluminal communication between the true and the false lumen in the descending thoracic aorta in the patient with a Type I dissection. (*Reprinted with permission: Wiet SP, McPherson DD. Role of transesophageal echocardiography in diagnosing diseases of the thoracic aorta. In: Yao JST, Pearce WH, eds. Aneurysms: New Findings and Treatments. Norwalk, CT: Appleton & Lange, 1994.*)

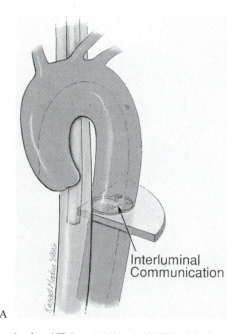

Figure 26–4. (A) Schematic of and [**B** (see color insert)]; TEE of the interluminal communication between the true and the false lumen in the descending thoracic aorta in a patient with a Type I dissection. The high velocity color-flow Doppler jet directs flow from the true lumen to the false lumen (A, *arrow*). (*Reprinted with permission: Wiet SP, McPherson DD. Role of transesophageal echocardiography in diagnosing diseases of the thoracic aorta. In: Yao JST, Pearce WH, eds. Aneurysms: New Findings and Treatments. Norwalk, CT: Appleton and Lange: 1994.*)

plished using TEE.[5,6] Table 26–1 lists the advantages and limitations of TEE for evaluation of aortic dissection.

Unsuspected thoracic aortic dissections and/or aneurysms can also be identified by TEE. Figures 26–6 and 26–7 illustrate examples from a patient of ours who presented postcoronary artery bypass grafting procedure with a large ascending aorta. A large anteriorly placed dissection and pseudoaneurysm was seen by TEE. Subsequent surgery identified this as originating within the location of the aortic cannulation site from the previous bypass surgery.

How does TEE compare to other techniques for evaluation of aortic dissection? It compares very favorably to vascular MRI in both sensitivity and specificity.[7-11] Vascular MRI, like TEE, can assess luminal flow and aortic insufficiency and demonstrate mural thrombus. However, vascular MRI requires the use of a scanner that, if available, is often far from the emergency room, causes claustrophobia, cannot be performed in hemodynamically unstable patients, and is somewhat costly. In patients with pacemakers, infusion pumps, and ventilators, the examination can often not be performed. Also, in some patients, there is difficulty visualizing the intimal flap when the false lumen is thrombosed. However, in spite of these limitations, vascular MRI has extremely good sensitivity and specificity with respect to diagnosis of aortic dissections.

TEE seems to have similar, if not better, sensitivity and specificity than CT in the evaluation of aortic dissection.[12,13] Computed tomography is generally widely available, reliable, and reproducible. However, it requires radiation and contrast exposure, cannot detect aortic valve dysfunction, is of limited value in unstable patients, cannot dynamically assess flow in the true or false lumen (including precise site of reentry), and, like TEE, may not always provide accurate identification of aortic branch involvement.

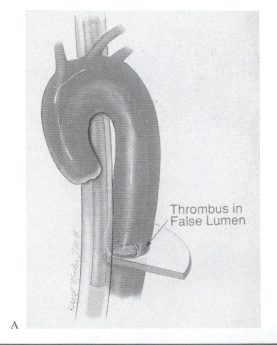

A

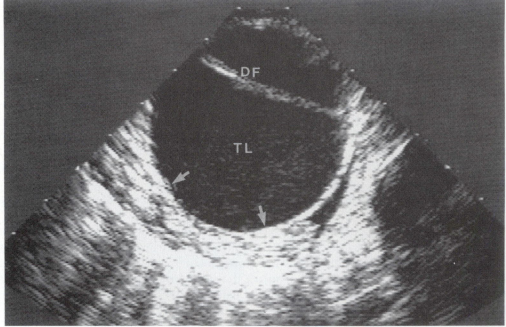

B

Figure 26–5. (A) Schematic of and **(B, C)** TEE of thrombus in the false lumen in a patient with a Type I aortic dissection. Part B demonstrates the transverse images corresponding to the schematic in part A. **(C)** The longitudinal images. The dissection flap (DF) is easily seen. The arrows point to a large bright thrombus in the false lumen, which has extended posteriorly around the true lumen (TL). (*A is reprinted with permission: Wiet SP, McPherson DD. Role of transesophageal echocardiography in diagnosing diseases of the thoracic aorta. In: Yao JST, Pearce WH, eds. Aneurysms: New Findings and Treatments. Norwalk, CT: Appleton and Lange: 1994.*)

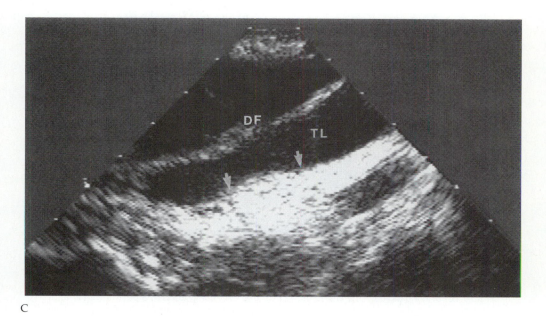

C

Figure 26–5. *Continued*

TEE is superior to aortography, as are both vascular MRI and CT imaging. This is due to the fact that the aortogram is essentially a "luminogram," which opacifies to greater or lesser extent both the true and false lumens, may obscure the dissection flap, may not be able to identify the false lumen if filled with thrombus, and cannot provide detail concerning the wall and the presence of a pericardial effusion. Therefore, angiog-

TABLE 26–1. TRANSESOPHAGEAL ECHOCARDIOGRAPHY ADVANTAGES AND LIMITATIONS

Advantages
1. Safe and rapid acquisition time—usually less than 15 minutes.
2. Can be done in the emergency room without having to move the patient and avoiding delays.
3. Can be performed at the bedside of unstable patients.
4. Avoids the comorbid events associated with angiography and CT scan (dye allergy, hematoma, perforation, exposure to x-rays).
5. High sensitivity and specificity.
6. Can be performed intraoperatively to assess surgical repair.
7. Can accurately assess aortic valve function with well-established criteria.
8. Accurately identifies communications between true and false lumens.
9. Accurately identifies pericardial and pleural effusions.
10. Sensitivity and specificity for ascending aorta and arch involvement enhanced with biplane and omniplane probes.
11. Can assess flow in both true and false lumens as well as thrombus.
12. Can be performed safely during pregnancy.
13. Reproducible in inpatients and outpatients at lower cost than MRI and CT scan.

Limitations
1. Cannot assess the abdominal aorta.
2. Lower sensitivity in the ascending aorta and arch with monoplane transesophageal probes.

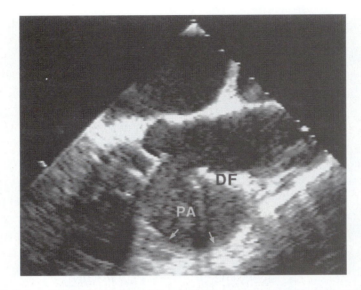

Figure 26–6. Longitudinal TEE image of the proximal ascending aorta in a patient with a large anteriorly placed dissection and pseudoaneurysm (see text for details). PA, pseudoaneurysm; DF, dissection flap; arrows outline pseudoaneurysm.

raphy in most studies is believed to be neither as sensitive nor as specific as other imaging techniques including TEE.[14]

In recent studies comparing TEE, CT, and vascular MRI, the sensitivity of TEE for aortic dissection ranges from 95% to 100%, CT from 80% to 100%, and vascular MRI from 96% to 100%.[15,16]

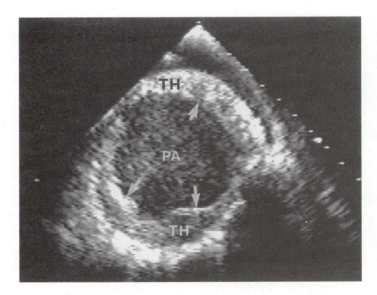

Figure 26–7. Transverse TEE image through the pseudoaneurysm (PA) of the patient shown in Fig. 26–6. Notice the layered thrombus (TH) encircling the pseudoaneurysm. The PA has dimensions of at least 5 cm (see text for details). Arrows outline intraluminal thrombus.

TABLE 26–2. PRACTICAL ASSESSMENT OF THE FOUR DIAGNOSTIC TECHNIQUES

Advantage	Aortography	CT	MRI	TEE[a]
Readily available	Fairly	Quite	Fairly	Very
Rapid	Fairly	Quite	Fairly	Very
Performed at patient's bedside	No	No	No	Yes
Noninvasive	No	Yes	Yes	Yes
Does not use IV contrast agent	No	No	Yes	Yes
Cost	High	Reasonable	Moderate	Reasonable

[a] TEE denotes transesophageal echocardiography.

Reprinted with permission from Cigarroa JE, Isselbacher EM, DeSanctis RW et al. Diagnostic imaging in the evaluation of suspected aortic dissection: old standards and new directions. *N Engl J Med.* 1993;328:35–43.

Table 26–2 summarizes the practical assessment of the four diagnostic techniques for evaluation of thoracic aortic dissection. With the widespread use of TEE to evaluate aortic dissection, it is not surprising that a recent study by Erbel et al.[17] demonstrated that preoperative mortality in aortic dissection appears to be reduced by TEE, allowing rapid initial treatment. Intraoperative and postoperative mortality remains high. This may be decreased if intraoperative echocardiography can better identify those requiring a second surgery or closure of entry sites to induce thrombus formation and reduce aortic wall stress.

Wiet et al.[18,19] reviewed the experience at our institution from July 1, 1989, to December 31, 1992. Using traditional criteria, 37 patients were referred for evaluation of suspected aortic dissection of which 20 patients were found to have dissection. Eleven of the 20 were Type I, 2/20 were Type II, and 7/20 were Type III. In all patients with the diagnosis of dissection, the dissection plane, the presence or absence of aortic insufficiency, and thrombus formation were seen. An interluminal communication was found in 14/20 patients. CT scans were performed in 15/37 patients, aortography in 3/37 patients, and surgical confirmation in 6/37 patients. One CT scan was false-positive for dissection and was ruled out by both TEE and aortography. There was concordance among studies from all other patients. Therefore, our experience is similar to that of others, indicating a high degree of accuracy for using TEE in the evaluation of aortic dissection.

In addition to helping in diagnosis, TEE can aid in evaluating the operative repair of aortic dissections. Figure 26–8 illustrates the Cabrol precedure with TEE images demonstrating good graft placement within the dissection. Complications such as dissection enlargement following graft placement, dissection extension beyond the graft site, aneurysm or pseudoaneurysm formation, rupture, progression of aortic insufficiency, and coronary and branch vessel compromise can also be assessed.

CONCLUSION

Transesophageal echocardiography is an excellent diagnostic imaging technique to evaluate disease of the thoracic aorta. It has been shown to correlate well with other imaging techniques (vascular MRI, CT, angiography) for the evaluation of aortic dissection and aneurysm formation. Due to its ease of use and rapid image acquisition, information is instantaneously obtained such that diagnostic decisions can be made at the time of the examination.

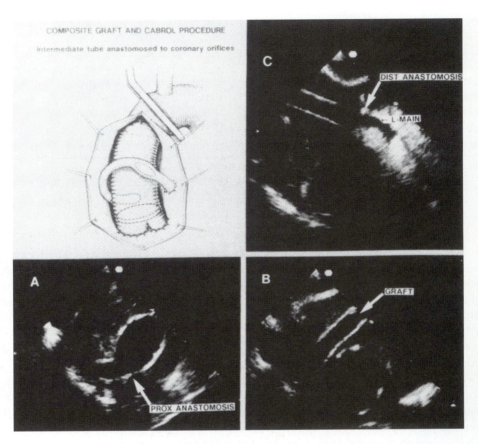

Figure 26–8. This is a diagram of the Cabrol procedure (top left) and three transesophageal echocardiographic images from a patient with the Cabrol. (**A**) The proximal anastamosis of the Cabrol graft to the aortic tube graft. (**B**) A longitudinal image of the Cabrol graft between the tube graft and the native aortic wrap. (**C**) The distal anastamosis of the Cabrol graft to the left main coronary artery (L-Main). (*Reprinted with permission: Goldstein SA, Mintz GS, Lindsay J Jr. Aorta: comprehensive evaluation by echocardiography and transesophageal echocardiography. J Am Soc Echo. 1993;6:652.*)

Acknowledgment

The authors wish to thank Bonnie Kane, BS, for her expert preparation of the illustrations and Cynthia Shane for her expert manuscript preparation.

REFERENCES

1. DeBaky ME, McCollum CH, Crawford ES, et al. Dissection and dissecting aneurysms of the aorta; twenty-year follow-up of five hundred twenty-seven patients treated surgically. *Surgery*. 1982;92:1118–1134.
2. Doroghazi RM, Slater EE, DeSanctis RW, et al. Long-term survival of patients with treated aortic dissection. *J Am Coll Cardiol*. 1984;3:1026–1034.
3. Haverich A, Miller DC, Scott WC, et al. Acute and chronic aortic dissections—determinations of long-term outcome for operative survivors. *Circulation*. 1985;72(suppl):II-22–II-34.
4. Eagle KA, DeSanctis RW. Aortic dissection. *Curr Prob Cardiol*. 1989;14:225–278.

5. Goldstein SA, Mintz GS, Lindsay J Jr. Aorta: comprehensive evaluation by echocardiography and transesophageal echocardiography. *J Am Soc Echo.* 1993;6:634–659.
6. Hashimoto S, Kumoda T, Osakada G, et al. Detection of the entry site in dissecting aortic aneurysm using transesophageal Doppler ultrasonography.
7. Neinaber CA, vonKodolitsch Y, Nicolas V, et al. The diagnosis of thoracic aortic dissection by noninvasive imaging procedures. *N Engl J Med.* 1993;328:1–9.
8. Cigarroa JE, Isselbacher EM, Desanctis RW, Eagle KA. Diagnostic imaging in the evaluation of suspected aortic dissection: old standards and new directions. *N Engl J Med.* 1993;328:35–43.
9. Neinaber CA, vonKlodlitsch Y, Siglow V, et al. Detection of dissection of the thoracic aorta: improved specificity by magnetic resonance tomography in comparison with echocardiography techniques. *Zeitschrift fur Kardiologie.* 1992;81:205–216.
10. Neinaber CA, Speilmann RP, Wiseheart JD. Diagnosis of thoracic aortic dissection. Magnetic resonance imaging versus transesophageal echo-cardiography. *Circulation.* 1992;85:434–447.
11. Amano W, Takenaka K, Sakamoto T, et al. Usefulness of transesophageal echocardiography in thoracic aortic disease: comparison with computed tomography and angiography. *J Cardiol Suppl.* 1991;26:45–56. Japanese.
12. Tottle AJ, Wilde P, Hartnell GG, Wiseheart JD. Diagnosis of acute thoracic aortic dissection using combined echocardiography and computed tomography. *Clin Radiol.* 1992;45:104–108.
13. Ballal RS, Nanda NC, Gatewooe R, et al. Usefulness of transesophageal echocardiography in assessment of aortic dissection. *Circulation.* 1991;84:1903–1914.
14. Shuford WH, Sabers RG, Weens HS. Problems in the aortographic diagnosis of dissecting aneurysm of the aorta. *N Engl J Med.* 1969;280:225–231.
15. Erbel R, Engberging R, Daniel W, et al. Echocardiography in the diagnosis of aortic dissection. *Lancet.* 1989;1:457–461.
16. Monacada R, Salinas M, Churchill R, et al. Diagnosis of dissecting aortic aneurysm by computed tomography. *Lancet.* 1981;1:238–241.
17. Erbel R, Oelert H, Meyer J, et al. Effect of medical and surgical therapy on aortic dissection evaluated by transesophageal echocardiography. *Circulation.* 1993;87:1604–1615.
18. Wiet SP, Pearce WE, McCarthy WJ, et al. Utility of transesophageal echocardiography in the diagnosis of disease of the thoracic aorta. *J Vasc Surg.* (in press).
19. Wiet SP, McPherson DD. Role of transesophageal echocardiography in diagnosing diseases of the thoracic aorta. In: Yao JST, Pearce WH, eds. *Aneurysms: New Findings and Treatments.* Norwalk, CT: Appleton and Lange; 1994.

27

Intraoperative Intra-Arterial Thrombolytic Therapy

Anthony J. Comerota, MD, FACS

Intra-arterial delivery of plasminogen activators is an important adjunct in the treatment of patients with acute limb ischemia. The principle of intra-arterial thrombolysis is based on the most important mechanism of action of plasminogen activators, which is activation of fibrin-bound plasminogen. Therefore, delivery of high concentrations of lytic agents into the arterial lumen should accelerate lysis of pathologic thrombi.

During the clinical use of regional catheter-directed thrombolysis in patients with peripheral vascular disease, significant clot dissolution has been observed prior to patients developing a systemic fibrinolytic response.[1] Likewise, acute arterial emboli to the distal arteries have been dissolved in the early postoperative period, following a short course of intra-arterial catheter-directed lysis, without bleeding complications.[2] These clinical observations indicated that direct intra-arterial infusion of lytic agents could dissolve blood clots within a short period of time without undue risk of hemorrhagic complications.

These were welcome observations in light of the uniform recognition that persistence of residual intra-arterial thrombi was the rule following both clinical and experimental balloon catheter thromboembolectomy for acute arterial occlusion. Greep et al.[3] showed that almost all patients treated with standard balloon catheter techniques had additional thrombus removed with a modified wire basket catheter retrieval system. Angiographic studies demonstrated that 36% of patients had residual thrombus extracted following the best attempts at balloon catheter thromboembolectomy for acute arterial occlusion.[4] Such data were subsequently corroborated in an experimental study demonstrating that 85% of dogs had angiographically demonstrable residual thrombi following balloon catheter thromboembolectomy.[5] The persistence of residual thrombi following the best attempts at mechanical removal provides a strong rationale to administer thrombolytic agents in the operating room. Moreover, in the intraoperative setting, the judicious use of lytic agents having a short half-life would likely minimize or avoid a systemic lytic effect persisting after wound closure.

Experimentally, canine hind-limb ischemia for more than 6 hours produces arteriolar thrombosis.[6] This extensive degree of thrombotic occlusion indicates that simple mechanical thrombectomy will not restore perfusion to nutrient vessels even if patency is restored to the main arteries.

In a controlled canine hind-limb perfusion study, Quinones-Baldrich et al.[5] demonstrated that thrombolysis following the best attempt at balloon catheter thromboembolectomy significantly improved angiographic results and was associated with a marked trend toward improved perfusion compared with control limbs. Belkin et al.,[7] in an isolated limb ischemic muscle preparation, demonstrated that urokinase infusion salvaged more ischemic muscle compared with a control group. In addition, significantly less injury, as demonstrated by reperfusion edema, was noted in the lytic group compared with the control group. This study also demonstrated a trend toward improved blood flow with lytic infusion. Therefore, experimental animal models confirm the clinical observations that balloon catheter thromboembolectomy frequently leaves residual thrombus. These data also demonstrate that arteriolar perfusion can be restored, tissue salvaged, and reperfusion injury reduced with the use of intra-arterial infusion of lytic agents.

CLINICAL EXPERIENCE

Despite an early report indicating that the infusion of intraoperative streptokinase was associated with significant bleeding complications,[8] clinicians found that intraoperative intra-arterial thrombolysis was valuable in the management of patients with acute limb ischemia. Quinones-Baldrich et al.[9] reported five patients with angiographically documented residual thrombi following balloon catheter thrombectomy who were treated with intra-arterial streptokinase (SK) over a 30-minute period. All five patients had successful lysis without bleeding complications.

Norem et al.[10] demonstrated that the infusion of SK following their best attempts at mechanical thrombectomy allowed retrieval of additional thrombus. After balloon catheter thromboembolectomy, intra-arterial SK was infused in the operating room. After a short waiting period, thrombectomy yielded additional thrombus removal, and all patients demonstrated angiographic improvement. Similar findings occurred with the use of intraoperative urokinase (UK) infusion.[11]

Parent et al.[12] treated 28 patients with intraoperative intra-arterial thrombolysis who had acute ischemia and residual thrombus following balloon catheter thrombectomy. Seventeen patients had operative arteriograms demonstrating thrombi. Of those 17, 15 had successful lysis when treated with intraoperative thrombolytic therapy. Both SK and UK were used and were shown to be equally effective (85% success with SK and 91% success with UK). However, bleeding complications were significantly greater with SK compared to UK (29% versus 5%, $p < 0.05$). Patients treated with SK had significantly greater fibrinogen depletion ($p = 0.054$), with 43% of SK treated patients having a fibrinogen less than 100 mg% compared to 5% of the patients treated with UK ($p < 0.05$).

Intraoperative intra-arterial thrombolytic therapy is part of the routine operative care of patients with acute limb ischemia at Temple University Hospital. A report of 53 patients with impending limb loss and occlusion of their runoff vessels demonstrated that this approach was clinically effective without significant bleeding complications.[13] The principle of short duration infusion of 250,000 to 500,000 IU of UK into the distal limb was initially based on clinical experience and outcome observation but now is supported by a prospective, randomized, placebo-controlled clinical trial.[14]

PROSPECTIVE, RANDOMIZED EVALUATION

Although the goal of intraoperative intra-arterial thrombolytic therapy was to deliver a plasminogen activator at high enough concentration to a thrombus, which would promote regional thrombolysis with minimal effects on plasma fibrinogen or clotting factors, little information was available about the regional effects compared with systemic effects of such an intraoperative infusion. Moreover, the dose–response relationship to the infused plasminogen activators had not been previously evaluated. Therefore, a prospective, multicenter, randomized, blinded, and placebo-controlled study was performed to address a number of these basic issues regarding intraoperative delivery of UK. The purposes of this study were to evaluate (1) the regional and systemic effects on plasma fibrinogen and the fibrinolytic system of intraoperative intra-arterial urokinase infusion; (2) whether there is a dose–response relationship to either plasminogen activation or fibrinogen depletion; (3) whether there is breakdown of cross-linked fibrin in a limb undergoing routine lower extremity revascularization (chronic limb ischemia) following a bolus dose of UK; and (4) whether there is an increased risk of excessive bleeding, operative blood loss, or wound hematomas.

One-hundred and thirty-four patients were prospectively randomized to receive one of three doses of UK or a saline placebo infusion in a blinded fashion into the distal arterial circulation during routine infrainguinal lower extremity revascularization for chronic limb ischemia. The end points analyzed were (1) the degree of plasminogen activation; (2) the regional and systemic breakdown of fibrinogen and fibrin; (3) the degree to which a dose–response relationship could be established; and (4) safety parameters that would be associated with intraoperative intra-arterial UK infusion. One of three doses of study drug or placebo was infused in a 30-cc volume as a bolus through the distal arteriotomy at the time of vascular reconstruction. Patient groups included (1) placebo (saline); (2) UK 125 (urokinase, 125,000 IU); (3) UK 250 (urokinase, 250,000 IU); and (4) UK 500 (urokinase 500,000 IU).

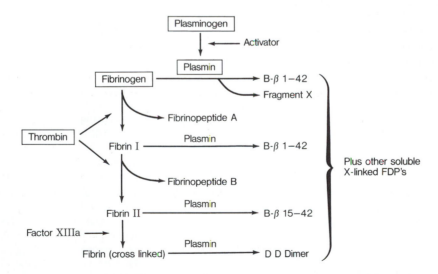

Figure 27–1. Schematic diagram of the markers of thrombin and plasmin-mediated proteolysis of fibrinogen and fibrin. [*Reproduced with permission: Comerota AJ, Rao AK, Throm RC, et al. A prospective, randomized, blinded and placebo-controlled trial of intraoperative, intra-arterial urokinase infusion during lower extremity revascularization: regional and systemic effects. Ann Surg. 1993;218(4):534.*]

Simultaneous blood samples were drawn from the ipsilateral femoral vein to evaluate regional effects and the arm (usually radial artery catheter) to evaluate systemic effects. Blood samples were analyzed for (1) plasminogen activity; (2) fibrinogen; (3) fibrin(ogen) degradation products (FDPs); (4) D-dimer; and (5) fibrinopeptide B-β_{15-42} breakdown products. Figure 27–1 demonstrates the rationale for using these end points as markers of thrombin and plasmin-mediated proteolysis of fibrinogen and fibrin.

RESULTS

Patient characteristics were similar among treatment groups, with the exception that those in the placebo group were somewhat younger than patients receiving UK ($p = 0.042$). There were no significant differences across treatment groups with respect to the distribution of associated risk factors, degree of ischemia at presentation, type of operative procedure, or anesthesia administered. The results of the regional and systemic blood tests are listed in Table 27–1 as maximal changes from baseline, and the patient morbidity and mortality data are listed in Table 27–2.

Compared with the placebo group, there appeared to be a dose-dependent decline in plasminogen that was significant ($p < 0.001$) only at the highest dose of UK (Fig. 27–2). Even at UK 500, however, the mean values were still within the normal range for plasminogen concentration. There was no significant decline in either the regional or systemic plasma fibrinogen following bolus UK infusion (Fig. 27–3). The plasma FDP levels were elevated in the treatment group in a dose-related fashion, with increases

TABLE 27–1. MAXIMAL CHANGES FROM BASELINE (VALUES REPORTED AS MEAN/MEDIAN) AFTER INFUSION OF STUDY DRUG INTO THE DISTAL ARTERIAL CIRCULATION

	Placebo ($n = 33$)	UK 125 ($n = 32$)	UK 250 ($n = 34$)	UK 500 ($n = 35$)
Regional				
Plasminogen (%)	NA	NA	NA	NA
Fibrinogen (mg/dL)	−30.72/−27.00	−28.62/−28.0	−20.35/−22.00	−38.97/−41.00
FDPs (μg/mL)	2.75/0.00	11.25/0.00	9.65/0.00	27.20/18.00 ($p < 0.001$)[a]
D-Dimer (μg/mL)	−0.106/−0.003	0.035/0.008 ($p < 0.001$)	0.100/0.029 ($p < 0.001$)	0.401/0.127 ($p < 0.001$)
B-β_{15-42} (pmol/mL)	−0.305/−0.226	0.461/0.143	0.595/0.136 ($p = 0.021$)	0.952/0.296 ($p = 0.017$)
Systemic				
Plasminogen (%)	−4.62/−6.50	−9.53/−10.50	−13.03/−15.00 ($p = 0.052$)	−27.46/−23.00 ($p < 0.001$)
Fibrinogen (mg/dL)	−43.78/−30.00	−30.52/−28.00	4.34/−10.00 ($p = 0.018$)	−50.91/−56.00
FDPs (μg/mL)	3.45/0.00	9.12/0.00	7.74/8.00 ($p = 0.005$)	18.00/10.00 ($p < 0.001$)
D-Dimer (gmg/mL)	0.066/0.003	0.026/0.003	0.069/0.035 ($p = 0.005$)	0.288/0.111 ($p < 0.001$)
B-β_{15-42} (pmol/mL)	−0.249/−0.075	0.572/0.125	0.199/0.234 ($p = 0.025$)	0.552/0.301 ($p = 0.001$)

[a]*Note:* p values refer to comparisons to placebo and were calculated using the Wilcoxon rank sum analysis. $p < 0.05$ values are listed, but significance is assigned at $p \leq 0.01$.
Reproduced with permission from Comerota AJ et al.[14]

TABLE 27–2. PATIENT MORBIDITY AND MORTALITY ACCORDING TO TREATMENT GROUP

	Placebo	UK 125	UK 250	UK 500	Total
Blood loss (mL)					
Mean	306.1	420.7	355.2	368.1	361.2
Median	250.0	350.0	325.0	300.0	300.0 ($p = 0.12$)
Blood replaced (mL)					
Mean	146.9	150.0	140.9	187.6	156.8
Median	0.0	0.0	0.0	0.0	0.0 ($p = 0.89$)
Excessive operative bleeding (% of patients)	5.9	9.7	2.9	2.9	5.2 ($p = 0.56$)
Wound hematoma (% of patients)					
None	91.2	86.7	87.5	94.1	90.0
Mild	5.9	6.7	12.5	5.9	7.7 ($p = 0.71$)
Moderate–severe	2.9	6.6	0.0	0.0	2.3
Death (%)	12.1	0.0	5.9	0.0	4.5 ($p = 0.034$)
Length of stay (postoperative days)					
Mean	10.8	22.7	15.7	16.2	16.3
Median	9.5	16.0	9.0	11.0	10.0 ($p = 0.06$)

Significance $p \leq 0.05$.
Reprinted with permission from Comerota AJ et al.[14]

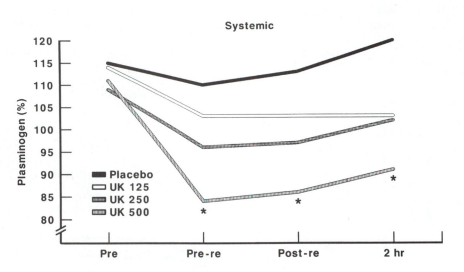

Figure 27–2. Mean plasma plasminogen levels in the systemic circulation for each time period and dose of UK infused. There appeared to be a dose-related decline in plasminogen, which was significantly different from placebo in the UK 500 group. *Reflect $p < 0.001$. Presample taken after heparin infusion but before arteries clamped. Pre-re (pre-reperfusion) blood samples obtained immediately before reperfusion. Post-re (post-reperfusion) blood samples obtained approximately 1 minute following reperfusion. Two-hour blood samples obtained from the arm 2 hours after reperfusion. [*Reproduced with permission: Comerota AJ, Rao AK, Throm RC, et al. A prospective, randomized, blinded and placebo-controlled trial of intraoperative, intra-arterial urokinase infusion during lower extremity revascularization: regional and systemic effects. Ann Surg. 1993;218(4):534.*]

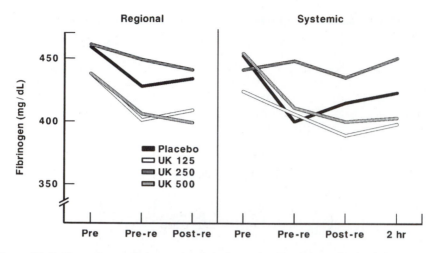

Figure 27–3. Mean plasma fibrinogen levels in the regional and systemic circulations by time period and dosage level. There was no significant change in any of the UK treatment groups compared to placebo. [*Reproduced with permission: Comerota AJ, Rao AK, Throm RC, et al. A prospective, randomized, blinded and placebo-controlled trial of intraoperative, intra-arterial urokinase infusion during lower extremity revascularization: regional and systemic effects. Ann Surg. 1993;218(4):534.*]

becoming significant ($p < 0.001$) in the UK 250 and UK 500 groups regionally and the UK 500 group systemically ($p = 0.01$). There were significant elevations of D-dimer regionally at each UK dose ($p < 0.001$), which increased in a dose–response fashion (Fig. 27–4). Systemic levels of D-dimer became significantly elevated at UK 250 and

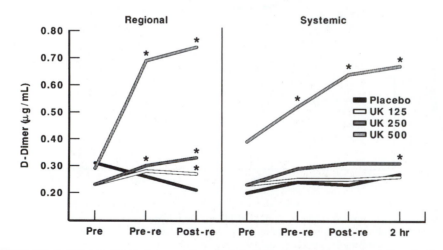

Figure 27–4. Mean levels of plasma D-dimer in the regional and systemic circulations by time period and dose of urokinase. Note significant and dose-related elevations at all doses of UK, regionally, and at UK 250 and UK 500, systemically. [*Reproduced with permission: Comerota AJ, Rao AK, Throm RC, et al. A prospective, randomized, blinded and placebo-controlled trial of intraoperative, intra-arterial urokinase infusion during lower extremity revascularization: regional and systemic effects. Ann Surg. 1993;218(4):534.*]

UK 500 ($p < 0.001$). Finally, fragment B-β_{15-42} levels showed a trend toward elevation at the higher doses of UK but achieved significance only at UK 500 ($p = 0.009$).

There was no difference in blood loss, the amount of blood replaced or the assessment of operative bleeding for any patient group. There was no difference in the frequency of wound hematomas comparing patients receiving UK with those receiving placebo. There was a trend toward a shorter hospital stay in the placebo group compared with the treatment groups ($p = 0.06$), although this was the result of a small number

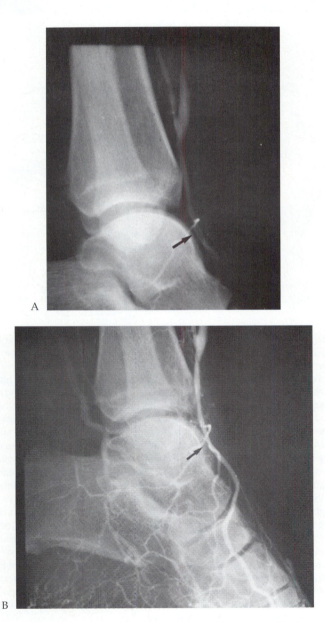

Figure 27–5. Completion arteriogram following a femoral-distal anterior tibial artery bypass for gangrene of the great toe. (**A**) Acute thrombus (?embolus) in the dorsalis pedis artery (*arrow*). (**B**) Following a 30-minute infusion of 250,000 U urokinase in 60 cc of saline, the repeat arteriogram shows that patency is restored to the dorsalis pedis with complete lysis of the thrombus.

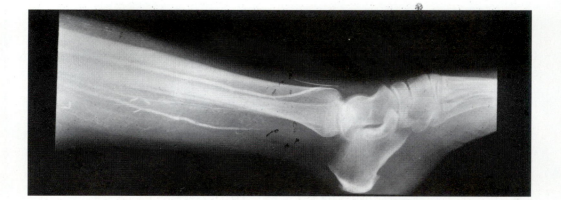

A

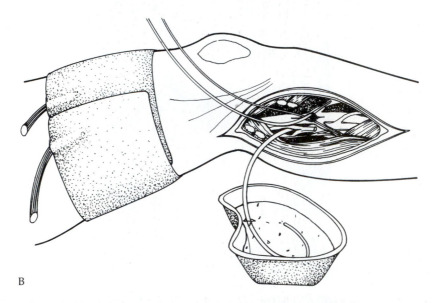

B

Figure 27–6. Technique of high-dose isolated limb perfusion of a thrombolytic agent in a patient who was at risk of bleeding from systemic fibrinolysis (having had a coronary artery bypass 2 days earlier) and who had acute multiple-vessel distal arterial occlusion that was unlikely to resolve with a single bolus of a fibrinolytic agent. The patient had an acute embolic/thrombotic arterial occlusion after percutaneous removal of an intra-aortic balloon, which was required following her emergency coronary artery bypass. Shown is the intraoperative arteriogram after balloon catheter thrombec-tomy of her popliteal and tibial vessels. Additional thrombus could not be mechanically removed. Catheters were placed into the origin of the posterior tibial and anterior tibial arteries, and the arteriogram (**A**) was performed with this selective injection technique. There was no evidence of contrast material entering the foot. Since additional thrombus could not be retrieved, we believed the patient would suffer a major amputation. (**B**) The patient's limb was elevated and the venous blood exsanguinated with a rubber bandage. A sterile blood pressure cuff (tourniquet) was placed on the distal thigh and inflated to 250 mm Hg. The popliteal vein was cannulated with a red rubber catheter and drained into a basin. One million units of UK were infused into the lower leg in a volume of 1 L of saline (500,000 IU in each of the anterior tibial and posterior tibial arteries) over 20 minutes. Following completion of the UK infusion, the limb was flushed with a heparin–saline solution. The venotomy was closed primarily, and the arteriotomy closed with a patch. (**C**) A postinfusion arterio-gram documented significant improvement of perfusion to the foot. The patient had a palpable dorsalis pedis pulse and a pink foot following wound closure. [*Reproduced with permission: Comer-ota AJ, Rao AK, Throm RC, et al. A prospective, randomized, blinded and placebo-controlled trial of intraoperative, intra-arterial urokinase infusion during lower extremity revascularization: regional and systemic effects. Ann Surg. 1993;218(4):534.*]

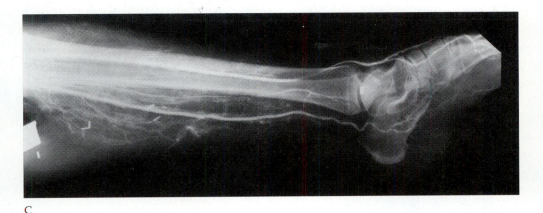

C

Figure 27–6. *Continued*

of outliers. An unexpected finding was the higher mortality in the placebo group (12.1% in placebo compared with 2.0% in patients receiving UK; $p = 0.033$). There were no significant differences between the maximal changes noted in the systemic and regional circulations for any of the plasma measurements.

DISCUSSION

Intraoperative intra-arterial thrombolytic therapy is now an important part of the treatment of patients with acute limb-threatening ischemia in which distal intra-arterial thrombus is part of the pathophysiology of the patient's ongoing ischemia. Experimental and clinical observations of catheter-directed thrombolysis support the use of intraoperative intra-arterial infusion of plasminogen activators.

A single or double bolus intra-arterial infusion or a short (20- to 30-minute) infusion of 250,000 units of UK may be all that is required to lyse a small thrombus occluding the outflow from a distal tibial bypass (Fig. 27–5). However, in patients with multiple-vessel acute thrombosis causing critical limb ischemia, a single bolus may not be sufficient for limb salvage. If systemic thrombolysis is contraindicated, an isolated limb perfusion with a high dose of plasminogen activator infused intra-arterially with drainage of the venous effluent can maximize clot lysis in addition to protecting the patient from any systemic lytic effect (Fig. 27–6). Quinones-Baldrich and colleagues[15] have taken the isolated limb perfusion technique one step farther, by incorporating the extracorporeal pump in the management of these patients with acute limb ischemia. They reported the use of high-dose plasminogen activators, UK (1 to 2 million units), or tissue plasminogen activator (125 mg) infused into the distal arterial circulation with an extracorporeal pump. A tourniquet was placed proximal to the cannulation site and inflated above systolic pressure in order to maintain isolation of the circulation of the extremity. These authors noted that while maintaining perfusion pressures at a physiologic level, the volume of flow increased as lysis progressed. After restoring patency of the distal circulation, lower extremity bypass procedures could then be performed. This resulted in limb salvage of 70% of these acutely ischemic patients. Unfortunately, pretreatment and post-treatment arteriograms were not obtained; therefore, objective evidence of lumenal dissolution of thrombus was not demonstrated.

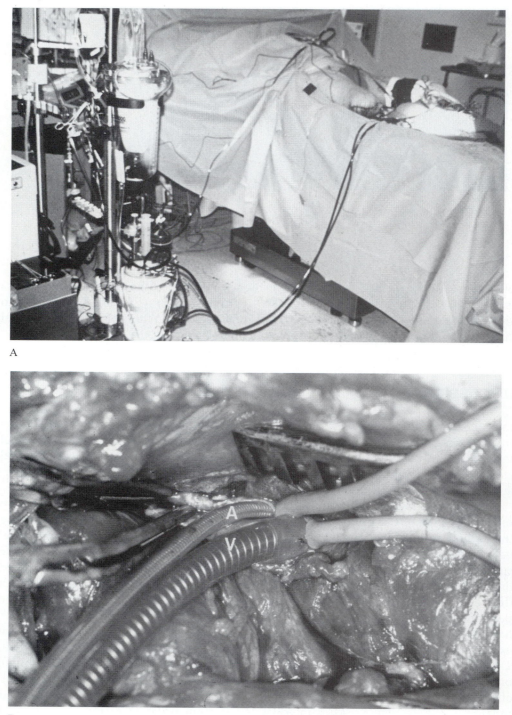

A

B

Figure 27–7. Illustration of the use of a membrane pump oxygenator with high concentrations of UK added to the reservoir for isolated limb perfusion for extensive thrombosis of a left leg. (**A**) The patient had a right above-knee amputation performed as a life-saving maneuver for extensive muscle necrosis due to distal thrombosis of his right leg. (**B**) Photograph of arterial cannula (A) and venous cannula (V), which were inserted into the popliteal artery and vein, respectively.

This concept of using a membrane pump oxygenator with high concentrations of a plasminogen activator added to the system for perfusion of an isolated limb was recently used at Temple University Hospital. A 57-year-old male suffered extensive, bilateral, lower extremity thrombosis following a femoral–femoral bypass. After multiple attempts at thrombectomy and after a failed bypass, both lower extremities remained critically ischemic. Upon arrival it was evident that the patient's right leg was not salvageable. Therefore a right above-knee amputation was performed. Although perfusion could be restored to the left popliteal artery, all infrapopliteal arteries were occluded, without arteriographic visualization of arteries to the lower leg or foot. A membrane pump oxygenator was used for a 75-minute isolated limb perfusion of 2 million units of UK, adding 250,000 U to the reservoir every 15 minutes (Fig. 27–7). A 24 French catheter drained the popliteal vein and a 14 French arterial cannula was inserted into the distal popliteal artery. A mean infusion pressure of 100 mm Hg was used throughout the infusion. Interestingly, the initial flow rate of 44 mL/min increased to 170 mL/min during the course of the infusion, indicating a marked drop in peripheral resistance. Unfortunately, this was not accompanied by significant improvement as evidenced by the post-treatment arteriogram. The patient's leg had improved perfusion postoperatively, however, it deteriorated with time such that a below-knee amputation was required.

This aggressive, organ-preservation approach to salvage of the ischemic limb is in its infancy. Much more attention is required to address reperfusion injury, appropriate perfusion pressures, doses of plasminogen activators, and many more variables. The near future will offer highly effective options for antithrombotic treatment, which will assist in maintaining patency following successful lysis.

Although the acutely ischemic limb with suspected distal thrombi is the most frequent indication for intraoperative fibrinolytic therapy, plasminogen activators may be of some benefit in patients with chronic lower extremity ischemia. In the prospective, randomized, placebo-controlled trial previously discussed, it was evident that complexed fibrin in the distal circulation was broken down. There appeared to be a dose-related elevation of D-dimer, suggesting that lysis of fibrin in the distal circulation occurred. If this is indeed the case, small distal vessel thrombosis may be part of the pathophysiology of progressive chronic limb ischemia. Since bleeding complications were not observed with bolus doses of up to 500,000 units, it seems reasonable to consider distal infusion of urokinase in patients undergoing operations for chronic but severe limb ischemia. Clearly, additional randomized trials are required to clarify this important issue.

TABLE 27–3. APPLICATIONS FOR INTRAOPERATIVE INTRA-ARTERIAL THROMBOLYSIS

Indication	Goal of Infusion	Suggested Technique
1. Following native artery or bypass graft thromboembolectomy	Lyse residual/ adherrent thrombus	Bolus dose $\times$ 1–2 100–500 $\times$ 10^3 IU UK 10–20 mg rt-PA
2. Open single tibial artery to provide runoff for bypass	Restore patency or dissolve residual thrombus	Bolus dose $\times$ 1–2, or short duration infusion 100–500 $\times$ 10^3 IU UK 10–20 mg rt-PA
3. Multivessel, extensive distal arterial thrombosis	Dissolve occlusive clot/thrombus	High-dose isolated limb perfusion ($\pm$extracorporeal pump) 1,000–2,000 $\times$ 10^3 IU UK 100–125 mg rt-PA

The utility of intraoperative intra-arterial lytic therapy is summarized in Table 27–3. Judicious use of plasminogen activators in the operating room is safe and may make the important difference in achieving reperfusion in patients with limb ischemia. Newly developed thrombin inhibitors and advances in the treatment of reperfusion injury will extend our ability to salvage the critically ischemic limb.

REFERENCES

1. Comerota AJ, Rubin R, Tyson R, et al. Intra-arterial thrombolytic therapy in peripheral vascular disease. *Surg Gynecol Obstet.* 1987;165:1.
2. Chaise LS, Comerota AJ, Soulen RL, et al. Selective intra-arterial streptokinase therapy in the immediate postoperative period. *JAMA.* 1982;247:2397.
3. Greep JM, Allman PJ, Janet F, et al. A combined technique for peripheral arterial embolectomy. *Arch Surg.* 1972;105:869.
4. Plecha RF, Pories WJ. Intraoperative angiography in the immediate assessment of arterial reconstruction. *Arch Surg.* 1972;105:902.
5. Quinones-Baldrich WJ, Ziomek S, Henderson TC, et al. Intraoperative fibrinolytic therapy: experimental evaluation. *J Vasc Surg.* 1986;4:229.
6. Dunnant JR, Edwards WS. Small vessel occlusion in the extremity after periods of arterial obstruction: an experimental study. *Surgery.* 1973;75:240.
7. Belkin M, Valeri R, Hobson RW. Intra-arterial urokinase increases skeletal muscle viability after acute ischemia. *J Vasc Surg.* 1989;9:161.
8. Cohen LJ, Kaplan M, Bernhard VM. Intraoperative fibrinolytic therapy: an adjunct to catheter thromboembolectomy. *J Vasc Surg.* 1985;2:319.
9. Quinones-Baldrich WJ, Zierler RE, Hiatt JC. Intraoperative fibrinolytic therapy: an adjunct to catheter thromboembolectomy. *J Vasc Surg.* 1985;2:319.
10. Norem RF, Shrot DH, Kerstein MD. Role of intraoperative fibrinolytic therapy in acute arterial occlusion. *Surg Gynecol Obstet.* 1988;167:87.
11. Garcia R, Saroyan RM, Senkowsky J, et al. Intraoperative, intra-arterial urokinase infusion as an adjunct to Fogarty catheter embolectomy in acute arterial occlusion. *Surg Gynecol Obstet.* 1990:171:201.
12. Parent NE, Bernhard VM, Pabst TS, et al. Fibrinolytic treatment of residual thrombus after catheter embolectomy for severe lower limb ischemia. *J Vasc Surg.* 1989;9:153.
13. Comerota AJ, White JV, Grosh JD. Intraoperative, intra-arterial thrombolytic therapy for salvage of limbs in patients with distal arterial thrombosis. *Surg Gynecol Obstet.* 1989;169:283.
14. Comerota AJ, Rao AK, Throm RC, et al. A prospective, randomized, blinded and placebo-controlled trial of intraoperative, intra-arterial urokinase infusion during lower extremity revascularization: regional and systemic effects. *Ann Surg.* 1993;218(4):534–540.
15. Quinones-Baldrich WJ, Deaton DH, Ahn SS, et al. Isolated fibrinolytic limb perfusion with extracorporeal pump in the management of acute limb ischemia. Paper presented at eleventh annual meeting of the Western Vascular Society; January 22, 1996.

28

Adjunctive Use of Intravascular Shunts in Management of Arterial and Venous Injuries

Aires A. B. Barros D'Sa, MD, FRCS, FRCSEd

Over the millenia the treatment of vascular injuries was aimed solely at saving life. Apart from a few anecdotal reports, the concept of vascular repair directed at preserving organ and limb only emerged during the early part of the twentieth century. Anastomotic techniques and vein grafting in vascular injuries of the limbs caused by high explosives and missiles during the bitter operational conditions of World War I proved impracticable and an amputation rate of 72.5% was recorded.[1] In casualties of World War II, vascular repair 10 hours after injury was seen to be demonstrably superior to ligation, and the amputation rate fell to 35.8%.[2] The time lag dropped to 6 hours in the Korean War during which reconstruction dramatically reduced the amputation rate to 13%.[3] This incidence remained unchanged at 12.7% during the Vietnam War and, as documented in the Vietnam Vascular Registry, improved long-term results were attributed to evacuation by helicopter within 3 hours of injury and to excellent surgical facilities staffed by surgeons experienced in vascular repair and vein grafting.[4,5] Experimental studies on the wounding capacity of missiles contributed significantly to the way in which these wounds were managed.[6]

Although wars on a global scale have not occurred during the second half of this century, civil wars and flashpoints of terrorism have been almost endemic. The endless toll of accidents on the road and at work inevitably means that complex vascular injuries will continue to occur. Violence has been a feature of life and the traditional use of knives and handguns has escalated in recent years to the use of automatic weapons and assault rifles, often by juveniles, and has matched the mounting traffic in illicit drugs and the accompanying culture of gangsterism. The glamorization of brutality and acts of inhumanity and the depiction in the media and films of gratuitous violence as a "normal" ingredient of human existence stimulate increasing debate on the harm done to the young mind. Freedom of expression and libertarian values must be tempered by the tenets of a universal sense of morality, and societies and governments have a duty to legislate against abuses.

In Northern Ireland indiscriminate assault by terrorists armed with sophisticated weapons, massive bombs, and incendiary devices has taken a toll of more than 3,500 dead and more than 37,000 injured; during a quarter of a century an estimated 1,500 injured vessels were treated in this province. A resilient people and those defending them have endured physical suffering and grief with unparalleled dignity and spirit, even as the fabric of their lives has been blighted by the systematic destruction of their homes and their places of work and leisure. Belfast's largest university hospital, the Royal Victoria, assumed the main responsibilities of a front-line evacuation center for casualties, often from major disasters. Vascular injuries caused by low- and high-velocity bullets, and shrapnel from bombs, mines, mortar shells, and rockets were treated.[7-11] Against this background of penetrating trauma, deceleration accidents on the roads and injuries sustained in industry and elsewhere accounted for complex vascular damage. Any dividends in management arising from experience the Royal Victoria remain a tribute to all these victims.[12-21]

ADJUNCTIVE INTRAVASCULAR SHUNTING

The concept of temporary or adjunctive intravascular shunting has been applied in the past to coronary artery perfusion and continues to be used by a majority of surgeons performing carotid endarterectomy and by some during operations for thoracic aortic aneurysm or injury.

The critical influence of the passage of time on the outcome of arterial repair is best illustrated in vascular injuries of the limbs and especially those of the lower limb. After a period of warm ischemia exceeding 6 hours, the incidence of amputation of the lower limb rises steeply.[22] A rich collateral network protects the upper extremity in proximal arterial injury, but it may not be helpful in brachial artery trauma, particularly in combat wounds that have damaged the deep brachial artery.

During World War I silver tubes were used by French[23] and British[1] surgeons, the first to conceive of the idea of employing some form of conduit to temporarily bridge an arterial gap to maintain distal flow. Glass tubes in limb injuries were employed in World War II by British and Canadian[24] as well as American[2] surgeons to maintain tissue perfusion with the objective of giving time for collateral flow to develop. In wartime when specialist vascular experience may not be available in forward positions, the placement of an intravascular shunt before transfer to a base hospital has obvious advantages. In 1971, a report from the Middle East described the use of a temporary polythene shunt in a small series of patients with peripheral artery injuries.[25]

For 18 years the Royal Victoria intravascular shunts have been used immediately on exploration not only to restore flow in the injured artery but, very importantly, in the vein as well[12-21] (Fig. 28–1). In high-energy penetrating and blunt trauma of the limb they have played a central role in the management of complex injuries, minimizing complications and limiting limb loss. These shunts arrest ischemia time, reduce the degree of reperfusion injury, and introduce a disciplined and logical sequence of operative steps (Fig. 28–2), which can be taken unhurriedly and diligently with greatly improved results. Intravascular shunts also have a place in the management of penetrating trauma of brachiocephalic arteries, intrathoracic and carotid in particular, and, more controversially, in the management of caval trauma.

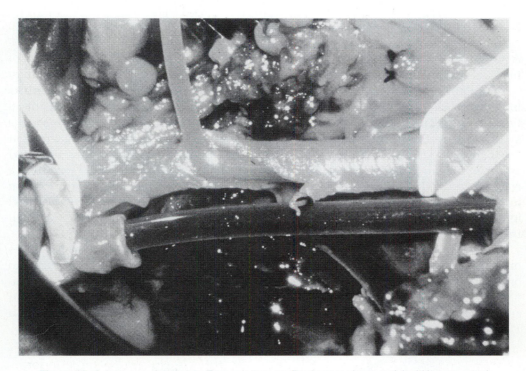

Figure 28–1. Intravascular shunts: Brener in torn popliteal artery above and Javid in transected popliteal vein below preparatory to vein graft replacement of each vessel. (*Reproduced with permission: Barros D'Sa AAB. How do we manage acute limb ischaemia due to trauma? In: Greenhalgh RM, Jamieson CW, Nicolaides AN, eds. Limb Salvage and Amputation for Vascular Disease. London: WB Saunders; 1988:143.*)

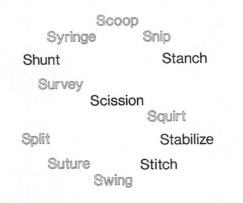

Figure 28–2. Aide-mémoire for the *Sequence* of *Steps* in the operative management of complex limb vascular injury: *stanch* the bleeding, *snip* damaged ends of vessels, *scoop* out clot, *syringe* in heparinized saline, *shunt* both artery and vein, *survey* the wound and identify nerve injury, perform *scission* of nonviable soft tissue, *squirt* saline to irrigate wound, *stabilize* fractured bones, *stitch* or repair both artery and vein, *swing* tissue for cover, *suture* the wound (delayed primary if contaminated), and, if necessary, *split* fasciae (fasciotomy). (*Reproduced with permission: Barros D'Sa AAB. Complex vascular and orthopaedic limb injuries. J Bone Joint Surg. 1992;74-B:178. Editorial.*)

MECHANISMS OF VASCULAR INJURY

A knife or low-velocity bullet damages a vessel lying in its path but a missile of high velocity, dissipating its energy at right angles to its trajectory, causes temporary "cavitation" approximately 30 to 40 times its cross-sectional area, a process that sucks in pieces of clothing, debris, and bacteria. These forces exceed the elastic limits of all tissues, displacing and tearing them far from the actual path of the bullet to produce a large exit wound; fragmented bones forming secondary missiles cause further soft tissue trauma (Fig. 28–3). An apparently benign exit wound conceals severely disrupted and contaminated tissues. Similarly, a shotgun discharged at close range produces a concentrated "spread" of damage, the depth of which is often underestimated on inspection. Shrapnel and secondary missiles from a bomb explosion cause widespread internal injuries. Following explosions or any major accident, falling masonry will frequently cause a crush syndrome and renal failure.

In road, rail, mining, and air disasters, sudden deceleration places avulsive forces on certain vessels, which are either relatively fixed or form the vascular pedicles to organs of substantial mass. The isthmus of the thoracic aorta, the origin of the innominate artery, less frequently the origins of the left subclavian and left common carotid arteries, the renal artery, especially on the left side, and the mesenteric vessels of a

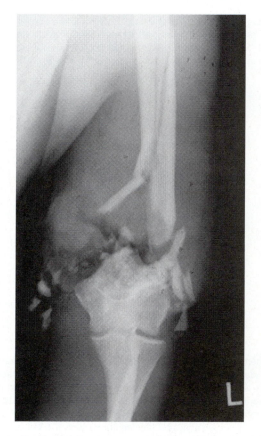

Figure 28–3. High-velocity missile injury: gross comminution of humerus, transection of brachial artery and ulnar nerve. (*Reproduced with permission: Barros D'Sa AAB. Arterial injuries. In: Eastcott HHG, ed. Arterial Surgery. London: Churchill Livingstone; 1992:358.*)

heavily loaded segment of bowel can all be injured indirectly. Direct trauma from a steering wheel may fracture the clavicle and upper ribs and in the process injure the subclavian artery. The immense shearing forces generated by sudden violent angulation and fracture of long bones can damage adjacent vessels, especially at points of relative fixity, or they may be injured directly by sharp bone fragments. A 10% to 40% incidence of vascular injury and correspondingly high amputation rates of 32% to 85% accompany these injuries.[26,27] In posterior dislocations of the knee, the tissues are stretched and torn, as are the layers of the artery, which beginning with the intima outward disrupt progressively; notoriously, a popliteal artery injury may remain unrecognized because the dislocated knee tends to reduce spontaneously. In severe and often contaminated limb injuries, classically in Type IIIc open fractures of the tibia, both arteries and veins may be damaged in association with comminuted fractures, periosteal stripping, and severe muscle and skin loss.[28] Injuries to two or more crural arteries, problems of bony union, and complications such as compartment syndrome and sepsis inevitably lead to high amputation rates.

PATHOPHYSIOLOGY OF VASCULAR INJURY

When the main artery to a limb has been transected, arrest of distal flow results in ischemia, tissue hypoperfusion, and hypoxia, further compromised by hypovolemic shock, rising afterload, and falling stroke volume. Cell membrane permeability increases, causing interstitial and some cellular edema. The vulnerability of striated muscle to continued warm ischemia beyond 6 to 8 hours, depending on the degree of injury and availability of collateral flow, leads to myonecrosis and to amputation in the majority of cases.

Paradoxically the restoration of flow causes ischemia-reperfusion injury (IRI), which represents an additional assault on cell membranes and is manifested by muscle edema, necrosis, and loss of function.[29,30] The extent of IRI is directly proportional to the duration of preceding ischemia and also has wider systemic implications for the lungs, liver, heart, and kidneys. The complex biochemical and cellular pathophysiology of IRI has been appreciated to a degree only during the last decade. The generation of oxygen-derived free radicals (ODFRs), activation of neutrophils, and the production of arachidonic metabolites are of central importance in mediating IRI.

Ischemia initiates a catabolic process in endothelial cells in which hypoxanthine is produced and energy losses and derangement of cell membrane ionic pumps are associated with increased cytosolic calcium concentration, which in turn activates proteases, bringing about the conversion of xanthine dehydrogenase to xanthine oxidase. With restoration of flow and reintroduction of molecular oxygen, xanthine oxidase acts on its substrate hypoxanthine, generating the superoxide (O_2^-), which is an ODFR.[29,30] Under the action of superoxide dismutase, this ODFR forms H_2O_2 with which it reacts further to form the toxic (^-OH) free radical.[31] This particular radical may also be released in a reaction between ODFRs and nitrous oxide (NO), otherwise known as the endothelial-derived relaxing factor or EDRF.[32] All these free radicals promote lipid peroxidation of reperfused muscle cell membranes, further raising their permeability with the formation of arachidonic acid and lipid peroxyl radicals.[32,33] These events induce chemoattraction of neutrophils and their activation releases ODFRs to cause more microvascular injury. Intimately involved in this destructive process is a sharp drop in cellular energy reserves, disruption of calcium homeostasis, and release of myoglobin, potassium, and hydrogen ion. Arachidonic acid is metabolized under the action of phospholipase

A_2, producing thromboxane A_2, prostaglandins, and leukotrienes, which are potent vasoactive eicosanoids[34] that strongly mediate in the pathophysiology of IRI.

These complex responses and interactions result in edema and raised interstitial pressure within the confines of inelastic fascial compartments, particularly if an injured vein is clamped or ligated, or if bone and soft tissues are also injured; exudation will raise compartment pressure to a level that may even obliterate the main arteries. The sequelae of compartment syndrome, microvascular stasis and thrombosis, aseptic muscle necrosis, ischemic nerve palsy, Volkmann's contracture, and amputation will follow unless timely and effective fasciotomy is undertaken.

The remote effects of IRI on the lungs, heart, brain, and bowel will also influence outcome. Pulmonary injury is manifested by raised microvascular permeability, neutrophil sequestration, and pulmonary hypertension.[35] Myocardial depression, hyperkalemic dysrhythmias, and even cardiac arrest may ensue. ODFRs generated by the endothelium of cerebral microvasculature are implicated in IRI,[36] bringing about cerebral vasodilatation, resistance to the vasoconstrictive effects of hypocapnia, and inactivation of EDRF. The effects of acute mesenteric ischemia following aortic or mesenteric arterial injury are especially evident in the gut mucosa where xanthine oxidase is freely available.[29,30] The gut mucosa is also firmly implicated in the consequences of lower limb ischemia reperfusion.[37] The injurious effect on gut mucosa produces bacterial translocation and a general release of cytokines, the remote effects of which may bring about multisystem organ failure and fatality.[38]

The adverse effects of IRI are aggravated by contamination by a wide spectrum of organisms including gram-positive cocci, gram-negative cocci, and bacilli, some of which may act synergistically to cause cellulitis or fasciitis, leaving an underlying repair open to breakdown and secondary hemorrhage. The anaerobic environment of ischemic tissue facilitates the regeneration of clostridial spores (*Clostridium welchii, C. novyii,* and *C. septicum*) to produce gas gangrene with its classical features of tense edema, crepitus, frothy brown watery exudate, brick-red necrotic muscle, toxemia, and cardiovascular collapse. Conditions that favor such an outcome are prolonged ischemia due to delayed exploration, lapses in the essentials of wound care in complex injuries, ligation rather than repair of vessels and unrelieved compartment hypertension. Fasciotomy incisions to relieve the effects of IRI are themselves open to superinfection, particularly by *Pseudomonas aeruginosa,* which heightens the possibility of amputation later.[39]

LIMB VASCULAR INJURY

The Importance of Time

In the multiply injured patient, life-threatening injuries of the head, chest, and abdomen receive deserved priority, while definitive repair of limb vascular injury is usually delayed, the duration of ischemia being pivotal to outcome. The tolerance to ischemia depends on the level of arterial injury, concomitant vein injury, the quality of collateral flow, the degree of hypotension, and the extent of associated soft tissue and bone injuries. The relentless effect of warm ischemia time on striated muscle and of IRI following renewed flow herald the onset of various complications including limb loss. To shorten the period of ischemia and to minimize IRI in complex limb vascular injuries, control of bleeding, resuscitation, and definitive surgery ought to be overlapping rather than sequential stages of management. Even then, a finite and sometimes unacceptable period of time is required for the exposure of injured artery and vein, wound care, stabilization of bone injuries, and the repair of artery and vein.

A heightened awareness of the importance of time and the understandable desire to proceed expeditiously may cause regrettable lapses in principles of operative technique. Wound care may be cursory, inviting septic complications and amputation. In this climate of urgency, an artery may be repaired before stabilizing a fracture, and that repair may fail because expedient techniques are used, namely, lateral suture causing stenosis, end-to-end anastomosis under tension, and interposition vein grafting of incorrect length. To save time, an essential main vein may be ligated, causing venous hypertension, which compounds IRI and compromises an adjacent arterial repair. The subsequent robust manipulations necessary to reduce the fracture may disrupt a delicate vascular repair. If, however, fixation of the fracture precedes vascular repair, damage to soft tissues and vessels by bone fragments is averted, and vein grafts of optimal length are used and will remain undisturbed. Nonetheless, the orthopedic surgeon, conscious of the dangers of extending ischemia time, may be hurried into a less than ideal and possibly technically imperfect fixation, which could compromise the vascular repair and perhaps lead to delayed union or nonunion.

Clearly, time plays a crucial and challenging role in these complex injuries and therefore must be used profitably. If intravascular shunts are placed in both artery and vein at the outset (Fig. 28–1), a considered and logical sequence of operative maneuvers can be adopted with no need to cast an anxious eye on the clock.[20] At this center the repair of an artery before bone fixation, or indeed the treatment of any complex injury in random fashion, is virtually obsolete. Instead, during the last 18 years, the implementation of a policy formulated around the early use of intravascular shunts to restore perfusion and drainage has fostered a harmonious and multidisciplinary approach, reduced the need for fasciotomy, lowered the incidence of complications such as sepsis, ischemic nerve palsy, and amputation, and facilitated early discharge.

Initial Exploration

Standard incisions are employed to approach and control injured vessels. Initial control of bleeding by digital pressure is followed by sharp and blunt dissection to expose a sufficient length of segment of artery and vein above and below the injured site before clamping. The injured artery is trimmed back to a point where the wall is intact. The upper clamp is released to allow thrombus to be washed out or removed by balloon catheter. When back bleeding is poor or absent, distal balloon exploration is usually productive, aided if necessary by vigorous upward milking of the limb to express propagated clot. Poor back bleeding in the younger patient may mean that collateral circulation is not well established, making arterial repair even more essential. The distal artery is best perfused with heparinized saline (20 U/mL) though systemic heparinization is acceptable in the absence of other injuries.

Shunting and Operative Discipline

An indwelling shunt that reconnects the ends of a transected femoral or popliteal artery immediately arrests ischemia, revitalizes the limb, and by minimizing IRI in proportion to the preceding period of ischemia, keeps compartment pressures within a safe range and significantly reduces the need for fasciotomy. Very importantly, it buys the necessary time for a precise approach to the rest of the operation. When lengthy segments of vessel are destroyed in extensive wounds, an outlying shunt will keep the distal limb alive[17] (Fig. 28–4). It is important to reestablish venous drainage and to discourage thrombosis, particularly when collateral veins also appear to be damaged, by placing a shunt in a severed vein. If the distal limb is perfused via an intact artery or an injured

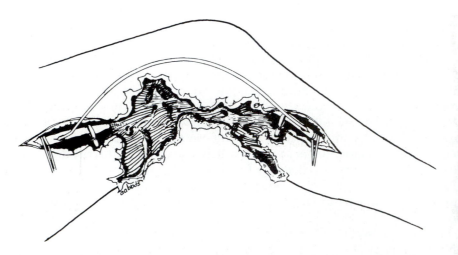

Figure 28–4. In extensive injury outlying shunt picks up flow proximal to the injured segment and revitalizes the limb distally. (*Reproduced with permission: Barros D'Sa AAB. Upper and lower limb vascular trauma. In: Greenhalgh RM, ed. Vascular Surgical Techniques. London: WB Saunders; 1989:54.*)

one that has been shunted, a clamped main vein will cause an acute and unacceptable rise in compartment pressure. When life-saving head or chest surgery is in progress in the multiply injured patient, and should circumstances allow, a vascular surgeon can unobtrusively expose and shunt injured vessels of the lower limb for later definitive repair.

If commercially available shunts are not on the shelf, an eminently acceptable alternative would be silicone elastomer or plastic tubing of suitable consistency, length, and caliber. A smooth-nosed atraumatic umbilical or similar catheter, the ends of which have been tailored to prevent intimal damage, works very well. Based on experience in Northern Ireland, the ideal design for a shunt specifically intended for use in vascular trauma was conceived,[14] stimulating experimental studies by armed forces medical establishments on a temporary shunt.[40] The side arm of a Brener shunt placed in an artery (Fig. 28–5) is a convenient portal for blood gas and other tests, injection of heparinized saline, and contrast for on-table angiography.[14] Placed in a vein, the side arm of a Brener shunt offers an outlet to flush out stagnant blood, which is of low pH and rich in potassium ion and products of reperfusion, which are harmful to the myocardium and other organs.[19,20]

Intravascular shunting allows the surgeon ample time to inspect the wound, identify nerve injury, remove debris, and irrigate the tissues. Reestablished circulation provides sharper demarcation between dead and viable tissue,[20] enabling precise debridement and better hemostasis, which is desirable in high-energy penetrating or blunt injuries. Dark muscle that does not bleed or contract is excised, and bone fragments, dirt, and other foreign bodies are removed, and the wound is copiously irrigated to lower the concentration of bacterial inoculum. Although scoring systems[41,42] are helpful in predicting outcome in the critically injured limb, temporary restoration of flow by thrombectomy and insertion of one or more intravascular shunts permits a more objective evaluation of the potential viability of distal tissues. These measures also help to dampen excessive zeal, which may be misdirected in attempting to salvage a mutilated and irreparable limb; this scenario commits both surgeon and patient to a protracted

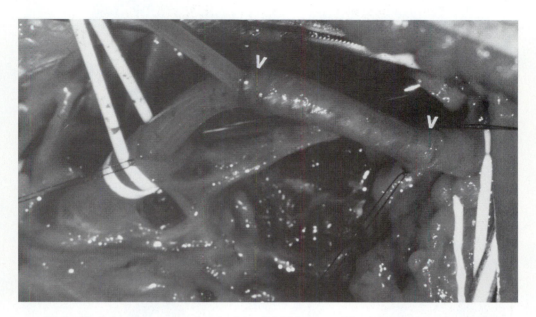

Figure 28–5. An interposed reversed vein graft (VV) borne on intravascular Brener shunt (with side arm) bridging popliteal artery. Two anchoring sutures inserted at commencement of distal anastomosis. In the background intravascular Javid shunt bridging adjacent vein.

series of injudicious operations, inviting complications of sepsis, secondary hemorrhage, poor rehabilitation, and in the longer term amputation of an insensate appendage.

Agreed incisional approaches between vascular and orthopedic surgeon and adherence to a clear sequence of steps (Fig. 28–2) has allowed each specialist to work unhindered.[20] The restoration of skeletal integrity, either by internal or external fixation of the realigned limb, prepares the way for definitive vascular repair. Long intravascular shunts of the Javid type leave sufficient slack for bone reduction[14] (Fig. 28–6A). Those who advocate vascular repair before ensuring skeletal stability cannot reasonably dispute the view that to establish bone fixation first is sound practice, permitting optimal repair of both artery and vein, secure in the knowledge that they will not be disrupted (Fig. 28–6B).

Arterial Repair

When an artery and vein are concomitantly injured, shunting of each vessel dispels debate as to the order of their repair. While the type of arterial repair depends on the circumstances of each case, intravascular shunts encourage optimal choices. For example, lateral suture, which can cause stenosis and thrombosis of critical vessels such as the brachial and popliteal, thereby endangering an extremity, is avoided. Such an outcome may also result from direct end-to-end anastomosis carried out under tension, possibly even after division of useful collaterals. The general availability of good-quality donor vein and the presence of shunts gives the surgeon all the time needed to excise an injured artery adequately, leaving pristine ends for vein graft reconstruction. The upper long saphenous vein, preferably from the contralateral limb, and indeed absolutely if the deep vein is injured, is usually of adequate caliber for most interposition grafts.

In larger vessels, the shunt serves conveniently as a stent so that a continuous suture commenced at diametrically opposite points does not cause purse-stringing at

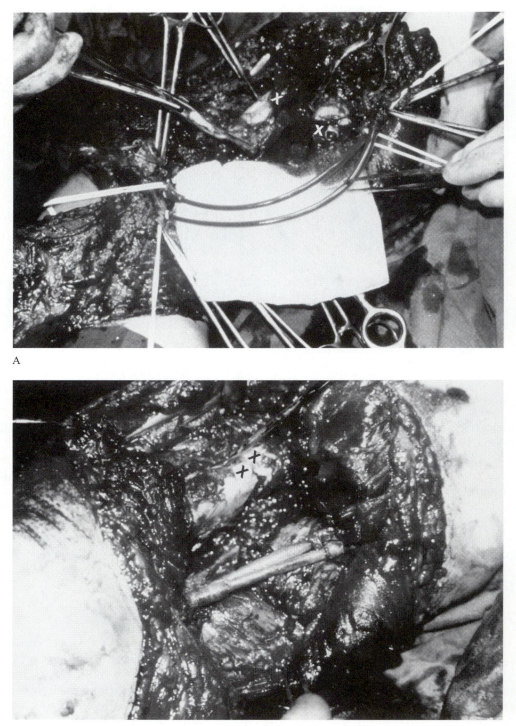

A

B

Figure 28–6. (A) A virtually dismembered leg at midthigh: Javid shunt bridging lengthy gap in femoral artery and perfusing distal limb; another such shunt bridging adjoining femoral vein and draining the limb. Ends of a fractured femur (XX) being manipulated prior to fixation. **(B)** After stabilization of fracture (XX) three interposed vein grafts restore flow through femoral artery and vein and the deep femoral vein. (*Reproduced with permission: Barros D'Sa AAB, Moorehead RJ. Combined arterial and venous intraluminal shunting in major trauma of the lower limb. Eur J Vasc Surg. 1989;3:579.*)

the anastomoses. In vessels of less than 3 mm in diameter, accurate coaptation of obliquely cut and spatulated ends over a soft silastic shunt prevents adventitial intrusion and allows eversion of intimal surfaces for placement of fine interrupted sutures that will retain vessel diameter. Shunts are not required by surgeons with impeccable technique, but if they are used, great care is required during insertion and removal. The precept of ensuring a satisfactory cross-sectional area of lumen at the anastomosis is important, particularly in a child's limb, the future growth and development of which are dependent on good flow.

When outlying shunts are used to restore flow in severe injuries involving lengthy, and especially atherosclerotic, arterial segments, an extra-anatomic vein bypass graft, if necessary unreversed, with its valves disrupted, may be tunneled through clean tissues to reestablish distal flow[17] (Fig. 28–7).

Blood flow is a rigorous taskmaster that punishes disruption of laminar flow following repair by causing thrombotic failure. This is likely if the caliber of a vein graft is much smaller than that of the host artery. Intravascular shunts remove constraints of time so that a compound vein graft of larger diameter and with good prospects of long-term patency can be fashioned.[16–19] In one well-tried technique, two and, if neces-

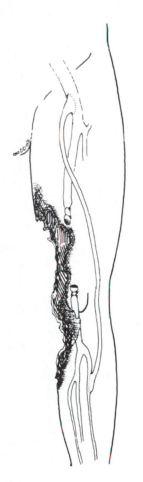

Figure 28–7. Extra-anatomic vein bypass for extensive contaminated wound. (*Reproduced with permission: Barros D'Sa AAB. Upper and lower limb vascular trauma. In: Greenhalgh RM, ed. Vascular Surgical Techniques. London: WB Saunders; 1989:59.*)

sary, three equal segments of vein of suitable length are opened longitudinally to form panels and after excising any valves are sewn together side by side to create a panel compound vein graft (Fig. 28–8). This graft can either be constructed over a shunted vessel or slipped over the shunt after it has been put together on the bench. Alternatively, a longitudinally slit length of vein, bereft of valves, is wound spirally over a bridging shunt of a bore matching the host artery; the adjoining margins of artery and vein are then sutured to produce a spiral compound graft[17] (Fig. 28–9).

Polytetrafluoroethylene (PTFE) may be safe and effective in closed vascular injuries and those caused by knives and low-velocity missiles, particularly if vessel cover for a vein is unreliable. In wounds caused by bomb explosions, however, the potential risk of infection, including secondary hemorrhage and amputation, should not be obscured lest it lead to complacency. While a vein graft is liable to break down under the action of bacterial collagenase,[43,44] a prosthetic graft remains immune, but it should be recognized that necrosis can still occur at the point of anastomosis of the prosthesis with the host vessel.

Vein Repair

The early objectives of vein repair, as opposed to ligation, are arrest of bleeding, preservation of flow, and enhancement of patency of an adjacent arterial repair. Other

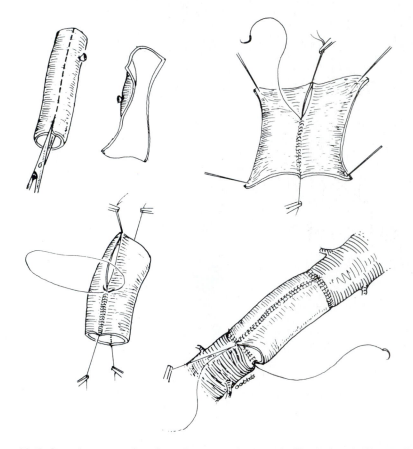

Figure 28–8. Steps in construction of panel compound vein graft. (*Reproduced with permission: Barros D'Sa AAB. Upper and lower limb vascular trauma. In: Greenhalgh RM, ed. Vascular Surgical Techniques. London: WB Saunders; 1989:59.*)

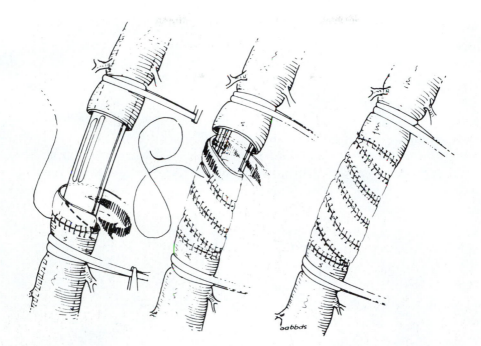

Figure 28–9. Steps in construction of a spiral compound vein graft. (*Reproduced with permission: Barros D'Sa AAB. Upper and lower limb vascular trauma. In: Greenhalgh RM, ed. Vascular Surgical Techniques. London: WB Saunders; 1989:60.*)

secondary aims are prevention of thromboembolism, chronic edema, venous insufficiency, and the small chance of venous gangrene and amputation. Vein ligation is reasonable in life-endangering situations but this view should not give succor to the apologists of vein ligation who claim, often on very little basis, that vein repair is usually followed by thrombosis, that venous collaterals are adequate for limb survival, or indeed that ligation is not necessarily harmful. While a limb vein is of larger caliber and tolerates lateral suture better than the adjacent artery, it is less tolerant of an interposition vein graft of smaller diameter. Shunting of the vein buys time for the creation of an arteriovenous fistula, which might enhance the long-term patency of a graft and, better still, for reconstruction using a panel compound vein graft (Fig. 28–10). If time allows, a large ligated vein can be shunted and repaired in this manner, successfully reversing venous hypertension.

Fasciotomy

The insertion of intravascular shunts in an artery to arrest ischemia and in a vein to restore drainage, will limit the extent and degree of IRI and its consequences, significantly decreasing the need for fasciotomy. The benefits of mannitol, once ascribed almost entirely to its osmotic properties, are now recognized to be largely due to the accelerated inactivation of ODFRs[45,46]; a slow infusion over a 12- to 24-hour period is worthwhile. In the upper limb the muscle compartments of the lower forearm and palm, and in the lower leg the anterior compartment that lies within rigid osseous and fascial boundaries, are especially vulnerable to increased pressure. The traditional indications for fasciotomy can often be ignored when shunts are employed. Simultaneous artery and vein injury or delay in completing vascular repair cease to be of concern when both vessels are routinely shunted. Obviously, fasciotomy will still be required

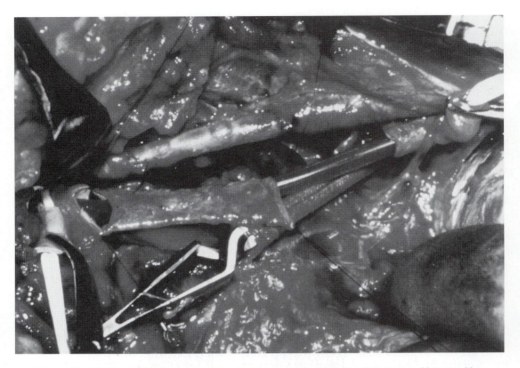

Figure 28–10. Popliteal artery above (previously shunted) repaired using reversed interposition vein graft. Popliteal vein below being repaired by panel compound vein graft. (*Reprinted with permission: Barros D'Sa AAB. Vascular injuries of the limb. In: Chant ADB, Barros D'Sa AAB, eds. Emergency Vascular Practice. London: Arnold; 1996.*)

when there is significant soft tissue injury with muscle edema, patchy muscle necrosis, and compartment hypertension.

Wound Closure

The practice of arterial and venous shunting at the first operation has enabled better wound care and has given the surgeon some assurance about the quality and viability of residual tissue for vessel cover. It has also reduced the need to swing over local muscles to ensheath a graft, but the skills of a plastic surgeon in constructing free vascularized flaps are still required (Fig. 28–6B).

Postoperative Care

Experience with contaminated wounds over 25 years has confirmed the value of delayed primary suture no earlier than 5 to 7 days. Good care of the wound at the outset, best undertaken without haste and ideally achieved when shunts are in place, has reduced the number of subsequent anaesthetics for reinspection or secondary debridement of necrotic and septic foci.

Close vigilance of pulses, capillary refill time, and Doppler pressures and pulse waveforms will register a drop in distal flow. Thrombotic occlusion of a vessel repair usually reflects the use of less than optimal methods of reconstruction constrained by the exigencies of time. An intravascular shunt permits generous excision of a damaged vessel, enables the liberal use of vein graft of appropriate caliber, and as a stent it encourages good suture technique. The incidence of reexploration and revision of grafts fell sharply after the introduction of a policy of routine shunting.

EXTRACRANIAL CEREBROVASCULAR INJURIES

The majority of those who sustain injuries of brachiocephalic arteries in the chest and neck succumb to exsanguination and the sequelae of associated organ injury. The few who survive do so only when evacuation time to hospital is brief and if operation is immediately undertaken for control and definitive reconstruction. Neurologic impairment due to arrested flow and aggravated by hypovolemia is minimized and possibly reversed by the early insertion of intravascular shunts.

Most of these patients require emergency surgery without the luxury of angiography or enhanced spiral computed tomography (CT) scans. A median sternotomy offers a swift approach to the great vessels and other mediastinal structures. Haemorrhage at the origin of the great vessels is controlled by a partially occluding C clamp or by cross-clamping of the innominate and left common carotid arteries. Standard cervical incisions are employed to gain access to the carotid arteries, the first and second parts of the vertebral arteries, and the subclavian vessels. Intravascular shunts will maintain maximal cerebral perfusion in the hypotensive patient and limit the equivalent of cerebral IRI.[36] Shunts are not necessary routinely but it is wiser to use at least one shunt when the innominate and left common carotid artery are simultaneously injured. Because ligation of these vessels can cause fatal cerebral ischemia, it seems logical to assume that clamping is also unacceptable, ergo, flow should be maintained until reconstruction is complete. The ends of these great vessels tend to retract and a prosthetic graft is generally necessary. Alternatively, the stem of a bifurcated graft is sutured to a fresh aortotomy on the ascending aorta and the limbs anastomosed to the distal innominate and left common carotid arteries. Postoperatively, a case may be made for mannitol infusion to prevent cerebral edema and to limit IRI.

The overwhelming majority of carotid artery injuries are penetrating and in the absence of a closed head injury must be held responsible for a neurologic deficit, especially if the patient is fully conscious. The duration, extent, and progression of the deficit are of importance in their management. If cerebral ischemia is already present, maintenance of good respiratory function will influence outcome. Coexisting carotid and laryngotracheal injury demands immediate endotracheal intubation and inflation of the cuff to protect the airway. Volume replacement and restoration of cerebral perfusion are essential.

Surgical intervention is imperative in cases of hemorrhage, neurologic deficit, or injury to the adjacent aerodigestive structures. In the case of developing neurologic deficit, exploration must not be deferred until a CT brain scan becomes positive because by then it will be too late. In the hemodynamically and neurologically stable patient, a more selective approach has been recommended to reduce the incidence of negative explorations.[47] In these patients, angiography sharpens the selective process in zone I injuries at the root of the neck and in zone III injuries above the angle of the mandible. In zone II injuries at the carotid bifurcation, angiography can be helpful but is not essential and certainly at this center most of these are explored straight away.

The view that ligation is preferable to repair to avert mortality when neurologic signs are present has fortunately been superceded by evidence that early vascular repair gives better results. In cases of fixed neurologic deficit and absence of retrograde flow from the distal internal carotid artery, vascular repair may result in fatality. If back flow is absent, a balloon catheter is carefully advanced to remove clot. If back flow, preferably pulsatile and at a pressure of 60 to 70 mm Hg, is restored, cerebral perfusion is probably satisfactory.[48] After flushing the proximal artery, a shunt bearing a vein graft is inserted, facilitating precise suture technique while cerebral perfusion continues to be maintained.

ABDOMINAL VASCULAR INJURIES

Very few of those who sustain major abdominal vascular injury survive to be admitted, partly due to associated trauma to organs in the abdomen and chest. Suprarenal truncal injuries, because of their relative inaccessibility for control, carry a higher mortality rate. Immediate operative control is an essential component of resuscitation. Cross-clamping of the abdominal aorta and mesenteric arteries for a time is admissible if collateral flow is adequate. This does not hold true for renal artery injury because kidneys have a low tolerance of warm ischemia.

Injuries of the inferior vena cava result in rapidly exsanguinating losses. The caval system is devoid of valves and receives the entire flow from the systemic circulation below the diaphragm, from the portal venous system and from the liver itself. The application of cross-clamps has the effect of denying venous return to the right heart and in the shocked hypotensive patient can lead to terminal arrest. A shunt of suitable caliber positioned by snugged tapes eliminates this concern. It is sometimes advocated that a segment of infrarenal cava should be removed to reconstruct an injured suprarenal segment of cava but that seems an unnecessarily destructive solution. Instead, a spiral compound graft can be constructed over the shunt, which also serves as a stent (Fig. 28–9).

Access to the retrohepatic cava is tricky enough in the midst of torrential bleeding, often from the liver itself, and is not greatly diminished by Pringle's maneuver. Packs and pressure are used to reduce bleeding while the coronary and triangular ligaments are divided to allow the liver to be mobilized forward and downward to expose the upper part of the retrohepatic cava.

A variety of elegant techniques have been described to isolate the hepatic bed while maintaining venous return, but the concept of atriocaval shunting makes the most sense. An Argyle chest drain, inserted through a purse-stringed opening in the right atrial appendage that has been exposed through a median sternotomy, is guided into the inferior vena cava to the level of the renal veins; bleeding from the snugged and isolated section of injured cava is controlled while venous return continues unhindered. The upper end of this shunt, clamped outside the atrium, could also be used as a portal for direct infusion as long as special care is taken to exclude the risk of air embolism. A further device inserted transfemorally and advanced and positioned within the retrohepatic cava by inflating occluding balloons also incorporates a channel for venous return. A recent successful technique has been the use of a venovenous femoroaxillary bypass using an extracorporeal pump, which allows the cava to be clamped.[49] Given the urgency with which these measures have to be implemented in casualties sustaining shrapnel and gunshot wounds, their success at this center must be regarded as no more than modest.

REFERENCES

1. Makins GH. Injuries to the blood vesels. In: *Official History of the Great War Medical Services. Surgery of the War.* Vol 2. London: HMSO; 1922:170–296.

2. De Bakey ME, Simeone FA. Battle injuries of the arteries in World War II. *Ann Surg.* 1946;123:534–579.

3. Hughes CW. Arterial repair during the Korean War. *Ann Surg.* 1958;147:555–561.

4. Rich NM, Hughes CW. Vietnam vascular registry: preliminary report. *Surgery.* 1969;65: 218–226.

5. Rich NM, Baugh JH, Hughes CW. Acute arterial injuries in Viet Nam: 1000 cases. *J Trauma.* 1970;10:359–369.

6. De Muth WE. Bullet velocity makes the difference. *J Trauma.* 1969;9:642–643.

7. Livingston RH, Wilson RI. Gunshot wounds of the limbs. *Br Med J.* 1975;1:667–669.

8. Barros D'Sa AAB, Hassard TH, Livingston RH, et al. Missile-induced vascular trauma. *Injury.* 1980;12:13–30.

9. Barros D'Sa AAB. Management of vascular injuries of civil strife. *Injury.* 1982;14:51–57.

10. Johnston GW, Barros D'Sa AAB. Injuries of civil hostilities. In: Carter DC, Polk HC, eds. *International Medical Reviews. Surgery, Vol. 1 Trauma.* London: Butterworths; 1981.

11. Graham ANJ, Barros D'Sa AAB. Missed arteriovenous fistulae and false aneurysms in penetrating lower limb trauma: relearning old lessons. *Injury.* 1991;22:179–182.

12. Barros D'Sa AAB. A decade of missile-induced vascular trauma. *Ann R Coll Surg Engl.* 1981;64:37–44.

13. Barros D'Sa AAB. How do we manage acute limb ischaemia due to trauma? In: Greenhalgh RM, Jamieson CW, Nicolaides AN, eds. *Limb Salvage and Amputation for Vascular Disease.* London: WB Saunders; 1988;Chp 13:135–150.

14. Barros D'Sa AAB. The rationale for arterial and venous shunting in the management of limb vascular injuries. *Eur J Vasc Surg.* 1989;3:471–474.

15. Barros D'Sa AAB, Moorehead RJ. Combined arterial and venous intraluminal shunting in major trauma of the lower limb. *Eur J Vasc Surg.* 1989;3:577–581.

16. Elliott J, Templeton J, Barros D'Sa AAB. Combined bony and vascular limb trauma: a new approach to treatment. *J Bone Joint Surg.* 1984;66-B:281.

17. Barros D'Sa AAB. Upper and lower limb vascular trauma. In: Greenhalgh RM, ed. *Vascular Surgical Techniques.* London: Balliere Tindall; 1989:47–65.

18. Barros D'Sa AAB. Arterial injuries. In: Eastcott HHG, ed. *Arterial Surgery.* London: Churchill Livingstone; 1992:355–411.

19. Barros D'Sa AAB. Shunting in complex lower limb trauma. In: Greenhalgh RM, Hollier L, eds. *Emergency Vascular Surgery.* London: WB Saunders; 1992;Chap 27:331–344.

20. Barros D'Sa AAB. Complex vascular and orthopaedic limb injuries. *J Bone Joint Surg (Br).* 1992;74:176–178. Editorial.

21. Barros D'Sa AAB. Twenty-five years of vascular trauma in Northern Ireland. *Br Med J.* 1995;310;1–2.

22. Miller HH, Welch CS. Quantitative studies on the time factor in arterial injuries. *Ann Surg.* 1949;130:428–438.

23. Tuffer P. French surgery in 1915. *Br J Surg.* 1917;4:420–432.

24. Matheson NM, Murray G. Recent advances and experimental work in conservative vascular surgery. In: Hamilton-Bailey, ed. *Surgery of Modern Warfare.* Vol 1. Baltimore, MD: Williams and Wilkins; 1941:324–327.

25. Eger M, Goleman L, Goldstein A, et al. The use of a temporary shunt in the management of arterial vascular injuries. *Surg Gynecol Obstet.* 1971;132:67–70.

26. Lefrak BA. Knee dislocation. *Arch Surg.* 1976;111:1021–1024.

27. Alberty RE, Goodfried G, Boyden AM. Popliteal artery injury with fracture dislocation of the knee. *Am J Surg.* 1981;142:36–40.

28. Gustilo RB, Mendoza RM, Williams DN. Problems in the management of Type III (severe) open fractures: a new classification of Type III open fractures. *J Trauma.* 1984;24:742–746.

29. McCord JM. Oxygen-derived free radicals in post-ischaemic tissue injury. *N Engl J Med.* 1985;312:159–163.

30. Granger DN, Hollwarth ME, Parks DA. Ischaemia-reperfusion injury: role of oxygen-derived free radicals. *Acta Physiol Scand.* 1986;54B(suppl 1):47–63.

31. Halliwell B, Gutteridge SMC. Oxygen toxicity, oxygen radicals, transition medals and disease. *Biochem J.* 1984;219:1.

32. Beckman JS, Beckman TW, Chen J, et al. Apparent hydroxyl radical production by peroxynitrite: implications for endothelial injury from nitric oxide and superoxide. *Proc Natl Acad Sci USA.* 1990;87:1620–1624.
33. Ernester L. Biochemistry of reoxygenation injury. *Crit Care Med.* 1988;16:947–953.
34. Meerson FZ, Kagan VE, Kozhor YP, et al. The role of lipid peroxidation in the pathogenesis of ischaemic damage and the antioxidant protection of the heart. *Basic Res Cardiol.* 1982;77:465–485.
35. Anner H, Kaufman RP, Vateri CR, et al. Reperfusion of ischaemic lower limbs increases pulmonary microvascular permeability. *J Trauma.* 1988;28:607–610.
36. Armstead WM, Mirro R, Bursija DW, Leffler CW. Postischaemic generation of superoxide anion by newborn pig brain. *Am J Physiol.* 1988;255:H401–H403.
37. Yassin MMI, Barros D'Sa AAB, Parks TG, et al. Lower limb ischaemia-reperfusion alters gastrointestinal structure and function. *Br J Surg.* 1996 (in press).
38. Carrico CJ, Meakins JL, Marshall JC, et al. Multiple organ failure syndrome. *Arch Surg.* 1986;121:196–208.
39. Drapanas T, Hewitt RL, Weichert RC, et al. Civilian vascular injuries, a critical appraisal of three decades of management. *Ann Surg.* 1970;172:351–360.
40. Walker AJ, Mellor SG, Cooper GJ. Experimental experience with a temporary intraluminal heparin-bonded polyurethane arterial shunt. *Br J Surg.* 1994;81:195–198.
41. Gregory RT, Gould RJ, Peclet M, et al. The mangled extremity syndrome (MES): a severity grading system for multisystem injury of the extremity. *J Trauma.* 1985;25:1147–1150.
42. Johansen K, Daines M, Howey T, et al. Objective criteria accurately predict amputation following lower extremity trauma. *J Trauma.* 1990;30:568–573.
43. Shah DM, Leather RP. Polytetrafluoroethylene grafts in the rapid reconstruction of acute contaminated peripheral vascular injuries. *Am J Surg.* 1984;148:229–233.
44. Feliciano DV. Use of prosthetic vascular grafts in civilian vascular trauma. In: Flanagan DP, ed. *Civilian Vascular Trauma.* Philadelphia: Lee and Febiger; 1992:36–43.
45. Buchbinder D, Karmody AM, Leather RP, Shah DM. Hypertonic mannitol. Its use in the prevention of revascularization syndrome after acute arterial ischaemia. *Arch Surg.* 1981;116:414–421.
46. Shah DM, Naraynsingh V, Leather RP, et al. Advances in the management of acute popliteal vascular blunt injuries. *J Trauma.* 1985;25:793–797.
47. Casbares HV. Selective surgical management of penetrating neck trauma: 15 year experience in a community hospital. *Am J Surg.* 1982;48:355–358.
48. Ehrenfeld WK, Stoney RJ, Wylie EJ. Relation of carotid stump pressure to safety of carotid artery ligation. *Surgery.* 1983;93:299.
49. Baumgartner F, Scudamore C, Nair C, et al. Venovenous bypass for major hepatic and caval trauma. *J Trauma.* 1995;39:671–673.

VIII

Reoperative
Surgery

29

Reoperation for *In Situ* Bypass

Benjamin B. Chang, MD, Robert P. Leather, MD,
R. Clement Darling III, MD, Philip S. K. Paty, MD,
and Dhiraj M. Shah, MD

The use of the *in situ* bypass for infrapopliteal arterial reconstruction has become standard practice for many vascular surgeons. After earlier pioneering efforts by Rob and Hall, the *in situ* technique was largely abandoned in favor of reversed-vein techniques.[1,2] Later work in the 1970s led to the development of a reliable, clinically practical, and reproducible technique that produced excellent patency results.[3,4] These results were most impressive with bypasses to infrapopliteal arteries and with smaller veins; reproduction of these results by several other groups led to the widespread adoption of the *in situ* technique as a standard method of vein preparation by many surgeons.[5–7]

The proliferation of the *in situ* concept has led to the development of several types of instrumentation for rendering the valves incompetent. Unfortunately, unlike human beings, valvulotomes are not all created equal. The modified Mills valvulotome[8] remains the single safest and, in many ways, simplest tool for rendering the valves incompetent by valve incision with the least potential for vein injury. Use of this instrument, however, requires an incision along the entire length of the bypass ("open technique"); this is not only time consuming, but also produces a surgical wound that carries with it the potential for infection, breakdown, and necrosis.

The use of the intraluminal cutter as described by Leather et al.[9] allows the operator to incise the valves within the saphenous vein in the thigh without a continuous incision ("closed technique"). While potentially saving time and avoiding complications, this instrument is used blindly and requires the operator to be familiar with a myriad of potential technical issues and pitfalls. Others have developed similar instruments,[10–12] but these generally carry limitations, such as introduction via distal divided end of the greater saphenous vein, that make their use potentially hazardous, especially with smaller diameter veins (<4.0 mm) reflected in a 30-day failure rate of 20%.[13]

In an effort to visualize the valve incision process, others have employed the angioscope in conjunction with a valvulotome.[14] Although theoretically attractive, the use of the angioscope certainly requires more time, has the potential for vein injury by the angioscope itself, and may not actually improve results over conventional techniques; this technique will require further analysis in the future.

PERIOPERATIVE COMPLICATIONS

Early Postoperative Bleeding

Bleeding in the immediate postoperative period usually comes from unsecured vein branches. To avoid this problem, smaller branches are suture ligated with 5-0 or 6-0 monofilament suture. Larger branches are ligated with larger suture (3-0), which is usually reinforced with a hemoclip. In no case is a branch secured with only a hemoclip, because these may slip off under arterial pressure.

Anastomotic bleeding may sometimes be produced if the vein is anastomosed under tension; this may not be apparent until the hip or knee is extended. Prevention requires the operator to leave sufficient length of vein to accommodate joint extension.

The vein preparation, the subsequent arterialization of the saphenous vein, and the construction of the distal anastomosis require only minimal systemic heparinization (i.e., approximately 30 mg/kg or 2,000 to 3,000 units intravenously); thus, bleeding caused by excessive heparin (5,000 to 10,000 units) is avoided. In addition, the necessity for reversal by the administration of protamine, which in itself may be productive of significant complications, is unnecessary.

Residual Fistulas

A complication unique to the *in situ* technique is the creation of arteriovenous fistulas. Although some investigators have attributed bypass failure to such fistulas, this is rarely, if ever, the case.[15] Instead, most residual fistulas will spontaneously thrombose over the first postoperative year.[16] Thrombosis of a fistula may sometimes produce an area of superficial phlebitis but this is usually self-limited and requires only symptomatic treatment. Central necrosis of the phlebitic area has been reported, but has been seen only twice in more than 2,000 cases in our series.[17]

Approximately 1% of the time, fistula flow may significantly decrease distal arterial perfusion. At worst, there may even be reversal of flow at the distal anastomosis. Clinical evidence of poor limb perfusion may be confirmed with pulse volume recordings and segmental pressures. Duplex ultrasound may then be used to confirm the diagnosis as well as localize the offending fistula(s). These fistulas may be ligated under local anesthesia with intravenous sedation.

In less than 5% of cases, fistula flow after discharge may produce or aggravate postrevascularization edema. Duplex scanning may be used to localize the fistulas and assess the relative amount of flow going out the fistulas. If more than 200 to 300 mL/min of fistula flow occurs along with significant unresolving edema of the limb, outpatient ligation under local anesthesia may be performed.

Wound Infection and Breakdown

Significant wound complications may be seen in 2% of *in situ* bypasses. Prevention, as with most complications, is more effective than treatment. Skin incisions are performed sharply and lymphatics are either preserved or ligated. Liberal use of perioperative antibiotics will help decrease postoperative wound infection. Incisions are placed such that the vein does not directly underlie the incision; conversely, skin flaps should be kept at a minimum to prevent devascularization. Proper incision placement is greatly facilitated with the use of preoperative duplex vein mapping.

Incision placement is especially critical when performing an *in situ* bypass to the dorsalis pedis artery. This usually produces two parallel incisions, one overlying the artery and the other the former bed of the distal vein. The incision for exposure of the dorsalis pedis artery should be placed 3 to 5 mm lateral to its axis and should be as short as possible to limit the length of this bipedicle flap. In addition this type of incision will keep it as wide based as possible and the distal anastomosis will be covered by the flap. Care should be taken not to undermine the skin between these two incisions. Both incisions should be closed with suture because this produces less skin tension across the incisions than staples. The incision adjacent to distal anastomosis should be closed first; if the other incision cannot be closed without producing tension on the flap, it should be left open and the defect covered with a meshed split-thickness skin graft.

Patients should be cautioned to elevate their operated limb when they are not actually walking, at least until the incisions are completely healed. Postrevascularization edema left unchecked not only increases tension across the skin closure but also causes the leakage of fluid through the wound, predisposing to wound infection and necrosis.

Minor degrees of wound cellulitis may be managed with oral antibiotics; actual purulence may necessitate admission for leg elevation, intravenous antibiotics, and local care of the incision.

Flap necrosis may be managed differently depending on the location of the bypass relative to the necrosis. If the affected area is superficial and there is still viable tissue overlying the bypass, home treatment with dressings and periodic office debridement is usually sufficient. If the necrotic area is in direct contact with the bypass, operative debridement of the necrotic area followed by immediate skin grafting will prevent bypass hemorrhage from infection. When possible, as in the calf, the bypass may be mobilized and covered with gastrocnemius or soleus to gain coverage. Actual pedicled flap coverage is rarely necessary and is best done in conjunction with plastic surgery assistance.

LATE POSTOPERATIVE COMPLICATIONS

Most late postoperative complications involve the development of a stenosis of the arterial tree of the affected limb, sometimes with actual bypass thrombosis. These complications include the development of proximal and distal arterial lesions presumably due to progression of atherosclerosis and to the development of bypass stenoses, usually as a sequela of injury to the vein at the time of the original operation ("neointimal hyperplasia") or much more infrequently, due to the development of atheromatous-type lesions in the bypass.

Surveillance

The concept of bypass surveillance has gained considerable support during the past decade.[18,19] Conceptually, detection of stenoses in bypasses prior to actual occlusion allows for elective correction of easily treated lesions. This is especially important in view of data that suggests that graft thrombosis followed by either surgical thrombectomy or catheter-delivered thrombolytic therapy is associated with very poor long-term patency. Conversely, correction of prestenotic lesions is associated with long-term patency rivaling that of nonrevised patent bypasses. With current surveillance programs, a 15% increase in patency rates (secondary) may be obtained.[20]

Our current surveillance program consists of physical examination, segmental pressures, pulse volume recordings, and, if indicated, duplex ultrasound of the entire bypass. These examinations are performed within the first 30 days postoperatively, followed by repeat examination every 3 months for the first year and every 6 months thereafter. Bypasses believed subjectively to be at greater risk due to small vein size, poor vein quality, poor outflow, or any other factors may be reviewed more frequently. In any case, the highest frequency of bypass stenosis occurs within the first year postoperatively, and surveillance programs should be designed with this in mind.

Progression of Inflow Disease

The development of stenosis cephalad to the proximal *in situ* anastomosis is most often due to the progression of atherosclerotic lesions. These may often be difficult to localize only with duplex examination and often require contrast arteriography for preoperative localization. Less frequently, narrow stenoses developing immediately proximal to the upper anastomosis may be related to overly aggressive clamping during the original procedure. Interestingly, *in situ* bypasses are remarkably resistant to thrombosis in the face of inflow occlusion.

Treatment of inflow lesions may be performed in the usual manner with bypass or endarterectomy. No special precautions need be taken with regards to the *in situ* bypass. To avoid previous dissection around the common femoral artery, use of the proximal *in situ* bypass as the distal anastomotic site is probably acceptable although not necessarily preferred.

Perianastomotic Stricture

Stenoses can often occur in and around either the proximal or distal anastomosis. If the stenosis involves primarily the vein, the etiology is probably related to vein injury at the time of preparation. During the original procedure, sufficient vein should be mobilized at either end to allow for debridement of the ends, which are, by the necessity of the valve incision technique, the most handled and therefore the most likely to sustain injury. Although the pathogenesis of neointimal hyperplasia has been the subject of innumerable studies, it is clear that vein injury is an important inciting factor. The anastomoses should be constructed with a "no-touch" technique: No instrument should touch the inside of the vein or artery. Circumferential injury, such as that induced by the introduction of dilators or sounds, is especially onerous.

Detection of such lesions can usually be accomplished with duplex ultrasonography, although some anastomoses are too deep for accurate imaging. Contrast arteriography is therefore sometimes necessary for diagnosis as well as operative planning.

The treatment of these lesions remains largely surgical, because the fibroproliferative nature of these lesions tends to simply stretch and contract when balloon angioplasty is attempted. Most investigators have found less reliable results with balloon angioplasty compared with surgical correction, but not uniformly so.[20] The use of stents in this situation is not well studied and should be regarded as experimental at this time.

Operative correction of perianastomotic strictures may be generally accomplished with two principal techniques: the jump bypass and direct vein angioplasty. We generally regard the use of a short segment of vein, when available, to jump between the preexisting bypass and the neighboring artery. This allows the surgeon to avoid the scarring around the anastomosis itself and to suture into undiseased vessels.

Alternatively, a diamond-shaped patch may be constructed at the anastomosis across the stenosis; this requires careful dissection of the anastomosis, not always a simple proposition, especially in a deep distal anastomosis. Patching does, however, carry the benefit of requiring only a very short vein segment for completion.

Midgraft Stenoses

If the ends of the vein are properly prepared and debrided at the time of the original operation, stenoses can still occur along the length of the bypass. These should occur relatively randomly, but often with a predilection for the sites of valves. In the early to intermediate postoperative period, these stenoses are again related to intraluminal injury and have a fibroproliferative nature. In the late postoperative period, degenerative lesions similar to arterial atheromas may develop in the vein wall.

Because of the largely subcutaneous position of the *in situ* bypass, such bypass stenoses are readily localized with duplex ultrasound. Clinical examination is sometimes useful where the distal vein segment is easily palpable because a weak pulse in this area is suggestive of a more proximal stenosis. Patients can be taught to monitor their bypasses daily by feeling for a strong pulse in this area. Segmental pressures and pulse volume recordings are unfortunately quite insensitive to moderate degrees of bypass stenosis; a decrease in one of these studies is usually indicative of a greater than 80% stenosis of the bypass. Routine duplex ultrasound is therefore necessary to detect such lesions reliably before they become critical.

Although arteriography is usually not necessary, the operator may feel more comfortable with this information. The management of these lesions is best performed with a segmental replacement of the affected area with autogenous vein. Initially the vein should be opened over the stenosis. The hyperplastic response may often extend proximally or distally for a surprisingly long distance depending on the nature of the original vein injury. If the available vein is of good quality, the entire affected area may be removed. Alternatively, a shorter segment may be replaced, but the bypass should be closely monitored for progression of the remaining hyperplasia. Anastomoses may be performed in either end-to-side or end-to-end fashion; we prefer the latter unless there is a marked mismatch in vein diameter.

Vein patch angioplasty can also be performed for these lesions, but may not function as well over the long term. The reasons for this may involve continuing progression of the hyperplastic lesion with eventual restenosis or occlusion. In addition, if the patch is more than 1 cm in length, patching will involve more suturing than two short end-to-end anastomoses.

Bypass Occlusion

Occlusion of an *in situ* bypass can occur at any time within the postoperative period. Although embolism, patient hypercoagulability, extrinsic compression, and other factors may sometimes cause occlusion, the most frequent identifiable cause is the development of a bypass stenosis leading to thrombosis. In the immediate postoperative period, vein injury may lead to the accumulation of platelets; less often, a missed valve leaflet may lead to early occlusion. Later occlusions are attributable to the progression of hyperplastic lesions to a critical degree.

Bypass occlusion is usually an easily detectable event, most often with the onset of recurrent clinical symptoms. A lack of pulse in the bypass and poor segmental studies lead to confirmation by duplex ultrasonography. It is critical to try to define the exact time of occlusion; in many cases, thrombosis of one segment does not immediately cause thrombosis of the remainder, or the thrombus that propagates may not be adherent to the bypass wall itself similar to the central propagation associated with embolic arterial occlusions. Significant portions of the bypass may thus remain patent and useful for up to 2 weeks. In some cases of distal thrombosis, the bypass occludes only as far as the next open fistula. In these cases, early reintervention may save large portions of the bypass. Conversely, if the bypass has occluded several weeks previously, the bypass is likely to be unsalvageable in any way; if the patient is asymptomatic, observation is probably the best policy.

After diagnosis, arteriography is indicated in most cases. Occult inflow lesions should be searched for and dilated when possible. Distal outflow vessels should be imaged and compared with prebypass arteriograms when possible; often the acute nature of the bypass occlusion makes visualization of patent tibial and pedal vessels difficult. The surgeon should not be discouraged if no vessels are seen on the arteriogram; exploration of the leg should be undertaken.

The use of thrombolytic agents is controversial. Certainly use of these agents is reasonable if the leg is viable and there is no available autogenous conduit. In some cases, a course of thrombolysis may open the bypass and reveal a short stenotic lesion that can be directly repaired. However, unless the thrombus has not yet become adherent to the wall of the bypass, the long-term patency of such conduits is generally poor.

Direct operative exploration is usually necessary. Prior to this, effort should be given to identifying all sources of usable autogenous vein. Duplex ultrasonography is again useful in imaging and mapping these veins before bypass.[21] In particular, the lesser saphenous veins and residual greater saphenous vein in the ipsilateral leg should be sought. Careful husbanding of available autogenous conduit will result in a higher percentage of successful redo operations.

The occluded bypass may be opened distally. If the thrombus is not adherent, it may be extracted without instrumentation and the conduit used. If, as is usually the case, the thrombus is clearly organized and involving the bypass wall, a Fogarty catheter may be passed proximally to extract thrombus. Occasionally this may be sufficient, but generally such thrombectomized conduits rethrombose frequently.

Rebypass with autogenous vein should ideally be performed in these cases. If the other leg is not critically ischemic itself, harvest of its saphenous vein is the most effective course. Alternatively, ipsilateral residual saphenous vein and the ipsilateral lesser saphenous may be spliced together. Other limb veins may be pieced together with good results, but only if the operating team has the experience and patience to do this in a careful manner.

If the proximal bypass is open, a short segment of vein may be harvested to splice with this; the distal anastomosis is performed distal to the previous anastomosis or in another, unscarred area when possible.

When insufficient autogenous conduit is available, polytetrafluoroethylene bypass may be performed. Patency with this is usually poor, however, and modifications such as distal arteriovenous fistulas, the Miller cuff, and Taylor patch may be undertaken in an effort to improve on this dismal track record.

CONCLUSION

The primary goal of the surgeon is to avoid the need for reoperative procedures whenever possible. Careful and meticulous performance of the *in situ* technique and the careful selection of instruments will help minimize the number of difficult redo operations. A thorough and diligent follow-up program with duplex ultrasonography of the entire bypass will roughly halve the incidence of bypass thrombosis. Finally, an awareness of alternative vein sources will allow the surgeon to offer the patient the best chances of a successful rebypass if this becomes necessary.

REFERENCES

1. Hall KV. The great saphenous vein used *in-situ* as an arterial shunt after extirpation of the vein valves: a preliminary report. *Surgery.* 1962;51:492.

2. Barner HB, Judd DR, Kaiser GC, et al. Late failure of arteriologic "*in situ*" saphenous vein. *Arch Surg*. 1969;99:781.

3. Leather RP, Powers SR, Karmody AM. A reappraisal of the "*in-situ*" saphenous vein arterial bypass. *Surgery*. 1979;86:453–460.

4. Leather RP, Shah DM, Karmody AM. Infrapopliteal artery bypass for limb salvage: increased patency and utilization of the saphenous vein used *in situ*. *Surgery*. 1981;190:1000–1008.

5. Carney WI, Balko A, Barrett U, et al. *In situ* saphenous vein femoralpopliteal and infrapopliteal bypass. *Arch Surg*. 1985;120:812–816.

6. Bergamini TM, Towne JB, Bandyk DF, et al. Experience during 1981 to 1989: determinant factors of long-term patency. *J Vasc Surg*. 1991;13:137–149.

7. Fogle MA, Whittemore AD, Couch NP, et al. A comparison of *in situ* and reversed saphenous vein grafts for infrainguinal reconstructions. *J Vasc Surg*. 1987;5:46.

8. Mills N, Oschner JL. Valvulotomy of valves in saphenous vein grafts before coronary artery surgery. *J Thorac Cardiovasc Surg*. 1976;71:878.

9. Leather RP, Shah DM, Corson JD, Karmody AM. Instrumental evolution of the valve incision method of "*in-situ*" saphenous vein bypass. *J Vasc Surg*. 1984;1:113–123.

10. Gruss JD, Bartels D, Vargas H, et al. Arterial reconstruction for distal disease of the lower extremities by the *in-situ* vein graft technique. *J Cardiovasc Surg*. 1982;23:231–234.

11. Acher CW, Turnipseed WD. *In situ* distal saphenous vein bypass using the intraluminal valve-disruption technique. *Arch Surg*. 1985;120:933–935.

12. Lemaitre GD, Arakelian MJ. *In situ* grafting made easy: modification of a technique. *Arch Surg*. 1988;123:101–103.

13. Moody AP, Edwards PR, Harris PL. *In situ* versus reversed femoropopliteal vein grafts: long-term follow-up of a prospective, randomized trial. *Br J Surg*. 1992;79:750–752.

14. Mehigan JT. Angioscopic control of *in situ* bypass: technical considerations. *Semin Vasc Surg*. 1993;6:176–179.

15. Leather RP, Shah DM. *In situ* saphenous vein arterial bypass. In: Rutherford RB, ed. *Vascular Surgery*. 3rd ed. Philadelphia, PA: WB Saunders; 1989:414–425.

16. Leather RP, Leopold PW, Kupinski AM, et al. *In situ* bypass hemodynamics: the effect of residual A-V fistulae. *J Cardiovasc Surg*. 1989;30:843–847.

17. Shah DM, Darling RC III, Chang BB, et al. Long-term results of *in situ* saphenous vein bypass: analysis of 2058 cases. *Ann Surg*. 1994;222:438–448.

18. Bandyk DF, Kaebnick HW, Bergamini TM, et al. Hemodynamics of *in situ* saphenous vein arterial bypasses. *Arch Surg*. 1988;123:477–482.

19. Leather RP, Shah DM, Chang BB, Kaufman JL. Resurrection of the *in situ* saphenous vein bypass 1000 cases later. *Ann Surg*. 1988;208:435–442.

20. Bergamini TM, Towne JB, Bandyk DF, et al. Durability of the *in situ* bypass following modification of abnormal vein segment. *J Surg Res*. 1993;54:196–201.

21. Kupinski AM, Evans SM, Khan AM, et al. Ultrasonic characterization of the saphenous vein. *J Cardiovasc Surg*. 1993;1:513–517.

22. Chang BB, Darling RC III, Bock DEM, et al. The use of spliced vein bypasses for infrainguinal arterial reconstructions. *J Vasc Surg*. 1996;21:403–421.

30

Repetitive Bypasses for Critical Limb Ischemia

Anthony D. Whittemore, MD

Continued advances in vascular surgical techniques have provided marked improvement in graft patency and limb salvage rates associated with infrainguinal arterial reconstruction. Primary graft patency rates for autogenous reconstruction approximate 70% at 5 years and secondary patencies of 80% are routinely anticipated. Thirty percent of grafts, therefore, fail during the first 5 years from a variety of causes, some of which were initially brought to our attention by Dr. Emerick Szilagyi et al.[1] more than 20 years ago. Persistent studies addressing the mechanisms of failure have led to an improved understanding of methods for both avoiding those failures as well as coping with them when they arise.

Fifteen years ago in a small series from the Peter Bent Brigham Hospital we were able to determine the cause of graft failure in 70% of 109 infrainguinal arterial reconstructions and found, as anticipated, the group of early failures resulted primarily from technical errors or optimistic overestimation of the runoff capacity.[2] The delayed failures were associated with the inevitable progression of distal atherosclerotic disease. An important observation, however, was the finding that the most common cause of failure was perianastomotic or vein graft stenosis occuring within 18 months of initial implantation (Fig. 30–1). A second major observation was that the 5-year assisted patency rate associated with simple patch angioplasty of these lesions carried out prior to graft thrombosis was significantly greater (80%) than if the same patch angioplasty was carried out following balloon catheter thrombectomy of a graft presenting with initial occlusion (20% to 27%). These observations have proven reproducible as reported by several groups, including our own again in 1992 reviewing our experience with primary *in situ* saphenous vein bypasses in 455 consecutive patients.[3] Once again, of 104 causes contributing to primary failure of 85 *in situ* saphenous vein grafts, 40% consisted of vein graft stenoses occurring either in the perianastomotic or midgraft segments. The peak interval in which these lesions exerted their maximal impact was 6 to 12 months following initial bypass. That the development of these stenoses is associated with a higher incidence of ultimate graft occlusion has also been established, thereby justifying prophylactic surveillance ensuring the identification of these lesions prior to graft thrombosis and subsequent intervention to optimize sustained patency.[4,5] Initial surveillance depended on recurrent symptoms and, later, the hemodynamic

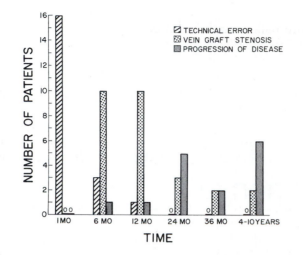

Figure 30–1. The temporal distribution of the three most frequent failure modes for femoro-popliteal vein graft. The majority (80%) of technical errors occurred during the first month after original bypass; vein graft stenoses were encountered most often during the first year; and an increasing incidence of progressive atherosclerosis was responsible for vein graft failure after 1 year. (*Reprinted with permission: Whittemore AD, Clowes AW, Couch NP, Mannick JA. Secondary femoropopliteal reconstruction. Ann Surg. 1981;193:39.*)

assessment in a noninvasive lab, both of which have proven unreliable in the majority of patients in whom hemodynamically significant vein graft stenoses have been documented by duplex scan. Thus, color-flow duplex surveillance utilizing high-flow criteria allows the rapid identification of these lesions and the efficacy of such protocols has been justified by an augmentation of the primary patency rate by 12% to 25% to provide assisted patency rates of 85% to 88%.[6,7] A simple vein patch angioplasty for these focal lesions often suffices, or alternatively, excision of the segment with an interposition vein graft.

Unfortunately, in spite of such protocols, a majority of patients still return with occluded vein grafts and require secondary intervention for limb salvage.[3] In our initial experience 15 years ago, we found that secondary bypasses employing either saphenous vein, lesser saphenous or arm vein, or utilizing a portion of the thrombectomized original vein graft yielded 5-year patency rates ranging from 35% to 40% and overall limb salvage rates of 50%.[2] Although not optimal, at least half of limbs clearly threatened following initial graft occlusion were salvaged. These results were inferior to those associated with an entirely new bypass, and established the policy followed by most surgeons of abandoning a thrombosed graft in favor of a new autogenous conduit where possible.

With the advent of balloon angioplasty, we had hoped that focal vein graft stenoses might be amenable to simple balloon angioplasty, thereby avoiding a secondary operative procedure. Although technically successful initially, balloon angioplasty did not prove any more durable in stenotic patent grafts than in occluded grafts that required initial thrombolysis; only 22% of such vein bypasses remained patent for 4 years.[8] The superior results with reoperative patch angioplasty or interposition graft prior to graft occlusion remain unchallenged.

As thrombolytic therapy emerged as a therapeutic reality, lysis of occluded grafts offered the potential for better results than those achieved with conventional balloon thrombectomy at the time of reexploration. In theory, thrombolytic therapy would avoid repetitive trauma to the endothelial surface; remove thrombus more completely than is possible with balloon catheter thrombectomy; ensure more adequate lysis of thrombus in the outflow vessels; and conserve ectopic autogenous conduit. Once again, while often initially successful, long-term durability fell shy of the mark with only 20% of such thrombosed grafts remaining patent after 3 years.[9] It has thus been repeatedly established that the optimal method for managing a thrombosed primary bypass is an entirely new autogenous conduit.

In spite of a rigorous surveillance protocol, only 25% of grafts failing within 5 years in our experience were seen with a patent but stenotic conduit amenable to a simple graft revision.[3] The majority of such grafts were occluded at the time of presentation, necessitating a secondary procedure. We recently reviewed 300 consecutive secondary interventions in 251 patients operated on during the past two decades.[10] Of these, 272 bypasses represented the first secondary reoperation; there were 20 second time and 8 multiple reoperations. Sixty-seven percent of patients were male and the mean age was 65 years. The demographics were characteristic for this patient population and included tobacco use in 76%, diabetes in 34%, hypertension in 52%, and coronary artery disease in 47%. The majority of patients (84%) required secondary reoperation for limb-threatening critical ischemia. As detailed in Tables 30–1 and 30–2, 213 conduits were autogenous and 87 prosthetic, most of which consisted of expanded polytetrafluo-

TABLE 30–1. GRAFT CHARACTERISTICS OF 213 AUTOGENOUS GRAFTS

	No.	%
Conduits		
In situ greater saphenous vein (GSV)	24	11.3
Nonreversed GSV	36	16.9
Reversed GSV	61	28.6
Composite GSV	12	5.6
Arm vein	36	16.9
Arm–GSV composite	9	4.2
Arm–arm composite	1	.5
Lesser saphenous vein (LSV)	21	9.9
LSV–GSV composite	12	5.6
LSV–LSV composite	1	.5
Inflow Artery		
Common femoral	125	58.7
Deep femoral	10	4.7
Superficial femoral	42	19.7
Popliteal	36	16.9
Outflow artery		
Above-knee popliteal	22	10.3
Below-knee popliteal	51	23.9
Tibioperoneal trunk	8	3.8
Anterior tibial	36	16.9
Posterior tibial	48	22.5
Peroneal	40	18.8
Dorsal pedal	8	3.8

From Belkin M, Conte MS, Donaldson MC, et al. Preferred strategies for secondary infrainguinal bypass: lessons learned from 300 consecutive reoperations. *J Vasc Surg.* 1995;21:284. Used with permission.

TABLE 30–2. GRAFT CHARACTERISTICS OF 87 PROSTHETIC GRAFTS

	No.	%
Conduits		
PTFE	69	7
Umbilical vein	16	18
Dacron	2	5
Inflow Artery		
Common femoral	79	91
Superficial femoral	8	9
Outflow Artery		
Above-knee popliteal	34	39
Below-knee popliteal	38	44
Tibial vessels	15	17

From Belkin M, Conte MS, Donaldson MC, et al. Preferred strategies for secondary infrainguinal bypass: lessons learned from 300 consecutive reoperations. *J Vasc Surg.* 1995;21:284. Used with permission.

roethylene (PTFE). Composite grafts included two or more segments anastamosed by primary venovenostomy or, as illustrated in Figures 30–2 and 30–3, longer segments harvested from contiguous limbs of the greater saphenous or arm vein system.[11,12] The majority (59%) of secondary autogenous reconstructions originated from the common femoral artery. In addition, nearly 40% of prosthetic reconstructions terminated in the above-knee popliteal location, while the majority (90%) of autogenous reconstructions were carried below the knee. Common strategies employed in secondary procedures included the utilization of more distal inflow sources in order to accommodate shorter segments of available autogenous conduit and the use of nonanatomic tunnels. As illustrated in Table 30–3, a single fatal myocardial infarction resulted in the 30-day operative mortality of 0.3%. Significant morbidity includes a 6% early amputation rate associated with autogenous reconstruction and a 10% rate for prosthetic bypass. In comparing the results of autogenous reconstruction with those achieved with prosthetic bypass, note that 80% of the prosthetic reconstructions were carried out during the first decade of this series, reflecting a more deliberate attempt to utilize autogenous tissue in the latter decade as a result of earlier disappointing results. After five years, the secondary patency rates associated with autogenous vein grafts was 52%, nearly twice that achieved with prosthetic bypasses (27%) (Fig. 30–4). Interestingly enough, despite the disparate secondary patency rates, the 5-year limb salvage rate of 54% achieved with prosthetic reconstruction did not differ significantly from the 59% overall salvage rate associated with autogenous bypass, a rate that increased, however, to 72% during the more recent decade. The 5-year patient survival rate was 72% for both groups.

Since early primary graft failure reflects different mechanisms than those resulting in later failure, we were interested in comparing the two groups with regard to graft patency rates. Those who sustained early primary graft failure within 3 months of initial bypass yielded primary and secondary patency rates approximating 30% after 5 years, significantly lower than that achieved with secondary bypass following a delayed failure (52% and 61%, respectively). This is not surprising since many of the early failures result from an attempt to salvage an extremity in the face of marginal outflow or conduit, a situation remaining unchanged when confronted with the necessity for a secondary bypass. The overall 43% primary patency for autogenous reconstruction does not do justice to the technical improvements achieved during the past two decades. The 5-year primary patency rate associated with secondary reconstruction

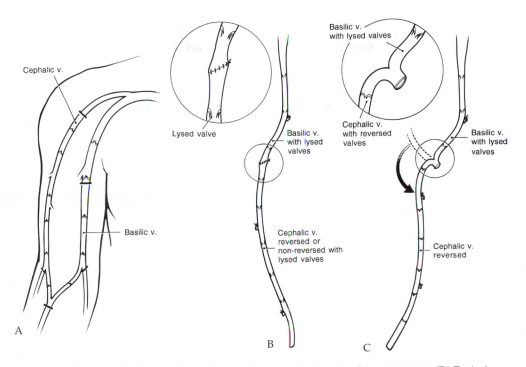

Figure 30–2. (A) Typical anatomy of the basilic and cephalic veins of the upper arm. **(B)** Typical configuration of a composite arm vein bypass graft constructed of basilic and cephalic veins. Nonreversed basilic vein with lysed valves forms the proximal portion of the graft. The distal portion is completed with either reversed or nonreversed cephalic vein with lysed valves. **(C)** Arm vein bypass graft consisting of a proximal nonreversed basilic vein with lysed valves. The distal portion of the graft consists of reversed cephalic vein that is in continuity with a basilic vein through their natural junction at the medial antecubital vein. (*Reprinted with permission: Belkin M, Whittemore AD. Reoperative approaches for failed infrainguinal vein grafts. Sem Vasc Surg. 1994;7:162.*)

during the latter decade was 59%, a marked improvement over the 38% rate observed during the previous decade (Fig. 30–5). Whether the graft terminated in a popliteal or tibial anastomosis did not affect overall patency or limb salvage results.

Five-year primary graft patencies resulting from secondary procedures employing greater superficial saphenous vein were clearly superior (60%) to those achieved with alternative sources (35%). The secondary patency rates demonstrated a similar trend with 69% of greater saphenous veins remaining patent as compared to 48% with ectopic sources ($p < 0.09$). The 5-year limb salvage rate, however, was significantly superior with greater saphenous vein (78%) when compared with alternative conduits (54%, $p < 0.05$). When ectopic sources were required, lesser saphenous vein and arm vein provided similar results with respect to both graft patency and limb salvage.

Provided the failing reconstruction is identified and corrected prior to graft thrombosis, sustained graft patency and limb salvage can be anticipated in the vast majority of patients. Unfortunately, a significant number of individuals continue to return with thrombosed grafts for which surgical thrombectomy or interventional thrombolytic therapy have provided equally dismal results.[13,14] Both measures have proven temporizing at best with 5-year patency rates ranging from 0% to 37%.[2,9] It is generally agreed, therefore, that the most durable limb salvage procedure following graft thrombosis consists of an entirely new autogenous conduit. The 27% 5-year secondary patency

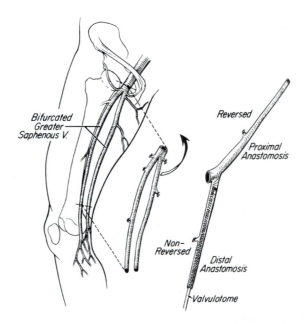

Figure 30–3. Short duplicated greater saphenous vein removed intact and prepared to create a long vein graft. (*Reprinted with permission: Thompson RW, Mannick JA, Whittemore AD. Arterial reconstruction at diverse sites using nonreversed autogenous vein. Ann Surg. 1987; 205:750.*)

rate we achieved with prosthetic bypass primarily in the first decade of our experience does not compare favorably with results reported by Yang et al.[15] who achieved a 55% patency rate at the same interval in a series of 73 secondary PTFE reconstructions. While other authors have consistently reported poor results with prosthetic secondary reconstructions, it may well be that more favorable results can be achieved with the incorporation of adjunctive methods such as the Taylor patch, Miller cuff, or arterio-venus fistulas. Based on current results, however, we believe our rigorous adherence to an all autogenous policy for secondary reconstruction is justified by 5-year secondary patency rates approximating 60% with limb salvage rates of 75%.

To achieve these results, several alternatives are available and incorporate a number of technical improvements in our ability to work successfully with smaller, more distal outflow vessels, nonanatomic tunnels, and alternate sources of conduit, which, given an individual patient's anatomy, may tax our most creative ingenuity. Contralateral greater saphenous vein, residual ipsilateral saphenous vein, lesser saphenous vein, arm vein, and duplicated segments of vein can all prove useful sources in a variety of configurations. The appropriate location for the distal anastomosis should therefore be determined by the length of available conduit and may require a more distal inflow source to provide the lowest resistance outflow, whether it be in the popliteal or distal tibial vessel. While our results with secondary reconstruction are not as favorable as those achieved with primary procedures, a 75% overall limb salvage rate after 5 years justifies the secondary effort in the vast majority of patients. Given the fact that these individuals have failed the initial primary bypass, it is unrealistic to expect comparable results with a secondary reconstruction. Those individuals whose initial graft fails are frequently characterized by more severe systemic atherosclerosis affecting both the inflow and distal outflow, by a more vigorous intimal hyperplastic response, by a higher incidence of hypercoagulothopies, and by suboptimal autogenous conduits.

TABLE 30–3. PERIOPERATIVE MORBIDITY AND MORTALITY RATES IN 300 CONSECUTIVE SECONDARY INFRAINGUINAL BYPASSES

	No.	%
Mortality		
Fatal myocardial infarction	1	0.3
Morbidity		
Myocardial infarction	5	1.7
Congestive heart failure	6	2
Arrhythmia	23	7.7
Renal failure	7	2.3
Transient ischemic attack	1	0.3
Pneumonia (by culture and x-ray)	4	1.3
Graft infection	2	0.7
Wound infection	12	4
Hematoma	8	2.6
Coagulopathy	2	0.7
Gastrointestinal bleed	1	0.3
Liver failure	1	0.3
Deep venous thrombosis	1	0.3
Pulmonary embolus	2	0.3
Total	75	25
Early Graft Failure		
Autogenous: 30-day amputation	29	13.6
	12	5.6
Prosthetic: 30-day amputation	25	28.7
	9	10.3

From Belkin M, Conte MS, Donaldson MC, et al. Preferred strategies for secondary infrainguinal bypass: lessons learned from 300 consecutive reoperations. *J Vasc Surg.* 1995;21:285. Used with permission.

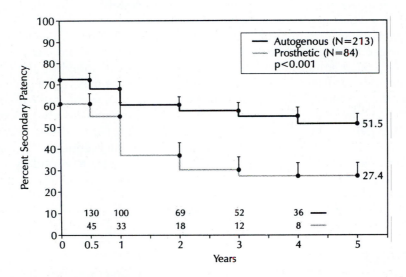

Figure 30–4. Life table analysis of secondary patency rates of secondary autogenous vein graft versus prosthetic bypass grafts. (*Reprinted with permission: Belkin M, Conte MS, Donaldson MC, et al. Preferred strategies for secondary infrainguinal bypass: lessons learned from 300 consecutive reoperations. J Vasc Surg. 1995;21:286.*)

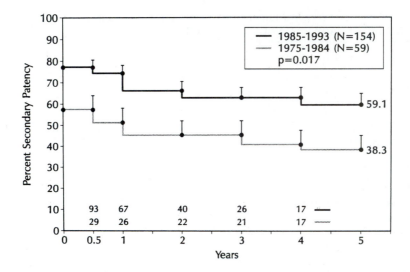

Figure 30–5. Life table analysis of secondary patency rates of autogenous vein secondary bypass grafts performed in 1975–1984 time interval versus 1985–1993 time interval. (*Reprinted with permission: Belkin M, Conte MS, Donaldson MC, et al. Preferred strategies for secondary infrainguinal bypass: lessons learned from 300 consecutive reoperations. J Vasc Surg. 1995;21:289.*)

Nevertheless, the improvements during the past 20 years have provided an increase in limb salvage rates from 50% to 75% and continue to justify an aggressive posture.

There is no doubt that limb salvage does not translate into preservation of limb function in all instances. There is little more discouraging than a patient who has weathered a secondary reconstruction only to be left with a chronically swollen and painful dysfunctional lower extremity. Fortunately, these individuals represent the minority, yet it is important to recognize that amputation does indeed play a part in the management of recurrent critical ischemia. Both patient and surgeon must be willing at some point to use amputation wisely as a means of restoring rather than obliterating functional survival.

Occlusion of an infrainguinal autogenous bypass graft continues to present the vascular surgeon with an intellectual and technical challenge. From our recent experience, an aggressive strategy favoring repetitive bypass is justified by the 60% 5-year graft patency rate resulting in continued limb salvage for the majority of patients (73%). The proper management in any given instance depends on a number of considerations, among which is the potential functional status of the limb. An elderly patient leading a relatively sedentary life, without significant ischemic pain or tissue necrosis, may very well remain stable without the need for further intervention. The majority of patients, however, will develop critical ischemia and require a secondary procedure for limb preservation and/or relief of pain. While amputation is always an expeditious alternative, secondary bypass seems warranted given the low operative mortality rate and favorable rate of limb preservation anticipated for the majority of patients.

REFERENCES

1. Szilagyi DE, Elliott JP, Hageman JM, et al. Biologic fate of autogenous vein implants as arterial substitutes. *Am Surg.* 1973;178:232–246.

2. Whittemore AD, Clowes AW, Couch NP, et al. Secondary femoropopliteal reconstruction. *Ann Surg.* 1981;193:35–42.
3. Donaldson MC, Mannick JA, Whittemore AD. Causes of primary graft failure after *in situ* saphenous vein bypass grafting. *J Vasc Surg.* 1992;15:113–120.
4. Bandyk DF, Schmitt DD, Seabrook GR, et al. Monitoring functional patency of *in situ* saphenous vein bypass: the impact of a surveillance protocol and elective revision. *J Vasc Surg.* 1989;9:286–296.
5. Erickson CA, Towne JB, Seabrook GR, et al. Ongoing vascular laboratory surveillance is essential to maximize long-term *in situ* saphenous vein bypass patency. *J Vasc Surg.* 1996;23:18–27.
6. Mattos MA, van Bemmelen PS, Hodgson KJ, et al. Does correction of stenoses identified with color duplex scanning improve infrainguinal graft potency? *J Vasc Surg.* 1993;17:54–66.
7. Mirza IM, Blankenstein JD, deGier P, et al. Impact of a color flow duplex surveillance program on infrainguinal vein graft patency: a five-year experience. *J Vasc Surg.* 1993;17:42–53.
8. Whittemore AD, Donaldson MC, Polak JF, et al. Limitations of balloon angioplasty for vein graft stenosis. *J Vasc Surg.* 1991;14:340–345.
9. Belkin M, Donaldson MC, Whittemore AD, et al. Observations on the use of thrombolytic agents for thrombotic occlusions of infrainguinal vein grafts. *J Vasc Surg.* 1990;11:289–296.
10. Belkin M, Conte MS, Donaldson MC, et al. Preferred strategies for secondary infrainguinal bypass: lessons learned from 300 consecutive reoperations. *J Vasc Surg.* 1995;21:282–295.
11. Belkin M, Whittemore AD. Reoperative distal bypass surgery. *Semin Vasc Surg.* 1994;7:158–164.
12. Thompson RW, Mannick JA, Whittemore AD. Arterial reconstruction at diverse sites using nonreversed autogenous vein. *Ann Surg.* 1987;205:747–751.
13. Graor RA, Risus B, Young JR, et al. Thrombolysis of peripheral arterial bypass grafts: surgical thrombectomy compared with thrombolysis. *J Vasc Surg.* 1988;7:347–355.
14. Parent FN, Prowski JJ, Bernhard VM, et al. Outcome of intraarterial urokinase for acute vascular occlusion. *J Cardiovasc Surg.* 1991;32:680–690.
15. Yang PM, Wengerter KR, Veith FJ, et al. Value and limitations of secondary femeropopliteal bypasses with polytetrafluoroethylene. *J Vasc Surg.* 1991;14:292–298.

31

Postoperative Neurologic Deficit

William H. Baker, MD, and M. Ashraf Mansour, MD

The aim of carotid endarterectomy is to prevent stroke. Unfortunately, stroke, both in the immediate postoperative period as well as late after carotid endarterectomy, still occurs. This chapter attempts to outline the methods of prevention, etiology, and treatment of these disorders.

POSTOPERATIVE STROKE

Stroke that occurs within the first 30 days of operation is rightly assigned directly to the operative procedure. These strokes may occur as the patient awakes in the operating room, in the recovery room, during hospitalization, or any time during the first 30 postoperative days. Strokes occurring later than 30 days postoperatively are addressed in the second half of this chapter.

The incidence of postoperative stroke is highly variable. Ideally, the risk of stroke should be less than 5% and perhaps as low as 1% or 2%. The North American Symptomatic Carotid Endarterectomy Trial (NASCET) had an operative stroke rate of 5.5%.[1] The European Carotid Surgery Trial (ECST) had a higher stroke rate of 7.5% within 30 days of operation.[2] In 1988, the Rand study found a 9.8% incidence of postoperative stroke and death.[3] The Rand study suggested that this incidence of mortality and morbidity was virtually identical in different parts of urban and rural America. These latter two studies have an unacceptable rate of mortality and morbidity by 1996 standards. The Asymptomatic Carotid Atherosclerosis Study (ACAS) had an enviable perioperative stroke rate of only 1.2% (2.3% including stroke related to angiography).[4] However, the surgeons in this study were chosen on the basis of their excellent results. Surgeons of lesser ability were not allowed to participate. Thus, it appears that the postoperative stroke rate following carotid endarterectomy is operator dependent.

There are three general causes of stroke following operation. Intraoperative embolization may occur at any time during the procedure. The carotid bifurcation harbors friable atherosclerosis that may be accompanied by intraluminal thrombus. If this bifurcation is unduly manipulated before the clamps are applied, an intraoperative embolization and neurologic deficit may occur. When the carotid is clamped, the brain that depends on this artery will become relatively ischemic. Thus, many surgeons use a temporary indwelling shunt during the time of carotid clamping.

The shunt itself may be inserted in such a manner as to snowplow atherosclerotic debris. This debris and/or air bubbles may embolize during the process of shunting. Finally, the recently operated carotid artery may thrombose.[5] Although all surgeons have had perfectly excellent operations thrombose, most of these thrombotic episodes are the result of a roughened endarterectomy surface, an imperfect end point, or an imperfect closure.

The best treatment of postoperative stroke is its prevention. Technical perfection is required to avoid postoperative problems. As previously mentioned, the carotid bifurcation should not be manipulated before the placement of clamps. We take special care to apply clamps before the back wall of the carotid is dissected to minimize the chance of embolization. The judicious use of a temporary indwelling shunt will prevent ischemic stroke.[6] Whereas some surgeons use a shunt for all of their patients, most surgeons use the shunt selectively. The rationale for selective shunt usage is beyond the scope of this chapter and the reader is encouraged to look elsewhere to delve into this problem. If a temporary indwelling shunt is used, the arteriotomy must be of sufficient length to allow the operator to see the end of the atherosclerosis. In that way, the risk of snowplowing of atherosclerotic debris will be minimized. The introduction of the shunt without inadvertently introducing air should not be a problem.

A complete endarterectomy needs to be performed, ensuring that all the little fronds of retained media and atherosclerosis are removed. The end point should be adherent even if this requires the placement of tacking sutures. The closure should not compromise the lumen. We advocate the liberal use of a patch angioplasty. Following the completion of the closure, flow is directed first into the external carotid artery before directing blood and potential emboli to the internal carotid artery.

Intraoperative Duplex Scanning

We believe that the endarterectomy site should be evaluated in the operating room so that any technical problems can be corrected. We prefer to use a duplex scanner. The machine that is used in the Peripheral Vascular Laboratory is wheeled into the operating room and a small (10-MHz) probe is encased in a sterile sheath. The probe can interrogate the entire surface of the carotid quite easily. By varying the angle of the probe, almost all of the walls can be seen. In general, we have reexplored the artery on very few occasions. Most of the reexplorations have been for a compromised proximal end point that had not been tacked down. We have seen free-floating thrombus as well as multiple fronds waving during diastole and systole.[7] On one occasion, an artery was reopened on the basis of turbulent flow alone.[7] We should mention that other authors use the hand-held Doppler probe to listen for disturbed frequencies. Operative arteriography is easily obtained in most operating rooms. The quality of these pictures, however, is highly variable.

Diagnosis

Ideally, the patient should awaken in the operating room and a gross neurologic examination should be performed. Many times, however, the patient cannot be adequately evaluated until he or she awakens more fully in the recovery room. This is especially true in patients who have had a preoperative neurologic deficit. Sometimes any patient with a deficit who undergoes a general anesthesia (even for a cholecystectomy) may awaken with a temporary deficit. However, these temporary deficits should improve within minutes, not hours. If the operating surgeon has not performed a complete neurologic examination preoperatively, he or she will have a difficult time deciding whether or not a hand incoordination is new or old. Patients who have a preexisting contralateral internal carotid artery occlusion and who occlude the ipsilateral carotid artery are especially difficult to evaluate. Although some of these patients will awaken with an easy-to-detect profound deficit, many others will be merely "slow to awake." These patients may or may not demonstrate lateralizing neurologic signs. If this scenario occurs and the anesthesiologist is as puzzled as the surgeon regarding the slow emergence from the anesthetic, these patients should be considered to have an occluded carotid artery until proven otherwise.

Treatment

The goals of treatment of postoperative stroke are easy to outline. If the patient has suffered an embolic event, the surgeon cannot remove the emboli. More recently, such a case was treated with intraoperative lytic therapy with a good clinical result. This case report will have to be followed by many others before this form of treatment becomes standard.[8] The surgeon cannot revive brain that has been damaged as a result of intraoperative ischemia. If, indeed, there has been a prolonged clamp time or a needed shunt was not used for technical reasons, the surgeon cannot remedy the situation. The surgeon's main hope is to find a totally occluded internal carotid artery. In this case, a thrombectomy can be performed to restore flow to the ischemic, but not necrotic, brain. If indeed flow can be restored within 1 or at most 2 hours of the onset of a neurologic deficit, isolated anecdotal reports suggest that many patients will show neurologic improvement.[9] Thus, it is the surgeon's main goal to identify those patients who have an internal carotid artery occlusion and who can have flow restored within 1 or, at most, 2 hours.

If stroke occurs in the operating room, the most expeditious maneuver is to reopen the wound and explore the operative carotid artery.[10] If indeed a pulse is present, we insist that the carotid be further interrogated. This may involve a repeat duplex examination, an operative arteriogram, or a direct inspection through an open arteriotomy. Under most circumstances the latter is preferable. When the carotid is explored and after the thrombus (if any) is removed, a temporary indwelling shunt is inserted so that the brain will not be further stressed. An operative arteriogram through the shunt should diagnose intraoperative embolization.

There are many exceptions to the preceding rule. We have seen patients who have had prolonged intraoperative cerebral ischemia because of a complex operation. Their duplex scans were perfectly normal 15 minutes before the discovery of a neurologic deficit. In these patients reexploration has not been undertaken. We have not, to our knowledge, missed any internal carotid artery occlusions. All of our patients have had the internal carotid artery patent when examined on later duplex or arteriographic examinations. If a neurologic deficit occurs in the recovery room, the same principles apply. Those patients who enter the recovery room neurologically intact and later develop an obvious deficit are rushed back to the operating room. We presume the carotid artery has freshly occluded. We do not obtain any procrastinating test such as duplex scanning or arteriography because these examinations will delay the restoration of flow if indeed the carotid is totally occluded. The few duplex examinations that we obtained were in special circumstances where a patient develops a neurologic deficit and the scanner is immediately available, or their return to the operating room was delayed for logistical reasons.

Depending on the degree of cooperation from the patient, the reexploration may be performed under local anesthesia. However, we prefer general anesthesia. When stroke occurs in the hospital after the patient leaves the recovery room, but before discharge, the same principles apply. However, it is sometimes difficult to return the patient to the operating room in an expeditious manner so that flow is restored within the arbitrary 1 to 2 hours. If indeed an undue delay has occurred, we believe the exploration should not be undertaken.

Some patients have a postoperative transient attack, that is, the physician is called to examine the patient, who has had an obvious neurologic deficit. Upon reexamination the deficit disappears before one's eyes. These patients probably have had an embolic episode. However, an occasional patient will exhibit such signs and symptoms even with a total internal carotid artery occlusion. Our approach to these patients is to immediately assess the internal carotid artery. This can usually be done most expeditiously with a duplex scanner. Those patients who have total occlusion are taken back to the operating room under most, but not all, circumstances. Patients who have had an embolic event, but who do not have any visualized thrombus in the operated artery, are usually treated with anticoagulants. Prior to discharge, the anticoagulation is discontinued and aspirin is begun. Early in the course of anticoagulation, a computed tomography (CT) scan is obtained to ensure that the patient has not had a bleed into an ischemic area of the brain.

Urgent Reexploration After Endarterectomy

In selected cases, immediate reexploration was not performed for several reasons. Sometimes the patient does not report the transient ischemic attack until rounds the next morning. Under these circumstances there would be a 6- to 12-hour delay between the onset of symptoms and the discovery of a total occlusion. In addition, patients who have a completely patent contralateral internal carotid and vertebral arterial system, and who are known to have a high stump pressure, are sometimes not reexplored. This is especially true if there are other medical events occurring at the same time.

A year ago, we reported our 10-year experience with stroke after carotid endarterectomy.[11] In a review of our records, 16 patients were found with a stroke within 30 days of operation (2.7%). In addition, 5 patients had transient ischemic attacks. Eight of these combined events occurred in the immediate postoperative period, 10 within the same hospitalization, and 3 after discharge, but within 30 days of surgery. Of the 8 immediate deficits, 5 were not reexplored. As stated previously, no internal carotid occlusions were knowingly missed.

Among the three vessels that were reexplored, no thrombus was found in any patient. Ten patients had symptoms after leaving the recovery room, but before discharge from the hospital. Four of these patients had transient ischemic attacks and 6 had a stroke. Two of these patients had proven occlusions. One of these patients underwent reexploration, although this reexploration occurred more than 2 hours after the onset of symptoms. His dense hemiparesis did not improve. The second patient had an internal carotid artery occlusion that was not recognized in a timely fashion. He did not undergo reexploration and eventually died of neurologic complications. Of the 5 patients who had transient ischemic attacks, 3 had normal angiographic findings. One was not studied with angiograms, but had a normal duplex scan. He died, many months later, of a stroke that was difficult to characterize. The fifth patient had a kink of her internal carotid artery that was treated with aspirin. Three of our patients had the onset of neurologic symptoms after they were discharged from the hospital. One patient had a typical transient ischemic attack with a normal internal carotid artery angiographically. The second patient had a seizure with an abnormal CT scan that was consistent with this clinical picture. The third patient had a retinal infarct that was recognized postoperatively, although it may have occurred earlier in the patient's course.[11]

RECURRENT CAROTID STENOSIS

Incidence

Whereas early postoperative stroke is due to a technically flawed operation or intraoperative ischemia, late recurrence is due to an anatomic obstructive lesion. There are two distinct clinicopathologic patterns of recurrence after 30 days. Recurrent carotid stenosis (RCS) occurring in the first 2 years after carotid endarterectomy (CEA) is most likely due to myointimal hyperplasia (MIH) while later recurrence is due to atherosclerosis.[12–14] Long-term surveillance studies have shown that the incidence of RCS varies from 6% to 37%. Careful analysis of the literature, however, reveals that the incidence of hemodynamically significant stenosis (>50%) averages 14%.[15] Several authors have reported that early restenosis usually runs a benign course, could regress, and may represent the poorly studied phenomenon of plaque remodeling.[16] Although these lesions less commonly cause symptoms, they have been known to do so. Conversely, hemodynamically significant RCS occurring after 2 years may or may not give rise to clinically important symptoms of cerebrovascular insufficiency, as would any other atherosclerotic lesion.[17–22]

Pathology

Endothelial cells are found lining the luminal surface of both early and late RCS lesions. The histologic characteristic of *early* stenosis is that of neointimal hyperplasia. These lesions appear grossly as grayish white, glistening smooth lesions involving a varying portion of the endarterectomy site. Microscopic examination reveals MIH with an abundance of smooth muscle cells. Immunocytochemical stains confirm the presence of actin and desmin. However, *late* recurrent atherosclerosis usually appears as a yellow friable lesion.[12,18] The site of recurrence tends to be more pronounced at the proximal or distal end point, but could be anywhere in the endarterectomized segment. Although several authors have suggested that recurrent lesions due to atherosclerosis are more likely to be symptomatic than MIH, it may well be that physicians were attracted to these patients because of their symptoms.[16] Microscopic features of these lesions include needle-shaped cholesterol clefts, foam cells, and identifiable cholesterol and other fats within the specimen.[14]

Is MIH a precursor of atherosclerosis? Although some authors believe this to be true, it is difficult to prove. Rapp et al.[23] from the San Francisco VA Hospital have demonstrated that patients with MIH following CEA tended to have an increase in risk factors for atherosclerosis. Clearly cholesterol and other lipids can be found within these early plaques. Regardless, their gross appearance and characteristics require that they be treated differently in the operating room.

Diagnosis

Color-flow duplex scanning is the most widely used noninvasive test to monitor disease of the carotid bifurcation. Postoperative scans are performed in the same fashion as preoperative ones and criteria for detection of a stenotic lesion are unchanged. In our laboratory, a peak systolic velocity of 250 cm/s is used to identify significant stenoses (≥75% area stenosis). Other laboratories obviously use different velocity criteria as well as turbulent flow, spectral broadening, and the B-mode image. Early RCS may be identified by the absence of the double line on B-mode scanning after CEA.[24]

Routine surveillance after CEA is indicated. The precise schedule of postoperative studies continues to be debated on the basis of cost effectiveness. The rationale for advocating a relaxed schedule is the low incidence of stroke associated with early recurrent stenosis.[25,26] Conversely, these lesions may progress and total carotid occlusion may cause a stroke in up to 25% of patients.[27] In addition, CEA patients have diffuse atherosclerosis and the contralateral carotid is often the seat of progressive disease. Initially, we perform a color-flow duplex scan intraoperatively after completion of the endarterectomy. Any technical defects are, of course, immediately repaired prior to leaving the operating room. This study is used as a baseline scan and is augmented by another duplex scan the next day prior to discharge.[7] Patients are routinely scanned at 6 months postoperatively, and those with a normal duplex scan are then followed yearly. Patients with stenoses are followed at shorter intervals depending on the nature of the abnormality.

Angiography

Patients with recurrent transient ischemic attacks including amaurosis fugax or minor strokes have a repeat duplex scan. Assuming that their carotid artery is patent, an angiogram is obtained. We have not yet established a policy of operating on RCS without such a study. This is in contradistinction to our usual clinical algorithm.[28]

The asymptomatic patient with RCS is an enigma. Those patients who have a contralateral internal carotid artery occlusion are more urgently shepherded toward angiography and subsequent repeat carotid reconstruction. It is our habit to measure an internal carotid artery stump pressure at the time of the original endarterectomy. Those patients with low stump pressures who may be at an increased risk of stroke with internal carotid artery occlusion are likewise encouraged to undergo angiography and repair. Angiography under these circumstances should be similar to angiography in patients with primary stenoses. Although an arch view is helpful to identify proximal lesions in the vessels as they arise from the aorta, most arch lesions can be identified by physical examination or by decreased velocities in the respective common carotid arteries.

Indications for Operation

Patients with temporary hemispheric symptoms, temporary monocular blindness, or nondisabling strokes are offered reoperation. These indications are the same regardless of primary or secondary pathology. Asymptomatic patients with early recurrence, thought to represent a smooth myointimal lesion, are usually watched unless the lesion is progressive or the patient has a galaxy of other lesions. Patients who have late RCS are thought to have atherosclerosis as the basic pathologic finding. These patients are offered prophylactic re-endarterectomy per the guidelines of the ACAS.[4]

Technical Considerations

The patient is prepared for operation much like any other CEA candidate. We prefer general anesthesia for almost all patients. Although regional anesthesia has been used in some patients with primary operation, we have never used it for RCS. We use intraoperative cerebral protection electively based on stump flow measurements.[29]

Reoperations are technically more demanding because the vessels and cranial nerves are often encased in dense scar tissue.[21,23] In general, the most proximal common carotid artery is identified primarily. The dissection is then carried on top of the carotid artery, unroofing the carotid bifurcation and elevating the hypoglossal nerve medially and superiorly. If it is possible to find a clean, undissected plane distally around the internal carotid artery this vessel is next encircled. Finally, taking care to neither grasp the vagus nerve nor significantly manipulate the carotid artery, we attempt to identify a plane between the vagus and the carotid artery. Although this maneuver has the potential disadvantage of dislodging emboli, we believe it to be important to avoid injury to the vagus nerve. This dissection is a knife dissection in order to minimize the complication mentioned.

Once the artery has been controlled, heparin is administered and a stump pressure is measured. A shunt is selectively employed based on this pressure. A longitudinal arteriotomy is performed. If a previous prosthetic graft has been used in the original closure, this must be excised. Myointimal hyperplasia will not be separated easily from the wall of the artery and these lesions are usually left in place. Sometimes excrescences of this fleshy tissue are individually excised using knife dissection. The arteriotomy is then closed using a generous, but not aneurysmal, patch.[30] Patients who have recurrent atherosclerosis that occurs late after the original endarterectomy are often re-endarterectomized. Patients with difficult plaques that are adherent and difficult to endarterectomize are treated as patients who have MIH. Atherosclerotic recurrences are also universally closed using a patch angioplasty technique. We currently prefer Dacron as the material of choice.

In a recent review of our experience with RCS, the incidence of redo endarterectomy was 7%. Reoperations were performed for symptomatic recurrence in 68%, and the majority of the closures were performed with vein patches or grafts. However, in our most recent nine cases, we have replaced the internal carotid artery using polytetrafluoroethylene. Raithel et al.[31,32] reported excellent results using this technique primarily, with a very low incidence of recurrent stenosis. Since 10% of our patients undergoing operation for RCS have a second recurrence, we have adopted this latter technique in an effort to reduce this figure.[33]

Operative Results

Redo CEAs for recurrent stenosis have been performed for 20 years. Most series report an acceptable perioperative stroke rate. The most common surgical complication is either a transient or permanent cranial nerve injury (Table 31–1). Transient nerve paresis is usually due to overzealous retraction and affects the hypoglossal or marginal mandibular branch of the facial nerve. Paresis may last up to 3 months with full return of function.[17–21] Permanent cranial nerve injuries occur during dissection to gain control of the artery. The vagus nerve may be intimately adherent to the common carotid artery where it might be injured by a clamp or dissection. The hypoglossal nerve is injured when distal dissection is carried out to reach a relatively normal distal segment of the internal carotid artery. Other postoperative complications include transient ische-

TABLE 31–1. SUMMARY OF REPORTS ON MANAGEMENT OF RECURRENT STENOSIS

Reference	N =	Incidence (%)	Symptomatic (%)	Pathology: MIH (%)	ASO (%)	Second Restenosis (%)	Operative Stroke (%)	Death (%)	Cranial Nerve Injury (%)
Das et al.,[20] 1986	65	3.8	51	43	57	NR	1.5	3.1	9.2
Piepgras et al.,[17] 1986	57	NR	NR	25	47[a]	NR	10.5	0	NR
Bartlett et al.,[19] 1987	116	NR	70	41	59	5.8	4.3	1.7	17[b]
Shurriway et al.,[13] 1987	66	2	89	17	72[c]	7.5	1.5	0	3
Kazmers et al.,[34] 1988	14	1.3	100	28	36[c]	NR	0	0	14
AbuRahma et al.,[21] 1994	46	5	72	24	76	2	7	0	6.5
Coyle et al.,[18] 1995	69	6.4	54	NR	NR	NR	1.4	2.9	NR

NR, not reported; MIH, myointimal hyperplasia; ASO, atherosclerosis.
[a] Included aneurysm, thrombus, and proximal scarring.
[b] Some cranial nerve injuries were transient with subsequent full recovery.
[c] Shumway had 11% and Kazmers had 28% of lesions with a combination of MIH and ASO.

mic attacks or stroke. The incidence of stroke varies between 1.4% and 10.5% (Table 31–1). Wound hematomas can also occur.

CONCLUSION

The treatment aim for patients with a neurologic deficit, manifested early after operation, is to identify the ones with a totally occluded carotid artery and to restore flow within an hour. This plan gives the best chance of salvaging potentially viable brain. RCS manifested 30 days or more following endarterectomy is an uncommon problem. Early restenosis (<2 years) is usually due to MIH and runs a benign course. Late restenosis (>2 years) is due to recurrent atherosclerosis. Symptomatic patients in each category are shepherded toward operation. Asymptomatic patients with atherosclerosis are treated based on the tenets of ACAS. Asymptomatic patients thought to have MIH are usually closely followed nonoperatively unless special circumstances are present.

REFERENCES

1. North American Symptomatic Carotid Endarterectomy Trial Collaborators. Beneficial effect of carotid endarterectomy in symptomatic patients with high-grade stenosis. *N Engl J Med.* 1991;325:445–453.
2. European Carotid Surgery Trialists' Collaborative Group. European Carotid Surgery Trial: interim results for symptomatic patients with severe (70–99%) or with mild (0–29%) carotid stenosis. *Lancet.* 1991;337:1235–1243.
3. Winslow CM, Solomon DH, Chassin MR, et al. The appropriateness of carotid endarterectomy. *N Engl J Med.* 1988;218:721–727.
4. Executive committee for the Asymptomatic Carotid Atherosclerosis Study. Endarterectomy for asymptomatic carotid stenosis. *JAMA.* 1995;273:1421–1428.
5. Riles TS, Imparato AM, Jacobowitz GR, et al. The cause of perioperative stroke after carotid endarterectomy. *J Vasc Surg.* 1994;19:206–216.
6. Littooy FN, Halstuk KS, Mamdani M, et al. Factors influencing morbidity of carotid endarterectomy without a shunt. *Am Surg.* 1984;50:350–353.
7. Baker WH, Koustas G, Burke K, et al. Intraoperative duplex scanning and late carotid artery stenosis. *J Vasc Surg.* 1994;19:829–833.
8. Barr JD, Horowitz MB, Mathis JM, et al. Intraoperative urokinase infusion for embolic stroke during carotid endarterectomy. *Neurosurgery.* 1995;36:606–611.
9. Kwaan JHM, Connolly JE, Sharefkin JB. Successful management of early stroke after carotid endarterectomy. *Ann Surg.* 1979;190:676–678.
10. Edwards WH Jr, Jenkins JM, Edwards WH Sr, Mulherin JL. Prevention of stroke during carotid endarterectomy. *Am Surg.* 1988;54:125–128.
11. Baker WH. Treatment of perioperative neurologic deficits after carotid surgery. Presented at the 21st Annual Symposium Current Critical Problems in Vascular Surgery; November 1995, New York.
12. Javid H, Ostermiller WE Jr, Hengesh JW, et al. Natural history of carotid bifurcation atheroma. *Surgery.* 1970;67:80–86.
13. Shumway SJ, Edwards WH, Jenkins JM, et al. Recurrent carotid stenosis. *Am Surg.* 1987; 53:61–65.
14. Schwarcz TH, Yates GN, Ghobrial M, Baker WH. Pathologic characteristics of recurrent carotid artery stenosis. *J Vasc Surg.* 1987;5:280–288.
15. Sumner DS, Mattos MA, Hodgson KJ. Surveillance program for vascular reconstructive procedures. In: Yao JST, Pearce WH, eds. *Long-Term Results in Vascular Surgery.* Norwalk, CT: Appleton & Lange; 1993:33–59.

16. Washburn WK, Mackey WC, Belkin M, O'Donnell TF. Late stroke after carotid endarterectomy: the role of recurrent stenosis. *J Vasc Surg.* 1992;15:1032–1037.

17. Piepgras DG, Sundt TM, Marsh WR, et al. Recurrent carotid stenosis. *Ann Surg.* 1986;203:205–213.

18. Coyle KA, Smith RB III, Gray BC, et al. Treatment of recurrent cerebrovascular disease. *Ann Surg.* 1995;221:517–524.

19. Bartlett FF, Rapp JH, Goldstone J, et al. Recurrent carotid stenosis: operative strategy and late results. *J Vasc Surg.* 1987;5:452–456.

20. Das MB, Hertzer NR, Ratliff NB, et al. Recurrent carotid stenosis. *Ann Surg.* 1985;202:28–35.

21. AbuRahma AF, Snodgrass KR, Robinson PA, et al. Safety and durability of redo carotid endarterectomy for recurrent carotid artery stenosis. *Am J Surg.* 1994;168:175–178.

22. Edwards WH Jr, Edwards WH Sr, Mulherin JL, Martin RS III. Recurrent carotid artery stenosis. *Ann Surg.* 1989;209:662–669.

23. Rapp JH, Stoney RJ. Recurrent carotid stenosis. In: Bernhard VM, Towne JB, eds. *Complications in Vascular Surgery.* New York: Grune & Stratton; 1985:763–773.

24. Caps MT, Hatsukami TS, Bergelin RO, et al. A clinical marker for arterial wall healing: the double line. The International Society for Cardiovascular Surgery, North American Chapter; 1995. Abstract.

25. Mattos MA, Shamma AR, Rossi N, et al. Is duplex follow-up cost effective in the first year after carotid endarterectomy? *Am J Surg.* 1988;156:91–95.

26. Cook JM, Thompson BW, Barnes RW. Is routine duplex examination after carotid endarterectomy justified? *J Vasc Surg.* 1990;12:334–340.

27. Strandness DE. Recurrent carotid artery stenosis following endarterectomy. In: Ernst CB, Stanley JC, eds. *Current Therapy in Vascular Surgery.* St. Louis, MO: CV Mosby; 1995:76–78.

28. Horn M, Michelini M, Greisler HP, et al. Carotid endarterectomy without angiography: the preeminent role of the vascular laboratory. *Ann Vasc Surg.* 1994;8:221–224.

29. Hirko MK, Morasch MD, Burke K, et al. The changing face of carotid endarterectomy. *J Vasc Surg.* 1996;23:622–627.

30. Hertzer NR, Beven EG, O'Hara PJ, Krajewski LP. A prospective study of vein patch angioplasty during carotid endarterectomy. *Ann Surg.* 1987;206:628–635.

31. Raithel D. Choice of graft material in carotid surgery: vein vs. PTFE. In: Veith FJ, ed. *Current Critical Problems in Vascular Surgery.* St. Louis, MO: Quality Medical Publishing; 1994:259–263.

32. Raithel D. Recurrent carotid disease: optimum technique for redo surgery. *J Endovasc Surg.* 1996;3:69–75.

33. Mansour MA, Kang SS, Baker WH, et al. Carotid endarterectomy for recurrent stenosis. Midwest Vascular Surgical Society; 1996. Abstract.

34. Kazmers A, Zierler RE, Huang RW, et al. Reoperative carotid surgery. *Am J Surg.* 1988;156:346–352.

32

Surgery for Recurrent Aortic Aneurysms

Sunil S. Menawat, MD, and Kenneth J. Cherry, Jr., MD

Aortic aneurysms that occur following previous aortic aneurysm repair pose many challenges for vascular surgeons. The aneurysms may be true or false. They may be in proximity to or in continuity with the previous repair, or they may arise in different segments of the aorta. Perioperative morbidity and mortality are increased in comparison with those figures for primary operations.[1–3] Coronary artery disease remains the most likely cause of late death in patients with aneurysmal disease who have undergone repair, followed by cancer. Recurrent aneurysmal disease is the third leading cause of death in these patients and the most frequently encountered vascular complication in the long term.[4] Aneurysms may arise in the body of prosthetic grafts[5,6]; however, in this chapter, we address the more common problems of recurrent true and anastomotic aneurysms of the aorta.

INCIDENCE

The true incidence of recurrent aortic aneurysms is not known for a variety of reasons: many patients are not followed; others remain asymptomatic and undergo no or inadequate testing, despite follow-up; and of those followed, not all undergo imaging studies that provide complete visualization of the thoracic and abdominal aorta. Recurrent aortic aneurysms are not as accessible to physical diagnosis as are pseudoaneurysms in the groin, and the sophisticated diagnostic methods currently used to study the suprarenal abdominal aorta and the thoracic aorta were not available in the past. Estimates of the incidence of recurrent true aortic aneurysms and aortic pseudoaneurysms in the past were, therefore, in all likelihood, low and representative of a select group of symptomatic or worrisome patients. Several retrospective studies addressed the problem in the past. Szilagyi and associates[7] reported the incidence of aortic pseudoaneurysms in their 4,114 patients followed from 1 month to 14 years (mean 3.4 years) to be 0.2%. The incidence of iliac pseudoaneurysms was 1.2%. Crawford and colleagues[8] looking at infrarenal abdominal aortic aneurysms in 920 patients seen over a 25-year period, found 23 pseudoaneurysms and 32 true aneurysms at other sites. Plate et al.[4] from the Mayo Clinic reported on recurrent aneurysms following abdominal aortic aneurysm repair in 1,112 patients. Forty-nine true, 14 anastomotic (4 of the aorta), and 5 dissections were described in 55 patients (5.4%). Of those aneurysms, there were 24 thoracic, 5 thoracoabdominal, 11 abdominal aortic, and 6 iliac artery aneurysms. The probability of finding a new aneurysm was 3% at 5 years and 11% at 10 years. Patients with hypertension had a threefold increased risk of developing further aneurysms, and 8.4% of the late mortality in this series was due to related vascular complications.

Van den Akker et al.[9] reported a 4.8% incidence of aortic pseudoaneurysms and a 6.3% incidence of iliac pseudoaneurysms in a group of more than 500 patients undergoing aortic reconstruction for aortoiliac occlusive disease.[9] There was a statistically significant increase in aortic pseudoaneurysms following end-to-side proximal anastomoses.

Several groups recently have followed their patients aggressively to determine the frequency of recurrence of abdominal aortic aneurysms. Sieswerda and colleagues[10] found a 2.6% rate of aortic anastomotic aneurysms in 122 patients. They found a 12.3% incidence of iliac artery pseudoaneurysms. This group used ultrasonography and intravenous digital subtraction angiography. Interestingly, they found that the latter technique was more useful to them.

Edwards et al.[11] in 1992 reported 111 patients having aortic reconstructions who were followed by serial ultrasonography. Ten percent were found to have recurrent intra-abdominal para-anastomotic aneurysms a mean of 144 months following operation. There were 7 anastomotic aneurysms and 4 true aneurysms. Three of these 11 aneurysms occurred within 3 years, whereas the other 8 occurred between 7 and 28 years postoperatively. Life table analysis of their data indicated an incidence of 27% at 15 years. The incidence of *thoracic* aortic aneurysms in these two reports is not known.

Coselli et al.[12] recently reviewed 123 patients who had aneurysms of the proximal aorta following repair of an infrarenal aortic aneurysm. The mean time between first and second operations was 8.2 years. Eighty-two percent of the aneurysms were in continuity with the previously placed prosthetic graft, and 76.4% involved the thoracoabdominal aorta.

PRESENTATION

Symptomatic recurrent aortic aneurysms may present with abdominal or chest pain, a palpable mass, embolization, or rupture. The majority of recurrent aneurysms, however, are probably asymptomatic. Curl et al.[3] reported 21 patients with aneurysmal changes above previous aortic anastomoses in patients undergoing infrarenal reconstruction (14 for aneurysmal disease and 7 for occlusive disease). They found 12 false and 9 true aneurysms. Fourteen of these 21 patients were asymptomatic, except for an abdominal mass. Seven patients had symptoms of acute expansion and, of these, 3 patients presented with rupture and 1 with thrombosis. Gautier et al.[13] performed a study of 13 patients with infrarenal anastomotic aneurysms and found 4 presenting with abdominal pain, 2 with distal embolization, and 1 with intestinal hemorrhage. We recently identified another 19 patients with recurrent aortic aneurysms operated on between January 1989 and December 1995. The denominator for these patients is unknown, as many of the patients were referred. There were 10 aortic pseudoaneurysms and 10 true aortic aneurysms, 1 patient having both. The time between the two operations averaged 5 years with a range of 3 months and 12.2 years. Interestingly enough, 13 of the 19 patients were symptomatic with 4 ruptures in this group.

DETECTION

The importance of strict and prolonged follow-up, early detection of recurrent aortic aneurysms, and elective repair is emphasized by the poor results of operation for ruptured recurrent true and false aortic aneurysms. Twenty-five patients in the Mayo Clinic series with recurrent aortic aneurysms presented with rupture and died.[4] Thoracic aortic aneurysms occurred in 24 of these patients and was the cause of death of 20. All 15 patients presenting with ruptured thoracic aortic aneurysms died. Three patients presented with recurrent ruptured thoracoabdominal aortic aneurysms and all died. Of 11 abdominal aortic aneurysms, 6 were ruptured at presentation, and all of these patients died. In Cronenwett's compilation of three large series, rupture of other aneurysms accounted for 12% of late mortality in patients having had previous abdominal aortic aneurysm repair.[14]

Gloviczki et al.[2] reported a 47% mortality for emergent repairs of recurrent aortic aneurysms. Further, 4 of 55 patients presenting with synchronous aneurysms experienced rupture of the second aneurysm following repair of the first while awaiting their next elective operation.

Treiman et al.[1] reported a 67% mortality for ruptured para-anastomotic aneurysms of the aorta and iliac arteries. Eriksson et al.[15] reported on patients with rupture of pararenal aortic aneurysms. Although none of the patients had *recurrent* aneurysms, there was a 20% mortality for urgent operations (nonruptured) and a 42.8% mortality for patients with rupture.

Thus, the single most important step in treating recurrent aortic aneurysms is that of diagnosis. Although ultrasonography can clearly image the infrarenal abdominal aorta, it does not demonstrate well the suprarenal abdominal or thoracic aorta and may fail to reveal iliac artery aneurysmal disease, especially in overweight patients. Recurrent aortic aneurysms present late, occurring as late as 20 years postoperatively. Routine annual reexamination of these patients is paramount. The abdominal aorta and thoracic aorta are best visualized by computed tomography (CT) scanning. CT scans of the thorax, abdomen, and pelvis every third or fourth year during follow-up without contrast would seem a reasonable method of following these patients. Admittedly, the frequency for obtaining such examinations remains empiric. The use of magnetic resonance imaging and magnetic resonance angiography, especially with gadolinium enhancement, is under investigation and shows great promise.[16–18] More clinical correlation in comparison with conventional techniques will be needed before the value of these newer technologies is known.

RECONSTRUCTION

Recurrent aortic aneurysms require direct aortic reconstruction. Endovascular techniques may have promise for some of these aneurysms, especially true aneurysms of the thoracic aorta not in continuity with previously placed grafts.[19] Long-term data concerning endovascular repair of these aneurysms are not yet available, but in some of these poor risk patients, the concept of endovascular repair is appealing. For the present, conventional repair is the treatment of choice. Appropriate decisions concerning sites of incision, method and extent of exposure, clamp placement, and methods of repair are influenced by the previous repair, the site of recurrence, the type of recurrence, and the presence of concomitant occlusive as well as aneurysmal disease. The patient's overall health is critical to the decision-making process.

Size criteria for operation on true aortic aneurysms, whether primary or recurrent, is dealt with in detail elsewhere in this book. In general, the same size criteria are used to help determine the need for intervention for these recurrent *true* aortic aneurysms as for primary aortic aneurysms. A more aggressive stance is justified for recurrent aortic *anastomotic* aneurysms, because these aneurysms are prone to rapid expansion and rupture.[1]

Infrarenal abdominal aortic aneurysms arising following repair of thoracoabdominal or thoracic aortic aneurysms are treated in the usual manner. Similarly, thoracic or thoracoabdominal aneurysms arising in patients who have undergone repair of abdominal aortic aneurysms are handled in standard manner. If the recurrent aneurysms are contiguous with the old graft, the appropriate anastomosis may be made to that graft. If there is normal, healthy aorta interposed between the two aneurysms, it may be preferable to preserve that portion of the aorta, especially so if visceral, intercostal, or lumbar arteries arise from that segment. Fox and Berkowitz[20] found no difference in mortality or morbidity for repair of thoracoabdominal aneurysm repairs in patients who had had previous infrarenal abdominal aortic aneurysm repair and in those who had not undergone previous abdominal aortic reconstructions. Recurrent thoracic aortic aneurysms may be approached by standard posterolateral thoracotomy. In a variation of that, Walterbusch et al.[21] report repair of distal arch and proximal thoracic aortic lesions via an anteroaxillary thoracotomy. This approach was used in 14 patients, 3 of whom had false aneurysms. They reported 2 deaths, both in patients presenting with rupture. The patient is positioned at a 45-degree angle on a slightly flexed table. The skin incision begins in the axillary groove at the edge of the latisimus dorsi muscle and curves toward the submammary line. The thoracic cavity is entered through the fourth intercostal space.

Interestingly, patients presenting with thoracic aneurysms are more likely to develop a second aneurysm than those patients presenting with abdominal aortic aneurysms. Gloviczki et al.[2] found that 2% of patients having repair of abdominal aortic aneurysms underwent eventual repair of a second or third aneurysm in contrast to 18% of patients seen initially with thoracic aortic aneurysms. Bickerstaff et al.[22] in their study of thoracic aortic aneurysms found associated abdominal aortic aneurysms in one-quarter of their patients. Crawford and Cohen[23] reported 68% of their patients with descending thoracic aneurysms had multiple aneurysms in contrast to 12% of their patients with abdominal aortic aneurysms.

JUXTARENAL VERSUS SUPRARENAL AORTIC ANEURYSMS

The greatest technical demands made of vascular surgeons in dealing with recurrent aortic aneurysms are those faced when repairing thoracoabdominal aortic and pararenal (juxtarenal and suprarenal) aortic aneurysms. The repair of thoracoabdominal aortic aneurysms is described elsewhere.

Juxtarenal abdominal aortic aneurysms may be approached through an abdominal incision. If the aneurysm is not a suprarenal one, exposure may usually be obtained through a standard midline transperitoneal infracolic approach. Some authors have advocated routine retroperitoneal exposures through flank or low-lying thoracoabdominal incisions.[24–26] The experience of my colleagues and myself is that these incisions are not routinely necessary for juxtarenal abdominal aortic aneurysms. Even if the aneurysm extends to the level of the superior mesenteric artery, supramesenteric clamping through the standard approach can usually be achieved. Body habitus especially and previous operation influence these choices to a great extent and must be individualized. Division and ligation of the left renal vein may be helpful in exposing juxtarenal and suprarenal aneurysms. If there is associated left renal artery occlusive disease that requires reconstruction, we prefer, if at all possible, to mobilize the vein rather than divide it. Division of the diaphragmatic crura cephalad to the renal arteries aids in mobilization of the pararenal aorta and the renal arteries, and allows for easier dissection and clamping of the supramesenteric aorta. If this approach proves difficult, subdiaphragmatic clamping of the supraceliac aorta, as described by Crawford et al.,[27] may be used. A certain percentage of patients referred with "suprarenal" abdominal aortic aneurysms have in fact juxtarenal or indeed infrarenal aneurysms. Computed tomography scans may be misleading. The aorta elongates as well as expands and its upper extent may appear to involve the renal arteries when, in reality, the aneurysm is simply "bulging" superiorly. A lateral aortogram demonstrates this relationship accurately.[27,28] Growing familiarity with CT scanning has allowed more accurate preoperative assessment of the true anatomy by that modality.[29]

Suprarenal aortic aneurysms pose a greater challenge than do juxtarenal aortic aneurysms. They are usually not well approached through a standard midline transperitoneal infracolic exposure. Medial visceral rotation, however, will provide excellent exposure of the entire subdiaphragmatic aorta. In most instances, the left kidney and adrenal gland are mobilized medially with the other viscera. If reconstruction of the superior mesenteric artery is necessary, it is probably better to leave the left kidney in its bed or have it mobilized in such a way that it can be rotated medially and placed back in its bed as necessary. A retro-aortic left renal vein may also mitigate against mobilization of the left kidney. If the aneurysm extends to the level of the diaphragm (Crawford Type IV thoracoabdominal aortic aneurysm), medial visceral rotation is sometimes applicable and has been employed recently at our institution. In most instances, a low thoracoabdominal incision is preferable.

Qvarfordt et al.[30] from the University of California–San Francisco (UCSF) reporting their experience with pararenal aneurysms in 77 patients had only a 1.3% mortality. Seventy percent of those patients required renal artery reconstruction for aneurysmal involvement or occlusive disease. Their morbidity was 28% and was usually transient renal insufficiency. B-mode transesophageal cardiac monitoring was used in these patients. Clamping levels were supraceliac in 13 patients, supramesenteric in 17 patients, suprarenal in 45 patients, and above 1 renal artery only in 2 patients. The standard transperitoneal infracolic approach was employed in 92% of the patients and a thoracoabdominal retroperitoneal approach in the other patients. Since that time, that group has employed medial visceral rotation in preference to both other approaches.[31,32]

Crawford et al.[27] reporting on 101 patients with juxtarenal aneurysms had a 7% mortality. They included patients presenting with rupture. In the majority of cases they employed a midline approach with subdiaphragmatic clamping. Most deaths were secondary to renal and cardiac complications.

Tordoir et al.[25] reported 15 patients with pararenal aortic aneurysms, for whom they employed a thoracoabdominal approach with retroperitoneal exposure. Twelve of their 15 patients were clamped suprarenally and the others infrarenally. There were no deaths but 1 permanent renal failure.

Eriksson and colleagues[15] reported 46 patients having pararenal aortic aneurysms. A transabdominal approach was used in 45 of these patients. In the other patient, a thoracoabdominal incision was employed. Two patients were clamped at the supraceliac level, 1 at the supramesenteric level, 20 at the suprarenal level, and 23 above 1 renal artery. Their mortality was 7.4% for elective operations.

Poulias and colleagues[28] reported a more recent experience with juxtarenal aneurysms in 38 patients and had a 5% mortality. They employed a midline approach with suprarenal clamping.

The excellent results reported by Qvarfordt et al.[30] for their primary pararenal aneurysms may not be attainable for recurrent aortic aneurysms. Because these recurrences present late in the patient's follow-up, usually into the second decade postoperatively, the patients are older. The previous dissection and reconstruction make reoperation more technically difficult. These factors undoubtedly contribute to the higher mortality reported with recurrent aortic aneurysm repair. Isolated series, however, such as that from Sato and colleagues[33] on 11 aortic pseudoaneurysms report no mortality. Many of the patients in Sato's series had Takayasu's arteritis rather than atherosclerosis, and the mean age was 55 years. That disease entity and the relative youth of the patients probably favorably influenced the results, in contrast to the figures for older atherosclerotic patients.

Gloviczki and colleagues[2] at the Mayo Clinic reporting on operations for multiple aortic aneurysms had an 8% mortality for elective repairs of both thoracic and abdominal aortic aneurysms. Mortality increased with the number of procedures performed: 4.7% for the first operation, 10.4% for the second, and 33.3% for the third.

Treiman et al.[1] reporting on 18 patients with anastomotic aneurysms of the aorta and iliac arteries had an 8% elective mortality. Small pseudoaneurysms initially observed by them expanded rapidly over a short period and one of these ruptured.

Curl et al.[3] reported their experience with 21 patients having abdominal aortic aneurysms proximal to a previous aortic reconstruction. Twelve had anastomotic aneurysms and 9 true aneurysms. Their mortality was 24%, including those patients presenting with rupture and those with suprarenal aneurysms. The mortality for elective infrarenal reconstructions in this group of patients was 11%. Coselli et al.[12] from Baylor, in a recent series of 123 recurrent aortic aneurysms seen in patients previously treated for infrarenal abdominal aortic aneurysms, reported hospital mortality of 12.2% and renal failure of 11.4%. Seventy-six (76.4%) of their patients had thoracoabdominal aneurysms. Hospital mortality for 17 patients with juxtarenal aortic aneurysms was 5.9%.

INCISIONS

The choices for incisions through which to approach recurrent aortic aneurysms are many as the previously cited articles demonstrate, and fortunately quite good. Shepard and his colleagues at both the New England Medical Center[24] and the Henry Ford Hospital[26] described excellent results with an extended left flank incision and a retroperitoneal approach mobilizing the left kidney anteriorly. In the earlier report, 23 high-risk patients with abdominal aortic aneurysms were reported.[24] Fourteen of these patients required suprarenal or supraceliac clamping for pararenal aortic aneurysm or associated occlusive disease. There was only 1 death in this group (4%). In the later report, this approach was used in 85 complex aortic reconstructions, 70 of which were for aneurysmal disease.[26] One-half of these latter patients had pararenal aortic aneurysms. Suprarenal and supraceliac clamping was performed in 43 of the patients. Elective mortality was 1.2%.

In the left flank retroperitoneal approach, the patient is placed on the operating room table in a modified left thoracotomy position with the shoulder at a 70- to 80-degree angle relative to the table and the hips as flat as possible.[21] The patient's left flank is centered over the break in the table and the table extended to widen the exposure. An oblique incision is made from the lateral edge of the rectus abdominus muscle midway between the umbilicus and the symphysis pubis and extended into the appropriate intercostal space depending on the proximal extent of the aneurysmal aortic or visceral anatomy and the reconstruction intended. This exposure is very similar to the modified thoracoabdominal exposure advocated by Stoney and Wylie.[34]

The UCSF group as noted earlier has had excellent results with midline approaches and with thoracoabdominal approaches like that described earlier.[30] Subsequently, they have utilized a medial visceral rotation through a midline incision more frequently.[31,32] The patient is approached through a midline incision. The dissection is extraperitoneal, if possible. The spleen is dissected from its posterior and diaphragmatic attachments and the viscera rotated and mobilized medially. This allows easy visualization and control of the subdiaphragmatic aorta and the visceral branches. If higher exposure is needed, an incision of the crura or the medial portions of the diaphragm allows exposure of the low lying thoracic aorta. If extensive dissection of the superior mesenteric artery is necessary, the left kidney and adrenal are better left in their beds. Our experience would echo that of the San Francisco group: Medial visceral rotation allows excellent exposure of the entire abdominal aorta in most patients.

All of these exposures—thoracoabdominal, flank, and midline with medial visceral rotation—are excellent, providing thorough visualization and control of the involved aorta. The flank incision and the abdominal incision with visceral rotation are probably less morbid than the thoracoabdominal incision, especially in those patients with chronic obstructive pulmonary disease. However, all of the incisions are employed depending on the surgeon's preference, the patient's disease and body habitus, coexistent intra-abdominal pathology, and the overall status of the patient.

The placement of proximal clamps in the reconstruction of recurrent pararenal abdominal aortic aneurysms is a vital matter. The University of Rochester found supra-renal clamping to have a higher mortality than supraceliac clamping (32% versus 3%) with a higher incidence of frank renal failure (23% versus 3%).[35] It was believed that embolization of atherosclerotic debris accounted for these differences. Breckwoldt and colleagues[36] at the New England Medical Center found suprarenal clamping safe in their experience when compared to infrarenal clamping. Mortality was 1.2% for the patients having infrarenal clamping and 2.6% for the patients with suprarenal clamps. Transient renal insufficiency was more marked in the suprarenal group (28%) than in the infrarenal group (10%), but dialysis rates were not different for the two groups (3% and 2%).

Nypaver and colleagues[37] at the Henry Ford Hospital found supraceliac clamping to be well tolerated *unless* concomitant mesenteric or renal artery occlusive disease necessitating repair was present. There was a significant incidence of ischemic visceral complications when these concomitant reconstructions were necessary. Cross-clamp time was increased when these additional reconstructions were performed. The morbidity was 25% in those patients requiring concomitant repairs versus 0% in those patients not.

Allen and colleagues[38] from Washington University detailed excellent results in 65 patients undergoing repair of pararenal aortic aneurysms. They used all of the approaches mentioned earlier and placed their clamps selectively—suprarenal in 40%, supramesenteric in 18.5%, and supraceliac in 41%. They could find no difference in mortality as a result of site of clamp placement. There was only 1 death in this series. Only 3 of the 65 patients were operated on for recurrent abdominal aortic aneurysms.

Supramesenteric clamping is often a good choice as evidenced by the reports from San Francisco[30] and Saint Louis.[38] That has been our experience. In appropriately chosen patients exposure is excellent. There are probably fewer cardiac effects with supramesenteric clamping as opposed to supraceliac clamping because of the maintenance of gastric, splenic, and hepatic blood flow. The sustained flow helps unload the heart and reduces liver and gut ischemia. Patients have to be selected properly. Lateral aortograms are particularly vital in this selection process as severe posterior plaquing of the aorta above an aneurysm is not infrequently encountered. The use of all the approaches mentioned and of all the various clamp sites, individualized to the patient at hand, yields superior results as demonstrated by the report from Washington University.[38]

Stenting of the ureters has been advocated by the Northwestern group for redo operations.[39] The UCSF group does not employ them in their extensive reoperative practice.[32] Both have excellent results. Potential ureteral problems are more problematic when reconstructions are performed for secondary occlusions or aneurysmal disease *distal* to a previously placed aortic graft. We have employed selective stenting of ureters at our institution. This is usually done for patients with hydroureter, fixed points of kinking or stenosis, or other identified pathologic features.

CONCLUSION

The extent of repair for recurrent aortic aneurysms is determined by the extent of the recurrent aneurysm itself, the status of the previous repair, and other concomitant vascular problems, including distal aneurysmal or occlusive disease. The most important step in treating these aneurysms is in detecting them. Serial follow-up, including periodic CT scans of the chest and abdomen, of all patients having had an aortic aneurysm repair is to be encouraged. Patients having had thoracic aortic aneurysm repairs are much more likely to develop a second aneurysm than those having had abdominal aortic aneurysm reconstructions. Patients with hypertension are more likely to develop a second aneurysm than normotensive patients. The indications for operation on recurrent true aortic aneurysms, especially those not contiguous with the previously placed prosthesis, are essentially the same as for primary aortic aneurysms in the respective locations. Recurrent false aneurysms should be repaired in all but the most high-risk patients because these aneurysms have a propensity for rapid expansion and rupture with high reported operative mortality. Repair of recurrent aortic aneurysms has a higher morbidity and mortality than that of primary aneurysms. The choice of incision and exposure and the site of clamp placement are made on an individual basis. These decisions are related to the surgeon's preference, patient's body habitus, the extent of disease, both aneurysmal and occlusive, and the reconstruction anticipated.

REFERENCES

1. Treiman GS, Weaver FA, Cossman DV, et al. Anastomotic false aneurysms of the abdominal aorta and the iliac arteries. *J Vasc Surg.* 1988;8:268–273.
2. Gloviczki P, Pairolero PC, Welch T, et al. Multiple aortic aneurysms: the results of surgical management. *J Vasc Surg.* 1990;11:19–28.
3. Curl GR, Faggioli GL, Stella A, et al. Aneurysmal change at or above the proximal anastomosis after infrarenal aortic grafting. *J Vasc Surg.* 1992;16:855–860.
4. Plate G, Hollier LA, O'Brien P, et al. Recurrent aneurysms and late vascular complications following repair of abdominal aortic aneurysms. *Arch Surg.* 1985;120:590–594.
5. Watanabe T, Kusaba A, Kuma H, et al. Failure of Dacron arterial prostheses caused by structural defects. *J Cardiovasc Surg.* 1983;24:95–100.

6. Ratto GB, Truini M, Sacco A, et al. Multiple aneurysmal dilatations in a knitted Dacron velour graft. *J Cardiovasc Surg.* 1985;26:589–591.

7. Szilagyi DE, Smith RF, Elliott JP, et al. Anastomotic aneurysms after vascular reconstruction: problems of incidence, etiology, and treatment. *Surgery.* 1975;78:800–816.

8. Crawford ES, Saleh SA, Babb JW III, et al. Infrarenal abdominal aortic aneurysm: factors influencing survival after operation performed over a 25-year period. *Ann Surg.* 1981;193:699–709.

9. Van den Akker PJ, Brand R, van Schilfgaarde R, et al. False aneurysms after prosthetic reconstructions for aortoiliac obstructive disease. *Ann Surg.* 1989 210:658–666.

10. Sieswerda C, Skotnicki SH, Barentsz JO, Heystraten FM. Anastomotic aneurysms—an under-diagnosed complication after aorto-iliac reconstructions. *Eur J Vasc Surg.* 1989;3:233–238.

11. Edwards JM, Teefey SA, Zierler E, Kohler TR. Intraabdominal paraanastomotic aneurysms after aortic bypass grafting. *J Vasc Surg.* 1992;15:344–350.

12. Coselli JS, LeMaire SA, Buket S, Berzin E. Subsequent proximal aortic operations in 123 patients with previous infrarenal abdominal aortic aneurysm surgery. *J Vasc Surg.* 1995;22(1):59–67.

13. Gautier C, Borie H, Lagneau P. Aortic false aneurysms after prosthetic reconstruction of the infrarenal aorta. *Ann Vasc Surg.* 1992;6(5):413–417.

14. Cronenwett JL. Factors influencing the long-term results of aortic aneurysm surgery. In: Yao JST, Pearce WH, eds. *Long-term Results in Vascular Surgery.* Norwalk, CT: Appleton & Lange; 1993:171–179.

15. Eriksson I, Bowald S, Karacagil S. Surgical treatment of pararenal abdominal aortic aneurysms. *Int Angiol.* 1988;7:7–13.

16. Kaufman JA, Yucel EK, Waltman AC, et al. MR angiography in the preoperative evaluation of abdominal aortic aneurysms: a preliminary study. *J Vasc Interv Radiol.* 1994;5(3):489–496.

17. Petersen MJ, Cambria RP, Kaufman JA, et al. Magnetic resonance angiography in the preoperative evaluation of abdominal aortic aneurysms. *J Vasc Surg.* 1995;21(6):891–899.

18. Prince MR, Narasimham DL, Stanley JC, et al. Gadolinium-enhanced magnetic resonance angiography of abdominal aortic aneurysms. *J Vasc Surg.* 1995;21(4):656–668.

19. Parodi JC. Endovascular repair of abdominal aortic aneurysms and other arterial lesions. *J Vasc Surg.* 1995;21(4):549–557.

20. Fox AD, Berkowitz HD. Thoracoabdominal aneurysm resection after previous infrarenal abdominal aortic aneurysmectomy. *Am J Surg.* 1991;162:142–144.

21. Walterbusch G, Marr U, Abramov V, Fromke J. The antero-axillary thoracotomy for operations of the distal aortic arch and the proximal descending aorta. *Eur J Cardiothor Surg.* 1994;8:79–81.

22. Bickerstaff LK, Pairolero PC, Hollier LH, et al. Thoracic aortic aneurysms: a population-based study. *Surgery.* 1982;92:1103–1108.

23. Crawford ES, Cohen ES. Aortic aneurysm: a multifocal disease. *Arch Surg.* 1982;117:1393–1400.

24. Shepard AD, Scott GR, Mackey WC, et al. Retroperitoneal approach to high-risk abdominal aortic aneurysms. *Arch Surg.* 1986;121:444–449.

25. Tordoir JHM, van de Pavoordt HDWM, Eikelboom BC, et al. Thoracoabdominal aortic approach for the treatment of pararenal aneurysm. *Neth J Med.* 1988;40:1–5.

26. Shepard AD, Tollefson DFJ, Reddy DJ, et al. Left flank retroperitoneal exposure: a technical aid to complex aortic reconstruction. *J Vasc Surg.* 1991;14:283–291.

27. Crawford ES, Beckett WC, Greer MS. Juxtarenal infrarenal abdominal aortic aneurysm: special diagnostic and therapeutic considerations. *Ann Surg.* 1986;203:661–670.

28. Poulias GE, Doundoulakis N, Skoutas B, et al. Juxtarenal abdominal aneurysmectomy. *J Vasc Surg.* 1992;3:324–330.

29. Rubin GD, Dake MD, Napel S, et al. Spiral CT of renal artery stenosis: comparison of three-dimensional rendering techniques. *Radiology.* 1994;190(1):181–189.

30. Qvarfordt PG, Stoney RJ, Reilly LM, et al. Management of pararenal aneurysms of the abdominal aorta. *J Vasc Surg.* 1986;3:84–93.

31. Sauer L, Stoney RJ. Management of juxtarenal aortic occlusive disease by transabdominal exposure of the pararenal and suprarenal aorta by medial visceral rotation. In: Ernst CB, Stanley JC, eds. *Current Therapy in Vascular Surgery.* 2nd ed. Philadelphia: Decker; 1991.

32. Stoney RJ. Strategies for reoperation of the abdominal aorta. *Perspect Vasc Surg.* 1991;4:31–47.
33. Sato O, Tada Y, Miyata T, Shindo S. False aneurysms after aortic operations. *J Cardiovasc Surg.* 1992;33:604–608.
34. Stoney RJ, Wylie EJ. Surgical management of arterial lesions of the thoracoabdominal aorta. *Am J Surg.* 1973;126:157–164.
35. Green RM, Ricotta JJ, Ouriel K, DeWeese JA. Results of supraceliac aortic clamping in the difficult elective resection of infrarenal abdominal aortic aneurysm. *J Vasc Surg.* 1989;9:124–134.
36. Breckwoldt WL, Mackey WC, Belkin M, O'Donnell TF Jr. The effect of suprarenal cross-clamping on abdominal aortic aneurysm repair. *Arch Surg.* 1992;127:520–524.
37. Nypaver TJ, Shepard AD, Reddy DJ, et al. Supraceliac aortic cross-clamping: determinants of outcome in elective abdominal aortic reconstruction. *J Vasc Surg.* 1993;17:868–876.
38. Allen BT, Anderson CB, Rubin BG, et al. Preservation of renal function in juxtarenal and suprarenal abdominal aortic aneurysm repair. *J Vasc Surg.* 1993;17:948–959.
39. Yao JST, Flinn WR, Rizzo RJ, et al. Recurrent aortic and anastomotic aneurysms. In: Bergan JJ, Yao JST, eds., *Aortic Surgery.* Philadelphia: WB Saunders; 1989:305–316.

33

Redo Operations for Renal or Visceral Artery Occlusions

Darren B. Schneider, MD, and Ronald J. Stoney, MD

Revascularization of the major paired (renal) and unpaired (visceral) branches of the upper abdominal aorta can successfully relieve manifestations of ischemia in these critical vascular beds. The first reports describing renal endarterectomy were by Freeman et al.[1] in 1954, and mesenteric endarterectomy by Shaw and Maynard[2] in 1958 for atherosclerotic disease affecting this segment of the aorta and its branches. Soon bypass grafting with prosthetic materials and with autogenous vein were introduced as alternative techniques, which could also be applied to nonatherosclerotic renal or visceral artery lesions.[3,4] These procedures relied on simplified exposure of the infrarenal aorta, retrograde graft alignment, and distal exposure of the artery for graft attachment to provide improved renal or visceral blood flow. More recently the percutaneous, catheter-based interventions of balloon dilatation and stenting have been used for renal artery lesions caused by fibromuscular dysplasia as well as nonostial atherosclerotic lesions of the renal or visceral branches.[5]

Symptomatic visceral artery occlusive disease is caused by atherosclerosis in more than 95% of reported series. Atherosclerosis and fibromuscular dysplasia are the predominant causes of renal artery occlusive disease, while a variety of other disorders including congenital, inflammatory, traumatic, and other entrapment entities are occasionally seen. The widespread interest in detecting renovascular hypertension and the potential for its treatment by percutaneous interventions have altered the demographics of patients who ultimately require operative renal revascularization.[6] Most of the patients, like those requiring mesenteric revascularization, have atherosclerosis, but they are elderly with generalized atherosclerosis, and often hypertensive cardiomyopathy. Frequently, they have impaired renal function or ischemic nephropathy in addition to their multiple-drug-resistant hypertension.

Currently patients undergoing revascularization for symptomatic visceral or renal ischemia have advanced atherosclerotic occlusive disease of the paravisceral or pararenal aorta. Transaortic endarterectomy, an established, successful, and highly durable technique, is used frequently by those familiar and accomplished with this technically demanding procedure (Figs. 33–1 and 33–2). Most surgeons, however, prefer bypass grafting techniques that vary widely, although antegrade aortovisceral grafts (Fig. 33–3) and direct or extra-anatomic aortorenal grafts are popular. Prograde and retrograde

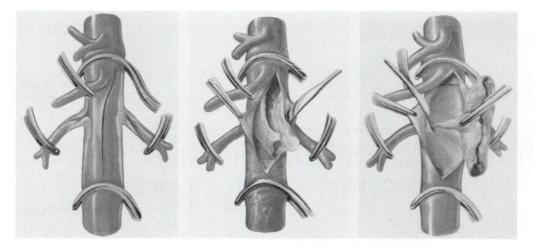

Figure 33–1. Diagrammatic representation of transaortic renal endarterectomy. Note the proximal and distal aortic clamp occlusion. The aortotomy extends proximal and lateral to the superior mesenteric artery (SMA).

graft alignment in selected experiences do produce satisfactory results.[7,8] The conduit used for grafting also varies, but, in the absence of contamination, prosthetic knitted Dacron tube or bifurcated graft configurations are preferred. Factors that influence the behavior of any aortic branch revascularization, and ultimately its long-term durability, involve the patient or the surgeon. In the remainder of this chapter we consider these factors, as well as the methods we employ to correct failed prior renal and visceral reconstructions, including the selection and use of revascularization techniques following failed angioplasty or stenting.

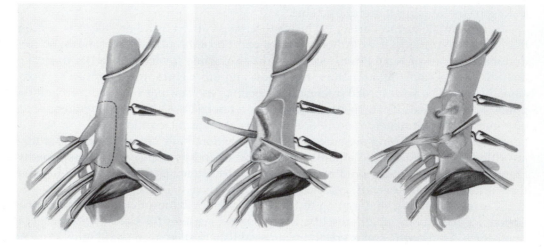

Figure 33–2. Diagrammatic representation of transaortic visceral endarterectomy using trapdoor aortotomy (*left*). The trapdoor is opened and hinged on the right aortic wall (*middle*). Note endarterectomy proceeding with removal of SMA lesion (*right*).

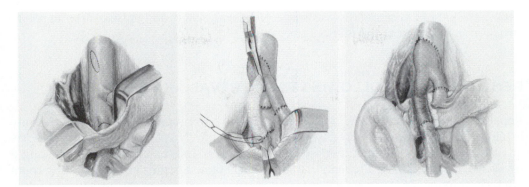

Figure 33–3. Diagrammatic representation of antegrade aortovisceral bypass using a bifurcated graft. Note location of the proximal anastomosis on the supraceliac aorta (*left*). After completion of the aortic anastomosis flow is restored through the aorta with the individual graft limbs clamped (*middle*). Completed bypass (*right*).

FACTORS INFLUENCING THE OUTCOME OF RENAL AND VISCERAL RECONSTRUCTIONS

To undertake reoperation successfully following failed renal or visceral operations the surgeon needs to understand the factors that are known to contribute to or cause early and late repair failures. The patient factors include the type, pattern, and distribution of disease for which the original operation was performed, and the precise type and conduct of the original operation. In any late repair failure, the patient's healing responses following the original operation, and the natural history and changes in the affected arteries are important.

The surgeon factors rest on the surgeon's experience in aortic branch revascularization, including proper selection and execution of the original repair and objectively determining the technical adequacy of the repair intraoperatively. The surgeon factors also include experience with aortic and aortic branch reconstruction failures, and the ability to identify unanticipated critical findings that warrant modification of the original surgical plan in order to achieve the objective of complete revascularization.

COMBINED AORTIC AND RENAL ARTERY DISEASE

A number of recent publications have focused on aortorenal revascularization in the presence of significant aortic occlusive or aneurysmal disease using a variety of different techniques.[9,10] Extra-anatomic renal revascularization has been advocated by some authors for the treatment of renovascular hypertension in patients with a severely diseased aorta.[11,12] While restoring renal blood flow, some of these techniques avoid treatment of the diseased aorta altogether. Following our success in treating combined aortic and renal branch lesions for more than four decades, we employ transaortic renal endarterectomy prior to anastomosis of a graft to the pararenal aorta for the treatment of combined severe aortorenal atherosclerosis with an acceptable operative mortality of 4%.[13] Using proven techniques for aortic and renal artery revascularization in combination, the patient's arterial disease is addressed completely and optimal arterial reconstruction is achieved at the original operation.

RENAL ISCHEMIA FOLLOWING RENAL REVASCULARIZATION

Renal revascularization using aortorenal bypass or transaortic renal endarterectomy achieves cure or improvement of hypertension in 85% to 95% of cases.[14,15] Early postoperative ischemia may produce persistent hypertension and/or azotemia, suggesting a revascularization failure. Prevention of a technical failure begins in the operating room after completion of the repair. Detection of an inadequate or incomplete operative repair using intraoperative duplex scanning is highly effective. Any major defects can be immediately corrected, producing an overall early patency rate of greater than 95%.[16]

Late ischemia, appearing many months to years following the repair, is due to adverse healing of the primary repair, or progression of the native disease. Late failures are now detected earlier by use of regular postoperative surveillance, including determination of blood pressure and renal function (BUN, creatinine), and transabdominal duplex ultrasonography.[17] Arteriography may define focal myointimal hyperplasia causing stenosis, and anastomotic or fibrotic strictures, which on occasion will respond to percutaneous balloon angioplasty or stenting. Diffuse lesions and more complex disease patterns require operative repair, sometimes including *ex vivo* renal preservation and microvascular repair when disease extends to the renal artery branches.[18] Progressive aortic atherosclerosis may compromise flow at the proximal end of an aortorenal graft and may be revised using aortic endarterectomy or limited aortic graft replacement at the origin of the renal graft.

VISCERAL ISCHEMIA FOLLOWING VISCERAL REVASCULARIZATION

Primary visceral revascularizations usually employ some form of aortovisceral bypass or, less commonly, transaortic visceral endarterectomy. Both techniques are comparable and achieve prolonged durability with low operative mortality.[19-24] Perioperative technical failures are preventable using meticulous, proven visceral revascularization techniques in combination with intraoperative duplex ultrasonography to confirm patency and high flow rates within the repair.[16] Identification of major defects that affect flow can be promptly corrected at the original operation. Early postoperative failure of mesenteric revascularization usually presents as acute mesenteric infarction. Unfortunately, this complication may be identified late because of the expected pattern of postoperative abdominal pain. Metabolic acidosis, peritonitis, and sepsis develop rapidly, so any change in a patient's routine postoperative course should arouse suspicion. Prompt reexploration can reveal extensive visceral infarction, but lesser degrees of ischemia may allow a revision of the revascularization and salvage crucial segments of compromised viscera.

Late failures following visceral repair are manifest by recurrent chronic visceral ischemia in about 75% of patients. These can be confirmed by duplex ultrasonography and aortography (anterioposterior and lateral views), which define the flow-limiting disease and status of the original repair (Fig. 33–4). Focal stenosis may possibly be improved by percutaneous balloon angioplasty or stent placement. Extensive disease causing occlusion requires reoperation, often with conversion to a technique that was not used with the original revascularization. For example, if the failed original revascu-

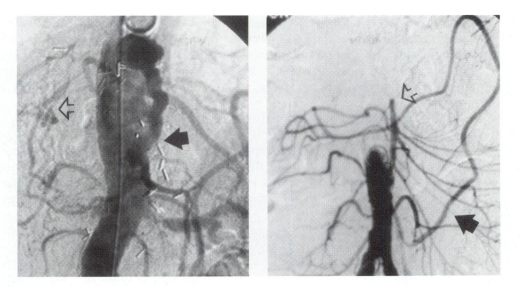

Figure 33–4. Anteroposterior angiographic views of a failed aortovisceral bypass procedure. (*Left*) Patent bypass graft from the supraceliac aorta to the proximal SMA (*solid arrow*) with SMA occlusion distal to the anastomosis. Occluded extra-anatomic hepatomesenteric graft (*open arrow*). (*Right*) Distal SMA (*open arrow*) circulation supplied via collaterals from the IMA (*solid arrow*).

larization was an antegrade aortovisceral bypass, conversion to a transaortic visceral endarterectomy would be an effective revascularization for the problem. The other 25% of patients presenting with late recurrent visceral ischemia following failed visceral repair develop acute visceral ischemia. This occurs when the repair fails rapidly due to sudden thrombosis or embolic occlusion, and a protective collateral circulation has not been established. End-organ visceral ischemia proceeds rapidly to infarction, precluding a successful reoperative revascularization for most of these critically ill patients.

OPERATIVE MANAGEMENT OF FAILED RENAL OR VISCERAL BRANCH REVASCULARIZATION

The surgical management of failed renal or visceral branch revascularization may be challenging for the vascular surgeon, and potentially threatening for the organs at risk. Patients are typically elderly and suffer from not only renal or mesenteric artery disease, but systemic atherosclerosis; concomitant coronary artery disease contributes importantly to the increased operative risk of these patients. Nonetheless, the consequences of nonoperative management of recurrent aortorenal or aortovisceral occlusive disease, renal failure or visceral gangrene, are not an option. The reoperative approach is aimed at complete revascularization of viscera at risk. There are no published standards regarding the surgical approach for failed renal or visceral revascularization, but two reports support redo renal revascularization.

Fowl et al.[25] from the Mayo Clinic reported 38 patients who underwent reoperation for recurrent renovascular hypertension. Approximately half the patients underwent revascularization of both kidneys or one kidney with contralateral nephrectomy, while the other half underwent unilateral nephrectomy with an overall hospital mortality of 7.9%. Redo revascularization improved or cured hypertension in 77% of patients and nephrectomy alone produced improvement or cure in 80% of patients. They concluded that redo renal revascularization was the treatment of choice whenever possible in patients with recurrent renal artery stenosis and that nephrectomy should be reserved for the rare patient in whom revascularization is not an option.

Stanley et al.[26] published the University of Michigan experience of 72 reoperations for renovascular hypertension. Only 18 of the reoperations were in patients with atherosclerotic disease, while the majority in this series were for fibromuscular disease, some occurring in pediatric patients. Altogether, there were 31 nephrectomies and 41 revascularization procedures. Hypertension was improved in 91% of all patients and the operative mortality rate was 1.4%. They concluded that although renal reoperation was difficult, it often yielded optimal results.

There are no published series of reoperations for recurrent visceral ischemia. At the University of California–San Francisco, we have performed repeat aortovisceral revascularizations in 18 patients. The majority of patients presented with symptoms of recurrent chronic visceral ischemia, namely, postprandial abdominal pain, weight loss, and altered intestinal motility. Fifteen of the 18 inpatients were treated with antegrade aortovisceral bypass, transaortic endarterectomy, or a combination of both procedures. Perioperative mortality was 5.6%, which is similar to the reported mortality for primary operations.[19] Approximately 80% of the patients were cured or significantly improved by repeat revascularization. The factors that appeared to correlate with failure of the primary operation were intraoperative modification of the intended primary operation or the use of revascularization procedures other than the preferred methods of antegrade aortovisceral bypass or transaortic visceral endarterectomy.

From a review of our experience with failed renal or visceral reconstruction during the past three decades as well as the few published reports it is obvious that recurrent renal or visceral ischemia resulting from a failed primary repair clearly mandate a secondary revascularization. Although reoperations are challenging, they are clearly indicated considering the consequences of renal failure or intestinal gangrene associated with nonoperative management. The principal goal of either primary or secondary aortic branch revascularizations is the same: Improve or restore perfusion to ischemic viscera and viscera at risk for ischemia. Since reoperation requires meticulous dissection in a reoperative field, a thorough preoperative evaluation must include reviewing original arteriograms and operative reports. Repeat aortography is essential, including lateral or oblique views, to define arterial anatomy and extent of disease.

Our operative strategy for failed renal revascularizations involves first avoiding nephrotoxic contrast agents within 72 hours of operation and establishing a diuresis intraoperatively prior to planned renal ischemia. The exposure through a transperitoneal midline incision usually involves the infracolic posterior peritoneal midline. Correction of focal lesions or placement of prosthetic grafts at the site of the native renal arteries may be accomplished through an infracolic exposure. Left medial visceral rotation is used to expose the supraceliac aorta and retropancreatic space. This permits attachment of a prosthetic straight or bifurcated graft to the supraceliac abdominal aorta and routing of the graft limb or limbs to the distal renal arteries for distal anastomosis (Fig. 33–5). This is used only when direct repair is not feasible. Medial visceral rotation (left or right) is also used if the pattern of disease and the repair failure necessitate *ex vivo* repair with perfusion preservation. These techniques with intraoperative duplex scanning should eliminate technical failure and salvage these patients' threatened kidneys.

Our operative approach for redo visceral reconstruction involves first obtaining optimal exposure of the abdominal aorta, usually via medial visceral rotation through a

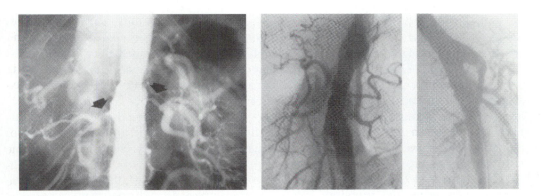

Figure 33–5. Preoperative (*left*) and postoperative views (*middle* and *right*) of a bilateral renal endarterectomy late failure treated successfully with antegrade aortorenal bypass using a bifurcated graft. Note distal anastomosis of graft to the renal arteries close to the hila (*middle*) and proximal aortic anastomosis to the supraceliac aorta (*right*).

full-length midline transabdominal incision. With the use of a self-retaining mechanical retractor system (Omni-Tract Surgical, Minneapolis, MN), unrestricted and safe exposure of the entire upper abdominal aorta and its branches, including the site of the prior repair, is regularly obtained.[27] Moreover, this exposure places no limitations on the choice of arterial reconstruction technique that may be selected. Once the upper abdominal aorta, the affected branches, and previous repair have been exposed the

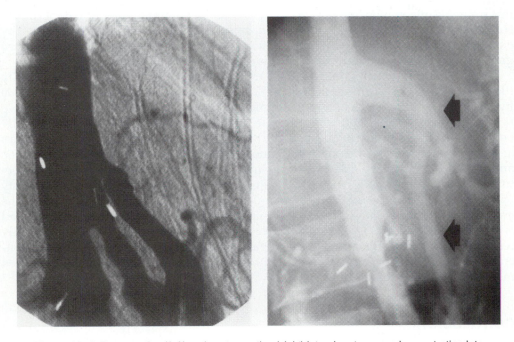

Figure 33–6. Preoperative (*left*) and postoperative (*right*) lateral aortograms demonstrating late reocclusion following transaortic visceral endarterectomy that was successfully revascularized by repeat endarterectomy.

secondary revascularization can be accomplished. Correctable localized defects may be simply repaired; for instance, patch angioplasty may correct a focal anastomotic stricture. If a simple correction is not possible, repeat aortic branch revascularization is employed using either transaortic endarterectomy or antegrade aortovisceral bypass grafting to convert the failed repair to a successful revascularization (Fig. 33–6). Both antegrade bypass and transaortic endarterectomy reliably achieve long-term patency and relief of ischemic symptoms in our experience.[19] Intraoperative duplex ultrasonography to visualize the reconstruction and flow within conduit and native arteries provides immediate assessment of reconstructions and virtually eliminates technical failures.

The preferred techniques of endarterectomy or prosthetic grafting can virtually always be accomplished, therefore, extra-anatomic bypass procedures are not required. Endarterectomy produces an anatomic reconstruction and is preferred for prior failed bypass. Antegrade aortovisceral or aortorenal bypass ensures proper graft inflow alignment and is preferred should a prior visceral endarterectomy fail. Using these guidelines and innovative revascularization techniques guided by the patient's operative findings, redo operation for failed renal and visceral repairs will achieve the goal of restoring blood flow to ischemic viscera or viscera at risk safely and durably.

OPERATIVE MANAGEMENT OF FAILED ANGIOPLASTY OR STENT PLACEMENT

Failure of a catheter-based intervention on either renal or visceral aortic branches may occur early, often immediately following the procedure. The etiology of early failures following percutaneous interventions is either ischemic or hemorrhagic. Hemorrhage usually occurs due to vessel disruption and may be life threatening, requiring urgent operative intervention. Unfortunately, salvage of the kidney by an arterial repair in this setting is uncommon and nephrectomy is usually required. Ischemic complications result from arterial dissection, embolization, or thrombosis of the artery being treated by endovascular procedures. These complications can be frequently corrected by standard grafting techniques or endarterectomy with salvage of the threatened kidney.

Late failures, occurring months to years following catheter-based intervention, in diseased visceral or aortic branches may result from adverse healing (myointimal hyperplasia) or the progression of incompletely treated atherosclerotic disease. These failures are usually detected clinically due to ischemic consequences in the vascular bed supplied by the artery in question. Further evaluation requires imaging techniques and aortography that will accurately define the extent of the lesion. Late restenosis is amenable to the primary operative techniques of prosthetic grafting and endarterectomy. Endarterectomy may be more difficult at the site of prior intervention (angioplasty or stenting), but a cleavage plane can be developed with meticulous dissection. The end point where the plaque terminates is usually beyond the site of intervention, and is therefore not affected. Occlusion of the vessel at the site of prior intervention usually results in thrombus formation, which propagates distally to established reentry collateral vessels. Prosthetic bypass combined with local thrombectomy is the preferred method of restoring blood flow.

CONCLUSION

Redo operation for renal or visceral artery occlusion (including failure of catheter-based interventions) requires an understanding of the factors that contribute to early and late revascularization failures. Life-threatening complications can be prevented by prompt recognition of patients with failed repairs and a thorough preoperative evaluation, followed by surgical correction. Using proven revascularization procedures and meticulous operative technique, the goal of restoring visceral blood flow can be achieved.

REFERENCES

1. Freeman NE, Leeds FH, Elliott WG, Roland SF. Thromboendarterectomy for hypertension due to renal artery occlusion. *JAMA.* 1954;156:1077.
2. Shaw RS, Maynard EP III. Acute and chronic thrombosis of the mesenteric arteries associated with malabsorption: a report of two cases successfully treated by thromboendarterectomy. *N Engl J Med.* 1958;258(18):874–878.
3. Morris CG Jr, Crawford ES, Cooley DA, DeBakey ME. Revascularization of the celiac and superior mesenteric arteries. *Arch Surg.* 1962;84:113–125.
4. Fry WJ, Kraft RO. Visceral angina. *Surg Gynecol Obstet.* 1963;117:417–424.
5. Working Group on Renovascular Hypertension. Detection, evaluation, and treatment of renovascular hypertension—final report. *Arch Intern Med.* 1987;147:820–829.
6. Bredenberg CE, Sampson LN, Ray FS, et al. Changing patterns in surgery for chronic renal artery occlusive diseases. *J Vasc Surg.* 1992;15(6):1018–1023.
7. Gentile AT, Moneta GL, Taylor LM Jr, et al. Isolated bypass to the superior mesenteric artery for intestinal ischemia. *Arch Surg.* 1994;129:926–932.
8. McMillian WD, McCarthy WJ, Bresticker MR, et al. Mesenteric artery bypass: objective patency determination. *J Vasc Surg.* 1995;21:729–741.
9. McNeil JW, String T, Pfeiffer RB Jr. Concomitant renal endarterectomy and aortic reconstruction. *J Vasc Surg.* 1994;20:331–337.
10. Cambria RP, Brewster DC, L'Italien G, et al. Simultaneous aortic and renal artery reconstruction: evolution of an eighteen-year experience. *J Vasc Surg.* 1995;21:916–925.
11. Reilly JM, Rubin BG, Thompson RW, et al. Long-term effectiveness of extraanatomic renal artery revascularization. *J Vasc Surg.* 1994;116:784–791.
12. Cambria RP, Brewster DC, L'Italien GJ, et al. The durability of different reconstructive techniques for atherosclerotic renal artery disease. *J Vasc Surg.* 1994;20:76–87.
13. Stoney RJ, Messina LM, Goldstone J, Reilly LM. Renal endarterectomy through the transected aorta: a new technique for combined aortorenal atherosclerosis—a preliminary report. *J Vasc Surg.* 1989;9:224–233.
14. Lawrie GM, Morris GC, Glaeser DH, DeBakey ME. Renovascular reconstruction: factors affecting long-term prognosis in 919 patients followed up to 31 years. *Am J Cardiol.* 1989;63:1085–1092.
15. Hansen KJ, Starr SM, Sands RE, et al. Contemporary management of renovascular disease. *J Vasc Surg.* 1992;16:319–330.
16. Okuhn SP, Reilly LM, Bennet JB III, et al. Intraoperative assessment of renal and visceral artery reconstruction: the role of duplex scanning and spectral analysis. *J Vasc Surg.* 1987;5:137–147.
17. Hudspeth DA, Hansen KJ, Reavis SW, et al. Renal duplex sonography after treatment of renovascular disease. *J Vasc Surg.* 1993;18:381–390.
18. Murray SP, Kent KC, Salvatierra O, Stoney RJ. Complex branch renovascular disease: management options and late results. *J Vasc Surg.* 1994;20:338–346.
19. Cunningham CG, Reilly LM, Rapp JH, et al. Chronic visceral ischemia: three decades of progress. *Ann Surg.* 1991;214:276–287.
20. Beebe HG, MacFarlane S, Raker EJ. Supraceliac aortomesenteric bypass for intestinal ischemia. *J Vasc Surg.* 1987;5:749–754.
21. Rheudasil JM, Stewart MT, Schellack JV, et al. Surgical treatment of chronic mesenteric arterial insufficiency. *J Vasc Surg.* 1988;8:495–500.

22. Hollier LH, Bernatz PE, Pairolero PC, et al. Surgical management of chronic intestinal ischemia: a reappraisal. *Surgery.* 1981;90:940–943.
23. Zelenock GB, Graham LM, Whitehouse WM, et al. Splanchnic arteriosclerotic disease and intestinal angina. *Arch Surg.* 1980;115:497–501.
24. Baur GM, Millay DJ, Taylor LM, Porter JM. Treatment of chronic visceral ischemia. *Am J Surg.* 1984;148:138–142.
25. Fowl RJ, Hollier LH, Bernatz PE, et al. Repeat revascularization versus nephrectomy in the treatment of recurrent renovascular hypertension. *Surg Gynecol Obstet.* 1986;162:37–42.
26. Stanley JC, Whitehouse WM Jr, Zelenock GB, et al. Reoperation for complication of renal artery reconstructive surgery undertaken for treatment of renovascular hypertension. *J Vasc Surg.* 2:133–144.
27. Reilly LM, Ramos TK, Murray SP, et al. Optimal exposure of the proximal abdominal aorta: a critical appraisal of transabdominal medial visceral rotation. *J Vasc Surg.* 1994;19:375–390.

IX

Venous Problems

34

Classification of Lower Extremity Venous Disease

Robert L. Kistner, MD, Bo Eklof, MD, PhD, and Elna M. Masuda, MD

Over the years venous maladies have been diagnosed as clinical entities with emphasis placed on the appearance of the clinical condition but with little attention given to the etiology, the pathogenesis, or the anatomic distribution of the venous abnormality. Because venous problems rarely cause loss of limb or life there has been a tendency to regard them as less important than arterial diseases, and this has resulted in a habit of diagnosis in venous disease that is far less precise than that of its arterial counterpart. As a result, the literature in venous disease lacks precision because the diagnoses are incomplete and in many instances frankly incorrect. This chapter highlights the importance of uniform classification and accuracy in diagnosis of venous abnormalities.

Until the advent of the continuous-wave (CW) Doppler, and the more accurate duplex scan, diagnoses by superficial inspection and bedside opinion were found acceptable as the basis for treatment decisions. The fallacy of this was made clear by Cranley et al.[1] who proved the clinical diagnosis in deep-vein thrombosis (DVT) to be wrong half of the time. Over the years, pure clinical diagnosis has been proven unreliable not only in DVT cases but also in pulmonary embolism[2] and in the "postphlebitic" leg.[3]

The need for accurate diagnosis and classification has been recognized for a long time in the deliberations of the Joint Councils of the SVS/ISCVS. Under the leadership of Robert Rutherford, a committee was chaired by John Porter to develop the original "Reporting Standards in Venous Disease," which was published in 1988 in the *Journal of Vascular Surgery*.[4] This original report was updated by Porter and Moneta[5] in 1995. As a part of this update report, which addressed the broad realm of venous disease, Porter and Moneta incorporated the new classification of chronic venous disease that had been developed by an ad hoc committee of the American Venous Forum. This chronic venous classification, which has been described as the CEAP classification, has also been published along with its own grading system for chronic venous disease as the full report of the consensus committee of the American Venous Forum.[6]

ACUTE VENOUS DISEASE

Classification in acute venous disease was presented in the update on reporting standards in venous disease.[5] The acute disease states are classified by degree of thrombosis and anatomic extent of involvement. The degree of thrombosis differentiates patent vessels from subsegmental nonocclusive thrombosis, from occlusive subsegmental thrombosis, and from occlusive thrombosis throughout the segment. In addition, the terms *phlegmasia alba dolens, phlegmasia cerulea dolens,* and *venous gangrene* are defined as progressive degrees of thrombosis in the limb.

The acute clinical states are described as superficial, deep, or combined. The lower extremity veins are divided anatomically into six deep segments and two superficial segments as follows: the deep segments are tibial-soleal, popliteal, common femoral or superficial femoral, iliac, and inferior vena cava; the superficial segments are greater or lesser saphenous vein, or unnamed cutaneous veins.

Each case of acute thrombophlebitis shall be classified anatomically as either superficial or deep phlebitis or both, consisting of either partially occluding mural thrombus or totally occluding thrombus, with a specific segmental distribution. Given this amount of detail, new information about acute venous disease can be developed. For instance, prospective studies of thromboses in any given segment can be compared to other segments to answer questions such as the late sequelae to be expected from a tibial thrombosis compared to those from a femoral-popliteal or an iliofemoral thrombosis, or the post-thrombotic development of reflux in a previously thrombosed segment can be followed. Knowledge of these and other observations will lend validity to the use of long-term elastic support in some cases, the duration of anticoagulant therapy, the documentation of recurrent new thromboses, and other facets of ongoing care.

CHRONIC VENOUS DISEASE

In medical practice today, the patient with chronic venous disease (CVD) is diagnosed in an essentially random fashion from one physician to another. The compelling reasons to agree on a standard classification of CVD flow from widespread confusion about the diagnosis and treatment of chronic venous problems. Three myths about CVD that require correction are that the venous problems are simple, that they are not very important in a clinical sense, and that they are not surgically correctable. These perceptions have been instrumental in leading physicians to underdiagnose chronic venous problems and have resulted in a lack of reliable scientific data in the overall field of CVD. Due to the lack of objective and reproducible diagnoses in chronic venous patients, we have failed to establish knowledge about the natural history and even about the basic disease processes that exist in primary and secondary insufficiency states.

To develop a reproducible knowledge base in CVD, it is essential to begin with accurate diagnoses based on reproducible objective testing methods and arrange the results of these tests in an orderly manner by proper and thorough classification. This step is a necessary prelude to the organization and conduct of prospective studies of carefully defined clinical problems managed by alternative treatment techniques that will clarify most of the controversies that exist presently in the management of CVD.

In a thoughtful presentation of the need to perform outcome analysis, Rutherford's presidential address to the International Society for Cardiovascular Surgery[7] in June 1995 recognized the basic nature of classification and reporting standards as the *sine qua non* from which outcome analysis can proceed. He referred to the necessity to address the pathophysiologic, etiologic, and anatomic aspects of CVD in addition to the clinical aspects, as developed in the CEAP classification.

The vagaries of CVD are such that long-term follow-up is needed to assess results. Compensatory mechanisms in the venous tree are different than those in the arterial tree. Because changes occur over longer periods of time, the venous system is prone to superb efforts at compensation for venous occlusive states while at the same time the effect of gravity in the erect individual leads to very slow but inexorable development of reflux states over time. Because of the chronicity of these changes, treatments need to be monitored by objective testing for long periods before their validity can be accepted.

The magnitude of the problem in CVD is very great. In one form or another, CVD has been found to affect 20% to 50% of the adult population.[8] Approximately 10% to 20% of these persons will be afflicted with a more severe degree of CVD, which will adversely impact their way of life and their ability to earn a living. The serious forms of the problem may affect 2% to 5% of the population at any given time.[8] These are huge numbers and constitute one of the major causes of loss of time from work in the United States. The precise magnitude of the social and economic impact of CVD has not yet been accurately studied. While it is true that CVD seldom causes limb loss and for this reason does not command the urgent attention that arterial insufficiency attracts in the lower extremity, the very chronic nature of venous disease and the very wide distribution of the disease does command great respect in the medical community and deserves accurate study and precise treatment.

The new approach to classification of CVD via the CEAP classification[6] utilizes objective diagnosis of CVD states to categorize clinical problems into standard groups. The essence of this approach is that it be both thorough and accurate: thorough by addressing the important aspects of each venous case including its etiology, pathogenesis, anatomic distribution, and clinical presentation, and accurate by utilizing standard testing methods. Prior classifications, which have been largely confined to delineation of the clinical condition, have led to confusion because the differentiation between primary and secondary disease, between reflux and obstructive disease, and between various anatomic distributions of disease have not been defined. The treatments prescribed for conditions that appear clinically the same but have different underlying features will have varying results depending on the case mix that happens to be involved in that particular series. If the problems are to be separated into their component parts, it is clear the analysis must begin with accurate diagnoses and definable classification into standardized groups.

Several steps are necessary to provide the basis for good clinical research that will lead to objective knowledge of CVD. To do this we must (1) define which patients are being treated by precise diagnoses; (2) define which tests to use in any given circumstance and thereby provide uniformity of diagnoses by insisting on adherence to recognized testing methods; (3) develop prospective studies based on thorough diagnoses and accurate objective testing; and (4) study the patients over an adequate follow-up time to allow the chronicity of venous disease changes to play its role.

THE CEAP CLASSIFICATION

In 1994, an international panel of experts gathered under the auspices of the American Venous Forum to develop a consensus statement on diagnosis and classification in CVD. This conference resulted in a new method of classification that has come to be

TABLE 34–1. CLINICAL CLASSIFICATION

Class 0: No visible or palpable signs of venous disease

Class 1: Telangiectases or reticular veins

Class 2: Varicose veins

Class 3: Edema

Class 4: Skin changes ascribed to venous disease (e.g., pigmentation, venous eczema, lipodermatosclerosis)

Class 5: Skin changes as defined above with healed ulceration

Class 6: Skin changes as defined above with active ulceration

The presence or absence of symptoms such as pain or aching, as contrasted to the above signs, which are enumerated as Classes 1–6, is denoted by use of a (asymptomatic) or s (symptomatic) to modify the class description.
Reprinted from Classification and grading of chronic venous disease in the lower limb. A consensus statement. *Vasc Surg.* 1995;21:635–645.

termed the *CEAP classification*.[6] The CEAP represents the clinical condition (C), etiology of the condition (E), anatomic distribution of the problem (A), and pathophysiologic mechanism of development of the problem (P). Each of these main categories of CEAP were subdivided into six clinical states varying from telangiectasia through severe recurrent ulceration; three etiologies of congenital, primary, and secondary causes of venous insufficiency; three major anatomic divisions of superficial, deep, and perforator, which were further subdivided into 18 anatomic segments; and the three pathophysiologic states of reflux, obstruction, and a mixed condition of combined reflux and obstruction (Tables 34–1 to 34–4). In addition to the classification itself, a scoring system (Table 34–5) for severity of venous insufficiency based on the individual signs and symptoms, and a disability score (Table 34–6) were devised in the consensus report.[6] The classification is expressed by a shorthand method that utilizes the C-E-A-P modified by numbers that refer to the tables within the classification. For example, C_{2-4-s}-E_p-$A_{s,p}$-$P_{R2,3,18}$ is the classification of a clinical case of varicose veins with skin changes ($C_{2,4}$) that is symptomatic with pain (-s-), whose etiology is primary vein disease (E_p), located in the superficial and perforator veins ($A_{s,p}$) and due to reflux in the greater saphenous of the thigh and calf and in the calf perforator veins ($P_{R2,3,18}$).

The consensus committee was concerned that the complexity of the CEAP classification would prove too daunting to the busy practitioner to allow it to ever achieve clinical usefulness. In spite of this concern, the basic elements of the CEAP classification were all deemed to be necessary in order to provide a meaningful classification method. The committee concluded that anything less than the final form of the classification would not be complete and would therefore defeat the effort to achieve reproducible diagnoses in CVD. The fault in CVD is not that the classification is overly complex but rather that

TABLE 34–2. ETIOLOGIC CLASSIFICATION

Congenital	(E_C)
Primary	(E_P)—undetermined cause
Secondary	(E_S)—known cause
	Post-thrombotic
	Post-traumatic
	Other

Reprinted from Classification and grading of chronic venous disease in the lower limb. A consensus statement. *Vasc Surg.* 1995;21:635–645.

TABLE 34–3. ANATOMIC CLASSIFICATION

Segment Number	
	Superficial Veins (A$_S$):
1	Telangiectases/reticular veins
	Greater (long) saphenous vein (GSV)
2	Above knee
3	Below knee
4	Lesser (short) saphenous vein (LSV)
5	Nonsaphenous
	Deep Veins (A$_D$):
6	Inferior vena cava
	Iliac
7	Common
8	Internal
9	External
10	Pelvic—gonadal, broad ligament, other
	Femoral
11	Common
12	Deep
13	Superficial
14	Popliteal
15	Crural—anterior tibial, posterior tibial, peroneal (all paired)
16	Muscular—gastrocnemial, soleal, other
	Perforating Veins (A$_P$):
17	Thigh
18	Calf

Reprinted from Classification and grading of chronic venous disease in the lower limb. A consensus statement. *Vasc Surg.* 1995;21:635–645.

the general perception that CVD is simple leads to misunderstanding. The committee recognized that CVD truly is complex and cannot be oversimplified if it is to be understood.

If the venous diagnosis were to be compared to diagnosis in arterial disease, it turns out that the same elements contained in the CEAP diagnosis have been customarily used in arterial disease. For example, in the clinical condition of an arterial foot ulcer, the routine diagnostic process includes its etiology as to whether it is due to atherosclerosis or other occlusive disease process or even embolization, the anatomic distribution of the disease in the femoral, popliteal, or tibial or iliac segments, and the pathophysiologic details such as stenosis of feeding proximal vessels or occlusive patterns with collateral arterial formation (Table 34–7). If it is obvious that we need this type of information

TABLE 34–4. PATHOPHYSIOLOGIC CLASSIFICATION

Reflux	(P$_R$)
Obstruction	(P$_O$)
Reflux and obstruction	(P$_{R,O}$)

The elements of reflux and obstruction may be reported by using the anatomic segments in Table 34–3 to accurately define the extent of the process segment by segment. Alternatively, obstruction can be simplified by using familiar segmental regions of occlusion, namely caval, iliac, femoral, popliteal, and crural (P$_{O\text{-}CAV}$, P$_{O\text{-}I}$, P$_{O\text{-}F}$, P$_{O\text{-}P}$, P$_{O\text{-}C}$).
Reprinted from Classification and grading of chronic venous disease in the lower limb. A consensus statement. *Vasc Surg.* 1995;21:635–645.

TABLE 34–5. CLINICAL SEVERITY

Pain	0 = none; 1 = moderate, not requiring analgesics; 2 = severe, requiring analgesics
Edema	0 = none; 1 = mild/moderate; 2 = severe
Venous claudication	0 = none; 1 = mild/moderate; 2 = severe
Pigmentation	0 = none; 1 = localized; 2 = extensive
Lipodermatosclerosis	0 = none; 1 = localized; 2 = extensive
Ulcer—size (largest ulcer)	0 = none; 1 = <2 cm diameter; 2 = >2 cm diameter
Ulcer—duration	0 = none; 1 = <3 months; 2 = >3 months
Ulcer—recurrence	0 = none; 1 = once; 2 = more than once
Ulcer—number	0 = none; 1 = single; 2 = multiple

This table can be simplified to denote severity of symptom/sign as 0 = absent; 1 = mild, moderate (localized, single); and 2 = severe (extensive, multiple).
Reprinted from Classification and grading of chronic venous disease in the lower limb. A consensus statement. *Vasc Surg.* 1995;21:635–645.

in the arterial system, then it follows that the same data are necessary in the venous system and we must change our attitude toward the disease rather than continuing to oversimplify and underestimate chronic venous problems.[9]

CLINICAL USE OF THE CEAP CLASSIFICATION

The CEAP classification has been tested in clinical practice in our vascular surgical service with two separate series, one of which consisted of 102 chronic venous patients[10] who presented with any complaint of chronic venous insufficiency and a second series of 56 consecutive proven venous ulcer cases.[9] In both series the cases were evaluated clinically by history and physical examination and CW Doppler, all performed by an experienced vascular surgeon. Duplex scanning was performed on everyone who had findings beyond telangiectasia or peripheral (branch) varicose veins; APG, venous pressure, and ascending and descending phlebography were applied selectively to the more complicated problems. Diagnostic workup was conducted until an accurate and objective diagnosis of etiology, pathophysiology, and anatomy was achieved in each case according to its clinical merits. The more extensive workup was done for the patients with more serious clinical levels of disease. The overriding factor in determining how much workup is appropriate to a given clinical case is related to the severity of the disease and the functional ability of the patient.

The results observed in these two series of cases are presented in Figures 34–1 and 34–2. In the series of 102 consecutive chronic venous patients (Fig. 34–1), there is a predominance of minor levels of venous findings and by far the most frequent finding

TABLE 34–6. DISABILITY SCORE

0	Asymptomatic
1	Symptomatic, can function without support device
2	Can work 8-hour day *only* with support device
3	Unable to work even with support device

Reprinted from Classification and grading of chronic venous disease in the lower limb. A consensus statement. *Vasc Surg.* 1995;21:635–645.

TABLE 34–7. ELEMENTS OF VASCULAR DIAGNOSES

Arterial	Venous	Classification
Foot ulcer	Leg ulcer	C
Atherosclerosis versus embolic	Primary versus post-thrombotic	E
Femoral-popliteal	Deep (fem-pop-tib)	A
Stenosis/occlusion	Reflux/obstruction	P

Reprinted from Kistner RL. Definitive diagnostic and definitive treatment in chronic venous disease: a concept whose time has come. *J Vasc Surg. 1996;24(5):703.*

was varicose veins. The 14% incidence of ulceration in this series probably reflects a referral population in this series rather than suggesting that 14% of all chronic venous insufficiency patients present with ulceration (Fig. 34–1). The predominance of primary insufficiency in the 102 unselected cases is to be expected because of the predominance of varicose veins and telangiectasia. It was not expected, however, that the ulcer series would show that 70% were due to primary causes and only 30% to secondary (post-thrombotic) disease.

A striking finding in the ulcer series (Fig. 34–2) was that the saphenous vein was the lone site of reflux in 29% of the ulcer cases that were due to primary disease and in none of the ulcer cases that were due to secondary disease. Of the primary cases, 32% presented with saphenous and perforator incompetence in the presence of a competent deep system as diagnosed by duplex scan criteria. This was an unexpectedly high frequency of this combination of reflux and a fortuitous one since it is amenable to relatively simple surgical treatment.

There are important surgical implications to the distribution of disease as noted in these tables. It has been our experience and that of others[11] that primary disease

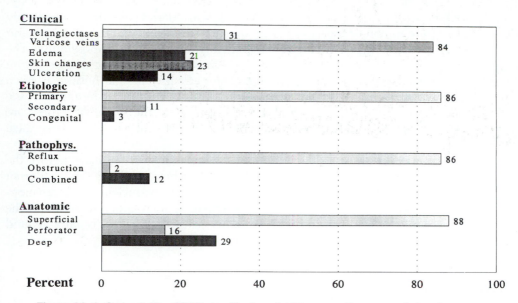

Figure 34–1. Series I. The CEAP classification of 102 consecutive cases of chronic venous disease. (*Reprinted from Kistner RL, Eklof B, Masuda M. Diagnosis of chronic venous disease: the CEAP classification. Mayo Clin Proc. 1996;71:338–345.*)

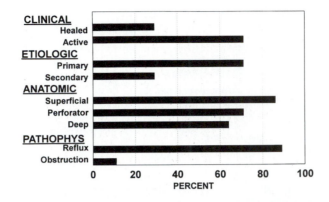

Figure 34–2. Series II. The CEAP classification in 56 cases of venous ulceration. (*Reprinted from Kistner RL. Definitive diagnosis and definitive treatment in chronic venous disease: a concept whose time has come. J Vasc Surg. 1996;24(5):703.*)

affecting the saphenous and perforator systems gives excellent results after surgical treatment when the deep system is competent. When the deep system is incompetent due to primary valve incompetence the surgical repair of valve incompetence at the superficial femoral level has still been accompanied by a 73% long-term (>10 years) rate of competence and freedom from recurrent ulceration.[12]

The value of knowing the anatomic distribution of venous abnormalities is reflected in the important finding that axial reflux in both thigh and calf was present in 51 of 53 ulcer cases. It appears that the extent of axial reflux (involving both thigh and calf) was a dominant factor in this series and that the length of the axial reflux (in thigh and calf) was more important than whether the reflux occurred in either the superficial or deep systems.

Knowledge of the etiology of the reflux is particularly important when considering the difference in therapeutic alternatives between primary and post-thrombotic deep-vein reflux. In post-thrombotic cases, the valves are scarred and sometimes completely destroyed and the lumen of the vessel is occupied by post-thrombotic synechiae and septae, which render surgical repair of valvular incompetence an impossibility. The degree of reflux in these veins is quite variable because the thrombotic masses within the veins may act as an obstructing element. The pathophysiologic finding is often one of mixed degrees of reflux and obstruction. This is entirely different than the pathophysiology of pure reflux in primary disease, where the valve structures are morphologically normal and the elongated valve cusps are still available for surgical reconstruction.

The importance of knowing the pathophysiology is to distinguish whether the problem is one of reflux or of obstruction because this is basic to the determination of surgical alternatives for any serious case of chronic venous insufficiency. The development of specific repair of venous reflux states makes it mandatory to separate the surgically repairable reflux cases from those reflux cases that are not repairable, and from the more unusual cases of venous obstruction.

CONCLUSION

Uniform classification of venous disease is a necessary basis for effective communication about details of venous disease. With the availability of noninvasive accurate testing methods, the specifics of anatomy and physiology can be routinely established in venous patients, and these can be used to set the basis for prospective interinstitutional studies and to identify accurately the pathologic processes in individual patients. Through this approach a new level of scientific validity can be established in the management of venous disorders.

REFERENCES

1. Cranley JJ, Canos AJ, Sull WJ. The diagnosis of deep venous thrombosis: fallibility of clinical signs and symptoms. *Arch Surg.* 1976;111:34–36.
2. Bergqvist D, Lindblad B. Incidence of venous thromboembolism in medical and surgical patients. In: Bergqvist D, Comeroto AJ, Nicolaides AN, Scurr JH, eds. *Prevention of Venous Thromboembolism.* London: Med-Orion; 1994:3–17.
3. Clinical diagnosis of postphlebitic leg. The calf pump failure syndrome: diagnosis and treatment. In: Browse NL, Burnand KG, Thomas ML, eds. *Diseases of the Veins. Pathology, Diagnosis and Treatment.* London: Edward Arnold; 1988:325–347.
4. Porter JM, Rutherford RB, Claggett GP, and NA-ISCVS/SVS Ad Hoc Committee on Reporting Standards in Venous Disease. (R. Rutherford, Chairman Ad Hoc Committee.) Reporting standards in venous disease. *J Vasc Surg.* 1988;8:172–181.
5. Porter JM, Moneta GL, and International Consensus Committee on Chronic Venous Disease. Reporting standards in venous disease: an update. *J Vasc Surg.* 1995;21:635–645.
6. Classification and grading of chronic venous disease in the lower limb. A consensus statement. *Vasc Surg.* 1996;30:5–11.
7. Rutherford RB. Presidential address: vascular surgery—comparing outcomes. *J Vasc Surg.* 1996;23:5–17.
8. Widmer LK. *Peripheral Venous Disorders. Prevalence and Socio-medical Importance. Observations in 4529 Apparently Healthy Persons. Basle III Study.* Bern: Hans Huber; 1978.
9. Kistner RL. Definitive diagnosis and definitive treatment in chronic venous disease: a concept whose time has come. *J Vasc Surg.* 1996;24(5):703.
10. Kistner RL, Eklof B, Masuda EM. Diagnosis of chronic venous disease of the lower extremities: the "CEAP" classification. *Mayo Clin Proc.* 1996;71:338–345.
11. Burnand K, O'Donnell T, Lea MT, Browse NL. Relationship between post-phlebitic changes in deep veins and results of surgical treatment of venous ulcers. *Lancet.* 1976;I:936–938.
12. Masuda E, Kistner RL. Long-term results of venous valve reconstruction: a 4- to 21-year follow-up. *J Vasc Surg.* 1994;19:391–403.

35

Understanding the Natural History of Deep-Vein Thrombosis

R. Eugene Zierler, MD, and Mark H. Meissner, MD

The principal purpose of a natural history study is to provide detailed information on the clinical outcome of a disease without any specific treatment. Since the primary goal of treatment is to improve on the natural history, such data are essential for evaluating the efficacy of therapeutic interventions. The characteristic feature of a natural history study is serial follow-up of patients to document both the initial severity of their disease and any subsequent changes that occur. Because natural history studies typically involve repeated evaluations of large numbers of patients, the risks, costs, and accuracy of the testing methods used are of critical importance. Based on these considerations, clinicians have been reluctant to use phlebography as a general screening and follow-up test for deep-vein thrombosis (DVT). Fortunately, noninvasive testing methods are ideally suited for natural history studies, and a variety of noninvasive methods have been developed for the evaluation of venous disease.

Early phlebographic and pathologic studies suggested that venous thrombi were dynamic structures that changed over time.[1-3] More recent observations based on the noninvasive technique of duplex ultrasound scanning have validated some of the early pathologic findings and provided new information about the evolution of venous thrombi.[4-8] Once formed, thrombi in the deep venous system may undergo organization, recanalization, extension, or rethrombosis. Which of these prevails at a particular site depends on interactions between the coagulation and fibrinolytic systems. The role of these processes in the production of valvular incompetence and persistent venous obstruction is critically important in the development of chronic venous insufficiency after an episode of DVT. If the determinants of valvular incompetence and persistent obstruction could be identified through natural history studies, it might be possible to devise specific therapies for DVT that would prevent those changes that contribute to a poor long-term outcome.

EVALUATION OF VENOUS ANATOMY AND FUNCTION

Although contrast phlebography or venography has served as the historical standard for documenting the presence of DVT, a number of features have limited its routine clinical use.[9–11] The major disadvantages of phlebography include patient discomfort, the requirement for radiographic contrast injection, relatively high cost, and risk of complications. The most significant complications associated with phlebography are extravasation of contrast material at the site of injection and initiation of thrombus formation. While the incidence of complications has been quite variable, they have been described in up to 9.5% of patients.[12] These features make phlebography unsuitable for screening large groups of patients or following patients over time with serial evaluations.

The invasive nature of phlebography has stimulated the development of a variety of noninvasive methods for evaluating the structure and function of the venous system. These methods can be considered as either indirect or direct, depending on the specific approach used (Table 35–1). In most vascular laboratories, the indirect techniques have been largely replaced by the direct evaluation with duplex scanning.

Plethysmography refers to a group of measurement techniques that monitor changes in the volume of a body part. In the clinical setting, these changes are primarily due to alterations in blood volume. Initial experience with plethysmographic techniques in the limbs emphasized the measurement of arterial flow during temporary venous occlusion.[13] Plethysmograpic approaches have also been extensively applied to the assessment of acute and chronic venous disease. While the details of the specific methods vary, they are all based on detecting the volume changes that occur as blood drains out of the lower extremity, typically after a brief period of venous occlusion. In the presence of a significant venous obstruction, high-resistance collateral venous pathways reduce the rate of outflow from the leg. An early clinical experience with venous plethysmography was reported in 1968 using a water-filled system.[14] Although this approach was accurate, it was relatively cumbersome and not practical for routine clinical use. The plethysmographic methods that have been widely applied for the diagnosis of DVT include strain gauge, impedance, and air-cuff plethysmography.[15–17] In the continuous-wave (CW) venous Doppler examination, the audible characteristics of venous flow are evaluated at multiple levels in the extremity. Important features include the spontaneous venous flow pattern, phasic variations with the respiratory cycle, and the response to proximal and distal compression maneuvers. Although the CW venous Doppler examination is quite subjective, an experienced examiner can obtain clinically useful information.[18]

Because the indirect tests rely on major alterations in venous flow patterns, they are most accurate when there is complete obstruction of the deep veins proximal to

---

TABLE 35–1. NONINVASIVE TESTS FOR VENOUS DISEASE

Indirect Tests

Plethysmography
   Strain gauge
   Impedance
   Phleborheography (air-cuff)
Doppler ultrasound
   Continuous-wave Doppler

Direct Tests

Duplex scanning
   B-mode imaging
   Pulsed Doppler flow detection
   Spectral waveform analysis
   Color-flow imaging

the level of the knee. Consequently, these tests are much less reliable in the presence of isolated calf vein thrombi or nonocclusive thrombi in the proximal deep veins. The indirect tests may give a false-negative result when DVT is associated with well-developed collaterals that provide an alternate path for venous drainage. A physiologic false-positive indirect test result can be obtained if there is extrinsic compression of the deep veins. The limitations of the indirect tests are largely overcome by the direct approach of duplex scanning, which permits the identification of both complete and partial venous obstruction, as well as valvular incompetence.

Venous duplex scanning is less subjective than the indirect tests because it provides a B-mode image of the vessel under study and a pulsed Doppler spectral waveform of the local flow pattern. The venous Doppler signal obtained during a duplex scan can be used to perform the same augmentation maneuvers required for the CW Doppler examination. In addition, the B-mode image enhances the effectiveness of Doppler flow detection by allowing direct visualization of specific venous segments and imaging of some thrombi. Duplex scanning is particularly useful for documenting the location and severity of valvular incompetence, information that is difficult to obtain by any other method, including venography.[19–21]

The specific criteria used for the diagnosis of DVT by duplex scanning include (1) visualization of thrombus by B-mode imaging; (2) incompressibility of a venous segment with direct probe pressure; (3) absence of spontaneous venous flow; and (4) absence of phasic flow with respiration. When these criteria were compared to contrast venography in 47 patients with suspected DVT, visualization of thrombus had a specificity of 92% and a sensitivity of only 50%, while incompressibility had a specificity of 67% and a sensitivity of 79%.[22] The Doppler criteria based on spontaneous and phasic flow had sensitivities and specificities that ranged from 76% to 100%. Errors related to visualization of thrombus were caused by failure to image 50% of the thrombi that were noted on venography. Echogenicity of thrombus appears to depend on the age of the clot, with most thrombi becoming less echogenic over time.[23] Combining both the B-mode image and Doppler criteria resulted in better overall accuracy, particularly when the imaging criteria were negative for thrombus.

A variety of methods have been used to identify and quantitate valvular incompetence and the resulting venous reflux. Although duplex scanning provides the capability to evaluate flow through individual venous valves and segments, the method used to elicit reflux is critically important. In normal supine subjects, venous valve closure occurs after the reverse flow velocity exceeds 30 cm/s. This velocity is achieved with a Valsalva maneuver only in the common femoral vein and is not reliably generated by manual limb compression.[20] The most effective and reproducible method for eliciting reflux at all levels of the lower limb appears to be distal cuff deflation in the standing position using a standardized pneumatic cuff. This simulates muscle relaxation and generates transvalvular pressure gradients in the same physiologic range as those associated with standing and walking. When this technique is used, the normal duration of reflux flow from the time of cuff deflation to valve closure is typically less than 0.5 seconds.[21]

MECHANISMS OF DEEP-VEIN THROMBOSIS

In 1856, Virchow described the now well-known triad of factors that contribute to the development of venous thrombosis: stasis, hypercoagulability, and vessel wall injury. However, the relative importance of these three factors is still not clearly established, and the multitude of clinical risk factors associated with DVT suggests that the role of the individual components of Virchow's triad vary from patient to patient. Hypercoagulability is now recognized as including abnormalities of both the coagulation and fibrinolytic systems. Vessel wall injury is perhaps the least important factor, since gross or microscopic endothelial injury appears to be neither a necessary nor sufficient condition for most cases of venous thrombosis.[24] There is also evidence that stasis alone is probably not an adequate stimulus for venous thrombosis.[25]

Although the initiation of DVT is multifactorial, clinical observations indicate that most venous thrombi originate in areas of relative stasis, either in the soleal veins of the calf or in valve sinuses.[26,27] The key event in venous thrombosis is probably thrombin generation in these areas leading to platelet aggregation and fibrin formation.[28] Thus, stasis can be viewed as a permissive factor for venous thrombosis. This concept is supported by experimental studies in which stasis and injury alone did not cause venous thrombosis in the absence of low levels of activated coagulation factors.[29] Many of the conditions associated with DVT involve either systemic activation of the coagulation system or imbalances between procoagulants, their inhibitors, and components of the fibrinolytic system.

The factors contributing to venous thrombosis can be studied by examining the formation and growth of thrombi formed in the valve sinuses of the lower extremity veins. In flow models, primary and secondary vortices are produced beyond the valve cusps that tend to trap red blood cells near the apex of the cusp.[30] Red cell aggregates formed within these vortices could provide the early nidus for thrombus formation; however, these aggregates are probably transient unless stabilized by fibrin formed by local activation of the coagulation system. Once early thrombi are present in the valve sinus they become adherent to the endothelium near the apex of the valve cusp.[27,31] Microscopically, these early thrombi consist of closely packed red cells and a variable number of leukocytes within a fibrin network. Further propagation of thrombi beyond the valve sinus probably depends largely on the relative balance between activated coagulation and thrombolysis. Once flow through the venous lumen is reduced, prograde and retrograde propagation of thrombus may be promoted by hemodynamic factors. Early thrombi may also fail to propagate and remain as endothelialized fibrin fragments within the valve sinuses. The processes of organization, recanalization, extension, and rethrombosis determine the ultimate anatomic and physiologic outcome after an episode of DVT.

RECANALIZATION AND RETHROMBOSIS

The terms *recanalization* and *thrombolysis* refer to the reestablishment of a venous lumen, which commonly occurs after an acute occlusive DVT. Both early venous patency and chronic sequelae are ultimately determined by a balance between thrombus organization and propagation, thrombolysis, and rethrombosis. Thrombus organization begins with the migration of surfacing cells over the thrombus from the adjacent venous endothelium.[31] These endothelial cells contribute to the activation of thrombus-bound plasminogen by release of tissue plasminogen activator, thereby promoting thrombolysis.[1] In the absence of thrombus propagation or rethrombosis, this results in a restored venous lumen with a slightly raised fibroelastic plaque where the initial thrombus was adherent to the vein wall.

From the clinical point of view, the most important events following initial thrombus formation are recanalization and rethrombosis. Impedance plethysmography was the first widely used noninvasive test suitable for serial evaluation of venous outflow obstruction following DVT. Although this test could not distinguish between true recanalization and flow through collateral venous pathways, such tests were found to normalize in 67% of patients by 3 months and 92% of patients by 9 months after initial detection of thrombus.[32] Recent studies based on duplex scanning have confirmed the occurrence of recanalization in previously thrombosed venous segments. Among 21 patients followed prospectively, recanalization was present in some involved segments by 7 days in 44% of patients and by 90 days in 100% of patients.[33] The percentage of initially involved segments that remained occluded decreased to a mean of 44% by 30 days and 14% by 90 days. In a similar study, an exponential decrease in thrombus load was noted over the first 6 months after femoropopliteal venous thrombosis.[34] Most recanalization occurred within the first 6 weeks, with restoration of flow in 87% of 23 completely occluded segments during this interval. The rate of thrombus clearance was not significantly different in the common femoral, deep femoral, superficial femoral, or popliteal venous segments. However, another study suggested more rapid clearance of thrombus from the posterior tibial veins, possibly reflecting the increased efficiency of thrombolysis in smaller venous segments.[4] In general, these studies indicate that recanalization begins early after an episode of DVT with the majority of thrombolysis occurring within the first 3 months. Further recanalization may continue at a slower rate for months and years after the acute event.[5]

Rethrombosis competes with recanalization in the natural history of DVT. Most clinical studies have included both recurrent DVT and pulmonary embolism as outcomes, with rates depending on type of treatment, location of thrombus, and duration of follow-up. Among patients with proximal DVT, recurrent thromboembolic events were observed in 5% of patients treated with a standard anticoagulation regimen for 3 months[35] compared to 47% of patients inadequately treated with a 3-month course of low-dose subcutaneous heparin.[36] In patients with isolated calf vein thrombosis, proximal propagation was reported in up to 23% of untreated patients and 10% of patients treated with intravenous heparin.[37]

As with recanalization, the process of rethrombosis has been examined with duplex scanning. Recurrent thrombotic events can occur in three forms: propagation of thrombus to initially uninvolved segments in the ipsilateral leg; thrombosis of segments in an initially uninvolved contralateral leg; and rethrombosis of a partially occluded or recanalized segment. Proximal thrombus propagation was noted in 38% of 24 patients being treated with intravenous heparin; such propagation was associated with smoking, but not with the initial level of thrombosis or the adequacy of anticoagulation.[38] In a larger series of 177 patients with DVT followed for a median of 9.3 months, recurrent thrombotic events (propagation, rethrombosis, or new contralateral thrombi) were observed in 52% of patients.[8] Among initially involved extremities, propagation of thrombus to new segments was documented in 30% and rethrombosis of partially occluded or recanalized segments in 31%. New thrombi were observed in 6% of initially uninvolved contralateral extremities. None of these events was associated with identifiable clinical risk factors. Propagation tended to occur in extremities with less extensive thrombosis at the time of presentation, while rethrombosis was significantly more common in limbs with more extensive initial involvement. Propagation to new segments in the ipsilateral limb was an early event, occurring within a median of 40 days after presentation. Rethrombosis and extension to the contralateral limb tended to occur more sporadically and at later times.

DEVELOPMENT OF VALVULAR INCOMPETENCE

Although damage to venous valves with subsequent incompetence and reflux is generally regarded as a consequence of DVT, up to one-third of patients remain free of chronic post-thrombotic symptoms after an acute lower extremity thrombotic event. Among 107 patients with 123 legs affected by DVT who were followed by duplex scanning for a mean of 341 days, reflux developed in 37% of legs by the end of the first month and 69% by the end of the first year.[5] The incidence of reflux in individual venous segments after 1 year was lower, ranging from 18% in the posterior tibial vein to 58% in the popliteal vein.

Reflux develops as flow is reestablished in a vein following an episode of acute DVT. In studies based on serial duplex scanning, the development of reflux appears to coincide with or slightly precede complete recanalization in most venous segments. As shown in Figure 35–1, median lysis times were shorter for venous segments without reflux compared to segments with reflux in all segments except the posterior tibial vein.[4] As for recanalization, the rate at which reflux develops is highest during the first 6 to 12 months after a DVT and slows considerably thereafter.[7] Such reflux may be transient in up to 23% of initially thrombosed segments.

There appear to be differences in susceptibility to reflux among the lower extremity venous segments. In particular, the incidence of reflux in the posterior tibial vein is lower than in other involved segments.[4,5] Both a more rapid rate of recanalization and the large number of valves in the posterior tibial venous segment may limit the development of reflux. Other possible determinants of valvular incompetence include the time required for complete recanalization, the occurrence of rethrombosis, the persistence of proximal thrombus, and differences in fibrinolytic activity between indi-

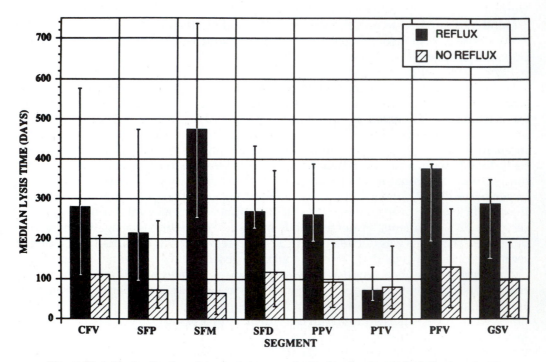

Figure 35–1. Median time from thrombosis to recanalization for all segments (lysis time), grouped according to reflux status at last visit. Error bars show interquartile range (25th to 75th percentile). Segments: CFV, common femoral vein; SFP, proximal superficial femoral vein; SFM, mid superficial femoral vein; SFD, distal superficial femoral vein; PPV, popliteal vein; PTV, posterior tibial vein; PFV, profunda femoris vein; GSV, greater saphenous vein. (*Reprinted with permission: Meissner MH, Manzo RA, Bergelin RO, et al. Deep venous insufficiency: the relationship between lysis and subsequent reflux. J Vasc Surg. 1993;18:596–608.*)

viduals. The relative importance of these factors will ultimately determine whether treatment measures such as thrombolytic therapy or a particular type, intensity, and duration of anticoagulation can decrease the incidence of post-thrombotic complications.

There is a growing body of evidence showing that early recanalization contributes to the preservation of valve function. In a series of 113 patients with 123 lower extremities affected by DVT, 88% of the patients were treated with standard anticoagulation measures.[4] During a mean follow-up period of 17.6 months, the time from thrombosis to recanalization was related to the ultimate development of reflux (Fig. 35–1). Complete recanalization required 2.3 to 7.3 times longer in segments developing reflux than in segments with return of normal valve function. The only exception was the posterior tibial vein, in which the time to complete recanalization was nearly identical for segments with and without reflux. These findings suggest that increasing the rate of recanalization with thrombolytic therapy may play a role in preserving valvular competence after an episode of acute DVT. However, despite the importance of the time required for complete recanalization, this is clearly not the only determinant of valve function. A few venous segments in this study developed reflux despite early lysis (<1 month), while others appeared to be protected from reflux despite relatively late lysis (>9 months).

Recurrent thrombotic events are also associated with the development of valvular incompetence. Propagation of thrombus to initially uninvolved venous segments places these segments at risk, and the incidence of reflux in such segments is nearly identical to that of initially involved venous segments.[8] In addition, rethrombosis of a partially recanalized venous segment further increases the risk of reflux. The incidence of reflux in segments with rethrombosis is in the range of 30% to 80%, considerably higher than in segments without rethrombosis (Fig. 35–2).

Abnormalities of the coagulation and fibrinolytic systems may contribute to both the initial development and late complications of DVT. Patients with hypercoagulable states appear to be at increased risk for recurrent thrombotic events that can result in valvular injury and incompetence. These considerations may be particularly important in patients with activated protein C resistance. Although hypercoagulable states related to deficiencies of antithrombin III, protein C, and protein S account for less than 10% of acute DVTs, resistance to activated protein C has been reported in between 33% and 64% of such cases.[39,40] An abnormal intravascular fibrinolytic response has been reported in up to 37% of patients with recurrent or idiopathic DVT.[41] This finding was related to increased plasminogen activator inhibitor (PAI) levels in approximately three-quarters of these patients and diminished tissue-type plasminogen activator (tPA) release in the remainder. Reduced tPA release is present in up to 10% of patients with idiopathic DVT and appears to be closely associated with recurrent thrombosis. If there is a relationship between abnormal fibrinolysis and recurrent DVT, such patients are likely to be at higher risk for development of valvular incompetence.

In a study of 35 patients with acute DVT who were followed with serial laboratory assays and duplex scanning, the plasma levels of various coagulation and fibrinolytic markers were correlated with the presence or absence of recanalization.[42] After 6 months of follow-up, 20 patients (57%) showed complete resolution of thrombus, while 15 patients (43%) had only partial recanalization, no change, or extension of thrombus. The levels of PAI were significantly lower at baseline and 1 week after diagnosis in patients with complete thrombus resolution compared to PAI levels in patients with other outcomes. Plasma levels of tPA were slightly higher at baseline and during follow-

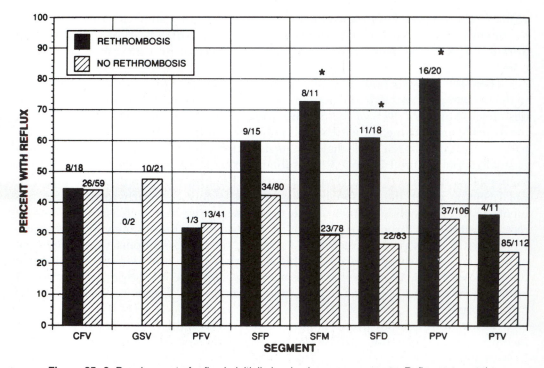

Figure 35–2. Development of reflux in initially involved venous segments. Reflux status at the last follow-up visit among those patients with and without rethrombosis. Numbers above bars indicate the number of segments in which reflux was observed over the number of segments in which reflux could be definitively assessed. Segments labeled as in Figure 35–1. Differences between segments with and without rethrombosis are statistically significant ($p < 0.005$) for the SFM, SFD, and PPV segments. (*Reprinted with permission: Meissner MH, Caps MT, Bergelin RO, et al. Propagation, rethrombosis and new thrombus formation after acute deep venous thrombosis. J Vasc Surg. 1995;22:558–567.*)

up in patients with complete thrombus resolution, but these differences were only statistically significant at the 4-week interval. These results suggest that certain plasma coagulation or fibrinolytic markers correlate with the process of recanalization. If this is true, then some of these markers might also correlate with the development of valvular incompetence following DVT.

CLINICAL IMPLICATIONS OF NATURAL HISTORY STUDIES

Although the long-term consequences of DVT can be attributed to the natural history events discussed earlier, the initial diagnosis remains a challenge. It is generally recognized that the clinical bedside diagnosis of acute DVT is relatively inaccurate, being correct only about 50% of the time.[43,44] Studies comparing duplex scanning with contrast venography have shown overall sensitivities and specificities in excess of 90% for the diagnosis of proximal DVT.[22] Based on this type of experience and the acknowledged disadvantages of venography, duplex scanning has become accepted as a diagnostic standard for the detection of DVT. Among 833 patients screened for suspected DVT by duplex scanning, 209 (25%) had a positive duplex scan.[45,46] The risk factors that correlated with a positive test were a previous episode of DVT or pulmonary embolism, cancer, and prolonged bedrest. The presence of limb swelling on physical examination was the only symptom or sign that was significantly associated with a positive test.[45] In the patients with a diagnosis of DVT the right leg was involved in 35%, the left leg in 48%, and both legs in 17%.[46] The venous segments most frequently affected by DVT were the superficial femoral in 74% of patients, popliteal in 73%, common femoral in 58%, and posterior tibial in 40%. The proximal or above-knee venous segments were involved in 95% of the patients, while the calf veins were involved in 40%. Thus, multisegment involvement was common. Isolated proximal DVT was present in 60% of patients and isolated calf thrombi were found in only 5%. These observations indicate that proximal DVT is much more frequent than isolated calf vein thrombosis among patients with suspected DVT referred to a vascular laboratory for screening. The relatively common finding of bilateral lower extremity venous involvement emphasizes the importance of examining both legs, even if only one is symptomatic.

Natural history studies have allowed the primary hemodynamic outcomes of DVT—valvular incompetence and persistent venous obstruction—to be correlated with the most significant clinical outcomes: the post-thrombotic syndrome and venous claudication. Valvular incompetence becomes apparent as recanalization occurs, while persistent obstruction represents a failure of the recanalization process. The post-thrombotic syndrome is the most common chronic complication of acute DVT, with as many as two-thirds of patients developing late symptoms of edema, hyperpigmentation, subcutaneous fibrosis, or ulceration. Ambulatory venous hypertension is regarded as the basic underlying physiologic mechanism for post-thrombotic signs and symptoms. Although both venous reflux and obstruction can contribute to abnormally high pressures in the deep venous system, there is evidence that the post-thrombotic syndrome results primarily from valvular incompetence. Furthermore, the manifestations of the post-thrombotic syndrome are related to the anatomic distribution of valvular incompetence. Reflux in the distal deep venous segments, particularly the popliteal and posterior tibial veins, is associated with post-thrombotic skin changes.[19,47,48] This relationship is supported by the observation that post-thrombotic symptoms are more closely correlated with a reduction in venous refilling time by photoplethysmography, suggestive of distal valvular incompetence, than with residual abnormalities of venous outflow.[49] In contrast, symptoms of venous claudication are related to persistent iliofemoral venous obstruction.[50] Incompetence of the greater and lesser saphenous veins is also common in patients with the post-thrombotic syndrome, probably as a result of the transmission of high venous pressures from the deep to the superficial system through incompetent perforating veins.[19]

In spite of the findings summarized here, there is evidence that residual venous obstruction combined with valvular incompetence may play a role in the development of post-thrombotic signs and symptoms.[6] Lower extremities with edema, hyperpigmentation, subcutaneous fibrosis, or ulceration are more likely to have a combination of reflux and residual obstruction than either abnormality alone (Fig. 35–3). Although reflux can be related to the initial presence of thrombus in the majority of incompetent venous segments, valves in uninvolved segments may also become incompetent after an episode of DVT. In one study, 29% of segments that developed reflux were uninvolved by the initial thrombotic process, and reflux in such initially uninvolved segments appeared to be related to persistent proximal obstruction.[7] Reflux in these segments was also more likely to be transient and resolve during follow-up than reflux in initially involved segments. The risk of developing reflux in segments involved by thrombus was more than twice that in uninvolved segments.

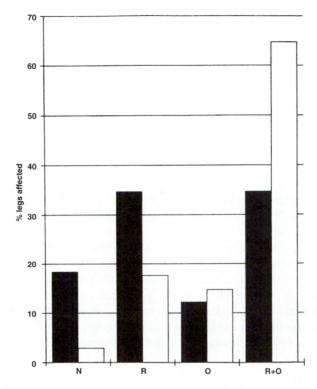

Figure 35–3. Proportion of limbs (% legs affected) demonstrating no abnormality (N), reflux alone (R), obstruction alone (O), and reflux with obstruction (R + O) after DVT. Dark bars indicate asymptomatic legs; white bars indicate legs with clinical features of post-thrombotic syndrome. (*Reprinted with permission: Johnson BF, Manzo RA, Bergelin RO, Strandness DE. Relationship between changes in the deep venous system and the development of post-thrombotic syndrome after an acute episode of lower limb deep vein thrombosis: a one- to 6- year follow-up. J Vasc Surg. 1995;21:307–313.*)

The goals of treatment for acute DVT are to prevent thrombus propagation, reduce the risk of pulmonary embolism, and promote recanalization and preservation of valve function. It has been noted that recurrent thrombotic events are relatively common during anticoagulant treatment, since 59% of patients showing propagation and 65% of patients showing rethrombosis are receiving anticoagulants at the time of the recurrent event.[8] However, the intensity of anticoagulant treatment is frequently inadequate in the acute setting, as demonstrated by monitoring of standard tests such as the partial thromboplastin time.[38] This issue is extremely important, because the incidence of recurrent thromboembolic events was observed to be 15 times higher among patients with inadequate early anticoagulation.[35] Determining the optimal duration of anticoagulation is complicated by the fact that most treatment protocols are directed toward reducing the acute risk of pulmonary embolism rather than the chronic morbidity of the post-thrombotic syndrome. Although a similar incidence of chronic venous insufficiency has been reported among patients treated with 4 weeks or 3 months of anticoagulation, a higher incidence of recurrent thromboembolism following a short course of anticoagulant treatment has also been reported.[51,52]

Thrombolytic therapy increases the lysis rates of venous thrombi compared to heparin alone, but it does not decrease the incidence of pulmonary embolism or overall mortality when compared with standard anticoagulant treatment.[53,54] In a meta-analysis of six randomized trials, streptokinase was 3.7 times more likely than heparin to produce some degree of thrombolysis.[55] However, despite the ability of thrombolytic therapy to restore a patent venous lumen, its role in the preservation of valve function is not clearly documented. Although some beneficial results have been reported, most studies have suffered from small numbers of patients, short follow-up periods, absence of objective hemodynamic data, and lack of a control group treated with standard anticoagulation.[56,57] In addition, there is an increased risk of bleeding associated with thrombolytic therapy that has led to the development of stringent criteria for its use.[58] Among 209 patients with a diagnosis of DVT, a contraindication to thrombolytic therapy was present in 194 or 93%.[59] Thus, only 7% of the patients were good candidates for this type of treatment. For those patients that can be treated with thrombolytic therapy, duplex scanning can be used to monitor the lytic process and determine the optimal duration of treatment.[60]

CONCLUSION

An episode of DVT can be considered as a dynamic balance between the coagulation and fibrinolytic systems, with the most dramatic changes occurring over the first 3 to 6 months after the initial thrombotic event. These competing processes have a direct impact on long-term outcome, because the rate of recanalization and the occurrence of rethrombosis clearly affect ultimate valve function. With respect to the rate of recanalization, thrombolytic therapy is extremely effective in promoting rapid and complete clearing of thrombus in some patients. However, there is still no conclusive evidence that thrombolytic therapy reduces the incidence of the post-thrombotic syndrome.

Finally, it appears that the risk of post-thrombotic sequelae may be predicted in some patients. Certain anatomic patterns of reflux, particularly those involving the popliteal and posterior tibial veins along with the superficial veins, appear to be associated with a higher incidence of the post-thrombotic syndrome. In contrast, since reflux rarely develops once recanalization is complete, a patient without reflux after complete recanalization is likely to be at lower risk for developing post-thrombotic signs and symptoms.

REFERENCES

1. Sevitt S. The mechanisms of canalization in deep vein thrombosis. *J Pathol.* 1973;110:153–165.
2. Sevitt S. The vascularization of deep-vein thrombi and their fibrous residue: a post-mortem angiographic study. *J Pathol.* 1973;111:1–11.
3. Thomas ML, McAllister V. The radiological progression of deep venous thrombosis. *Radiology.* 1971;99:37–40.
4. Meissner MH, Manzo RA, Bergelin RO, et al. Deep venous insufficiency: the relationship between lysis and subsequent reflux. *J Vasc Surg.* 1993;18:596–608.
5. Markel A, Manzo RA, Bergelin RO, Strandness DE. Valvular reflux after deep vein thrombosis: incidence and time of occurrence. *J Vasc Surg.* 1992;15:377–384.
6. Johnson BF, Manzo RA, Bergelin RO, Strandness DE. Relationship between changes in the deep venous system and the development of the postthrombotic syndrome after an acute episode of lower limb deep vein thrombosis: a one- to six-year follow-up. *J Vasc Surg.* 1995;21:307–313.

7. Caps MT, Manzo RA, Bergelin RO, et al. Venous valvular reflux in veins not involved at the time of acute deep vein thrombosis. *J Vasc Surg.* 1995;22:524–531.

8. Meissner MH, Caps MT, Bergelin RO, et al. Propagation, rethrombosis and new thrombus formation after acute deep venous thrombosis. *J Vasc Surg.* 1995;22:558–567.

9. Bauer G. A venographic study of thromboembolic problems. *Acta Chir Scand.* 1940;84(suppl):1–75.

10. Rabinov K, Paulin S. Roentgen diagnosis of venous thrombosis of the leg. *Arch Surg.* 1972;104:134–144.

11. Strandness DE Jr. Thrombosis detection by ultrasound, plethysmography, and phlebography. *Semin Nucl Med.* 1977;7:213–218.

12. Athanasoulis CA. Phlebography for the diagnosis of deep leg vein thrombosis. In: *Prophylactic Therapy for Deep Vein Thrombosis and Pulmonary Embolism.* DHEW Publication. National Institutes of Health. 1975;76:866.

13. Landowne M, Katz LN. A critique of plethysmographic method of measuring blood flow in extremities of man. *Am Heart J.* 1942;23:644–675.

14. Dahn I, Eriksson E. Plethysmographic diagnosis of deep venous thrombosis of the leg. *Acta Chir Scand.* 1968;398(suppl):33–42.

15. Barnes RW, Collicott PE, Mozersky DJ, et al. Noninvasive quantitation of maximum venous outflow in acute thrombophlebitis. *Surgery.* 1972;72:971–979.

16. Hull R, van Aken WG, Hirsh J, et al. Impedance plethysmography using the occlusive cuff technique in the diagnosis of venous thrombosis. *Circulation.* 1976;53:696–700.

17. Cranley JJ. Diagnosis of deep vein thrombosis by phleborheography. In: Bernstein EF, ed. *Noninvasive Diagnostic Techniques in Vascular Disease.* 3rd ed. St. Louis: CV Mosby; 1985:730–741.

18. Strandness DE Jr, Sumner DS. Ultrasonic velocity detector in the diagnosis of thrombophlebitis. *Arch Surg.* 1972;104:180–183.

19. Van Bemmelen PS, Bedford G, Beach K, Strandness DE Jr. Status of the valves in the superficial and deep venous system in chronic venous disease. *Surgery.* 1990;109:730–734.

20. Van Bemmelen PS, Beach K, Bedford G, Strandness DE Jr. The mechanism of venous valve closure. Its relationship to the velocity of reverse flow. *Arch Surg.* 1990;125:617–619.

21. Van Bemmelen PS, Bedford G, Beach K, Strandness DE Jr. Quantitative segmental evaluation of venous valvular reflux with duplex ultrasound scanning. *J Vasc Surg.* 1989;10:425–431.

22. Killewich LA, Bedford GR, Beach KW, Strandness DE Jr. Diagnosis of deep vein thrombosis: a prospective study comparing duplex scanning to contrast venography. *Circulation.* 1989;79:810–814.

23. Alanen A, Kormano M. Correlation of the echogenicity and structure of clotted blood. *J Ultrasound Med.* 1985;4:421–425.

24. Thomas DP, Merton RE, Wood RD, Hockley DJ. The relationship between vessel wall injury and venous thrombosis: an experimental study. *Br J Haematol.* 1985;59:449–457.

25. Thomas DP, Merton RE, Hockley DJ. The effect of stasis on the venous endothelium: an ultrastructural study. *Br J Haematol.* 1983;55:113–122.

26. Nicolaides AN, Kakkar VV, Field ES, Renney JT. The origin of deep vein thrombosis: a venographic study. *Br J Radiol.* 1971;44:653–663.

27. Sevitt S. The structure and growth of valve-pocket thrombi in femoral veins. *J Clin Pathol.* 1974;27:517–528.

28. Thomas DP, Merton RE, Hiller KF, Hockley D. Resistance of normal endothelium to damage by thrombin. *Br J Haematol.* 1982;51:25–35.

29. Aronson DL, Thomas DP. Experimental studies on venous thrombosis: effect of coagulants, procoagulants and vessel contusion. *Thromb Haemost.* 1985;54:866–870.

30. Karino T, Motomiya M. Flow through a venous valve and its implications for thrombus formation. *Thromb Res.* 1984;36:245–257.

31. Sevitt S. Organization of valve pocket thrombi and the anomalies of double thrombi and valve cusp involvement. *Br J Surg.* 1974;61:641–649.

32. Huisman MV, Buller HR, ten Cate JW. Utility of impedence plethymography in the diagnosis of recurrent deep-vein thrombosis. *Arch Intern Med.* 1988;148:681–683.

33. Killewich LA, Bedford GR, Beach KW, Strandness DE Jr. Spontaneous lysis of deep venous thrombi: rate and outcome. *J Vasc Surg.* 1989;9:810–814.

34. van Ramshorst B, van Bemmelen PS, Honeveld H, et al. Thrombus regression in deep venous thrombosis: quantification of spontaneous thrombolysis with duplex scanning. *Circulation.* 1992;86:414–419.

35. Hull RD, Raskob GE, Hirsch J, et al. Continuous intravenous heparin compared with intermittent subcutaneous heparin in the initial treatment of proximal vein thrombosis. *N Engl J Med.* 1986;315:1109–1114.

36. Hull R, Delmore T, Genton E, et al. Warfarin sodium versus low-dose heparin in the treatment of venous thrombosis. *N Engl J Med.* 1979;301:855–858.

37. Philbrick JT, Becker DM. Calf deep venous thrombosis: a wolf in sheep's clothing? *Arch Intern Med.* 1988;148:2131–2138.

38. Krupski WC, Bass A, Dilley RB, et al. Propagation of deep venous thrombosis by duplex ultrasonography. *J Vasc Surg.* 1990;12:467–475.

39. Svensson PJ, Dahlback B. Resistance to activated protein C as a basis for venous thrombosis. *N Engl J Med.* 1994;330:517–522.

40. Griffin JH, Evatt B, Wideman C, Fernandez JA. Anticoagulant protein C pathway defective in majority of thrombophilic patients. *Blood.* 1993;82:1989–1993.

41. Juhan-Vague I, Valadier J, Alessi MC, et al. Deficient t-PA release and elevated PA inhibitor levels in patients with spontaneous or recurrent deep venous thrombosis. *Thromb Haemost.* 1987;57:67–72.

42. Arcelus JI, Caprini JA, Hoffman KN, et al. Laboratory assays and duplex scanning outcomes after symptomatic deep vein thrombosis: preliminary results. *J Vasc Surg.* 1996;23:616–621.

43. Cranley JJ, Canos AJ, Sull WJ. The diagnosis of deep vein thrombosis: fallibility of clinical symptoms and signs. *Arch Surg.* 1976;111:34–36.

44. Barnes RW, Wu KK, Hoak JC. Fallibility of the clinical diagnosis of venous thrombosis. *JAMA.* 1975;234:605–607.

45. Markel A, Manzo RA, Bergelin RO, Strandness DE Jr. Acute deep vein thrombosis: diagnosis, localization, and risk factors. *J Vasc Med Biol.* 1991;3:432–439.

46. Markel A, Manzo RA, Bergelin RO, Strandness DE Jr. Pattern and distribution of thrombi in acute venous thrombosis. *Arch Surg.* 1992;127:305–309.

47. Gooley NA, Sumner DS. Relationship of venous reflux to the site of venous valvular incompetence: implications for venous reconstructive surgery. *J Vasc Surg.* 1988;7:50–59.

48. Rosfors S, Lamke LO, Nordstroem E, Bygdeman S. Severity and location of venous valvular insufficiency: the importance of distal valve function. *Acta Chir Scand.* 1990;156:689–694.

49. Killewich LA, Martin R, Cramer M, Beach KW, Strandness DE. An objective assessment of the physiological changes in the postthrombotic syndrome. *Arch Surg.* 1985;120:424–426.

50. Killewich LA, Martin R, Cramer M, et al. Pathophysiology of venous claudication. *J Vasc Surg.* 1984;1:507–511.

51. Schulman S, Lockner D, Juhlin-Dannfelt A. The duration of oral anticoagulation after deep vein thrombosis. *Acta Med Scand.* 1985;217:547–552.

52. Research Committee of the British Thoracic Society. Optimum duration of anticoagulation for deep-vein thrombosis and pulmonary embolism. *Lancet.* 1992;340:873–876.

53. Druckert F, Muller G, Nyman D. Treatment of deep vein thrombosis with streptokinase. *Br Med J.* 1975;1:479–481.

54. Ott P, Eldrup E, Oxholm P, et al. Streptokinase therapy in the routine management of deep vein thrombosis in the lower extremities: a retrospective study of phlebographic results and therapeutic complications. *Acta Med Scand.* 1986;219:295–300.

55. Goldhaber SZ, Buring JE, Lipnick RJ, Hennekens CH. Pooled analyses of randomized trials of streptokinase and heparin in phlebographically documented acute deep venous thrombosis. *Am J Med.* 1984;76:393–397.

56. Elliot MS, Immelmen EJ, Jeffery P, et al. A comparative randomized trail of heparin versus streptokinase in the treatment of acute proximal venous thrombosis: an interim report of a prospective trial. *Br J Surg.* 1979;66:838–843.

57. Arensen H, Hoiset A, Ly B, Godal HC. Streptokinase or heparin in the treatment of deep vein thrombosis: follow-up results of a prospective study. *Acta Med Scand.* 1982;211:65–68.

58. Sherry S, Bell WR, Duckert H, et al. Thrombolytic therapy in thrombosis: a National Institutes of Health consensus development conference. *Ann Intern Med.* 1980;93:141–144.
59. Markel A, Manzo RA, Strandness DE Jr. The potential role of thrombolytic therapy in venous thrombosis. *Arch Intern Med.* 1992;152:1265–1267.
60. Comerota AJ, Katz ML, White JV. Thrombolytic therapy for acute deep venous thrombosis: How much is enough? *Cardiovasc Surg.* 1996;4:101–104.

36

Imaging of Major Veins
by Computed Tomography
and Magnetic Resonance
Imaging Scanning

Anthony W. Stanson, MD, and Jerome F. Breen, MD

Computed tomography (CT) and magnetic resonance imaging (MRI) are complex imaging modalities that have made major contributions to the practice of medicine. Continued advancements in the spatial and temporal resolution capabilities of these machines have increased their clinical usefulness. Imaging of the venous systems is an area that has come under the domain of these diagnostic modalities.

COMPUTED TOMOGRAPHY

A CT scan is an x-ray image through a cross-section of the body. The body image is a computer-generated reconstruction of the attenuation of the transmitted x-ray beam. The resultant pictures demonstrate predictable shades of gray, black, and white; soft tissues are gray, gas is black, and bone is white as is contrast material. Oral contrast material serves to opacify the intestinal, and intravenous contrast material opacifies the vasculature and provides contrast enhancement of the organs through vascular perfusion. A CT image provides a much wider range of contrast densities than does a plain film. Intravenous (IV) contrast material makes the images especially sensitive in displaying anatomy and pathology. Also, the ability to detect the intrinsic high density of an acute hematoma and the ability to identify calcification of soft tissues and vessels further enhance the value of CT scanning.

The images of CT scanners are revealed as cross-sections of the body. This is a limitation of the technology. However, it is possible to perform off-line reconstructed images in a variety of other orientations: sagittal, coronal, oblique, and so on (Fig. 36–1). Usually, such reconstructed images have less spatial resolution than the primarily derived transaxial images. The reason for this is that the transaxial images are acquired at a body thickness of several millimeters, while the resolution of the images in the transaxial plane is much less than a millimeter. Another reason for the lack of resolution of the off-line reconstructed images is that with a conventional, slow scanner a new

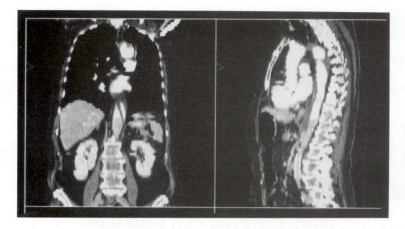

Figure 36–1. Reconstructed images from cross-section CT scans through the chest and abdomen. The left image is in the coronal view and the right image is a sagittal view. Note that the spatial resolution is less than that of a primarily acquired CT image (see Fig. 36–2).

breath hold is required for each single image and rarely is it possible for a patient to return to the original respiratory level for the subsequent acquisitions. This produces a reconstructed image with a staircase border making it particularly difficult to depict accurately anatomic detail in a coronal or sagittal format. By comparison, MRI is not limited to a single primary plane of acquisition; it can acquire primary images in almost any chosen plane.

Fast CT Scanners

Modern CT scanners acquire images much faster than was possible only a few years ago. The lastest generation of conventional scanners has a helical (or spiral) mode of function (all major manufacturers have their own model). In this capacity, the x-ray tube continuously spins around the patient while the table, on which the patient lies, moves at a constant rate, thus allowing a long axial segment of the body to be imaged during a single breath hold. The resultant image group represents a helical (or spiral) configuration. These machines function almost as rapidly in the standard incremental axial mode whereby each image is obtained separately for each table position. Either way, the main advantage of such rapid acquisition is that the IV contrast material is captured within the vascular bed uniformly throughout the body segments being examined. Indeed, it is possible to examine the entire chest, abdomen, and pelvis with a single infusion of IV contrast material. This improvement in temporal resolution represents a major advance over the last generation of conventional scanners. Now, images can be obtained in very thin sections with spiral/helical mode that allows for much higher quality off-line reconstruction in sagittal or coronal planes, further enhancing the anatomic display. Another benefit of these fast machines is the increase in examination throughput.

Since the mid-1980s, another type of fast CT scanner has been in use, but only in a few centers. It offers an electron-beam technology (Imatron, South San Francisco, CA). In this machine there is no x-ray tube that rotates around the patient, but rather an electron beam passes under the patient and strikes a strip of tungsten to produce the x-ray beam. This machine is very fast and the table can also be moved in a continuous mode, producing a spiral-like imaging sequence. The Imatron scanner is particularly valuable for studying aortic dissection, constrictive pericarditis, coronary artery calcification, pulmonary emboli, and cardiac masses.[1] The pulses of x-rays, and therefore the exposure time, can be as short as 0.1 second and can also be synchronized to the heartbeat thereby eliminating all cardiac motion artifacts, including aortic pulsation and even the motion artifact of breathing. This is not possible with spiral/helical machines where exposure times are relatively long, between 0.5 and 1.0 second, and cardiac motion artifacts are often problematic around the mediastinal structures, which include the superior vena cava (SVC) and the thoracic portion of the inferior vena cava (IVC).

In the abdomen and pelvis, arterial pulsation is minimal and does not contribute to motion artifacts. Even last-generation conventional CT scanners produce excellent images, except for the problem of not imaging fast enough to capture uniform IV contrast opacification of the arteries.

CT Scanning Technique

The major veins of the neck, thorax, abdomen, and upper thighs are large enough to allow a CT scan to distinguish between a disorder and a normal state. Those vessels oriented in the axial direction are seen best because they are viewed in cross-section. For venous segments that are oriented in other planes, off-line reconstructed imaging of thin section, spiral/helical acquisition will provide satisfactory anatomic display.

Venous Opacification

Usually, the study of the venous system by CT scanning requires IV contrast material. Indeed, it is unusual to obtain a preliminary set of scans without contrast material for a study of the veins. However, such a set of images would be valuable in detecting the high density of an acute hematoma either from hemorrhage or an intraluminal thrombus.[2,3]

Contrast material is usually administered through a peripheral vein of the upper extremity. In situations when a central venous line is in place, it is a good site for contrast injection. It is a more efficient site for delivery than is a peripheral location. The lag time in the effective circulation time is reduced because it does not travel the length of the arm and the thoracic inlet; therefore, somewhat less contrast volume would be necessary. This is especially important if a repeat injection is required to evaluate more than one vascular bed. Of course, caution must be exercised when injecting a central line so as not to risk the mechanical integrity of the catheter. For long, small catheters—5 French or less—injection rates are limited to 1 mL/s or less, which is usually too slow for adequate CT examination. On rare occasions, it may be necessary or desirable to use a foot vein to administer the contrast material. This would be when no upper extremity veins are available or when, for a specific reason, the pelvic veins or the low IVC must be evaluated. It is important to keep the leg elevated and to access the largest vein available, such as the saphenous, so that flow will not be impeded.

The ideal rate for infusion of contrast material must be sufficient to allow satisfactory density of the vessels on the images, but not so rapidly that the flow of contrast has ended long before the scanning has finished. Usually the rate of injection is between 1 and 3 mL/s; the older the patient, the lower the required rate. The allowable volume of contrast material for a single injection is approximately 2 mL/kg body weight assuming normal renal and cardiac function. Ideally, the volume of contrast material should be matched to the scanning requirements of the procedure without an excess amount being given. This is not a difficult task to accomplish once the circulation time is known, the rate of infusion is chosen, and the total time for the CT examination has been determined. The circulation time is measured with the CT scanner and is based on appearance of the contrast material into whatever organ or vessel is selected on a single, preliminary CT image. A 10-mL volume of contrast is injected and a temporal sequence of exposures is made over the predetermined body section. The scanner then automatically profiles the contrast density curve over the preselected anatomic site. The highest point of the CT generated flow curve represents the optimal circulation time.

The main problem involved with performing CT scanning for the major veins is that of coordinating the IV contrast opacification of the veins with the timing of the image acquisition. Unlike, the arterial system, which opacifies directly and predictably, the venous network is complex. The examination needs to be monitored for each venous bed. There is a great variation in the timing of contrast opacification among the SVC, upper and lower IVC, renal, superior mesenteric, portal, hepatic, pulmonary, and jugular veins. There are two levels of venous opacification: inflow venous and return venous.

The first level is the contrast material that is injected into an arm vein and drains through the ipsilateral innominate vein and into the SVC. It appears quickly and is densely opacified. The pulmonary arteries and veins opacify next, but are not as densely opacified as the SVC because of the dilution that occurs from IVC within the right atrium and ventricle.

The second level is the venous opacification that occurs as a result of venous return after arterial perfusion of organs and tissues. The appearance time of the various venous beds depends on their proximity to the aortic root and the blood flow to the organs and tissues. The jugular veins are the first systemic venous systems to fill with contrast material (Fig. 36–2). Soon, thereafter, the renal veins fill, followed in time by the upper IVC and the superior mesenteric and portal veins in turn. Several seconds later the hepatic veins opacify. Finally, the lower IVC fills. If the infrarenal IVC is found to be opacified early or densely, consider an arteriovenous fistula (AVF) either acquired from a postoperative complication or secondary to erosion through an aneurysm of the abdominal aorta (Fig. 36–3).

Obviously, it is not possible for a single series of CT acquisitions to capture the entire venous network. Therefore, coordination of the timing of contrast injection and

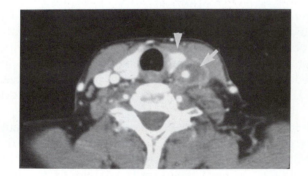

Figure 36–2. CT scan taken through the low neck shows a low density zone (*arrow*) around the left common carotid artery. This is an infection in the carotid sheath. Note that the internal jugular vein does not opacify because of occlusion. The high-density zone anterior to the left carotid artery is the thyroid gland (*arrowhead*). (*Reproduced with permission: Stanson AW, Breen JF. Computed tomography and magnetic resonance imaging in venous disorders. In: Gloviczki P, Yao JST, eds. Handbook of Venous Disorders. London: Chapman and Hall; 1996.*)

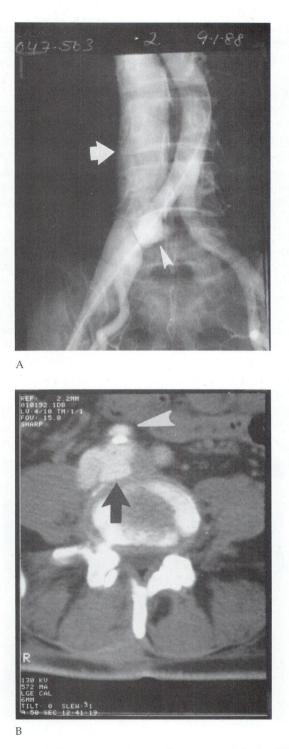

A

B

Figure 36–3. Postoperative AVF between the right iliac artery and the low IVC. (**A**) Aortogram demonstrates rapid filling of the cava (*arrow*) from a fistula arising from the right common iliac artery (*arrowhead*). (**B**) CT scan taken through this level shows opacification of the right common iliac artery (*arrowhead*) and simultaneous filling of the IVC (*arrow*). (*Reproduced with permission: Stanson AW, Breen JF. Computed tomography and magnetic resonance imaging in venous disorders. In: Gloviczki P, Yao JST, eds. Handbook of Venous Disorders. London: Chapman and Hall; 1996.*)

of the image acquisition needs to targeted to the specific area of interest. Furthermore, the examination must be monitored to be certain that the final images indeed accurately capture contrast material in the desired venous system.

Artifacts of Flowing Blood and Contrast Material

At the junctions of major veins, flow artifacts may be seen from the interface of contrast-laden blood in one vein and the wash-in from the adjacent vein that does not contain contrast material. The most demonstrative place where this occurs is at the junction of the innominate veins. Contrast material flowing from one upper extremity has a very dense CT appearance in the ipsilateral innominate vein and does not immediately mix with the venous return from the other innominate vein. This results in a filling defect throughout the course of the SVC (Fig. 36–4). This must not be misinterpreted as a mass or thrombus.

A similar, but less dense, filling defect appears within the IVC at the insertions of the renal veins and at the junctions of the hepatic veins (Figs. 36–5 and 36–6). The blood flow through the kidneys is high and contrast material appears in the renal veins quickly and densely. The low IVC demonstrates opacification later and only faintly because the blood return from the pelvis and the lower extremities is of a low volume and a low rate (Fig. 36–7). Flow artifacts will be seen in the low IVC at the junction of the iliac veins if contrast material is administered through a foot vein.

Indeed, even within the right atrium there is frequently an inhomogenous appearance of contrast material entering from the SVC mixing with fresh blood washing in from the IVC. However, within the right ventricle, contrast material is finally homogeneously mixed with blood and this homogeneity continues into the pulmonary circulation and out of the aorta.

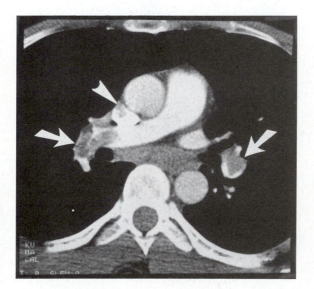

Figure 36–4. Electron-beam CT scan through the chest at the main pulmonary artery level. Contrast material within the SVC is present in the posterior portion only, indicating that only one arm was injected and the wash-in from the contralateral innominate vein results in incomplete mixing of contrast. This gives a false appearance of thrombus in the SVC (*arrowhead*). Also note the bilateral pulmonary embolism (*arrows*) in the lower lobe pulmonary arteries with a thin rim of contrast opacification peripherally. This is a typical appearance by CT scanning of acute pulmonary embolism.

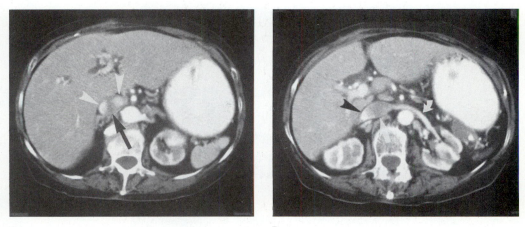

A   B

Figure 36–5. CT scan at the renal vein level shows incomplete opacification of the upper IVC. (**A**) Shows lateral zones of opacification (*arrowheads*) in the IVC, whereas the central portion is unopacified (*arrow*). (**B**) CT scan taken 2 cm caudal to part A shows right lateral opacification within the cava from the right renal vein (*arrowhead*). Note the opacification of the left renal vein (*curved arrow*). The majority of the IVC is devoid of opacification (*arrow*). (*Reproduced with permission: Stanson AW, Breen JF. Computed tomography and magnetic resonance imaging in venous disorders. In: Gloviczki P, Yao JST, eds. Handbook of Venous Disorders. London: Chapman and Hall; 1996.*)

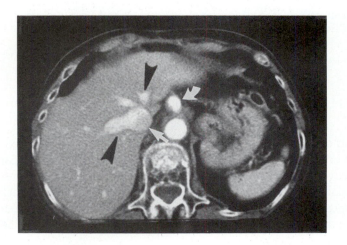

Figure 36–6. CT scan through the midliver shows hepatic vein opacification (*arrowheads*) with mixed density in the IVC from wash-in blood from the lower IVC (*arrow*). The scan was performed for evaluation of the celiac artery aneurysm (*curved arrow*). (*Reproduced with permission: Stanson AW, Breen JF. Computed tomography and magnetic resonance imaging in venous disorders. In: Gloviczki P, Yao JST, eds. Handbook of Venous Disorders. London: Chapman and Hall; 1996.*)

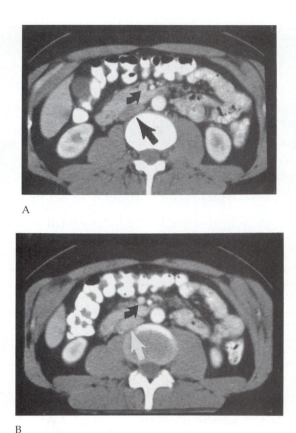

A

B

Figure 36–7. CT scan through the midabdomen. (**A**) At this level and time, the IVC (*arrow*) is not yet opacified with contrast material. Also note the opacification of the superior mesenteric artery and the lack of opacification of the mesenteric vein (*curved arrow*). (**B**) This scan is taken 1 cm caudal to part A and 2 seconds later. Note that now the IVC (*arrow*) and the mesenteric vein (*curved arrow*) have become opacified. (*Reproduced with permission: Stanson AW, Breen JF. Computed tomography and magnetic resonance imaging in venous disorders. In: Gloviczki P, Yao JST, eds. Handbook of Venous Disorders. London: Chapman and Hall; 1996.*)

CT Images

Vena Cava

The orientation of the superior and inferior vena caval segments is axial to the cross-section of the body, making it an ideal structure for evaluation by CT scanning. Because much of the cava is surrounded by fat, its outline is readily evident. However, IV contrast material is necessary for an accurate examination. As discussed earlier, the appearance times of contrast opacification within the SVC and IVC are much different. Indeed, appearance times of opacification within the high and low segments of the IVC are different.

Superior Vena Cava

Imaging applications of CT scanning of the SVC include persistence of the left SVC, extrinsic compression by mediastinitis, neoplasm, or aneurysm, thrombosis, tumor thrombus, and the normal postinterventional state and complications.

Persistence of the left SVC is an embryologic remnant of the primitive bilateral state.[4-6] On the CT image, it appears as a round or oval structure adjacent to the aortic arch, which then traverses caudally between the left artial appendage and the left superior pulmonary vein (Fig. 36–8). The terminal drainage is usually into the coronary sinus, which in turn drains into the right atrium, but, at times, drainage is into the hemiazygos vein. Sometimes the remnant is large and represents the complete venous drainage of the left innominate vein. Often, the left SVC is only partial, perhaps draining only the left subclavian vein or perhaps it is found to be only a prominent branch from the left innominate vein, while the innominate itself continues its course to join the right one to form the SVC.

A small, partial left SVC may be easily overlooked or misinterpreted as a small mass or lymph node, unless IV contrast material happened to have been injected into the left upper extremity. In cases of obstruction of the SVC, collateral venous development may present as a large highest intercostal vein, which may have a false

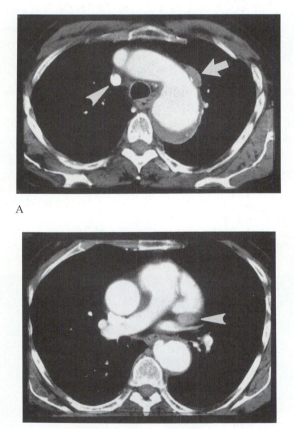

A

B

Figure 36–8. Left-sided SVC. (**A**) Electron-beam CT scan taken across the aortic arch shows a nonopacified vascular structure (*arrow*) representing the left SVC. This drains from the left innominate vein; however, the contrast material was injected from the right arm, which opacifies the right SVC (*arrowhead*). (**B**) CT scan taken a few centimeters caudal to part A shows the course of the left SVC (*arrowhead*) between the atrial appendage anteriorly and the pulmonary vein posteriorly. (*Reproduced with permission: Stanson AW, Breen JF. Computed tomography and magnetic resonance imaging in venous disorders. In: Gloviczki P, Yao JST, eds. Handbook of Venous Disorders. London: Chapman and Hall; 1996.*)

appearance of a partial left SVC. Bilateral upper extremity injections of contrast material will usually allow accurate distinction between an anomaly and collateral venous drainage secondary to SVC obstruction.

A very rare finding of the SVC and some other systemic veins of the thorax is aneurysm development for which CT, with IV contrast material, is an excellent diagnostic modality.[7]

Obstruction of the SVC is usually caused by extrinsic compression rather than intraluminal thrombus or tumor. This produces a syndrome of venous hypertension of the head, neck, face, and upper extremities.[8–11] The etiology of the compression is either inflammatory as caused by mediastinitis or secondary to neoplasm such as bronchogenic carcinoma. These conditions are ideally studied by CT scanning. For contrast administration it is important to make simultaneous infusions from each upper extremity. The standard dose and rate of injection can be divided. This technique allows maximum identification of the disease process and also demonstrates the collateral venous pathways. Also, the bilateral contrast injection prevents filling defects of wash-in blood from creating confusing artifacts.

The distinction between mediastinal tumor and inflammation is usually evident by CT. Tumor has a large bulk when it reaches the stage of causing SVC occlusion (Fig. 36–9), whereas mediastinitis presents as an infiltrative, edematous process that is mottled in its CT density. Although inflammatory adenopathy is often present, its bulk is not usually so great as to be expected to cause occlusion of the SVC (Fig. 36–10). Inflammation is a chronic condition and often is accompanied by calcific deposits when caused by histoplasmosis, which is endemic in the upper midwestern part of the United States. In addition, venous collaterals will be large and well developed in such a chronic condition, unlike the situation with a rapidly growing tumor.[10,12] Sometimes, with inflammatory obstruction of the SVC only a short segment above the azygos vein is occluded and the venous collaterals fill the azygos, which then drains into the caudal portion of the SVC. This can be determined by careful analysis of the CT images and would be more dramatically portrayed with off-line reconstruction in the coronal plane.

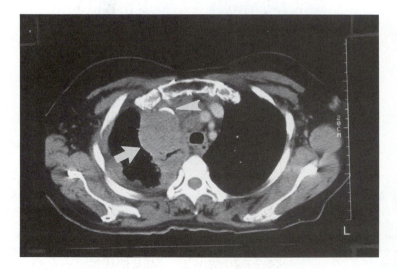

Figure 36–9. CT scan through the upper chest shows a mass (*arrow*) compressing and displacing the right innominate vein (*arrowhead*).

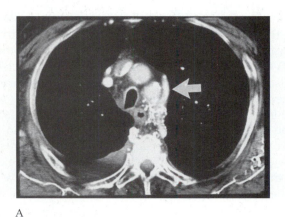

A

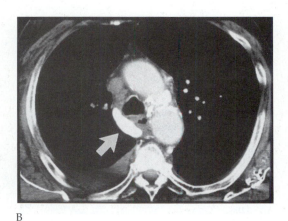

B

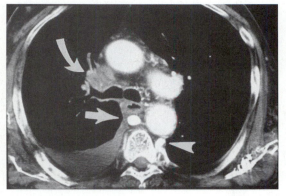

C

Figure 36–10. CT scan through the upper chest showing mediastinitis and occlusion of the SVC. Bilateral arm injections of contrast material were made. (**A**) Collateral venous drainage through the highest intercostal vein is indicated by the arrow. (**B**) A few centimeters caudal to part A, the azygos arch is densely opacified (*arrow*). It is flowing retrograde, bypassing the occluded SVC. (**C**) This section is caudal to part B and shows dense opacification of the azygos vein (*arrow*) and the hemiazygos vein (*arrowhead*). These veins are draining caudally into the IVC. Note the inflammatory mass (*curved arrow*) occluding the SVC.

Another cause of SVC compression is an aneurysm of the ascending aorta, with or without dissection (Fig. 36–11). Indeed the effect may be so severe that there is no evident flow within the SVC. In these cases the collateral venous drainage diverts to the azygos and hemiazygos veins with retrograde flow into the abdomen with subsequent drainage into the IVC. The CT images will demonstrate this clearly when contrast material is given. Also, the nature of the aneurysm and its extent can be fully evaluated if the imaging sequence is continued into the abdomen.

Thrombus within the SVC is not commonly found as an isolated entity but is usually an extension of thrombosis from one or both subclavian veins secondary to long-term catheter placement. The CT appearance is lack of contrast filling of the SVC. However, contrast material must be administered bilaterally to be certain of occlusion. In cases where the thrombus is not occlusive, the CT finding is a large central filling defect with a peripheral ring of contrast opacification. This is the appearance of early thrombosis, within 1 week.

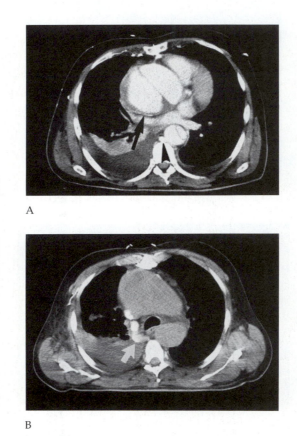

A

B

Figure 36–11. Dissection of the thoracic aorta with aneurysm of the ascending segment and marked effacement of the SVC. (**A**) CT scan shows the SVC to be a thin slit (*arrow*) compressed by the dissecting aneurysm of the ascending aorta. The azygos vein is densely opacified (*arrowhead*). (**B**) CT scan taken at the level of the azygos arch shows dense opacification of the azygos vein (*arrow*), which is draining the superior vena cava to a subdiaphragmatic site. (*Reproduced with permission: Stanson AW, Breen JF. Computed tomography and magnetic resonance imaging in venous disorders. In: Gloviczki P, Yao JST, eds. Handbook of Venous Disorders. London: Chapman and Hall; 1996.*)

Inferior Vena Cava

Disorders of the IVC include anomalies, thrombosis, tumors compressed by an adjacent mass or inflammation, and postprocedural conditions such as IVC filter placement and postoperative changes.

In a similar situation as the SVC, the anomalies of the IVC reflect persistence of embryologic pathways that often involve remnant left-sided structures. Usually, the persistent left-sided structure is only a partial remnant and involves the infrarenal segment and then enters into the left renal vein. Another IVC anomaly is an interruption between the renal and hapatic vein levels. This may be found with a single right-sided IVC or with double IVCs (Fig. 36–12).[13] In this congenital condition there are two drainages. The lower segments drain along the paraspinal regions into the thorax as the hemiazygos and azygos veins, while the upper abdominal segment drains normally into the right atrium. The CT evaluation of these anomalies requires multiple images so as not to misinterpret an abnormally located venous structure for an enlarged lymph node.

Thrombus within the IVC is easily detected as a filling defect provided the CT images capture the contrast-filled phase. Acute thrombus may have a high CT density that can be appreciated if scans are obtained before IV contrast material.[2,3] A secondary CT finding of acute thrombus or tumor within the cava is a distended, round shape as seen on cross-section. Normally the IVC is somewhat oval in shape, although, a sustained valsalva maneuver can also distend a normal cava into a round shape. Indeed, respiratory effort can induce considerable alteration in the shape of the IVC (Fig. 36–13). In the subacute state, thrombus has a retracted appearance and does not fill the entire cross-section of the cava, but rather appears as a tubular filing defect of small diameter

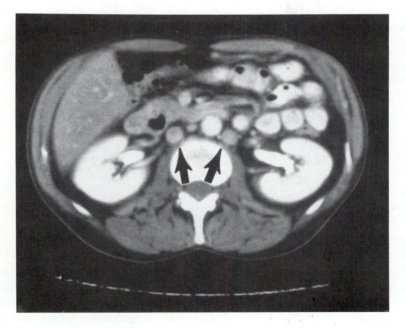

Figure 36–12. Duplication of the low IVC with azygos continuation into the thorax. Left and right IVCs are present (*arrows*). They drain into the chest through the hemiazygos and azygos veins (see Fig. 36–18). (*Reproduced with permission: Stanson AW, Breen JF. Computed tomography and magnetic resonance imaging in venous disorders. In: Gloviczki P, Yao JST, eds. Handbook of Venous Disorders. London: Chapman and Hall; 1996.*)

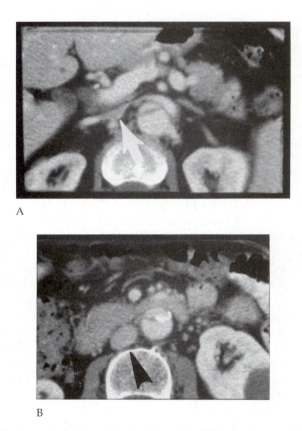

A

B

Figure 36–13. There is a large change in diameter of the IVC secondary to voluntary respiratory control. (**A**) CT scan shows the cava to be a narrow slit (*arrow*). (**B**) The cava has a much more rounded configuration (*arrowhead*) on this CT scan taken 3 cm caudal to part A. (*Reproduced with permission: Stanson AW, Breen JF. Computed tomography and magnetic resonance imaging in venous disorders. In: Gloviczki P, Yao JST, eds. Handbook of Venous Disorders. London: Chapman and Hall; 1996.*)

(Fig. 36–14). Chronic thrombosis of the IVC (or of any other vein) may eventually result in obliteration of the vessel into a fibrotic thread. It is important that this acquired condition not be misinterpreted as congenital absence of the IVC, because a history of previous thrombosis has important clinical implications. In rare circumstances, the consequence of thrombosis of the IVC may result in calcification of the organized thrombus (Fig. 36–15).

Tumors found within the IVC are usually secondary to extension and growth from adjacent organs and tributary veins, although, rarely, a primary leiomyosarcoma occurs. It is often impossible for a CT image to distinguish between intraluminal tumor and thrombus, unless a large tumor mass is present, making distinction from bland thrombus obvious. One possible diagnostic clue for tumor is contrast enhancement, but to be accurately detected there must be a precontrast scan for comparison. Determining CT density is an easy task to accomplish on the computer console. The most common intraluminal tumor is from renal cell carcinoma extending through the renal vein into the cava (Fig. 36–16).[14] This so-called "tumor thrombus" can extend cephalad into the heart (Fig. 36–16) and even a short distance caudally into the low IVC. Large adrenal tumors can demonstrate a similar phenomenon. Ovarian and uterine tumors may also

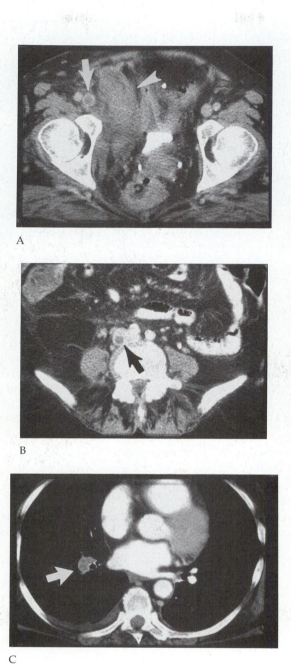

A

B

C

Figure 36–14. Thromboembolism. (**A**) CT scan taken through the femoral vein level shows acute thrombus within the right common femoral vein (*arrow*) with adjacent hematoma medially (*arrowhead*) secondary to complication of cardiac catheterization. (**B**) CT scan taken through the junction of the left and right common iliac veins shows thrombus (*arrow*) extending from the right common iliac vein up to the IVC. (**C**) Electron-beam CT scan through the midchest shows a large embolus in the right lower pulmonary artery (*arrow*). (*Reproduced with permission: Stanson AW, Breen JF. Computed tomography and magnetic resonance imaging in venous disorders. In: Gloviczki P, Yao JST, eds. Handbook of Venous Disorders. London: Chapman and Hall; 1996.*)

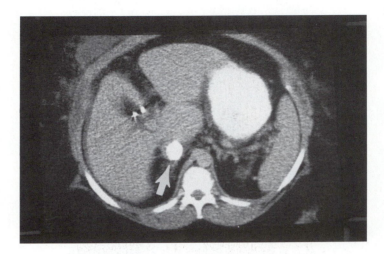

Figure 36–15. Old thrombosis of the IVC is densely calcified. The CT image is through the low hepatic portion of the IVC.

grow into their veins and extend eventually into the IVC. Rarely, other sources of retroperitoneal tumors may have venous extension into the IVC.[14]

Extrinsic compression of the IVC is often found with large retroperitoneal tumors. It can become so severe as to obliterate the caval lumen and even result in lower extremity edema. At times it may be impossible to locate the IVC on the CT scan, let alone to determine caval patency or to detect invasion by tumor. To facilitate the CT examination, it may be helpful to inject contrast material from a foot vein with leg elevation for rapid delivery. Extrinsic compression of the intrahepatic portion of the IVC often occurs with liver disease. This usually is secondary to enlargement of the caudate lobe but may also occur with polycystic liver disease and patients may become symptomatic from venous obstruction. A large aneurysm of the infrarenal aorta is another source of compression of the low IVC but should not cause symptoms of obstruction.

Certain types of retroperitoneal fibrosis can cause occlusion of the IVC.[15] The CT scan appearance is that of soft tissue thickening surrounding the aorta and IVC with indistinct borders. In the acute setting, the CT scan may show contrast enhancement of the inflammatory tissue. Periaortitis is an idiopathic inflammation of the adventitia of the aorta that presents as a rind of soft tissue thickening anteriorly and laterally and sometimes envelopes the IVC and obscures its borders. This particular type of retroperitoneal fibrosis does not obstruct the IVC, but it may obstruct the ureters. If an aortic aneurysm is also present, it is referred to as an inflammatory aneurysm. The CT scan shows a variable thickness of inflammatory tissue with distinct margins and contrast enhancement. The IVC may be difficult to identify without IV contrast material.

Inferior vena cava filter placement is readily identified by CT scanning (Fig. 36–17). All percutaneously placed filters are metallic and therefore are very opaque on all types of x-ray studies. A CT scan is a good method to evaluate them. Migration of the legs outside of the caval wall is easy to detect even without contrast material. To evaluate thrombus in and around the filter, the timing of the administration of IV contrast material and the scan acquisition must be accurately coordinated.

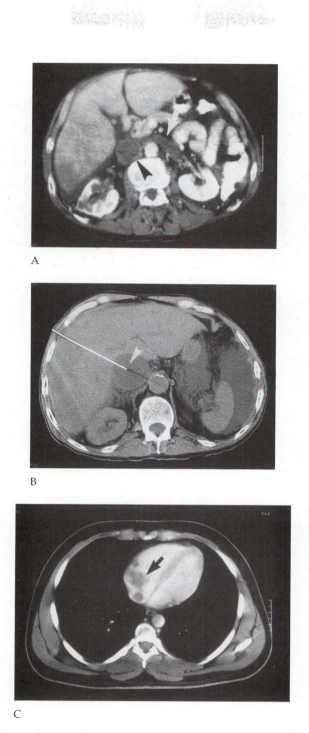

A

B

C

Figure 36–16. Tumor thrombus from a hypernephroma extending up to the atrium. (**A**) CT scan taken at the level of the kidneys shows extensive tumor thrombus within the left renal vein (*arrow*) extending across from the right renal vein (right hypernephroma is not visible on this scan level). The left renal vein and the cava (*arrowhead*) are dilated. The low-density area in the posterior aspect of the right lobe of the liver is edema secondary to obstruction of the right hepatic vein by the large tumor thrombus within the IVC. (**B**) The large tumor thrombus within the IVC extends cephalad. CT scan taken through the upper IVC with a biopsy needle (*arrowhead*) positioned in the center of the tumor thrombus. Note the marked dilation of the IVC. (*Reproduced with permission: Stanson AW, Breen JF. Computed tomography and magnetic resonance imaging in venous disorders. In: Gloviczki P, Yao JST, eds. Handbook of Venous Disorders. London: Chapman and Hall; 1996.*) (**C**) CT scan taken through the heart shows cephalad extension of the tumor thrombus into the right atrium (*arrow*).

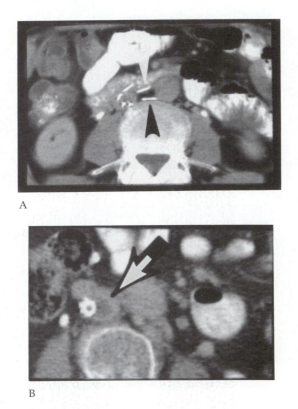

A

B

Figure 36–17. Inferior vena cava filter. (**A**) CT scan taken through the low IVC shows the legs of the caval filter (*arrowheads*) have penetrated through the wall of the cava. (**B**) CT scan at the level of the low IVC. The cava contains thrombus (*arrow*) alongside the cephalad tip of a caval filter indicating extension of thrombus beyond the filter. (*Reproduced with permission: Stanson AW, Breen JF. Computed tomography and magnetic resonance imaging in venous disorders. In: Gloviczki P, Yao JST, eds. Handbook of Venous Disorders. London: Chapman and Hall; 1996.*)

Other Thoracic Veins

Subclavian and Innominate Segments.   Identifying thrombus in the subclavian veins is somewhat difficult by CT scanning because the veins are not aligned in longitudinal axis, but are somewhat horizontally oriented. This is difficult to evaluate by the cross-section imaging of CT scanning. However, this obstacle can be overcome with thin section images and off-line reconstruction in the coronal plane. Thrombus within the right innominate vein is easily detected because its axis is the same vertical orientation as is the SVC. The left innominate vein has an oblique orientation in relation to the vertical axis, but detecting thrombus within is usually possible directly from the cross-section images.

When both innominate veins are occluded, the clinical presentation is the same as a SVC syndrome. Over time venous collaterals will improve and drainage will be evident through the azygos vein into the caudal portion of the SVC, which usually remains patent. The CT images of such thrombotic occlusion must be distinguished from the findings in mediastinitis.

Azygos and Hemiazygos Veins.   The azygos and hemiazygos venous systems are on the right and left sides of the thoracic spine, respectively, and have two crossover points where the hemiazygos drains into the azygos: One is near the level of the azygos

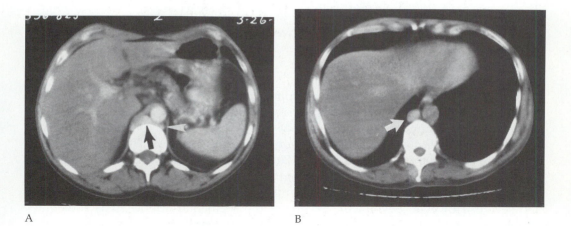

A   B

Figure 36–18. CT scans taken through the low thorax show a prominent azygos vein draining bilateral IVCs that are interrupted from the upper IVC (same case as Fig. 36–12). (**A**) The junction of the hemiazygos vein (*arrowhead*) and azygos vein (*arrow*). (**B**) This scan is a few centimeters cephalad to part A and shows a large azygos vein (*arrow*). (*Reproduced with permission: Stanson AW, Breen JF. Computed tomography and magnetic resonance imaging in venous disorders. In: Gloviczki P, Yao JST, eds. Handbook of Venous Disorders. London: Chapman and Hall; 1996.*)

arch and the caudal one is the lower thoracic region (Fig. 36–18). This system normally drains the regional intercostal and vertebral veins, which have small calibers. They become major sources of collateral drainage when there is obstruction of the SVC, IVC, or innominate veins, or in the presence of esophageal varices from portal hypertension (Fig. 36–19).[4,12] Computed tomography is an excellent method to evaluate this collateral pathway of venous drainage as well as to determine the site of obstruction and the nature of the disease process. A routine set of initial contrast-enhanced images may not include the proper time sequence to assess the entire pathologic process and sometimes a repeat series of images is necessary. But usually, with experience, the collateral drainage

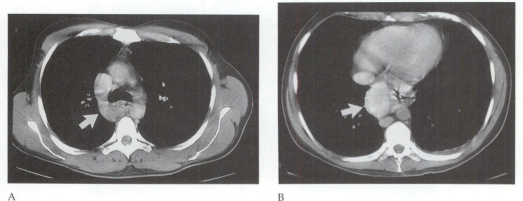

A   B

Figure 36–19. CT scan through the azygos arch. (**A**) The azygos vein (*arrow*) is enlarged secondary to high flow through the azygos system decompressing gastroesophageal varices from portal hypertension. (**B**) A CT scan taken several centimeters caudal to part A shows large esophageal varicies (*arrow*).

and the nature of the obstruction can be determined by detailed study of the initial images. It is important to distinguish between congenital abnormalities and acquired disease.

Pulmonary Embolism

In the past few years, fast CT scanning (spiral/helical and electron beam) has become an important method to diagnose pulmonary embolism.[16–18] The technique involves IV contrast material administered at a rate of 2 or 3 mL/s and a coordinated CT scan series to coincide with contrast opacification of the thoracic aorta. This is important so that both pulmonary veins and arteries are equally opacified; otherwise confusion would exist in distinguishing arteries from veins in many locations. Acute emboli in the larger pulmonary arteries are readily detected if cardiac motion artifacts are not too severe. However, beyond the origins of the segmental arteries, it is sometimes problematic to identify emboli. Also, pulmonary artery branches that are horizontal to the plane of the CT section and have a diameter less than the scan thickness are not easily evaluated.

Distinction between acute and chronic pulmonary emboli is made by the appearance of the embolus and is best seen in vessels that are oriented in the vertical axis of the body and therefore seen in cross-section. Acute embolus is seen as a filling defect in the central portion of the vessel, often surrounded by contrast material (Figs. 36–4 and 36–20) or as an occluded pulmonary artery that is dilated (Fig. 36–14). It usually fills the lumen, or if it only partially fills it, the embolus is seen as a tubular filling defect. Chronic emboli have the obverse appearance; a central lumen is patent while the defect of organized embolus is peripheral (Fig. 36–21). The central lumen is often irregular in outline and may be eccentric in position. It is the result of recanalization. Not all patients with chronic pulmonary embolism have this appearance. In about 10% of patients with surgically proved chronic pulmonary embolism, there is no laminated embolus to be seen on CT scan, but rather only a thin layer of fibrotic tissue. In these cases, the CT scan has a near normal appearance, while an angiogram shows extensive evidence of lumen irregularity and narrowing.

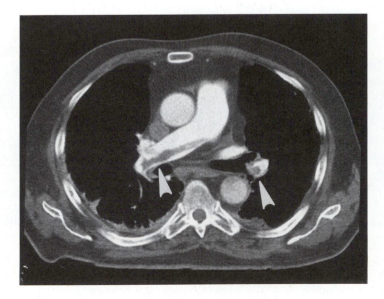

Figure 36–20. CT scan taken through the right pulmonary artery shows bilateral acute pulmonary embolism (*arrowheads*).

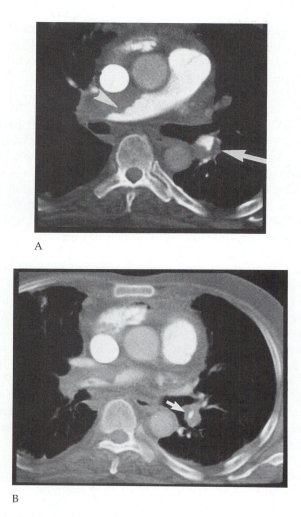

A

B

Figure 36–21. Electron-beam CT scan showing chronic pulmonary embolism. (**A**) The scalloped border of the right pulmonary artery (*arrowhead*) represents laminated thrombus. There is also laminated thrombus (*arrow*) in the left lower lobe pulmonary artery. (**B**) CT scan 2 cm caudal to part A shows a small, central recanalized lumen in the left lower pulmonary artery (*arrow*) with surrounding old laminated thrombus. This indicates recanalization of chronic pulmonary embolism. (*Reproduced with permission: Stanson AW, Breen JF. Computed tomography and magnetic resonance imaging in venous disorders. In: Gloviczki P, Yao JST, eds. Handbook of Venous Disorders. London: Chapman and Hall; 1996.*)

A CT scan for pulmonary embolism provides additional diagnostic information of the thorax. Indeed, it is essentially a complete CT examination of the chest; atelectasis, pneumonitis, other types of infiltrates, neoplasm, pneumothorax, aortic aneurysm or dissection, and coronary artery calcification can also be detected. In the evaluation of the patient with acute chest pain of unknown etiology, a chest CT scan before and after IV contrast material may prove valuable.

Other Abdominal Veins

CT scanning offers an excellent method to evaluate the abdominal contents and spaces. A noncontrast scan shows calcifications and high CT density hematomas. With contrast material, the perfusion of the organs is demarcated, and ascites and abscesses are easily detected. With attention to the timing of scan acquisition and administration of contrast material, major arteries and veins are also seen. In the case of venous thrombosis, a search can be made for collateral organ involvement, such as occult cancer, inflammatory bowel disease, fluid collections, and retroperitoneal fibrosis.

Renal Veins

The anatomic courses of the renal veins are different; the left one is horizontal, in coronal plane, to the cross-section of the CT section. It is seen well by CT, however, because it is large and has relatively high flow. The right one has a course that is obliquely vertical and is somewhat more cephalad than the left one; it is also seen well. The left vein crosses in front of the aorta in most cases and is usually a single structure. At times its course is retroaortic, and if there are two of them the more caudal one crosses posterior to the aorta. Another important anatomic finding associated with the left renal vein is an enlarged gonadal vein, which has a pathway similar to that of a left-sided low IVC. A variant of the right renal vein can present as a parallel structure to the adjacent IVC. All of these conditions can present as unusual small masses on the CT image and cause confusion in interpretation.

The two most frequently encountered disorders of the renal veins are thrombosis associated with membranous glomerulonephritis and extension of tumor thrombus from either hypernephroma or rarely from adrenal carcinoma.[11] The presence of these intraluminal masses causes a filling defect within the renal vein and distention of the diameter. Tumor thrombus may be massive and extend up and down the IVC and into the heart and across to the opposite renal vein (Fig. 36–16). CT evaluation of the junction of the IVC and renal veins must be performed carefully because of the high incidence of flow artifacts encountered in this area. For surgical planning, the CT scan can show the presence and extent of the tumor thrombus as well as provide staging of the neoplasm.

Superior Mesenteric Vein

Disorders of the superior mesenteric vein (SMV) most commonly involve either thrombosis or collateral drainage. Acute thrombosis can occur silently from a coagulopathy or be related to intra-abdominal sepsis or inflammatory bowel disease[2,19] (Figs. 36–20 and 36–22). Computed tomography scanning is an excellent method to detect thrombosis of the SMV because of its large size and vertical orientation. Collateral venous

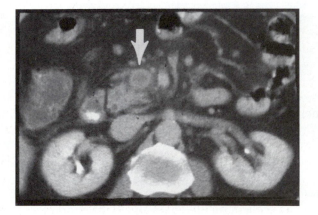

Figure 36–22. CT scan of the midabdomen shows acute thrombus within the SMV (*arrow*).

drainage of the mesenteric veins occurs in response to occlusion of the downstream drainage or secondary to portal hypertension. Dilated and tortuous veins in the region of the mesentery may be seen.

Portal Vein

The main portal vein is an extension of the superior mesenteric and splenic vein segments, although it is oriented in an oblique direction. However, thrombus or tumor invasion is readily detected by CT scanning if adequate contrast material is used. The development of collateral venous pathways in portal vein occlusion or hypertension is detected as tortuous, dilated veins along the lesser curvature of the stomach, which drain into esophageal varices (Figs. 36–22 and 36–23), as well as by enlargement of the umbilical vein within the falciform ligament.[20,21] Rarely, calcification in the walls of the splanchnic veins may be seen in patients with chronic portal hypertension.[22] Splenomegaly and atrophy of the liver are secondary changes of cirrhosis and portal hypertension and are also easily evaluated by CT. Overall, CT scanning is a very helpful tool in the evaluation of patients with portal hypertension.[21] The presence of gas within the portal vein and its branches is easily identified by CT and usually indicates ischemic bowel, liver abscess, or other causes of sepsis and rarely is associated with trauma.[23]

Splenic Vein

The splenic vein has a tortuous course that is rarely identified on a single CT image and is often difficult to assess by CT scanning. Most occlusions of the splenic vein are related pancreatic disease: pancreatitis or neoplasm. These diseases are usually evident on the CT images and alert the interpreter to the possibility of venous obstruction. A cluster of varicosities around splenic hilum and around the left renal vein is an indication of splenic vein obstruction or portal hypertension with a patent splenic vein.

Hepatic Veins

The manifestation of hepatic vein occlusion is the Budd-Chiari syndrome. Rarely is the occlusive process identified within the hepatic veins, but rather the abnormality is

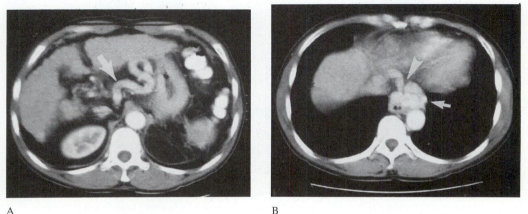

A   B

Figure 36–23. Massive varicosities secondary to portal hypertension. (**A**) CT scan through the upper abdomen shows a huge varicosity of the left gastric vein (*arrow*). There is also atrophy of the liver. (**B**) This CT section is a few centimeters cephalad to part A and shows the connection of the enlarged left gastric vein (*arrowhead*) to the massive esophageal varicosities (*arrow*).

detected in the edematous appearance of the liver, which, in the acute state, has a characteristic CT appearance of low parenchymal density in a peripheral zonal distribution corresponding to the subtended venous occlusion (Fig. 36–24).[3,24,25] The size of the zone depends on the extent of venous occlusion; sometimes the entire liver is involved. Often there is relative sparing of the caudate lobe because the hepatic veins from this region often drain separately into the IVC at a more caudal site than the main hepatic veins. When the occlusive process is secondary to obstruction of the adjacent IVC, the caval abnormality may be identified on the CT scan. However, if the site of the veno-occlusive disease is at the level of the microvasculature within the liver, then the hepatic veins and the adjacent IVC will appear normal.

Pelvic Veins

The anatomic alignment of the iliac veins is basically vertical to the CT imaging axis and therefore these segments are seen well especially if IV contrast material is used. It is important to allow an adequate length of time to pass after contrast material administration before scanning begins so as to capture the venous return from the legs and the pelvic structures. The disease processes to be considered are similar to those of the caval segments; however, anatomic variants are rarely seen.

Peripheral Veins

Because of the impact of Doppler ultrasound for diagnostic evaluation of the peripheral veins, the practical utility of CT is superseded. Also, except for the common femoral venous segments, peripheral veins are too small and the venous filling time is too unpredictable for CT to make a significant contribution.

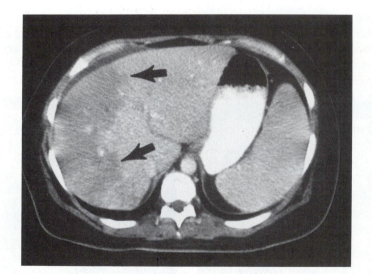

Figure 36–24. Budd-Chiari syndrome. CT scan through the liver—with contrast enhancement—shows mixed density parenchymal stain. The low density zone in the right lobe (*arrows*) demarcates the area of hepatic vein occlusion. The left lobe and caudate lobe are not involved and have normal density. (*Reproduced with permission: Stanson AW, Breen JF. Computed tomography and magnetic resonance imaging in venous disorders. In: Gloviczki P, Yao JST, eds. Handbook of Venous Disorders. London: Chapman and Hall; 1996.*)

MAGNETIC RESONANCE IMAGING

The nuclear magnetic resonance (NMR) phenomenon was first described in 1946 and has been used extensively as an analytic technique in organic chemistry. Imaging techniques were developed in the 1970s. The NMR phenomenon is a result of magnetic properties of mobile hydrogen nuclei or protons that, when placed in a magnetic field, act like small bar magnets and temporarily align themselves with the external magnetic field. When additional energy is applied at the "resonance frequency" the protons absorb this energy and become "excited" and resonate. This results in their magnetic moment deviating from alignment with the external field. These fluctuating magnetic moments can then be detected by an external antenna, and this constitutes the NMR signal. The signal produced by this process depends on the number and type of nuclei present within a volume element, the time for them to relax from their excited states (T1 and T2 relaxation times), and the time at which the signal is measured also known as the echo time, TE. The signal intensity from a specific tissue is also dependent on how often you repeat the NMR experiment, which is known as the TR or repetition time. Thus, the MR signal and MR contrast are dependent on inherent properties of the various tissues interrogated (T1, T2) and variables that can be manipulated by the imager (TE and TR). To generate images, it is necessary to apply additional magnetic (gradient) fields to encoded spatial position information into the NMR signal. A computer algorithm is used to decode all this complex information and then present it in a digital tomogram, which can be further manipulated. All the components of the MR imager are stationary. Imaging in any plane can be obtained by electronic switching of the various gradient fields without need to reposition the patient.

MR Scanning Technique

An MR image results from many repetitions from NMR phenomena and is not simply a "snapshot" like a conventional x-ray film or CT image. Imaging time with standard spin-echo techniques is therefore relatively long: Approximately 3 to 4 minutes are needed to obtain a typical volume through the chest or abdomen. Often in the chest, cardiac gating is utilized and a minimum of 128 to 256 heartbeats is utilized in signal acquisition. The spin-echo technique is the mainstay of morphologic imaging. It results in the highest resolution of stationary tissues, as well as typically good resolution of vascular structures as rapidly flowing blood results in a very dark signal or no signal, thus providing good contrast against stationary tissue. The potential for providing functional information imaging has been advanced by the development of "fast" MR techniques, which typically display flowing blood as a white or high-intensity signal. These faster acquisitions can be on the order of a single breath hold, thus greatly reducing image degregation caused by any patient motion. Various MR angiographic techniques have also been developed to selectively image vascular anatomy. This can be done totally noninvasively utilizing the natural contrast caused by flowing blood. Intravenous administration of paramagnetic contrast agents can result in near conventional contrast angiography quality images of medium and large vessels. The paramagnetic agents contain no iodine, and thus are safe to use in patients with iodine allergies or renal failure.[26–28] An MR angiographic technique known as phase angiography can measure both signal intensity and velocity of moving blood. Phase angiography can therefore be thought of as the MR equivalent of Doppler ultrasound technique.

Magnetic resonance imaging has few contraindications. Patients with pacemakers and internal cardiac fibrillators should not be imaged. Sternotomy wires, vascular clips, and valve prostheses are all common in the vascular patient population, but these are not contraindications. Vascular clips will cause some signal loss artifact and, therefore, care must be used in interpreting MR angiograms in the postoperative patient.

Magnetic resonance imaging is a powerful technology and has certain advantages over CT and conventional venography in venous imaging. The major advantage is the ability to demonstrate flow and flow dynamics without the need for intravenous iodinated contrast material in those patients with contrast contraindications. It shares the wide field of view and relative operator independence offered by these modalities that cannot be matched by ultrasound, especially in areas such as the thorax and pelvis. Spatial and contrast resolution is excellent and sufficient for most clinical situations. Imaging time has been significantly reduced in recent years, and is on par with other modalities, including the time to acquire the various planes of imaging offered with MRI. Scanners are becoming widely available with vascular imaging software typically supplied by the vendors.

Despite all that MRI can offer, use in our practice is somewhat limited compared to the other modalities. Ultrasound, which is also totally noninvasive, provides the majority of clinical information required in the extremities and in many abdominal applications. The cost of MRI exceeds that of CT or ultrasound. Clinician familiarity with MR vascular studies is less than that with CT or conventional venography. Interpretation of MR can be difficult for those not familiar with the various flow-related artifacts that are often present. In addition, while noninvasive, MRI is not an easy exam for many patients such as the obese, elderly, and the very ill patient. Fast imaging sequences and breath-hold techniques have shortened acquisition times, but patients are still required to remain motionless for several minutes at a time.

Our most common usage for MR in venous imaging is that of a "problem solver" role when other modalities fail to provide diagnostic information. Pelvis deep venous thrombosis (DVT) is a good example where MRI is typically superior to other methods (Fig. 36–25). Demonstrating flow dynamics and obtaining flow quantification in grafts or in the portal venous system, especially when serial evaluations are advantageous, are additional examples where MRI would be the method of choice (Fig. 36–26).

Vena Cava

Magnetic resonance imaging is an excellent modality to image the vena cava, especially in the coronal view where images can be quite striking in their clarity (Fig. 36–27). Congenital anomalies, thrombosis, extrinsic compression, and tumor involvement can be displayed replacing most cavograms in our practice when these specific diagnoses are sought.[29–31] In our practice, however, cavograms are most commonly performed in the setting of possible interventions such as stent or filter placement or balloon angioplasty. It is rare to image the cava noninvasively prior to such interventions. Tumor involvement of the cava is well demonstrated on coronal MRI; however, such a diagnosis is typically made at the time a CT scan is performed for initial clinical purposes (Fig. 36–28). When there is concern of tumor extension into the right atrium, MRI is typically superior to CT, which can present a confusing picture where unopacified blood mixes with contrast in the right atrium.

Simple "black blood" spin-echo imaging sequences in the coronal plane are usually adequate to display the cava without flow-related artifacts because of the

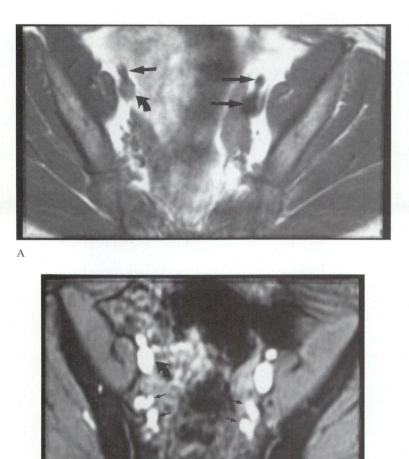

A

B

Figure 36–25. Magnetic resonance image of the pelvic veins. (**A**) Standard T1-weighted spin-echo imaging demonstrates flow void phenomenon in the external iliac arteries and left external iliac vein (*straight arrows*), but with intermediate signal intensity in right external iliac vein (*curved arrow*), indicating possible thrombosis. (**B**) Gradient echo image demonstrates patency of the right external iliac vein (*curved arrow*) as well as numerous patent branches of the internal iliac venous and arterial systems (*straight arrows*). (*Reproduced with permission: Stanson AW, Breen JF. Computed tomography and magnetic resonance imaging in venous disorders. In: Gloviczki P, Yao JST, eds. Handbook of Venous Disorders. London: Chapman and Hall; 1996.*)

relatively uniform and high flow. This also provides the greatest anatomic detail in the abdomen plus the added benefit of a short exam. To better demonstrate flow disturbances caused by stenoses or AVF communications, as well as filling defects such as thrombus, the addition of a "white blood" technique can be beneficial. Caval obstruction often results in extensive collateral formation, which can be very difficult to display with intravenous contrast techniques such as venography or CT because there is often very poor opacification of these numerous vessels. Magnetic resonance angiographic techniques are ideally suited to demonstrate these collaterals due to the sensitivity of these techniques to slow flow.[32,33] Detecting IVC thrombosis

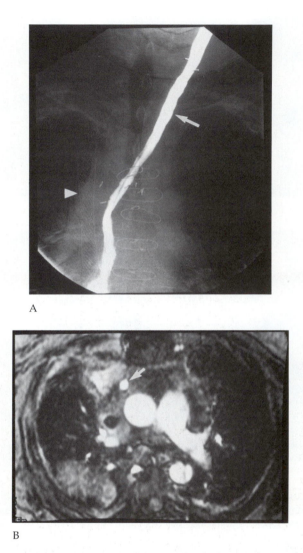

Figure 36–26. Left internal jugular vein—right atrial spinal vein graft. (**A**) Conventional venogram demonstrates patency of left internal jugular to right atrial appendage spiral vein graft (*arrow*). There is an occluded stent within the thrombosed superior vena cava (*arrowhead*). (**B**) Gradient echo image demonstrates the patency of the vein graft (*arrow*). There is signal loss in the superior vena cava, which is an artifact caused by the metallic stent resulting in the magnetic field disturbance. (**C**) Phase (*top*) and magnitude (*bottom*) images at the level of the lower neck demonstrate patency of the vein graft (*arrow*) located anterior to the left common carotid artery. The phase image contains both directional and velocity information. In this instance, flow toward the heart is set to give a high signal intensity. (**D**) Region of interest marker is placed around the vein graft and shows a typical venous flow plot and provides velocity and flow rates for future graft surveillance. (*Reproduced with permission: Stanson AW, Breen JF. Computed tomography and magnetic resonance imaging in venous disorders. In: Gloviczki P, Yao JST, eds. Handbook of Venous Disorders. London: Chapman and Hall; 1996.*)

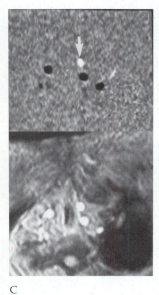

C

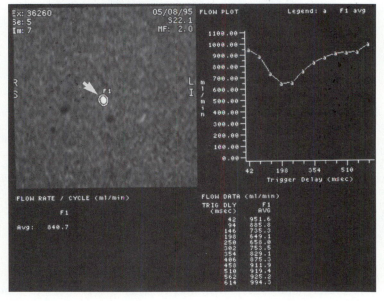

D

Figure 36–26. *Continued*

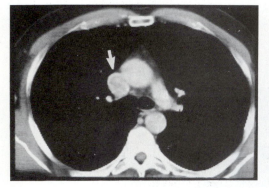

A

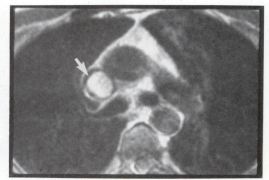

B

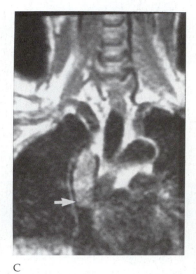

C

Figure 36–27. Tumor thrombus in the SVC. (**A**) Computed tomography with contrast, but with poor vessel opacification demonstrates filling defect within the superior vena cava (*arrow*). (**B**) Axial spin-echo MR image better depicts the tumor thrombus seen within the superior vena cava. Note that there is some signal void peripherally (*arrow*) indicating some residual patency. (**C**) Coronal spin-echo image demonstrating inferior aspect of the tumor thrombus (*arrow*). This was the result of metastatic renal cell carcinoma. (*Reproduced with permission: Stanson AW, Breen JF. Computed tomography and magnetic resonance imaging in venous disorders. In: Gloviczki P, Yao JST, eds. Handbook of Venous Disorders. London: Chapman and Hall; 1996.*)

can be done accurately and safely with the various caval filters in place without concern about filter migration.[34]

Peripheral Veins

Ultrasound has essentially replaced contrast venography for the majority of diagnoses of DVT in the extremities, however, clot detection within calf veins and extension into the pelvis and IVC is often unreliable. The MRI technique has been demonstrated to have similar sensitivity and specificity for calf DVT when compared to contrast venography.[35,36] An added advantage of MRI is its ability to study both limbs simultaneously (Figs. 36–29 and 36–30). Upper extremity venous obstruction is often at the level

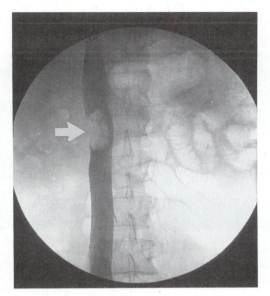

A

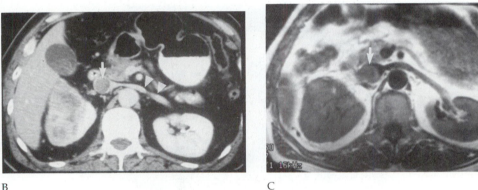

B

C

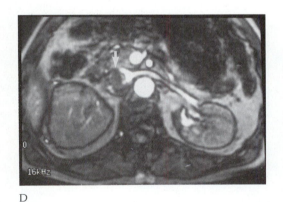

D

Figure 36–28. Tumor thrombus in the IVC. (**A**) Cavogram demonstrates a filling defect at the level of the right renal vein entrance (*arrow*). (**B**) Computed tomography with contrast demonstrating right hypernephroma as well as filling defect in the inferior vena cava (*arrow*). The left renal vein is patent (*arrowheads*). (**C**) Spin-echo and (**D**) gradient-echo images demonstrate the tumor thrombus in the inferior vena cava (*arrow*). (*Reproduced with permission: Stanson AW, Breen JF. Computed tomography and magnetic resonance imaging in venous disorders. In: Gloviczki P, Yao JST, eds. Handbook of Venous Disorders. London: Chapman and Hall; 1996.*)

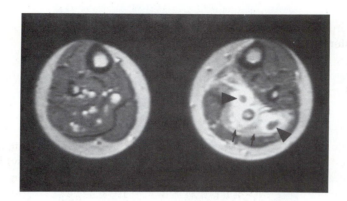

Figure 36–29. Left leg DVT. MRI at the level of the calves showed dilated veins (*arrowheads*) in the left calf. The surrounding muscles are edematous as shown by the high signal (*arrows*) compared to normal tissue.

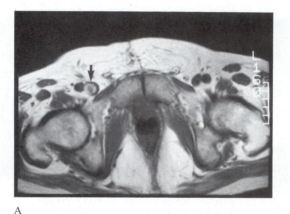

A

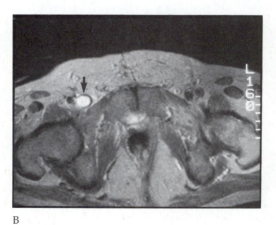

B

Figure 36–30. Thrombus in the right femoral vein. (**A**) T1-weighted spin-echo image demonstrates high signal within the right common femoral vein (*arrow*), which is mildly dilated. (**B**) T2-weighted image also demonstrates high signal with the right common femoral vein confirming the presence of thrombus (*arrow*). The remaining femoral vessels are patent. (*Reproduced with permission: Stanson AW, Breen JF. Computed tomography and magnetic resonance imaging in venous disorders. In: Gloviczki P, Yao JST, eds. Handbook of Venous Disorders. London: Chapman and Hall; 1996.*)

of the thoracic inlet. Ultrasound has difficulty displaying venous structures behind the clavicles and sternum. In the coronal, sagital, and oblique planes, MRI demonstrates not only the venous anatomy, but the surrounding anatomic structures in this complex area (Fig. 36–31). This multiplaner imaging capacity of MRI exceeds that of CT scanning, even with multiplaner reformatting.[37]

Portal, Mesenteric, and Hepatic Veins

Magnetic resonance phase angiography is ideally suited to demonstrate and quantitate venous flow within the abdomen.[38–41] Basically, phase angiography provides the equivalence of placing electromagnetic flow meters on vessels or grafts noninvasively. Direction of flow is easily demonstrated (Fig. 36–32). Detailed projections of portal and hepatic branch patterns in preoperative preparation for liver resections are provided by various MR angiographic sequences (Fig. 36–33).[42,43]

Pulmonary Veins

Gating the MR sequence to the cardiac cycle results in excellent demonstration of both systemic and pulmonary venous return to the heart (Figs. 36–34 and 36–35). Anomalous venous connections, as well as shunt calculations, can then be performed utilizing phase angiographic techniques.[44,45] Tumor invasion of the heart via pulmonary vein extension and pulmonary vein obstruction secondary to inflammatory or neoplastic conditions are readily identified. Large central pulmonary emboli are easily seen. Initial

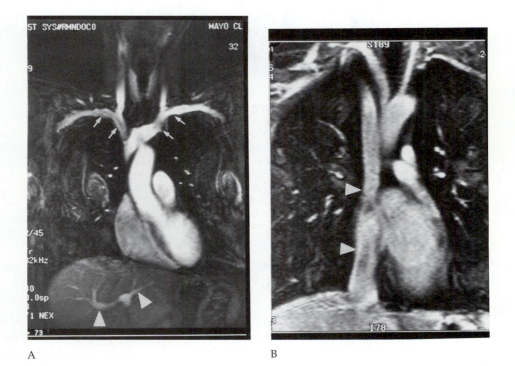

A   B

Figure 36–31. Gadolinium-enhanced imaging of thoracic veins: (**A**) Coronal tomogram demonstrating widely patent subclavian and innominate veins (*arrows*). Portal vein branches are also included (*arrowheads*). (**B**) Coronal projection including the junctions of the SVC and IVC (*arrowheads*) with the right atrium.

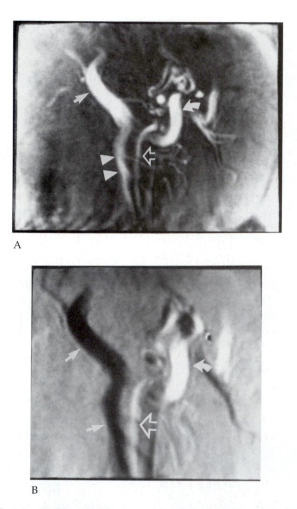

A

B

Figure 36–32. Portal vein flow. (**A**) Phase angiography without flow encoding demonstrates patency of the portal vein (*closed arrow*), superior mesenteric vein (*arrowheads*), and splenic vein (*curved arrow*). The superior mesenteric artery is also identified (*open arrow*). (**B**) With superior/inferior phase encoding, flow in a superior direction is shown as black signal as seen in the SMV and portal vein (*closed arrows*), flow in an inferior direction results in a white signal from the SMA (*open arrow*) and a segment of splenic vein (*curved arrow*). The area of the confluence of splenic and portal vein is poorly identified because flow is in mainly a left to right direction, which was not encoded for this sequence.

studies for identification of more distal pulmonary emboli indicate this may be feasible in the future.[46,47]

Klippel-Trenaunay Syndrome

Magnetic resonance imaging provides an excellent method for evaluating patients with Klippel-Trenaunay syndrome (KTS). The anomalous venous drainage is well seen and the location of the involvement can be identified. In the case of unilateral limb involvement, a comparison with the normal side is valuable to detect minimal abnormalities. The MRI findings are subcutaneous fatty hypertrophy, muscle atrophy, and abnormal veins both in the subcutaneous fat (especially laterally) and in the muscles (Fig. 36–36). In addition, remnants of the embryonic sciatic vein, partial or complete, are

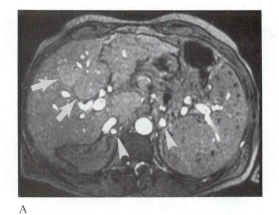

A

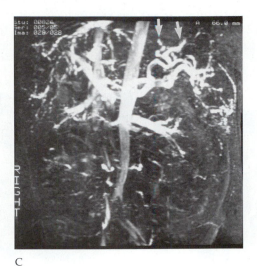

B

C

Figure 36–33. Portal hypertension with varicosities. (**A**) Axial view through the liver demonstrates cirrhotic appearing liver with regenerating nodules (*arrows*) and retroperitoneal venous collaterals (*arrowheads*). (**B**) Venous phase of splenic artery injection only faintly identifies the numerous varicosities (*arrows*). (**C**) Phase MR angiography more readily demonstrates the large gastric varicies (*arrows*).

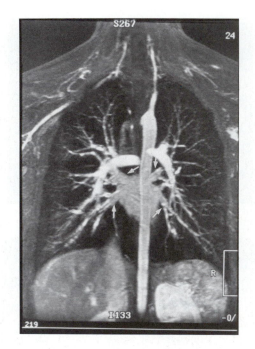

Figure 36–34. Normal pulmonary veins. Gadolinium-enhanced coronal projections through the left atrium demonstrate normal entrance of the four pulmonary veins (*arrows*) in this patient with hypoplastic pulmonary arteries.

commonly seen.[48,49] An MR sequence of T2 weighting, second echo, displays the venous network as a high signal intensity making it easy to observe. Although T1 images display fat as a high signal, they are not necessary to perform because it is detected well enough on the T2 sequence. Venography is reserved for those cases where it is deemed important to know about underlying dysplastic development of the expected

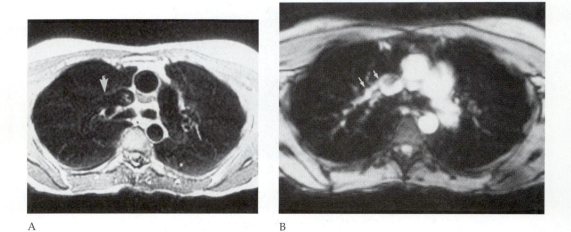

A   B

Figure 36–35. Partial anomalous pulmonary venous return. (**A**) Right upper pulmonary vein enters SVC (*arrow*). (**B**) The entrance into the SVC is better demonstrated with gradient echo (whiteblood) technique (arrows).

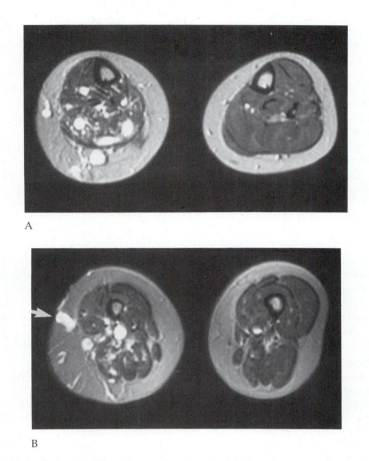

A

B

Figure 36–36. MRI of a patient with KTS affecting the right lower extremity shows some of the typical findings of this disorder. (**A**) CT scan taken through the mid lower legs shows an extensive venous malformation throughout the muscles and in the subcutaneous space of the right thigh displayed as high signal (= white) on the image. (**B**) CT scan taken through the mid thigh level shows findings similar to those of right calf. Lateral subcutaneous varicosities (*arrow*) are usually seen in this entity. Also, note that the right leg is larger than the left leg.

deep veins. The images of MR do detect these veins, but because of their small size and the axial orientation an adequate evaluation is not possible. Computed tomography is of limited value when compared to MRI for this disease.

CONCLUSION

Magnetic resonance imaging is a powerful tool for venous imaging. Advantages include multiplaner acquisitions, sensitivity to flow, quantitative capabilities, and excellent spatial resolution without need for iodinated contrast. Its current utilization largely depends on availability of both scanners and local expertise.

REFERENCES

1. Stanford W, Rooholamini SA, Galvin JR. Ultrafast computed tomography in the diagnosis of aortic aneurysms and dissections. *J Thorac Imag.* 1990;5:32–39.

2. Rahmouni A, Mathieu D, Golli M, et al. Value of CT and sonography in the conservative management of acute splenoportal and superior mesenteric venous thrombosis. *Gastrointest Radiol.* 1992;17:135–140.

3. Mori H, Maeda H, Fukuda T, et al. Acute thrombosis of the inferior vena cava and hepatic veins in patient with Budd-Chiari syndrome: CT demonstration. *Am J Roentgenol.* 1989;153:987–991.

4. Kellman GM, Alpern MB, Sandler MA, et al. Computed tomography of vena caval anomalies with embryologic correlation. *RadioGraphics.* 1988;8(3):533–556.

5. Dudiak CM, Olson MC, Posniak HV. Abnormalities of the azygos system: CT evaluation. *Roentgenology.* 1989;24:47–55.

6. Takada Y, Narimatsu A, Kohno A, et al. Anomalous left brachiocephalic vein: CT findings. *J Comput Assist Tomogr.* 1994;16:893–896.

7. Moncada R, Demos TC, Marsan R, et al. CT diagnosis of idiopathic aneurysms of the thoracic systemic veins. *J Comput Assist Tomogr.* 1985;9:305–309.

8. Schwartz EE, Goodman LR, Haskin ME. Role of CT scanning in the superior vena cava syndrome. *Am J Clin Oncol.* 1986;9:71–78.

9. Tatu WF, Winzelberg GG, Boller M, et al. Computed tomographic evaluation of compression of the superior vena cava and its tributaries. *Cardiovasc Intervent Radiol.* 1985;8:89–99.

10. Raptopoulos V. Computed tomography of the superior vena cava. *Crit Rev Diagn Imag.* 1986;25:373–429.

11. Chen JC, Bongard F, Klein SR. A contemporary perspective on superior vena cava syndrome. *Am J Surg.* 1990;160:207–211.

12. Trigaux JP, Van Beers B. Thoracic collateral venous channels: normal and pathologic CT findings. *J Comput Assist Tomogr.* 1990;14:769–773.

13. Cohen MI, Gore RM, Vogelzang RL, et al. Accessory hemiazygos continuation of left inferior vena cava: CT demonstration. *J Comput Assist Tomogr.* 1984;8:777–779.

14. Didier D, Racle A, Etievent JP, et al. Tumor thrombus of the inferior vena cava secondary to malignant abdominal neoplasms: US and CT evaluation. *Radiology.* 1987;162:83–89.

15. Rhee RY, Gloviczki P, Luthra HS, et al. Ilicocaval complication of retroperitoneal fibrosis. *Am J Surg.* 1994;168:179–183.

16. Remy-Jardin M, Remy J, Wattinne L, et al. Central pulmonary thromboembolism: diagnosis with spiral volumetric CT with the single-breath-hold technique—comparison with pulmonary angiography. *Radiology.* 1992;185(2):381–387.

17. Teigen CL, Maus TP, Sheedy PF, et al. Pulmonary embolism: diagnosis with electron-beam CT. *Radiology.* 1993;188:839–845.

18. Teigen CL, Maus TP, Sheedy PF, II, et al. Pulmonary embolism: diagnosis with contrast-enhanced electron-beam CT and comparison with pulmonary angiography. *Radiology.* 1995;194:135–140.

19. Vogelzang RL, Gore RM, Anschuetz SL, et al. Thrombosis of the splanchnic veins: CT diagnosis. *Am J Roentgenol.* 1988;150:93–96.

20. McCain AH, Bernardino ME, Sones PJ Jr, et al. Varices from portal hypertension: correlation of CT and angiography. *Radiology.* 1985;154:63–69.

21. Marn CS, Francis IR. CT of portal venous occlusion. *Am J Roentgenol.* 1992;159:717–726.

22. Ayuso C, Luburich P, Vilana R, et al. Calcifications in the portal venous system: comparison of plain films, sonography, and CT. *Am J Roentgenol.* 1992;159:321–323.

23. Aikawa H, Mori H, Miyake H, et al. Imaging and clinical significance of hepatic portal venous gas seen in adult patients. *Nippon Shokakibyo Gakkai Zasshi.* 1994;91:1320–1327.

24. Vogelzang RL, Anschuetz SL, Gore RM. Budd-Chiari syndrome: CT observations. *Radiology.* 1987;163:329–333.

25. Mathieu D, Vasile N, Menu Y, et al. Budd-Chiari syndrome: dynamic CT. *Radiology.* 1987;165:409–413.

26. Prince MR. Gadolinium-enhanced MR aortography. *Radiology.* 1994;191(1):155–164.

27. Prince MR, Narasimham DL, Stanley JC, et al. Breath-hold gadolinium-enhanced MR angiography of the abdominal aorta and its major branches. *Radiology.* 1995;197(3):785–792.

28. Revel D, Loubeyre P, Delignette A, et al. Contrast-enhanced magnetic resonance tomoangiography: a new imaging technique for studying thoracic great vessels. *Magn Reson Imag.* 1993;11(8):1101–1105.

29. Webb WR, Sostman HD. MR imaging of thoracic disease: clinical uses. *Radiology.* 1992;182:621–630.
30. Fisher MR, Hricak H, Higgins CB. Magnetic resonance imaging of developmental venous anomalies. *Am J Roentgenol.* 1985;145:705–709.
31. Levitt RG, Glazer HS, Gutierrez F, et al. Magnetic resonance imaging of spiral vein graft bypass of superior vena cava in fibrosing mediastinitis. *Chest.* 1986;90:676–680.
32. Finn JP, Zisk JH, Edelman RR, et al. Central venous occlusion: MR angiography. *Radiology.* 1993;187:245–251.
33. Sonin AH, Mazer MJ, Powers TA. Obstruction of the inferior vena cava: A multiple-modality demonstration of causes, manifestations, and collateral pathways. *RadioGraphics.* 1992;12:309–322.
34. Liebman LE, Messersmith RN, Levin DN, et al. MR imaging of inferior vena caval filters: safety and artifacts. *Am J Roentgenol.* 1988;150:1174–1179.
35. Evans AJ, Sostman HD, Knelson MH, et al. Detection of deep venous thrombosis: prospective comparison of MR imaging with contrast venography. *Am J Roentgenol.* 1993;161:131–139.
36. Siewert B, Kaiser WA, Layerm G, et al. MR venography in deep venous thromboses of the leg and pelvis. A comparison of 2D single layer images and 3D MIP reconstructions with phlebography. *Rofo Fortschr Geb Rontgenstr Neuen Bildgeb Verfahr.* 1992;156:549–554.
37. Weinreb JC, Mootz A, Cohen JM. MRI evaluation of mediastinal and thoracic inlet venous obstruction. *Am J Roentgenol.* 1986;146:679–684.
38. Arrivé L, Menu Y, Dessarts I, et al. Diagnosis of abdominal venous thrombosis by means of spin-echo and gradient-echo MR imaging: analysis with receiver operating characteristic curves. *Radiology.* 1991;181:661–668.
39. Applegate GR, Thaete FL, Meyers SP, et al. Blood flow in the portal vein: velocity quantitation with phase-contrast MR angiography. *Radiology.* 1993;187:253–256.
40. Burkart DJ, Johnson CD, Ehman RL. Correlation of arterial and venous blood flow in the mesenteric system based on MR findings. *Am J Roentgenol.* 1993;161:1279–1282.
41. Hricak H, Amparo E, Fisher MR, et al. Abdominal venous system: assessment using MR. *Radiology.* 1985;156:415–422.
42. Rodgers PM, Ward J, Baudouin CJ, et al. Dynamic contrast-enhanced MR imaging of the portal venous system: comparison and x-ray angiography. *Radiology.* 1994;191:741–745.
43. Kanematsu M, Imaeda T, Mochizuki R, et al. Analysis of three-dimensional imaging of the right hepatic vein and right portal vein branch using 2D-TOF MR angiography: evaluation of utility of MR angiography in determining puncture course on TIPS. *Nippon Igaku Hoshasen Gakkai Zasshi.* 1994;54:76–78.
44. Choe YH, Lee HJ, Kim HS, et al. MRI of total anomalous pulmonary venous connections. *J Compu Assist Tomogr.* 1994;18(2):243–249.
45. Hundley WG, Li HF, Lange RA, et al. Assessment of left-to-right intracardiac shunting by velocity-encoded, phase-difference magnetic resonance imaging. A comparison with oximetric and indicator dilution techniques. *Circulation.* 1995;91(12):2955–2960.
46. Erol C, Candan I. Non-invasive methods in the diagnosis of chronic major-vessel thromboembolic pulmonary hypertension. *Eur Heart J.* 1993;14(7):1004–1005.
47. Vinitski S, Thakur ML, Consigny PM, et al. Use of ferrum in MRI of lung parenchyma and pulmonary embolism. *Magn Reson Imag.* 1993;11(4):499–508.
48. Gloviczki P, Stanson AW, Stickler GB, et al. Klippel-Trenaunay syndrome: the risks and benefits of vascular interventions. *Surgery.* 1991;110:469–479.
49. Cherry KJ, Gloviczki P, Stanson AW. Persistent sciatic vein: the diagnosis and treatment of a rare condition. *J Vasc Surg.* 1995;23(3):490–497.

37

Endoscopic Ligation of Perforators

Peter Gloviczki, MD, Linda Canton, RN, BSN,
Sunil S. Menawat, MD, and Geza Mozes, MD

Subfascial ligation of incompetent perforating veins was first suggested by Linton[1] six decades ago to treat chronic venous stasis ulcers. His procedure included a long skin incision made on the medial aspect of the leg that allowed access to all perforating veins, including those located under the fascia of the deep posterior compartment. The original Linton operation is rarely performed today because of frequent wound complications and the need for prolonged hospitalization of these patients. Variations of his technique were developed in subsequent years. These included the use of short longitudinal or transverse skin incisions or blind avulsion of the perforators by passing a shearing instrument in the subfascial space to lessen the risk of wound complications.[2–7]

Endoscopic subfascial interruption of incompetent perforator veins was introduced in Europe in the mid-1980s by Hauer and by Fischer and Sattler.[8–10] Using a single scope for viewing and as a working channel, experience also has been accumulated by others in Europe.[11–13] The single-scope concept without gas insufflation has been further developed and used successfully in the United States by Bergan and associates.[14]

O'Donnell was the first to recognize the advantages of laparoscopic instrumentation used for nonvascular abdominal procedures. His group realized the potential limitations of the single-scope technique and the small working space and suggested water dissection of the subfascial space to enlarge the visual field.[15,16] In the United States, our group started to use CO_2 insufflation into the subfascial space to improve access to perforators and enlarge the working space for the operation. We use laparoscopic instrumentation with two or sometimes with three ports and apply a thigh tourniquet to obtain a bloodless field and to prevent gas embolism. We performed our first operation on August 5, 1993, and reported results of the first 11 procedures recently.[17] In this chapter, we review the surgical anatomy of the medial perforating veins of the leg and summarize our experience with endoscopic perforator vein surgery (SEPS) that now includes 30 procedures performed in 27 patients.

SURGICAL ANATOMY

In a recent study, we reviewed the available literature on perforating veins and summarized our findings obtained during anatomic dissections of 40 cadaver limbs.[18] Fifty-two percent of the medial perforators were direct perforators connecting the superficial system with the deep axial veins, 41% were indirect muscle perforators, and 7% were undetermined. We found five groups of medial distal perforating veins (Fig. 37–1). The distal leg perforators formed two clusters, one at 7 to 9 cm and one at 10 to 12 cm from the ankle (Fig. 37–2). These veins usually connected the posterior arch-vein with the paired posterior tibial veins. These groups correspond with the Cockett II and Cockett III perforators.[2,3] In our study, we did not perform dissection of the retromalleolar area, which frequently has an incompetent perforating vein in patients with chronic venous disease (Cockett I perforators). In the proximal half of the leg, direct paratibial perforating veins were identified within 1 cm from the medial edge of the tibia. These veins formed three clusters, at 18 to 22, 23 to 27, and 28 to 32 cm from the ankle. In cadaver studies performed in normal subjects, only 63% of the perforating veins were accessible from the superficial posterior compartment for endoscopic division. To gain access during operation to the paratibial veins or even to the Cockett II perforators, the incision of the paratibial area of the fascia of the deep posterior compartment may also be necessary (Figs. 37–3, and 37–4A–D).

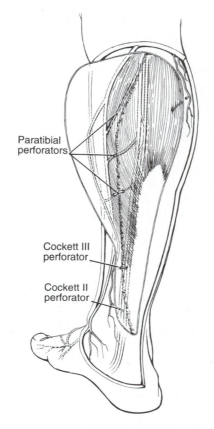

Paratibial perforators

Cockett III perforator

Cockett II perforator

Figure 37–1. Important medial perforating veins of the leg. [*Reproduced with permission: Mozes G, Gloviczki P, Menawat SS, et al. Surgical anatomy for endoscopic subfascial division of perforating veins. J Vasc Surg. 1996;24(S):800–808.*]

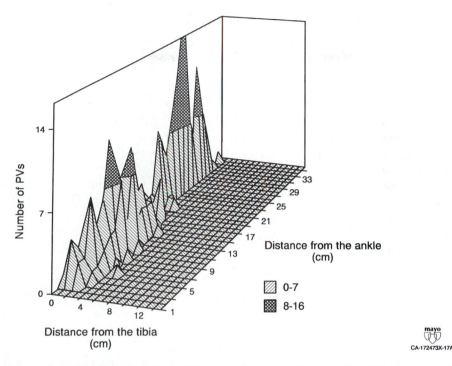

Figure 37–2. Number and location of 287 medial direct perforating veins in 40 legs. [*Reproduced with permission: Mozes G, Gloviczki P, Menawat SS, et al. Surgical anatomy for endoscopic subfascial division of perforating veins. J Vasc Surg. 1996 (in press).*]

PREOPERATIVE EVALUATION

Patients with advanced chronic venous insufficiency either due to previous deep venous thrombosis or due to primary valvular incompetence are considered for this operation. While some patients may belong to clinical Class 4 (lipodermatosclerosis, induration, or eczema), most are in Class 5 (healed ulcer) or Class 6 (active ulcer), using the updated classification of the Joint Vascular Societies.[19] Every patient should have undergone an

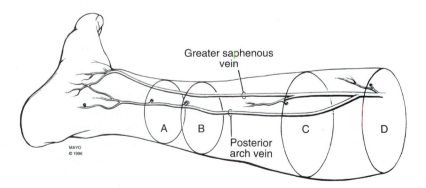

Figure 37–3. Superficial and perforating veins in the medial side of the leg. (Cross-sections at levels A–D are shown in Fig. 37–4). [*Reproduced with permission: Mozes G, Gloviczki P, Menawat SS, et al. Surgical anatomy for endoscopic subfascial division of perforating veins. J Vasc Surg. 1996;24(S):800–808.*]

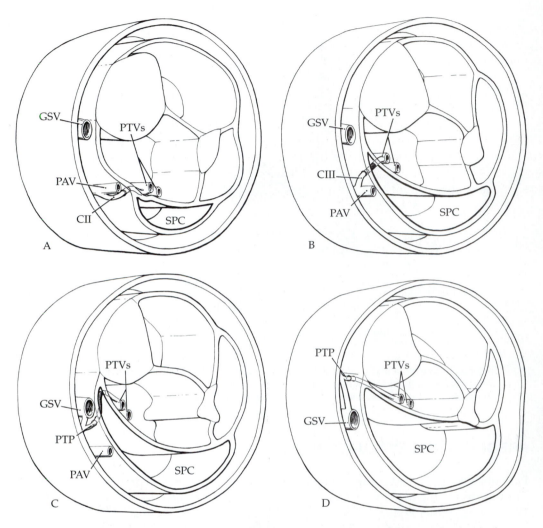

Figure 37–4. Compartments and medial veins of the leg. Cross-sections at the level of (**A**) Cockett II, (**B**) Cockett III, (**C**) 24 cm, and (**D**) more proximal paratibial perforating veins. GSV, greater saphenous vein; PAV, posterior arch vein; PTVs, posterior tibial veins; SPC, superficial posterior compartment; CII, Cockett II; CIII, Cockett III; PTP, paratibial perforator. [*Reproduced with permission: Mozes G, Gloviczki P, Menawat SS, et al. Surgical anatomy for endoscopic subfascial division of perforating veins. J Vasc Surg. 1996;24(S):800–808.*]

attempt to treat the ulcer nonoperatively before perforator ligations. The presence of an active ulcer, however, is not a contraindication to proceed with surgical treatment. However, infected ulcer, cellulitis, or eczema is first treated nonoperatively to decrease chances of wound complications. Adequate local care of the ulcer is complemented with graduated compression stockings, frequent elevation of the leg, and, in some cases, bedrest.

Our noninvasive venous evaluation includes strain gauge plethysmography to assess global venous function of the extremity, to confirm valvular incompetence of the superficial or deep system, and to exclude functional venous outflow obstruction. However, detailed duplex scanning of the venous system of the lower extremity has become the most important preoperative test of these patients. This includes examination of the greater saphenous vein and deep veins for obstruction and valvular incompetence. In patients who are surgical candidates, detailed examination of the medial perforating veins is performed to establish the diagnosis of valvular incompetence. Perforator vein incompetence is confirmed by bidirectional flow on duplex scan in a patient who is examined in the 70-degree semierect position on a tilted table, with full weight bearing on the contralateral lower extremity. If perforator incompetence is found with duplex scan, we proceed with the SEPS procedure. While ascending and descending venography was used in every patient in the first part of our experience, at this time we reserve venography for those rare patients who have evidence of significant deep venous occlusive disease.

CLINICAL MATERIAL

Between August 5, 1993, and March 10, 1996, 30 SEPS procedures were performed in 27 patients, 16 females and 11 males. Mean age of the patients was 47 years, ranging from 28 to 77 years. Eighteen limbs had active ulcers (Class 6) and 3 had healed ulcers (Class 5). Seven limbs had lipodermatosclerosis or other skin changes of chronic venous disease (Class 4) and 2 patients had pain and swelling of the leg without significant skin changes (Class 3). The etiology of chronic venous disease was previous deep venous thrombosis in 13 of the 30 limbs and primary valvular incompetence in 17.

SURGICAL TECHNIQUE

All perforator veins are mapped and marked on the skin preoperatively with the help of duplex scanning. We use an "X" to confirm location of incompetent and "O" to confirm the site of competent perforators. At present we interrupt all perforating veins of the medial aspect of the calf through the endoscope, from the ankle up to the proximal third of the calf and from the medial edge of the tibia to the posterior midline. Either general or epidural anesthesia is used to perform the operation. The affected lower extremity and groin are prepped and draped in a sterile fashion and Esmarque's bandage is used to exsanguinate the extremity. A bloodless field is obtained using a pneumatic tourniquet placed high on the thigh. The duration of the tourniquet inflation is continuously monitored and the pressure of the tourniquet is maintained at 300 mm Hg.

The most frequent port size that we use for the operation is 10 mm, although a 5-mm port is also available. The two ports have to be placed distant from the site of the ulcerations, but still close enough to reach the level of the ankle with the endoscopic instruments and the video camera. The ports should also be far away from each other to permit easy manipulation. The first incision is made about 10 to 12 cm distal to the level of the tibial tuberosity, about 3 cm medial to the medial edge of the tibia. The skin incision is limited to less than 12 mm to avoid air leak and the fascia is incised with an 11 blade knife.

A 10-mm laparoscopic port is inserted with the help of a blunt obturator to prevent placement of the port into the calf muscles (Fig. 37–5). Once the port is placed under the fascia, carbon dioxide is insufflated to obtain a pressure of 30 mm Hg (Fig. 37–6). A 10-mm video camera is inserted in the subfascial space to confirm correct port

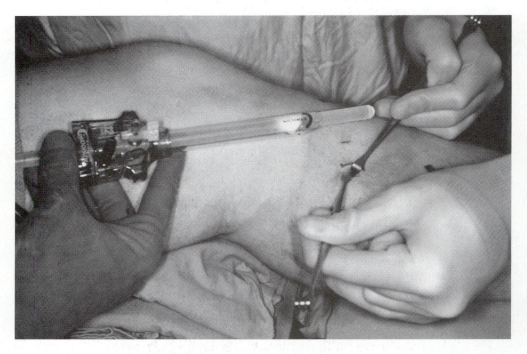

Figure 37–5. A 10-mm laparoscopic port is placed with help of blunt obturator into subfascial space. Note the small skin incision to permit an air seal around the port. (*Reproduced with permission: Gloviczki P, Cambria RA, Rhee YR, et al. Surgical technique and preliminary results with endoscopic subfascial division of perforating veins. J Vasc Surg. 1996;23:517–523.*)

position. The second 10-mm port is inserted 5 to 6 cm more posterior and 2 to 3 cm more distal to the first incision into the subfascial space. We use the video camera to guide placement of the trocar, which is inserted with the second laparoscopic port. Dissection is performed with laparoscopic forceps and scissors, which are placed through the second port (Fig. 37–7).

The most important veins that can be easily dissected from the superficial posterior compartment are the Cockett III perforators and most of the Cockett II perforators. These are located posterior to the edge of the tibia (up to 4 cm) and connect the posterior arch vein with the posterior tibial veins (Fig. 37–2). There is frequently a duplication of the fascia between the superficial and deep posterior compartment that may have to be incised to uncover the Cockett II perforators. They can also be completely covered by the thin fascia of the deep posterior compartment (Fig. 37–4A). To access most of the paratibial perforators, the deep fascia close to the tibia has to be incised with endoscopic scissors. Even Linton emphasized the need to incise the fascia of the deep posterior compartment to interrupt perforating veins that connect the posterior tibial veins with superficial veins immediately close to the tibia.[1] Incising the paratibial fascia is facilitated by the enlarged operating space available because of CO_2 insufflation into the subfascial plane.

We use 10-mm clips to occlude the veins and divide them with laparoscopic scissors to assist further dissection (Figs. 37–8 and 37–9). Small arteries or small nerves may accompany some of the perforating veins. Most of the time, these structures are divided without undue consequences.

After completion of the procedure, the videoscope, the dissecting instruments, and ports are removed and the remaining subfascial or subcutaneous gas is manually

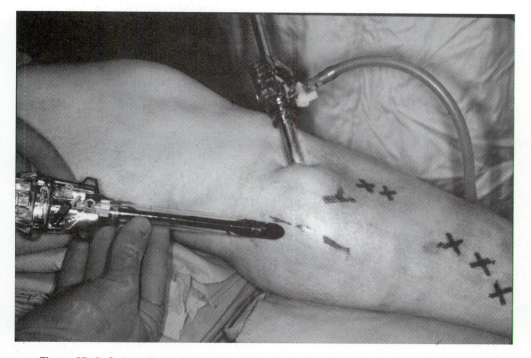

Figure 37–6. Carbon dioxide is insufflated through the first port, and placement of the second port is performed under video control. (*Reproduced with permission: Gloviczki P, Cambria RA, Rhee YR, et al. Surgical technique and preliminary results with endoscopic subfascial division of perforating veins. J Vasc Surg. 1996;23:517–523.*)

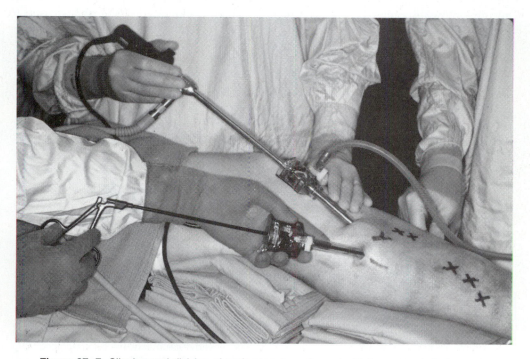

Figure 37–7. Clipping and division of perforators is performed with laparoscopic instruments through the second port; the first port is used for video control. (*Reproduced with permission: Gloviczki P, Cambria RA, Rhee YR, et al. Surgical technique and preliminary results with endoscopic subfascial division of perforating veins. J Vasc Surg. 1996;23:517–523.*)

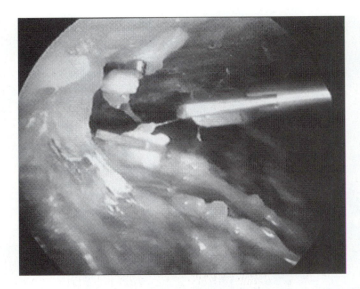

Figure 37–8. Division of a high Cockett perforator with endoscopic scissors after placement of vascular clips. (*Reproduced with permission: Gloviczki P, Cambria RA, Rhee YR, et al. Surgical technique and preliminary results with endoscopic subfascial division of perforating veins. J Vasc Surg. 1996;23:517–523.*)

expressed from the limb through the two small incisions. The tourniquet is then deflated. If the patient has an incompetent superficial system, high ligation and stripping of the saphenous vein is performed, together with varicose vein avulsion, which is done through small stab wounds. The port incision closer to the edge of the tibia is used to complete the saphenous vein stripping from the groin to below the knee. Longer

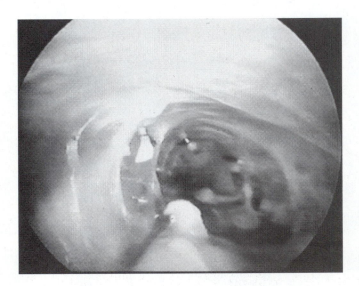

Figure 37–9. Full view of subfascial space after clipping and division of all medial perforating veins. (*Reproduced with permission: Gloviczki P, Cambria RA, Rhee YR, et al. Surgical technique and preliminary results with endoscopic subfascial division of perforating veins. J Vasc Surg. 1996;23:517–523.*)

incisions are closed with interrupted 2-0 subcutaneous Vicryl and the skin is closed with interrupted 4-0 subcutaneous Vicryl. The extremity is wrapped with an elastic bandage. Subcutaneous heparin, 5,000 units twice during the first 24 hours, is given to patients with recent episodes of deep venous thrombosis or with known coagulation abnormality. The patients are discharged usually within 24 hours after overnight observation. Ambulation is permitted within 3 hours after the operation.

RESULTS

Intraoperative Data

The number of perforating veins divided during the 30 SEPS procedure averaged 4.9, ranging from 2 to 10. Mean tourniquet time was 56 minutes, ranging from 25 to 75 minutes. Additional operations were performed in 26 limbs. These included stripping of the greater or lesser saphenous veins (17 limbs and 1 limb, respectively), high ligation of the greater saphenous vein (1 limb), and avulsion of varicose veins without operation on the saphenous veins (7 limbs). In 4 limbs, no additional procedures were performed other than the SEPS.

Clinical Results

Our follow-up averaged 8 months ranging from 1 to 26 months. Clinical outcome was excellent in 24 patients where the ulcer either healed or did not recur during the follow-up and the patients had no significant residual symptoms. However, all the patients continued to use elastic compression. The clinical status of 6 patients improved with fewer symptoms and/or smaller ulcers at last follow-up. In 1 of these 6 patients, the ulcer did not significantly change, but the symptoms of pain and swelling had clearly improved. Only 1 patient's clinical condition and ulcer size did not improve after the operation.

Complications

One patient developed a superficial wound infection at the groin at the site of high ligation of the greater saphenous vein. We did not observe wound infections at the site of the endoscopic port placement. One patient developed superficial thrombophlebitis within a few days after the operation proximal to the area of the port placement. Postoperative duplex scanning in this patient excluded deep venous thrombosis. This 46-year-old male had a history of recurrent deep venous thrombosis and he also had documented protein C deficiency. Two months after the operation, he developed recurrent popliteal vein thrombosis. Overall, his clinical condition did not improve after his operation. Two patients developed saphenous vein neuralgia; both underwent stripping of the greater saphenous veins in addition to perforator interruption. One of our patients with preoperative episodes of cellulitis developed one additional episode 6 months postoperatively that required hospitalization and intravenous antibiotic treatment.

DISCUSSION

Endoscopic subfascial division of the perforating veins is safe. Our preliminary results indicate that the use of an endoscope to divide subfascial perforating veins does not have a significant rate of morbidity or thromboembolic complications. Our technique, using carbon dioxide insufflation, laparoscopic instrumentation and a thigh tourniquet to obtain a bloodless field, had no significant side effect. One patient with post-thrombotic syndrome and high risk for thrombotic complications, however, developed deep venous thrombosis at 2 months after the operation. Preoperative thrombosis prophylaxis using subcutaneous heparin or low-molecular-weight heparin in patients with recent deep venous thrombosis or with known coagulation abnormalities appears essential.

The minimally invasive endoscopic Linton operation with the carbon dioxide insufflation is suitable to visualize and interrupt medial incompetent perforating veins. Paratibial fasciotomy with incision of the fascia of the deep compartment is also safe without apparent increase in complications to the neurovascular structures. The role of paratibial perforators in the pathomechanism of venous ulcers, however, is unclear at present.

In patients with severe lipodermatosclerosis of the subcutaneous tissue, it may be difficult to advance the endoscope all the way to the ankle. For this reason, division of the retromalleolar Cockett perforator with this technique is usually not possible. Increasing experience with ancillary techniques, such as the use of balloon dissectors, appears promising in facilitating distal dissection of perforators.

Preliminary results of the North American Subfascial Endoscopic Perforator Surgery (NASEPS) Registry were recently presented and they also indicate that SEPS is a safe procedure that can be performed with minimal morbidity and no mortality.[20] Clinically significant perioperative thromboembolism was not reported following 155 procedures, performed in 148 patients in 17 medical centers in the United States and Canada. The incidence of wound infection was 6%. Five patients had postoperative superficial thrombophlebitis, 4 developed cellulitis, 10 had saphenous neuralgia, and 1 developed skin necrosis at the site of the thigh tourniquet. The data indicated rapid ulcer healing with 88% of the ulcer healed in a subset of 85 patients. Mean days from surgery to healing was 42 days.

Our early clinical results confirm the findings of the NASEPS registry. Ulcer healing following the SEPS procedure has been rapid in most patients and patient satisfaction has been high. Future prospective trials, however, should assess late results and focus on recurrence rate, cost savings, return to work, and length of ulcer and pain free state of the patient. We have to assess the need for the SEPS procedure in these patients in addition to performing the conventional operations (high ligation, stripping, varicose vein avulsion) on the superficial veins. In addition to randomizing patients to these two surgical arms, future prospective studies will most likely need to include a third control group of patients who undergo best medical management without surgical treatment. In such studies functional improvement of the calf pump mechanism should also be assessed using plethysmographic techniques to document objective improvement. A prospective trial in larger numbers of patients in centers involved in the NASEPS registry is clearly warranted.

REFERENCES

1. Linton RR. The communicating veins of the lower leg and the operative technique for their ligation. *Ann Surg.* 1938;107:582–593.
2. Cockett FB, Jones DEE. The ankle blow-out syndrome: a new approach to the varicose ulcer problem. *Lancet.* 1953;1:17–23.
3. Cockett FB. The pathology and treatment of venous ulcers of the leg. *Br J Surg.* 1956;44:260–278.

4. Edwards JM. Shearing operation for incompetent perforating vein. *Br J Surg.* 1976;63:885–886.

5. De Palma RG. Surgical therapy for venous stasis. *Surgery.* 1974;76:910–917.

6. Wilkinson GE, Maclaren IF. Long-term review of procedures for venous perforator insufficiency. *Surg Gynecol Obstet.* 1986;163:117–120.

7. Cikrit DF, Nichols QK, Silver D. Surgical management of refractory venous stasis ulceration. *J Vasc Surg.* 1988;7:473–478.

8. Hauer G. The endoscopic subfascial division of the perforating veins—preliminary report (in German). *VASA.* 1985;14:59–61.

9. Fischer R. Surgical treatment of varicose veins; endoscopic treatment of incompetent Cockett veins. *Phlebologie.* 1989;1040–1041.

10. Fischer R, Sattler G, Vanderpuye R. The current status of endoscopic treatment of perforators (in French). *Phlebologie.* 1993;46:701–707.

11. Jugenheimer M, Junginger T. Endoscopic subfascial sectioning of incompetent perforating veins in treatment of primary varicosis. *World J Surg.* 1992;16:971–975.

12. Wittens CHA, Pierik RGJ, van Urk H. The surgical treatment of incompetent perforating veins. *Eur J Vasc Endovasc Surg.* 1995;9:19–23.

13. Pierik EGJM, Wittens CHA, van Urk H. Subfascial endoscopic ligation in the treatment of incompetent perforating veins. *Eur J Vasc Endovasc Surg.* 1995;9:38–41.

14. Bergan JJ, Murray J, Greason K. Subfascial endoscopic perforator vein surgery: a preliminary report. *Ann Vasc Surg.* 1996;10:211–219.

15. O'Donnell TF. Surgical treatment of incompetent communicating veins. In: Bergan JJ, Kistner RL, eds. *Atlas of Venous Surgery.* Philadelphia: WB Saunders; 1992:111–124.

16. Sullivan TR, O'Donnell TF. Endoscopic division of incompetent perforating veins. In: Gloviczki P, Yao JST, eds. *Handbook of Venous Disorders.* London: Chapman and Hall; 1996:482–493.

17. Gloviczki P, Cambria RA, Rhee YR, et al. Surgical technique and preliminary results with endoscopic subfascial division of perforating veins. *J Vasc Surg.* 1996;23:517–523.

18. Mozes G, Gloviczki P, Menawat SS, et al. Surgical anatomy for endoscopic subfascial division of perforating veins. *J Vasc Surg.* 1996;24(S):800–808.

19. Porter JM, Moneta GL, and an International Consensus Committee on Chronic Venous Disease. Reporting standards in venous disease: an update. *J Vasc Surg.* 1995;21:634–645.

20. Gloviczki P, Bergan JJ, Menawat SS, et al. Safety, feasibility and early efficacy of subfascial endoscopic perforator surgery (SEPS): a preliminary report from the North American Registry. Presented at the 50th annual meeting of the Society for Vascular Surgery; Chicago, IL, June 9–12, 1996.

38

Current Recommendation for Deep-Vein Thrombosis Prophylaxis

William R. Hiatt, MD

HEPARIN MECHANISM OF ACTION AND MONITORING

Heparin is a glycosaminoglycan with a molecular weight ranging from 5,000 to 30,000 (mean 15,000). Heparin has a high affinity for antithrombin III (ATIII), which then leads to an accelerated action of ATIII to inactivate thrombin (IIa), factor Xa, and factor IXa. At high doses, heparin acts through heparin cofactor II to inactivate IIa independent of ATIII.

The anticoagulant effects of heparin are quite variable. This is due to several factors including these: (1) The pharmacokinetics of heparin are not linear in that the half life of a dose of 25 μ/kg is 30 minutes, but at 100 μ/kg is 60 minutes; (2) heparin neutralizing plasma proteins, vascular endothelium, and elevated levels of factor VIII decrease its anticoagulant effect; and (3) differences in commercial activated partial thromboplastine time (APTT) reagents result in variability in the APTT values. Thus, several conditions such as pregnancy, malignancy, major surgery (cardiac), extensive thrombosis, and variability in APTT reagents may lead to a dissociation between heparin dose, heparin levels, and anticoagulant effects as assessed by the APTT.

Heparin is usually monitored by the degree of prolongation of the APTT. However, in the examples just listed, the APTT may not accurately reflect heparin effect.[1,2] Alternatively, heparin dosing can be monitored by the antifactor Xa heparin assay with a therapeutic range of 0.3 to 0.7 U/mL. Weight-based nomograms result in the most predictable means to achieve safe therapeutic anticoagulation in most patients. Currently an 80 μ/kg loading dose and 18 μ/kg/hour infusion are recommended, with monitoring of the APTT after 6 hours.[3]

HEPARIN SIDE EFFECTS

A concern with the use of heparin is the development of heparin-induced thrombocytopenia (HIT). This complication usually occurs after 5 to 15 days of therapy, is mediated by an IgG antibody, and results in a nadir in the platelet count of around 50,000.[2,4] The prevalence of HIT is 3%, with arterial and venous thrombosis occurring in 1% of patients. The thrombotic complications can be severe and fatal, with a ratio of venous to arterial of 4 : 1. Treatment includes stopping the heparin and administering Danaparoid, which inhibits factor Xa. Danaparoid is largely unavailable in the United States, but an alternative treatment is ReoPro, which is the antibody to the IIb/IIIa platelet receptor. This drug effectively prevents further platelet aggregation and has the potential to reverse HIT.

A second complication of chronic heparin therapy is osteoporosis. This is manifest as bone pain, rib, and spine fractures. Osteoporosis is very rare with doses less than 20,000 μ/24 hours and duration of therapy of less than 3 months. However, 5% to 15% of patients will develop osteoporosis when treated with 20,000 μ/24 hours for 6 months or more.[2]

A rare complication of heparin is inhibition of aldosterone synthesis resulting in hyperkalemia.

LOW-MOLECULAR-WEIGHT HEPARINS

Low-molecular-weight heparins (LMWHs) are derived by chemical or enzymatic depolymerization of standard unfractionated heparin. LMWH has a molecular weight of 1,000 to 10,000 (average 4,500). LMWH has less affinity for thrombin and therefore acts mainly through the inhibition of factor Xa. LMWH has much a higher bioavailability than standard heparin. This is because LMWH has less affinity for heparin neutralizing plasma proteins, vascular endothelium, and factor VIII. These properties of LMWH result in more predictable plasma heparin levels, longer plasma half-life, and more consistent anticoagulant effect than standard heparin. Therefore, LMWH may be administered once or twice daily at a weight-adjusted dose without need for laboratory monitoring or dose adjustment. LMWH appears to be associated with less bleeding and thrombocytopenia than standard heparin, and possibly less osteoporosis.

PROPHYLAXIS OF DEEP-VEIN THROMBOSIS

In hospitalized patients, venous thromboembolism is greatly underdiagnosed. In patients who died from pulmonary emboli, only 20% had clinically suspected thrombophlebitis. In patients older than the age of 40 who undergo major surgery, the incidence of deep-vein thrombosis (DVT) is 25% to 50%, and fatal pulmonary emboli occur 1% of the time. Pulmonary emboli account for 12% of all deaths in acute care hospitals.[5]

Risk factors for DVT include an age greater than 40 years, malignant disease, congestive heart failure, obesity, acute paraplegia, trauma, varicose veins and a history of thrombophlebitis, estrogens, hypercoagulable states, myocardial infarction, and immobilization.

Interventions to reduce the risk of DVT can be directed to intensive surveillance of high-risk groups with noninvasive techniques, or prophylaxis. Prophylaxis is favored because surveillance is expensive, pulmonary emboli may not be effectively prevented by anticoagulants once venous thrombosis is present, and some cases may be missed by the noninvasive techniques.

Mechanical

Early ambulation, leg elevation, and elastic stockings do not reliably reduce the risk of DVT. However, patients who are discharged from surgery within 4 days are at less risk of DVT than those who remain 5 days or more. This may be due to the nature of the underlying disease and the severity of illness rather than the effects of early ambulation.

External pneumatic compression stockings have been extensively studied and are of benefit in low- to moderate-risk general surgical, neurosurgical, urologic, and orthopedic patients. The results are similar to that of low-dose heparin with a threefold reduction in the incidence of DVT in treated patients. Pneumatic compression will decrease venous stasis and activate the fibrinolytic system.

Low-dose Heparin

Low-dose heparin therapy has been used for more than 20 years in both medical and surgical patients.[6–8] In low doses, heparin prevents the coagulation cascade by enhancing the action of ATIII. The results of several controlled trials of low-dose heparin in surgical patients show a threefold reduction in DVT (from 25% to 7%) and a tenfold reduction in pulmonary emboli (from 6.0% to 0.6%). The drug can be given as 5,000 units every 8 to 12 hours. The two dosing schedules are equivalent, but the more frequent dosing may result in more bleeding complications. Low-dose heparin is ineffective in orthopedic and urologic surgery and should be avoided in neurosurgery.

Low-molecular-weight Heparin

As described earlier, standard low-dose heparin prophylaxis following general surgery is safe and effective. Since LMWH is more expensive than standard heparin, in most cases standard heparin is preferred for prophylaxis against DVT. However in higher risk patients, several studies have compared LMWH to standard heparin. In patients undergoing abdominal or pelvic surgery for malignancy, LMWH and standard low-dose heparin are equally effective, but LMWH may have a reduced rate of bleeding.[9] Further clinical trials are needed to address the safety and efficacy of LMWH prophylaxis for DVT in patients with malignancies.

LMWH prevents DVT in patients undergoing total hip replacement with a risk reduction similar to warfarin therapy.[10] In most patients, LMWH can be administered subcutaneously twice daily beginning in the immediate postoperative period. In patients with a very high DVT risk, it is recommended that LMWH be started prior to surgery. In patients undergoing total knee replacement, LMWH is also effective when combined with external pneumatic compression stockings.[11,12]

Warfarin

Warfarin inhibits the synthesis of factors II, VII, IX, and X. It is the agent of choice in patients at high risk for DVT and in hip surgery. The drug is given in therapeutic doses to prolong the protime 1.5 times normal. It is usually started preoperatively, but is effective even if begun postsurgery. The major complication is bleeding, which may occur up to 20% of the time.

Dextran

Dextran decreases blood viscosity and platelet adhesiveness and promotes fibrin degradation. Dextran 40 is given as a 10% solution, 500 to 1,000 mL over 6 hours starting the day of surgery and then daily up to 5 days postoperatively. It is used mainly in hip surgery where it is not as effective as warfarin, but is better than other agents. Serious side effects include volume expansion and anaphylactic reactions.

Antiplatelet Agents

Aspirin (1.2 g/day) has been used in patients undergoing hip surgery, but is only effective in men at low risk for DVT. It therefore may be used in this subgroup of patients but is not as effective as dextran or warfarin.

MANAGEMENT OF ACUTE DVT

Thrombolytic Agents

Streptokinase and urokinase are plasminogen activators and induce a lytic state. They are most useful in extensive thrombotic disease, i.e., iliofemoral or subclavian vein thrombosis with extension into the vena cava. Studies have shown that these drugs are more effective than heparin in lysing clot, and preserving venous valves. The evidence that the postphlebitic syndrome is prevented is not yet conclusive. These drugs are contraindicated in patients with recent surgery, and intracranial neoplasms.

Heparin

Heparin remains the standard anticoagulant used in the initial treatment of acute, proximal DVT. Critical in the use of heparin is prompt and adequate anticoagulation of the patient presenting with a DVT. In a recent study, 120 outpatients with proximal vein thrombosis were randomized to initial anticoagulation with acenocoumarol (a warfarin drug) alone versus heparin followed by acenocoumarol.[13] As expected, 40% of the patients treated only with acenocoumarol had extension of the clot during the first week of therapy as compared to 8% in the heparin group. The recurrence rate of DVT in the patients anticoagulated with acenocoumarol alone was also unacceptably high over 6 months of follow-up. This study has important implications in the initial treatment of DVT. In a recent survey of physician practices, 60% of patients presenting with DVT or pulmonary emboli were inadequately anticoagulated with heparin during the first 24 hours of hospitalization.[14] Failure to adequately anticoagulate patients early in the course of the phlebitis may predispose them to clot extension and unacceptable rates of recurrence of DVT. The use of the weight-based nomograms described earlier (80 μ/kg loading dose and 18 μ/kg/hour infusion) result in the most predictable means to achieve safe therapeutic anticoagulation in most patients.

Once the patient is adequately anticoagulated on heparin, treatment needs to be continued for at least 5 days. In a recent study, 199 patients with DVT were randomized to 5 days versus 10 days of heparin.[15] The rates of bleeding complications and recurrent DVT over follow-up were the same in both groups, suggesting that 5 days of heparin is adequate and may also save hospital costs. When heparin is given for 5 days, it is important that warfarin is begun immediately after the patient is adequately anticoagulated on heparin. This is because it takes 4 to 5 days for warfarin to deplete activated clotting factors, particularly factor II.

LMWH may be more effective than standard heparin in the treatment of DVT. A recent meta-analysis suggests that LMWH resulted in greater reductions in thromboembolic complications, bleeding, and mortality than standard heparin.[16] Additional prospective trials are needed to confirm these results.

CHRONIC MANAGEMENT OF DVT

Warfarin

An important aspect of the monitoring of warfarin therapy is the use of the international normalized ratio (INR). The INR has been standard in Europe for many years, but has only recently become common practice in the United States. In a survey of coagulation laboratories, only 21% reported prothrombin times with the INR, but the INR is now more commonplace.[17]

In patients with DVT, recent work has shown that lower doses of warfarin are equally effective as the standard doses in preventing recurrent DVT, yet have a reduced risk of hemorrhage.[18] Current recommendations are to maintain the INR at 2.0 to 3.0 with chronic warfarin therapy.

Heparin

In patients who cannot tolerate warfarin, or are in the first trimester of pregnancy, chronic treatment with heparin is acceptable. Patients are treated with a BID dose given SQ, adjusted so that the partial thromboplastin time is 1.5 times the control value.[19] Under these conditions, heparin is as effective as full-dose warfarin for DVT.

CALF DVT

There remains a strong bias not to treat isolated calf DVT with long-term anticoagulation because these patients have a low risk of embolization. However, choosing to not anticoagulate patients with calf DVT may have serious consequences. In one study of patients with calf DVT, patients randomized to initial heparin therapy, followed by 3 months of warfarin, had a 2% rate of DVT recurrence when followed for 12 months.[20] In contrast, those on no therapy had a 29% rate of DVT recurrence, and a 4% rate of pulmonary emboli. In a review of the literature, it was concluded that anticoagulation of symptomatic calf DVT prevents clot extension, embolization, and recurrence.[21] Therefore, most patients with symptomatic calf vein DVT should be treated the same as those with proximal vein DVT.

REFERENCES

1. Barbour LA, Smith JM, Marlar RA. Heparin levels to guide thromboembolism prophylaxis during pregnancy. *Am J Obstet Gynecol.* 1995;173:1869–1873.
2. Hirsh J, Raschke R, Warkentin TE, et al. Heparin: mechanism of action, pharmacokinetics, dosing considerations, monitoring, efficacy, and safety. *Chest.* 1995;108:258S–275S.
3. Raschke RA, Reilly BM, Guidry JR, et al. The weight-based heparin dosing nomogram compared with a "standard care" nomogram. *Ann Intern Med.* 1993;119:874–881.
4. King DJ, Kelton JG. Heparin-associated thrombocytopenia. *Ann Intern Med.* 1984;100:535–540.
5. Anderson FA, Wheeler HB, Goldberg RJ, et al. A population-based perspective of the hospital incidence and case-fatality rates of deep vein thrombosis and pulmonary embolism. *Arch Intern Med.* 1991;151:933–938.
6. Russell J. Prophylaxis of postoperative deep vein thrombosis and pulmonary embolism. Surg *Gynecol Obstet.* 1983;157:89–104.
7. Hirsh J. Prophylaxis of venous thromboembolism. *Mod Concepts Cardiovasc Dis.* 1984;53:25–29.

8. Gallus AS, Hirsh J, Tuttle RJ, et al. Small subcutaneous doses of heparin in prevention of venous thrombosis. *N Engl J Med.* 1973;288:545–551.

9. Ficker JP, Vergnes Y, Schach R, et al. Low dose heparin versus low molecular weight heparin (Kabi 2165) in the prophylaxis of thromboembolic complications of abdominal oncological surgery. *Eur J Clin Invest.* 1988;18:561–567.

10. Levine MN, Hirsh J, Gent M, et al. Prevention of deep vein thrombosis after elective hip surgery. A randomized trial comparing low molecular weight heparin with standard unfractionated heparin. *Ann Intern Med.* 1991;114:545–551.

11. Hull RC, Raskob GE, Pineo GF, et al. Low-molecular-weight heparin (Logiparin) compared with less-intense warfarin prophylaxis against venous thromboembolism following total knee replacement. *Blood.* 1992;suppl 1:167a.

12. Hull R, Delmore T, Hirsh J. Effectiveness of intermittent pulsatile elastic stockings for the prevention of calf and thigh vein thrombosis in patients undergoing elective knee surgery. *Thromb Res.* 1979;16:37–45.

13. Brandjes DPM, Heijboer H, Buller HR, et al. Acenocoumarol and heparin compared with acenocoumarol alone in the initial treatment of proximal-vein thrombosis. *N Engl J Med.* 1992;327:1485–1489.

14. Wheeler AP, Jaquiss RDB, Newman JH. Physician practices in the treatment of pulmonary embolism and deep venous thrombosis. *Arch Intern Med.* 1988;148:1321–1325.

15. Hull RD, Raskob GE, Rosenbloom D, et al. Heparin for 5 days as compared with 10 days in the initial treatment of proximal venous thrombosis. *N Engl J Med.* 1990;322:1260–1264.

16. Lensing AWA, Prins MH, Davidson BL, Hirsh J. Treatment of deep venous thrombosis with low-molecular-weight heparins. A meta analysis. *Arch Intern Med.* 1995;155:601–607.

17. Bussey HI, Force RW, Bianco TM, Leonard AD. Reliance on prothrombin time ratios causes significant errors in anticoagulation therapy. *Arch Intern Med.* 1992;152:278–282.

18. Hull R, Hirsh J, Jay R, et al. Different intensities of oral anticoagulant therapy in the treatment of proximal-vein thrombosis. *N Engl J Med.* 1982;307:1676–1681.

19. Hull R, Delmore T, Carter C, et al. Adjusted subcutaneous heparin versus warfarin sodium in the long-term treatment of venous thrombosis. *N Engl J Med.* 1982;306:189–194.

20. Lagerstedt CI, Olsson CG, Fagher BO, et al. Need for long-term anticoagulant treatment in symptomatic calf-vein thrombosis. *Lancet.* 1985;2:515–518.

21. Philbrick JT, Becker DM. Calf deep venous thrombosis. A wolf in sheep's clothing? *Arch Intern Med.* 1988;148:2131–2138.

39

Acute Axillosubclavian
Venous Thrombosis

Twenty Years of Progress

Richard M. Green, MD

An aggressive approach to the treatment of axillosubclavian vein thrombosis (ASVT) has emerged during the last 20 years. ASVT may result from an anatomic abnormality at the thoracic outlet, related to the placement of a central venous catheter or it may occur in a hypercoagulable patient. Twenty years ago many researchers believed ASVT to be a benign, self-limiting condition and recommended conservative measures.[1] It is now generally accepted that if left untreated, 25% to 74% of the affected patients will have some limitations in activity,[2,3] as many as 12% of patients will have a pulmonary embolus,[4] and 1% of the patients will die. Those cases related to a thoracic outlet abnormality are often associated with strenuous activities and referred to as the Paget–Schroetter or "effort" thrombosis syndromes.[5,6] Noniatrogenic thrombosis of the axillosubclavian vein is an infrequent event with an estimated occurrence rate of 0.5% to 1.5% of all venous thromboses.[7] Catheter-induced thrombosis is an increasingly common event because of the more frequent utilization of central veins for access, nutrition, chemotherapy, and monitoring. Screening venography in patients with central venous catheters demonstrates that 33% to 60% of patients have thrombus in the axillosubclavian venous segment and 3% of these patients develop clinically evident ASVT.[8]

DIAGNOSIS

Patients with ASVT present with a bluish swollen arm and a pattern of upper extremity venous hypertension. Collateral veins are usually visible around the shoulder and the chest wall. A tender, palpable cord may be present. Patients typically describe an aching pain that is exacerbated by exercise. Venous color duplex studies are helpful but areas of the vein that lie behind the clavicle are difficult to image. Whereas the color duplex scan has virtually replaced venography in the diagnosis of lower extremity venous thrombosis, the exact opposite is true in the upper extremity. Venography has a greater

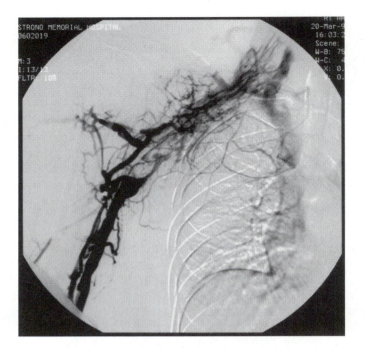

Figure 39–1. Axillosubclavian phlebogram performed with a catheter in the basilic vein and the arm in a resting position. This patient is an 18-year-old college athlete who recently started a vigorous upper body strengthening program. He presented 4 days after the onset of a blue, swollen painful arm. There is abundant thrombus with an extensive network of venous collaterals. Note that if the catheter had been placed in the cephalic vein, the area of thrombosis might have been overlooked.

diagnostic accuracy when performed properly. The catheter must be placed in the basilic vein because contrast injections into the cephalic system may bypass the involved segment of the axillosubclavian vein. Contrast should be injected initially with the arm at rest. This is usually sufficient for the diagnosis of thrombosis but may miss partial obstructions that require views with the arm abducted to 90 and 180 degrees. A typical acute ASVT is shown in Figure 39–1. This venogram was taken with a basilic vein catheter in an 18-year-old college athlete. He had recently begun an intensive upper body weight training program. He presented 4 days after his arm became blue, swollen, and painful. Extensive thrombus is seen as well as an abundant collateral venous network.

INITIAL MANAGEMENT

Current data support a role for conventional anticoagulation in all patients with ASVT. Becker et al.[9] reviewed the studies reported in the English literature between 1950 and 1990 that had at least 1 year of follow-up, stratified outcomes based on etiology and analyzed the results of treatment in 329 patients. This review concluded that conventional anticoagulation with heparin and warfarin is indicated for ASVT because of improved symptomatic results. Almost twice the number of patients remained symptomatic when anticoagulants were withheld (64%) compared to when they were administered (36%). Another indication for anticoagulation in the acute phase is prophylaxis against pulmonary embolism. Although the incidence of embolization from 5% to 10% is considerably lower than the 50% estimate associated with venous thrombosis of the proximal lower extremity vein,[10] ASVT does pose a significant risk for death. Patients with symptomatic thrombosis as a result of an indwelling catheter should have that catheter removed. Since indwelling catheters predispose to ASVT, consideration should be given to placing these patients on 1 mg of warfarin daily, which in a recent trial reduced the incidence of thrombosis to 9.5% compared to 37.5% in controls.[11]

TREATMENT BEYOND HEPARIN

Twenty years ago heparin followed by warfarin was considered aggressive therapy. This view changed in the early 1970s when DeWeese et al.[4] described their early experience with thrombectomies of recently occluded axillosubclavian veins. This challenged the extant management from one of, at the most, long-term anticoagulation and, at the least, watchful waiting to a consideration of clot removal and outlet decompression. Axillosubclavian venous thrombectomy with medial claviculectomy yielded anecdotal successes providing the operation was performed within 7 days. Even then with early intervention, many of the patients already had changes consistent with chronic venous thrombosis, that is, portions of the veins were cord-like, there were perivenous adhesions, organized synechiae, and thrombi within the vein making thrombectomy impossible. Despite this, many of the patients with nonreconstructible veins improved significantly. This led to the conclusion that complete clot removal is likely only in the true acutely affected patient and that decompression of the thoracic outlet by a medial claviculectomy by itself is an important element in the treatment of these patients. Later, Urschel and Razzuck[12] performed venous thrombectomy in association with a first rib resection through the axillary space. Because patients with chronically occluded veins often improved symptomatically, a debate ensued as to whether the bony operation necessary to provide exposure to the vein or the thrombectomy is the important aspect of treatment. Debate also occurred on whether any procedure was indicated given that, untreated, only 50% of the patients affected have significant morbidity. Most centers therefore adopted an algorithm that recommended operative intervention only in the patient with chronic ASVT and disabling symptoms and only to remove the clavicle or first rib. This has all changed with the recent experience with catheter-directed thrombolysis.

THROMBOLYSIS

Current treatment protocols suggest that catheter-directed clot lysis should be attempted in physically active patients with acute ASVT. These patients usually fall into the etiologic category of thoracic outlet abnormalities. The end point of this approach is recanalization of the occluded vein and identification and eventual correction of any underlying abnormality at the thoracic outlet. Roughly 50% of the patients treated with thrombolytic drugs and follow-up with venograms will have complete clot lysis.[13] It is important to recognize that removal of the thrombus alone without attention to the underlying cause will result in rethrombosis.[14] Some caution about thrombolytics is indicated however since a significant number of the reported cases of pulmonary emboli have occurred in these patients.[15]

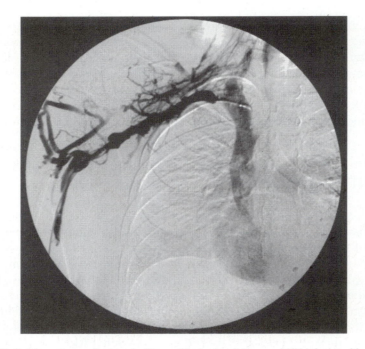

Figure 39–2. The same patient as in Figure 39–1 after 6 hours of UK infusion. Much of the thrombus load has been lysed and the catheter is through the stenosis at the costoclavicular space. The collateral network remains.

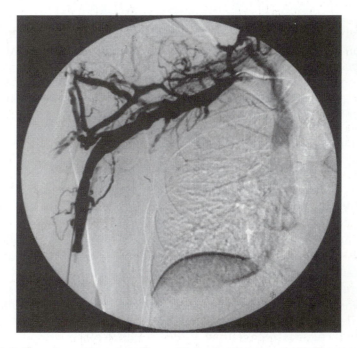

Figure 39–3. The same patient as in Figure 39–1 after 24 hours of UK. The clot has been lysed. The venous obstruction and collateral network remain.

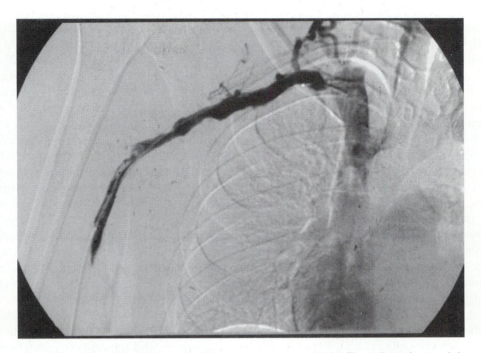

Figure 39–4. The same patient as in Figure 39–1 on day 2 of UK. The collateral network is gone and his arm is symptomatically better. The site of venous obstruction is clearly defined at the costoclavicular space.

It is generally accepted that catheter-directed thrombolysis is more effective than systemic lysis for ASVT. The catheter can be inserted through a percutaneous basilic approach at the time of the diagnostic venogram. Occasionally, a second catheter is required and can be placed retrograde via a femoral vein puncture. A guide wire should be placed through the thrombus prior to infusing the loading dose of urokinase (UK). An infusion catheter is placed over the guide wire into the thrombus and a loading dose of 250,000 IU of UK is given. The infusion is continued at a dose of 1,000 IU/min for up to 24 hours. Systemic heparin is administered concurrently to keep the partial thromboplastin at 1.5 times control values. Repeat venograms are necessary during the thrombolytic process to monitor progress. Figures 39–2 through 39–4 show the course of the patient in Figure 39–1 over 48 hours of UK. There is a progression from removal of thrombus, elimination in the collateral network, and eventual identification of the fibrous stenosis at the costoclavicular space responsible for the venous thrombosis. Some patients will not have a fixed lesion identified after thrombolysis and will require venograms with the arm abducted to identify the pathology. Their obstructions are extrinsic to the vein and further therapy to decompress the thoracic outlet will be required.

MANAGEMENT AFTER THE INITIAL PHASE

Treatment options at this point depend entirely on the result of the initial management. If a course of heparin and elevation was chosen, the patient is converted to oral warfarin and limited activity. The results of this approach depend on the resultant hemodynamics and the functional needs of the patient. There will be patients who will not have significant disability with this approach, which seems reasonable for elderly patients with catheter-related thromboses and those patients with malignancy and hypercoagulability. Complete recovery in patients with effort thrombosis is unlikely and 40% to 85% will have residual symptoms.[16] Those patients who develop functional limitations can then be evaluated for further therapy, which addresses the venous and any anatomic abnormalities. If thrombolysis was not successful, the post-treatment venogram will show persistent filling defects and large collateral veins. These patients are treated with oral warfarin and other conservative measures. Thoracic outlet decompression and/ or venous reconstruction are indicated for those patients with significant symptoms. Usually these patients will have large chest wall collateral veins that occlude when the arm is abducted. This can be determined by venography and if present can be corrected by a first rib resection.

If thrombolytic agents successfully restore patency, the post-treatment venogram shows no filling defects with the arms in a neutral position and no collaterals. Positional venograms are required to fully evaluate the patient at this point with the arms at 90 and 180 degrees. If extrinsic compression is identified, attention must be given to any structural abnormalities of the thoracic outlet. The axillary becomes the subclavian vein as it passes through the costoclavicular space. This space consists of the first rib as the floor, the clavicle as the ceiling, and the subclavius tendon and anterior scalene muscles as the walls. Two positions cause compression of the vein, those with the arm abducted and externally rotated and those with the shoulders back and the arms dependent, the so-called "military" position. Hyperabduction of the arm with external rotation causes the clavicle to rotate backward and downward toward the first rib with compression of the vein. The military position causes a scissors effect on the vein.[17]

The patient described earlier (Figs. 39–1 through 39–4) had a short stenotic lesion at the costoclavicular space, which requires both a thoracic outlet decompression and a venous reconstruction. Attempts at treating these short intrinsic vein lesions with percutaneous transluminal catheter dilatation have routinely failed.[18] Supplementing balloon dilatation with stents should not be done because the FDA has not approved them for this indication and they do not work. Rigid stents are susceptible to crushing from the scissoring action of the clavicle and first rib.

Resection of the medial third of the clavicle and transaxillary first rib resection eliminates the scissors mechanism at the thoracic outlet.[19,20] Claviculectomy provides the added benefit of excellent exposure of the axillosubclavian vein for both thrombectomy and reconstruction and also decompresses the costoclavicular space. This approach is not as popular as first rib resection[21] because of the cosmetic deformity and functional disability that may occur. Although reports are anecdotal, our institutional experience suggests that patients are able to do most physical activities after this operation without hindrance. These data have been corroborated by Dr. Jere Lord who has followed patients for more than 40 years and claims that there is little deformity and almost no functional limitation after claviculectomy. The claviculectomy is performed with an incision slightly above the bone from the sternal notch to the midsection of the clavicle. Once the bone is removed and the sternal-clavicular attachment disarticulated, the confluence of the subclavian and jugular veins can be seen (Fig. 39–5). A venotomy is made through the fibrous lesion into normal vein proximally and distally once the patient is heparinized. The venous web is identified (Fig. 39–6), excised, and then the subclavian vein is repaired with a saphenous vein patch. The postoperative venogram is shown in Figure 39–7. There is no longer any evidence of venous obstruction.

First rib resection also allows decompression of the costoclavicular space but is not a useful incision in the situation of a short stenosis that requires repair in the

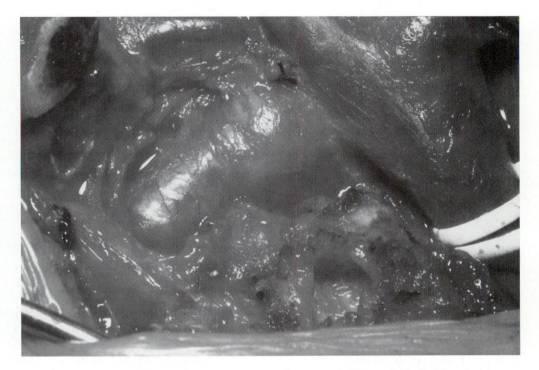

Figure 39–5. Operative photograph of patient in Figure 39–1. The medial half of the clavicle has been removed. The confluence of the jugular and subclavian veins is seen. The fibrous lesion is marked with an arrow and is directly under the head of the clavicle, on top of the first rib.

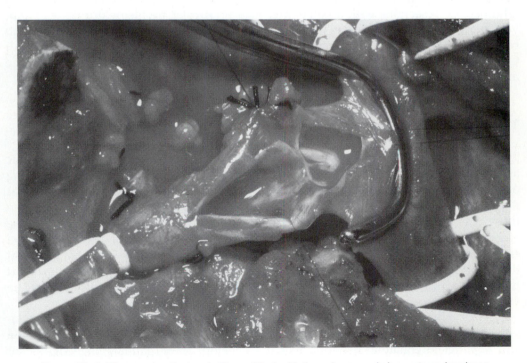

Figure 39–6. The same patient as in Figure 39–1 with the vein opened. A venotomy has been made through the fibrous lesion into normal vein proximally and distally. The web is then excised and the subclavian vein repaired with an autogenous vein patch.

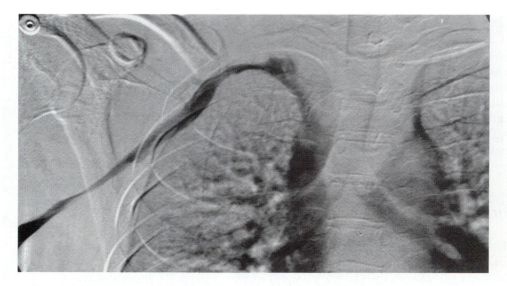

Figure 39–7. A postoperative venogram in the patient from Figure 39–1 3 days after repair. All the collateral veins are gone and the arm has returned to normal.

costoclavicular space. Strange-Vognsen et al.[22] performed first rib resections in 21 patients following lysis and used postoperative venograms to document the status of the vein. Persistent obstruction at the costoclavicular space was identified in 12 of these patients. Two of these patients reoccluded prior to first rib resection but 9 of the 10 who had rib resections with a patent vein had no further problems during a 1- to 6-year period. Our preference at the University of Rochester is to recommend first rib resection as the initial bony operation when direct operation on the vein is not required. Operative treatment of symptomatic patients with long persistent obstructions of the axillosubclavian vein should be deferred if possible.

TIMING THE OPERATION

The thrombolyzed axillosubclavian vein is at risk for rethrombosis. When an anatomic abnormality is detected, thoracic outlet decompression should be performed. The timing of the decompression is controversial, however. Kunkel and Machleder[18] found that patients operated on immediately after thrombolysis had a higher recurrence rate than those who were staged at a later date. This is counterintuitive to the notion that the earlier the decompression, the less likely a recurrent thrombosis will develop. Urschel et al.,[12] however, continues to recommend immediate decompression. Our policy at the University of Rochester accepts the principle of early operation when a short intrinsic venous abnormality can be repaired through a medial claviculectomy or an extrinsic lesion can be released through a transaxillary rib resection.

Some patients will require a more complicated reconstruction of the axillosubclavian vein. This situation occurs when thrombolysis is unsuccessful or not attempted and a sufficient collateral network does not develop. These patients have significant upper extremity venous hypertension and are limited in their activities. A variety of techniques using the ipsilateral jugular vein have been described.[23,24] These techniques utilize either a medial claviculectomy or a combined supraclavicular/infraclavicular approach. The internal jugular vein is dissected to the base of the skull and divided. It is turned down and anastomosed to the patient axillary vein. The limiting factor in successfully performing this procedure is an adequate axillary vein. This is another reason to attempt clot lysis early. Even if the entire vein is not salvaged, some extra length on the axillary vein is often achieved and this may be enough to allow for a subsequent reconstruction. Occasionally, the jugular vein is occluded in patients with catheter-related thromboses and this option is not available. Successful axillary to right atrial bypasses have been constructed with ringed polytetrafluorethylene. These patients often have a functioning hemoaccess fistula in the ipsilateral arm, which helps maintain patency of these prosthetic conduits.

CONCLUSION

The treatment of ASVT has changed during the past 20 years to one of anticoagulation and expectant operation to immediate attempts at clot removal with decompression of the thoracic outlet when necessary. Obviously, the therapeutic options in a patient with ASVT depend on the timeliness of the diagnosis and the status of the patient. All patients should be immediately anticoagulated with heparin. The treatment of a healthy young athlete who presents to the Emergency Room with a 12-hour history of a swollen arm should be very different from that of the elderly lady receiving chemotherapy via a subclavian venous catheter who develops a swollen arm over the course of her treatment. Both the functional demands and the likelihood of successful clot extraction whether by chemical or mechanical means are different. Aggressive early therapy with catheter-directed UK is therefore indicated in any patient without contraindications to clot lysis who anticipates an active lifestyle. Once the offending abnormality is uncovered, operative correction is indicated. An extrinsic stenosis is best relieved by first rib resection through the axilla. A short intrinsic lesion is best treated through a medial claviculectomy and open venoplasty. Treatment of a long occlusion by a jugular vein turndown procedure should be delayed until the magnitude of the patient's disability is evident.

REFERENCES

1. Ameli FM, Minas T, Weiss M, Provan JL. Consequences of 'conservative' conventional management of axillary vein thrombosis. *Can J Surg.* 1987;30:167–169.
2. Gloviczki P, Kazmier RJ, Hollier LH. Axillary-subclavian venous occlusion: the morbidity of a non-lethal disease. *J Vasc Surg.* 1986;4:333–337.
3. Tilney NL, Griffiths HFG, Edwards EA. Natural history of major venous thrombosis of the upper extremity. *Arch Surg.* 1970;101:792–796.
4. DeWeese JA, Adams JT, Gaiser DI. Subclavian venous thrombectomy. *Circulation.* 1970;16(suppl 2):158–170.
5. Hughes ESR. Venous obstruction in the upper extremity (Paget–Schroetter syndrome). *Int Abst Surg.* 1994;88:89–127.
6. Adams JT, DeWeese JA. Effort thrombosis of the axillary and subclavian veins. *J Trauma.* 1971;11:923–930.
7. Holzenbein T, Winkelbauer F, Teleky B, et al. Therapy and the natural course of axillary vein thrombosis—review of 765 patients and analysis of our personal patient sample. *Vasa-Supplementum.* 1991;33:107–108.
8. Brismar B, Hardstedt C, Jacobson S. Diagnosis of thrombosis by catheter venography after prolonged central venous catheterization. *Ann Surg.* 1981;194:779–783.

9. Becker DM, Philbrick JT, Walker FB. Axillary and subclavian venous thrombosis: prognosis and treatment. *Arch Intern Med.* 1991;151:1934–1943.

10. Doyle DJ, Turpie AG, Hirsh J. Adjusted subcutaneous heparin or continuous intravenous heparin in patients with acute deep vein thrombosis—a randomized trial. *Ann Intern Med.* 1987;107:441–445.

11. Bern MT, Lokich JJ, Wallach SR. Very low doses of warfarin can prevent thrombosis in central venous catheters. *Ann Intern Med.* 1990;112:423–428.

12 Urschel HC Jr, Razzuk MA. *N Eng J Med.* 1992;287:567. Letter.

13. Rogers LQ, Lutcher CL. Streptokinase therapy for deep vein thrombosis: a comprehensive review of the English literature. *Am J Med.* 1990;88:389–395.

14. Wilson JJ, Zahn CA, Newman H. Fibrinolytic therapy for idiopathic subclavian-axillary vein thrombosis. *Am J Surg.* 1990;159:208–211.

15. Druy EM, Trout HH III, Giordano JM, Hix WR. Lytic therapy in the treatment of axillary and subclavian vein thrombosis. *J Vasc Surg.* 1985;2:821–827.

16. Crowell LL. Effort thrombosis of the subclavian and axillary veins: review of the literature and case report with two year follow-up and venography. *Ann Intern Med.* 1960;52:1337–1343.

17. DeWeese JA. Management of subclavian venous obstruction. In: Bergan JJ, Yao JST, eds. *Surgery of the Veins.* New York: Grune and Stratton; 1985:365–372.

18. Kunkel JM, Machleder HI. Treatment of Paget-Schroetter syndrome. *Arch Surg.* 1989;125:1153–1158.

19. Lord JW Jr. Thoracic outlet syndromes: current management. *Ann Surg.* 1971;173:700.

20. Roos DB. Experience with first rib resection for thoracic outlet syndrome. *Ann Surg.* 1971;173:429.

21. Campbell CB, Chandler JG, Tegtmeyer CJ, Bernstein EF. Axillary, subclavian and brachiocephalic vein obstruction. *Surgery.* 1977;82:816–826.

22. Strange-Vognsen HH, Hauch O, Anderson J, Struckmann J. Resection of the first rib following deep arm vein thrombosis in patients with thoracic outlet syndrome. *J Cardiovasc Surg.* 1989;30:430–433.

23. Witte CL, Smith CA. Single anastomosis vein bypass for subclavian vein obstruction. *Arch Surg.* 1966;93:664–666.

24. Jacobson JSH, Haimov M. Venous revascularization of the arm. Report of three cases. *Surgery.* 1977;81:599–604.

40

Endovascular Metallic Stents for Treatment of Superior Vena Cava Syndrome

Robert L. Vogelzang, MD

The superior vena cava (SVC) syndrome is a well-known and described clinical entity resulting from obstruction of the large central veins, which causes regional venous congestion. Obstruction or stenosis of the SVC and/or brachiocephalic veins can produce the SVC syndrome. The reasons for obstruction include malignancy, central venous catheters, dialysis-related stenoses, and fibrosing mediastinitis among others.[1-5] The syndrome is usually characterized by marked swelling and venous distension of the upper torso including the head, neck, upper chest, and arms, which is usually exacerbated by lying down (Fig. 40–1). Cyanosis is often present as is headache, dyspnea, and blurred vision. Severe cases with acute onset or lack of significant development of collaterals can produce laryngeal and cerebral edema, as well. The large majority of patients (90% or greater) have malignancies such as lung cancer (with direct or metastatic involvement of the mediastinum), lymphomas, squamous cell carcinomas of the head and neck, or mediastinal metastases from a wide variety of sources. Important benign causes of the SVC syndrome include obliteration of the central veins by chronic central venous catheterization and/or development of venous endothelial scarring or hyperplasia as a result of local infusion of toxic or irritating substances, such as chemotherapy from a catheter positioned immediately adjacent to the SVC wall. Fibrosing mediastinitis, an inflammatory condition related to histoplasmosis or tuberculosis, can also present with complete obliteration of the central venous structures.[1-3]

In general, treatment for malignant causes of SVC syndrome has been palliative and predominantly directed at reduction of the malignant mass responsible for compression or obliteration of the superior vena cava. For most patients, this consists of mediastinal radiation with or without adjunctive chemotherapy. This approach will improve a considerable number of patients in the short term; however, not all will benefit. For these patients, endovascular stents are now clearly the treatment of choice since stenting produces a large functional venous conduit that will rapidly eliminate the findings of the SVC syndrome.

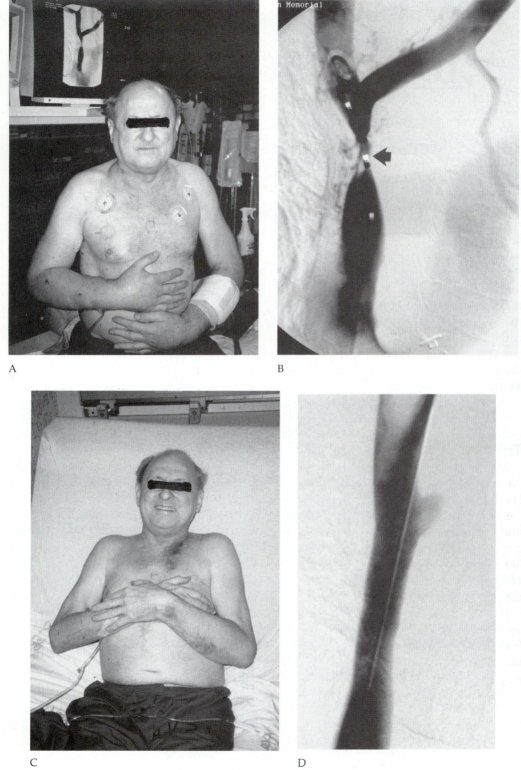

A

B

C

D

APPROACH TO SUPERIOR VENA CAVA OBSTRUCTION: IMAGING CONSIDERATIONS AND PERCUTANEOUS TECHNIQUES

For the patient with SVC syndrome, the initial diagnostic test should be cross-sectional imaging [either computed tomography (CT) or magnetic resonance imaging (MR)]. Cross-sectional imaging techniques are by far the most valuable modalities in determining the presence, nature, and level of the caval obstruction. The relative merits of CT versus MRI need not be debated here, but suffice it to say that both techniques produce excellent visualization and demonstration of the large central veins and the presence or absence of an obstructing mass (an important consideration in patients newly diagnosed with SVC syndrome). Both techniques can be used to produce three-dimensional reconstructed images in multiple planes, but for the most part, these ancillary imaging techniques are not necessary and careful inspection of the transverse sections usually suffices. MRI does have a number of advantages in terms of its ability to visualize flowing or stagnant blood, but our experience has been equally good with CT.

Venography is reserved for those patients in whom the nature, level, and/or extent of occlusion is not clear from cross-sectional imaging or in whom further therapy is planned. Venography of the central veins should be performed carefully and with good technique; a simple injection of contrast material through needles in forearm and antecubital veins is usually not sufficient to lay out the anatomy in the central veins and plan appropriate therapy. Rather, bilateral angiographic catheters should be inserted into upper extremity veins and power injection of contrast material made in order to produce an optimal image of the stenosis and its effects on local circulation. The jugular veins can also be used for venography, as can the femoral veins.

THROMBOLYSIS

Not all patients with central venous stenosis or occlusion have central venous thrombosis, but those who have such clots present an added challenge since thrombus can frequently obscure the exact nature of the underlying nature of the stenosis or occlusion and, in addition, poses a risk of embolization if stenting is performed. Therefore, we consider thrombolysis to be an essential component of treatment before stent placement is performed. Thrombolysis is performed in the usual manner with multiple side-hole catheters embedded in clot with urokinase (UK) infused at a rate of 60,000 to 240,000 units per minute. Thrombolysis takes longer in the central venous circulation than arterial thrombolysis; it may require up to 72 hours to produce clearing of the central veins. In some cases, stenting can be carried out in the presence of partial or incomplete lysis in order to produce better blood flow and/or more rapid thrombolysis but in these cases, thrombolysis should be continued after stent placement in order to prevent early failure.[6]

Figure 40–1. (A) Photograph of a 56-year-old man with lung cancer and superior vena cava syndrome. Note marked facial and upper extremity swelling. **(B)** High-grade stenosis in the superior vena cava (*arrow*). **(C)** Patient one day after stenting with markedly reduced facial and upper extremity edema when compared with preprocedural study. **(D)** Complete elimination of the stenosis after placement of a 14-mm Wallstent.

STENTS AVAILABLE FOR SUPERIOR VENA CAVA STENTING

A number of metallic stents are available in the United States in sufficient diameters for use in large central veins, such as the SVC. The majority of reports on the use of stents in the SVC and other large central veins are anecdotal with very little long-term clinical or imaging follow-up. Nevertheless, it is very clear to most investigators that transluminal angioplasty alone is rarely adequate for treatment of the vast majority of venous stenoses since benign venous stenoses tend to be resilient, resistant to angioplasty, and rapidly recurrent, and malignant lesions are subject to rapid regrowth and recurrence. Thus, stenting of large central veins such as the SVC has become widely accepted as the treatment of choice.

The stents available in adequate diameters (typically 12 to 20 mm) for SVC use include the following:

1. *Gianturco-Wallace Z stent.* This stent or one of its modifications as devised by Cesar Gianturco has been used in biliary, tracheobronchial, esophageal, and other tubular systems to restore patency. This stent, which consists of interconnected stent bodies with small barbs or hooks for secure attachment, has been fairly widely used in the SVC. The stent is quite radiopaque but the delivery device is large (up to 14 or 16 French) and the stent itself kinks readily at junction points between the stent bodies.[1,7,8] Despite these shortcomings, this stent produces excellent results (Fig. 40–2).

2. *Wallstent (Schneider; Plymouth, Minnesota, USA).* The Wallstent is available in multiple diameters and lengths and this device is rapidly becoming the treatment of choice for these lesions since the device is flexible and, therefore, can be inserted from a variety of approaches including the jugular, arm, and femoral veins (Fig. 40–1). The delivery system on which it is placed is relatively small in size (9 French) compared to the other devices. The Wallstent is also self-expanding, although the radial force applied by the device decreases rapidly with larger (greater than 10-mm-diameter) size. This may impair its ability to expand in rigid or resistant lesions such as those seen in fibrosis or in invasive carcinomas.[3,4,9–11]

3. *Palmaz stent.* The Palmaz stent was the first commercially available metallic stent and the device is radiopaque, can be easily seen, and has a significant advantage of markedly higher radial force application over the Wallstent since the balloon on which the stent is mounted provides the radial force to open the lesion and place the stent. The largest of the Palmaz stents can be deployed to up to 18 mm but the device has a significant disadvantage in that dilatation of the stent to that size results in marked shortening, which increases the likelihood of stent migration. Despite these limitations, the Palmaz stent is an excellent choice for stenting focal lesions of the central veins[4,12,13] (Fig. 40–3).

STENT PLACEMENT TECHNIQUE

Without going into extensive detail, suffice it to say that stent placement in central venous stenoses should be performed by an experienced operator who is cognizant of the problems that can occur in this particular location. In general, these devices are placed from brachial or femoral veins, although placement from subclavian or internal jugular venous approaches is relatively straightforward as well. The specific technique

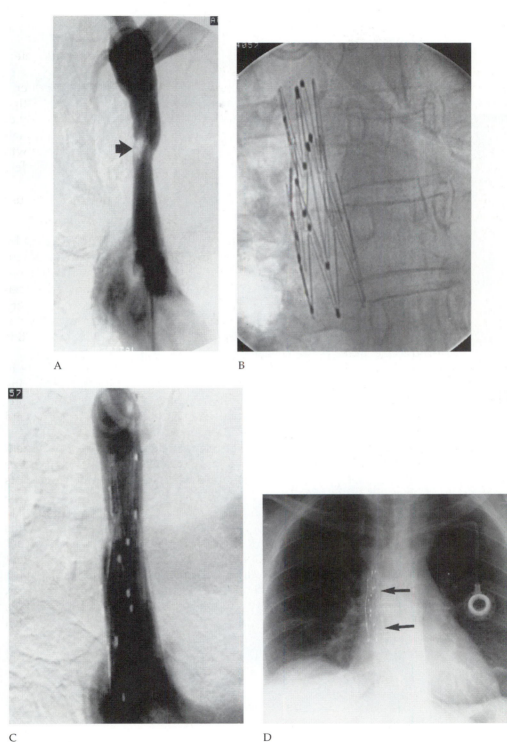

A

B

C

D

Figure 40–2. A 49-year-old woman with metastatic breast cancer as a cause of her SVC syndrome. (**A**) A pretreatment superior venacavagram demonstrating a high-grade stenosis (*arrow*). (**B**) Deployment of two Gianturco-Wallace Z stents. (**C**) Superior venacavagram after deployment of stents with elimination of stenosis. (**D**) Chest x-ray demonstrating stents in SVC (*arrows*).

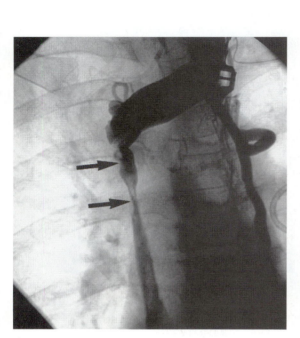

A

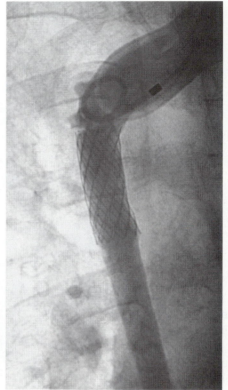

B

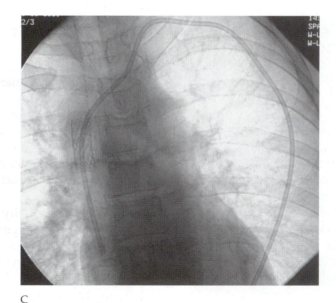

C

Figure 40–3. Benign central venous catheter-induced stricture of the SVC. This 23-year-old woman had a long history of central venous catheterization for feeding secondary to extensive Crohn's disease. She presented with dyspnea and facial swelling. (**A**) Superior venacavogram showing high-grade stenosis of the upper SVC (*arrows*). (**B**) After placement of 12-mm Palmaz stent with excellent anatomic result and elimination of all symptoms referable to the stenosis. (**C**) After stent deployment a new central venous catheter is placed through the stent. The stent is currently patent 13 months after initial placement.

is highly dependent on the stent used, but most workers believe that the lesion should be carefully localized and probably predilated with an angioplasty balloon in order to optimize stent placement and minimize migration.

PROBLEMS AND COMPLICATIONS WITH CENTRAL VENOUS STENTS

The three most common problems associated with central venous stents are failure to open due to resistant stenoses, recurrence of the stenosis or rethrombosis due to hypercoagulability, tumor ingrowth, or stent migration.

Failure to open is generally related to a high degree of resistance in a venous stenosis in patients with long-standing fibrotic lesions or with infiltrating aggressive malignancies, such as squamous cell carcinoma. In these patients, incomplete opening of stents may lead to early rethrombosis and aggressive anticoagulation should be carried out. Use of the Palmaz stent may be of benefit in this situation (Fig. 40–4).

Stent migration tends to occur predominantly with short focal stenoses in which the stent "squirts" or moves off the stenosis as it is being deployed. If the stent migrates superiorly (away from the heart), a new stent can generally be placed but if the stent migrates toward the heart, it must be retrieved through some percutaneous method.

Tumor ingrowth and rethrombosis recur as a result of either hypercoagualability of the patient or recurrence of disease. Rethrombosis is usually treated with thrombolysis or anticoagulation and tumor ingrowth is best treated with restenting.

RESULTS OF SUPERIOR VENA CAVA STENT PLACEMENT FOR MALIGNANT SUPERIOR VENA CAVA SYNDROME

Most reports of stent placement of SVC obstruction deal only with patients with malignant SVC syndrome. Most case series encompass small groups (20 or less) and have short intervals between stent placement and death of the patient due to underlying malignancy. For example, Rösch et al.[7] described the use of Gianturco-Rösch expandable Z stents in 20 patients. There was 100% immediate improvement and 95% long-term improvement but the average time to death was only 5.2 months. Gaines et al.[8] described immediate improvement of 90% in 20 patients treated for SVC obstruction with long-term improvement in 65% and 5-month median survival.

At Northwestern Memorial Hospital, we have had the opportunity to treat a total of seven patients with SVC syndrome. Six of these patients had malignant causes and one had a benign etiology for her disease. We performed thrombolysis in two of the seven prior to stenting; stenting was technically successful in all seven patients and resulted in completed elimination of symptoms referable to the SVC syndrome in all seven. There was one stent migration in which the Wallstent migrated off a short high-grade stenosis; this stent was successfully retrieved with a loop snare. Follow-up on these seven patients showed five deaths from underlying malignancy at a median of 3.4 months. One patient with pancreatic cancer is alive with a patent stent 10 months after stent deployment and the single patient with a benign central venous catheter-related stenosis of the SVC has a widely patent Palmaz stent in the superior vena cava 13 months after deployment.

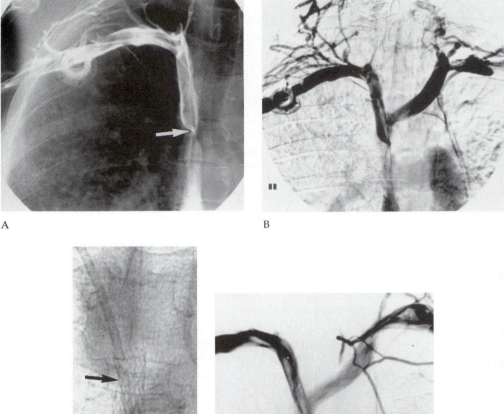

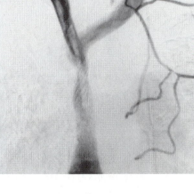

Figure 40–4. Malignant SVC obstruction secondary to lung cancer with extensive central venous thrombosis. A 46-year-old man with lung cancer presents with marked manifestations of the superior vena cava syndrome. (**A**) Venogram demonstrating extensive clot in the brachiocephalic veins and SVC and a high-grade SVC stenosis (*arrow*). (**B**) After 72 hours of bilateral thrombolysis performed through the antecubital veins with clearing of clot and persistence of stenosis. (**C**) After deployment of Palmaz stent, a persistent narrowing (*arrow*) was demonstrated related to highly resistant tumor. (**D**) This relative narrowing, however, did not limit flow on subsequent venography nor did the patient have any recurrent symptoms until his death from widely metastatic tumor 6 months later.

CONCLUSION

Stenting of the superior vena cava is a reliable, safe, and highly effective alternative to the much more morbid and generally less effective surgical alternative for patients with malignant SVC obstruction. We strongly recommend the use of cross-sectional imaging for initial evaluation of patients with signs and symptoms of the SVC syndrome; venography should be reserved for those patients in whom the cause of SVC syndrome is not clear or for those in whom therapy is contemplated. Thrombolysis of extensive venous thrombosis is recommended in order to most effectively treat central occlusions. The choice of stents appears to be operator dependent and all three available stents appear to work well in the short term. Long-term results are pending.

REFERENCES

1. Carasco CH, Charnsangavej C, Wright KC, et al. Use of the Gianturco self-expanding stent in stenosis of the superior and inferior venae cavae. *JVIR*. 1992;3:409–419.
2. Dondelinger RF, Goffette P, Kurdziel JC, Roche A. Expandable metal stents for stenoses of the vena cavae and large veins. *Semin Intervent Radiol*. 1991;8(4):252–263.
3. Antonucci F, Salomonwitz E, Stuckmann G, et al. Placement of venous stents: clinical experience with a self-expanding prosthesis. *Radiology*. 1992;183:493–497.
4. Trerotola SO. Interventional radiology in central venous stenosis and occlusion. *Semin Intervent Radiol*. 1994;11(4):291–304.
5. Kishi K, Sonomura T, Mitsuzane K, et al. Self-expandable metallic stent therapy for superior vena cava syndrome: clinical observations. *Radiology*. 1993;189:531–535.
6. Gray BH, Olin JW, Graor RA, et al. Safety and efficacy of thrombolytic therapy for superior vena cava syndrome. *Chest*. 1991;99:54–59.
7. Rösch J, Uchida BT, Hall LD, et al. Gianturco-Rösch expandable Z-stents in the treatment of superior vena cava syndrome. *Cardiovasc Intervent Radiol*. 1992;15:319–327.
8. Gaines PA, Belli AM, Anderson PB, et al. Superior vena caval obstruction managed by the Gianturco Z stent. *Clin Radiol*. 1994;49:202–208.
9. Dyet JF, Nicholson AA, Cook AM. The use of the Wallstent endovascular prosthesis in the treatment of malignant obstruction of the superior vena cava. *Clin Radiol*. 1993;48:381–385.
10. Oudkerk M, Heystraten FMJ, Stoter G. Stenting in malignant vena caval obstruction. *Cancer*. 1993;71:142–146.
11. Watkinson AF, Hansell DM. Expandable Wallstent for the treatment of obstruction of the superior vena cava. *Thorax*. 1993;48:915–920.
12. Elson JD, Becker GJ, Wholey MH, Ehrman KO. Vena caval and central venous stenosis: management with Palmaz balloon-expandable intraluminal stents. *JVIR*. 1991;2:215–223.
13. Solomon N, Wholey MH, Jarmolowski CR. Intravascular stents in the management of superior vena cava syndrome. *Cathet Cardiovasc Diagn*. 1991;23:245–252.

41

Impact of Duplex Ultrasound Scanning in Varicose Vein Surgery

Philip D. Coleridge Smith, DM, FRCS

The use of duplex ultrasonography in the assessment of patients with venous incompetence and varicose veins has become widespread in recent years. The availability of good-quality color duplex machines combined with a developing understanding of what they may show has led to their enthusiastic use in many Western countries. They may be used in the assessment of patients with primary varicose veins, recurrent varices, and venous leg ulcers. Surgeons may be helped to locate perforating veins, residual saphenous trunks, and veins in the popliteal fossa with the help of preoperative skin marking.

Published evidence shows that duplex ultrasonography detects more incompetent veins than clinical examination, hand-held continuous-wave (CW) Doppler ultrasound, or phlebography. Little data have been published to allow an objective judgment to be reached as to whether duplex ultrasonography improves the outcome of superficial venous surgery. Those who use this method as part of their practice immediately realize that no other technique can give them the same precision of information and do not need to be convinced by randomized clinical trials! The use of duplex ultrasonography will become more widespread in the future, and I believe that this will result in the improved management of patients with all types of venous disease.

INTRODUCTION

How Has Duplex Ultrasonography Modified the Management of Varicose Veins?

Color duplex ultrasonography is a technology that has been widely available since about 1990, although duplex ultrasonography offering pulsed Doppler analysis of blood flow has been available since the early 1980s. There has been a rapid expansion in its use for the investigation of patients with venous disease, as well as for patients with arterial problems. Although several papers have been published comparing angiographic techniques of investigating venous and arterial diseases, no study has so far addressed the question of whether an improvement in outcome of treatment can be expected following duplex assessment of either venous or arterial disease.

There are a number of reasons why this information has not become available for lower limb venous disease. Those who use duplex ultrasonography to assess patients with varicose veins realize that no other technique can provide such precise information about the anatomic distribution of veins and their function![1-4] Color duplex machines have only become widely used in the last 5 or 6 years, so few centers have had the opportunity to follow up patients for long enough to provide an answer. The design of varicose vein studies necessitates follow-up of at least 3 to 5 years for reliable data to be obtained, so these studies take a number of years to complete. Duplex ultrasonography rapidly received acceptance as the "gold standard" for investigation in venous disease. Evidence for its use comes from comparative studies to other techniques.

What Are the Alternative Methods of Investigation in Patients with Varicose Veins?

Clinical examination of the venous system has been widely used to assess varicose veins but it is well known that this technique is unreliable,[5] especially in patients with complex problems such as recurrent varices or leg ulceration. Many surgeons now employ hand-held CW Doppler ultrasound to detect venous valvular incompetence. The saphenofemoral junction can be reliably assessed in the majority of patients using this device. In many cases saphenopopliteal incompetence may also be detected. However, CW Doppler is not reliable in distinguishing deep from superficial venous incompetence, especially in the popliteal fossa.

Phlebography provides excellent anatomic information and may also be used to assess venous valvular incompetence. Until recently this investigation was widely used to assess all aspects of venous disease. Intravenous injection of contrast media and exposure to ionizing radiation are significant disadvantages. With the rapid expansion of duplex ultrasonography, phlebography is being used much less often.

Appropriate Use of Duplex Ultrasonography—In Which Clinical Situations Might It Be Useful?

Duplex ultrasonography is helpful in many stages of the management of varicose veins and venous disease. Preoperatively, this technique is used to identify the incompetent veins in primary venous disease. During the perioperative period it is useful in the identification of veins that cannot be easily localized by clinical examination. Examples of these include the saphenopopliteal junction, calf and thigh perforating veins, and residual segments of saphenous vein. Patients who have previously been operated on for their varicose veins may present with recurrent varices from many possible sources. These include a recurrence from the original site of ligation or from another source, as a consequence of progression of disease or failure to identify this source at the previous operation. Duplex ultrasonography is invaluable for this purpose. Many patients presenting with venous ulceration may be suitable for treatment by varicose vein surgery. Recent studies in which duplex ultrasonography has been used as the method of assessment have reported that up to 50% of patients with venous leg ulcers have superficial venous incompetence alone. This compares with as few as 10% of patients in which the diagnosis was achieved by earlier methods of diagnosis.

PREOPERATIVE ASSESSMENT

The outcome of varicose vein surgery is dependent on accurate preoperative assessment, as well as competent surgery, to achieve long-term cure of varicose veins. If, after clinical examination, the surgeon decided to ligate the saphenofemoral junction when the patient actually had saphenopopliteal junction incompetence, success is unlikely. The most important point at which duplex ultrasonography may modify management is at the assessment stage prior to surgery. An accurate diagnosis here will ensure that the correct operation is selected.

Clinical examination may be misleading. Varices apparently arising from the saphenopopliteal junction (SPJ) may come from the long saphenous system. Saphenofemoral junction (SFJ) and SPJ incompetence may coexist. A previous, unsuspected deep-vein thrombosis may have occluded or seriously damaged the deep veins. Removing the superficial veins may deprive the limb of a collateral route of venous drainage.

It is essential to assess each of these veins since valvular incompetence may occur in isolation at any of these, or at a number of sites: the SFJ, SPJ, long saphenous vein (LSV), short saphenous vein (SSV), perforating veins, and deep veins.

Clinical Examination, CW Doppler or Duplex Ultrasound?

Duplex ultrasonography has been compared against clinical assessment and CW Doppler ultrasound.[6-8] DePalma et al.[6] investigated 40 patients with varicosities in the distribution of the LSV. They compared clinical examination and CW Doppler with color duplex ultrasonography, which they used as the reference standard. Clinical examination and CW Doppler examination were equally sensitive (48%) in detecting LSV incompetence, missing a startling 26 of 50 incompetent LSVs. In 22 patients who had previously had saphenofemoral ligation, the groin recurrence present in 9 subjects on duplex was missed by CW Doppler. CW Doppler examinations in this study were carried out by an experienced vascular surgeon.

In a study carried out by McMullin et al.,[7] CW Doppler was compared with duplex ultrasonography in 136 patients with varicose veins. CW Doppler detected that 73% of the LSVs were found to be incompetent on duplex ultrasonography. Sensitivity in the popliteal fossa for saphenopopliteal incompetence was worse at only 33%, and 48% for deep-vein incompetence. The reason for inaccuracy in this region is that CW Doppler is poor at resolving complex anatomy (Fig. 41–1). The complexity has been highlighted by Somjen et al.[9] who studied 123 limbs with popliteal fossa venous incompetence. In 91 cases there was a single source of incompetence, but in the remaining limbs multiple sources of incompetence were found. In 48 of the cases reflux in the popliteal vein above the knee or superficial femoral vein was found, although in most cases the popliteal vein below the knee was competent.

The clinical advantage of duplex ultrasonography remains difficult to judge. A study in which patients were first examined by a surgeon using clinical examination and CW Doppler has been conducted in 48 patients, 10 of whom were being operated on for the second time.[8] An operation plan was devised for each patient based on this information. Patients were then examined by color duplex ultrasonography and the operation plan revised in 18 of 68 limbs. Escape points between the superficial and deep venous system would have been left intact in 14 limbs had duplex ultrasonography not been performed. This study shows that duplex ultrasonography is more reliable than CW Doppler, especially where complex anatomy is to be expected. It also suggests

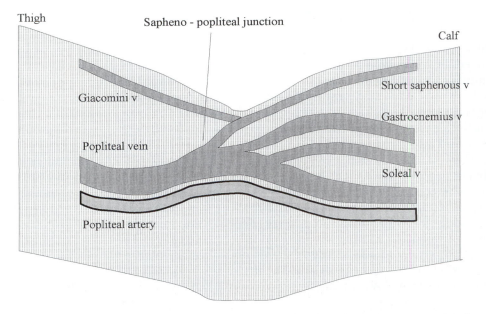

Figure 41–1. Longitudinal ultrasound anatomy of the popliteal fossa showing the complexity of the veins in this region.

that improved outcome of treatment might be expected with the use of duplex ultrasonography.

How Does Duplex Ultrasonography Compare with Phlebography?

Phlebography is not widely used for the investigation of primary varicose veins, but has been studied in comparison with duplex ultrasonography in the diagnosis of deep-vein incompetence. Duplex ultrasonography is as sensitive as phlebography in the femoral region and detects more cases of popliteal vein incompetence.[10] The difference here is that descending phlebography relies on demonstrating reverse flow in veins into which a hypertonic contrast medium has been injected. This investigation has to be performed at rest. Competent proximal valves may prevent the demonstration of incompetence in the (important) popliteal segment, since contrast medium never descends to this section of the venous system. Duplex ultrasonography relies on the flow of blood in veins and is not restricted by the need for injection of contrast material and is usually carried out with the patient standing, the position in which venous reflux is clinically significant.

The ability of duplex ultrasonography to reveal a wide range of patterns of venous valvular incompetence has led some authors to suggest that varicose vein surgery should be precisely tailored to each patient's needs.[11] Whether this actually improves the results of surgery has not been tested systematically.

Duplex Assessment of Patients with Recurrent Varicose Veins

Recurrent varicose veins are a difficult problem to assess clinically and the type of surgery performed by the previous surgeon may not be obvious from the skin incisions or recorded in the patient's hospital notes. The use of an imaging technique to determine their origin is widely accepted.[5] The most common source of recurrence following

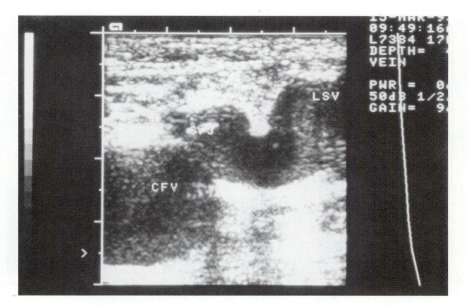

Figure 41–2. Ultrasound image of saphenofemoral recurrence.

surgery of the long saphenous system is the SFJ (Figs. 41–2, 41–3, and 41–4).[12–14] However, this only accounts for 40% of new varices, and investigation is necessary to establish whether veins fill from other sources.

In planning a further operation it is highly desirable to have the following information available:

1. Is there a recurrence at the SFJ or SPJ?
2. Was the LSV or SSV stripped previously?
3. Where do recurrent varices fill from?
4. Is incompetence present in a previously unoperated junction (SFJ or SPJ)?
5. Are the deep veins normal?

Clinical examination is as unreliable here as it is in other situations. Bradbury et al.[5] studied an unselected series of 36 patients who has previously undergone ligation of the SFJ. At operation three-quarters were found to have a patent SFJ. Of 26 cases with an operative diagnosis of a patent SFJ, 17 were identified clinically and 23 using CW Doppler. However, both these techniques identified further cases where a patent SFJ was not found at operation, resulting in poor specificity for these tests. CW Doppler examination may be unreliable in assessment of recurrent SFJ incompetence because in the groin, communications between the superficial abdominal veins and the thigh varices may simulate the sounds from a recurrent SFJ. Only an imaging technique can resolve this problem.

A frequently reported problem is persisting reflux in an unstripped LSV following earlier saphenofemoral ligation. The anatomy of this and its filling points cannot be resolved without an examination that provides imaging information. In fact, incompetence of the LSV trunk may occur in the presence of a competent SFJ, even before surgical intervention, in one-third of patients with primary LSV varices.[15]

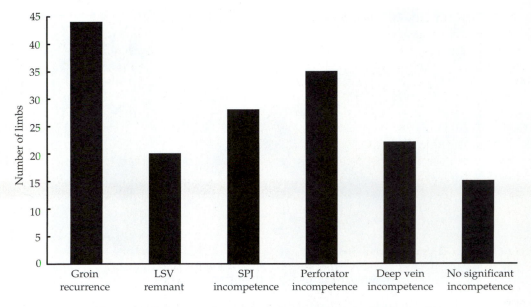

Figure 41–3. Sources of recurrent varices in a study by Quigley et al.[13]

Recurrent varices in the popliteal fossa are particularly difficult to treat. Inappropriate exploration may result in damage to important nerves or veins. An exact anatomic map is required before commencing an operation in this region. Duplex ultrasonography is very reliable when used to assess this area, giving 100% concordance with phlebography in a series of patients with recurrent SPJ varices.[16]

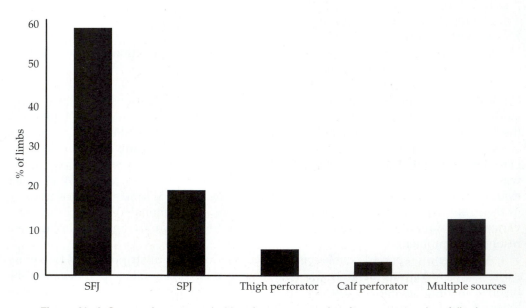

Figure 41–4. Source of recurrence in 36 patients reoperated on for recurrent varices following previous SFJ ligation.[5]

In many instances, recurrent varices are identified in a limb where previous surgery has been performed, but in a vein that was not operated on before. This is probably due to progression of disease into unaffected veins. This has been reported in one clinical study using an objective measure of outcome.[17] In this study 36 patients were examined clinically, by color Duplex scanning and photoplethysmography and 56 limbs with superficial venous incompetence identified. The same patients were re-examined after 20 months in which no treatment was given and an additional 10 sources of superficial venous reflux identified.

Many authors recommend the use of duplex ultrasonography for assessment of recurrent varicose veins. Interpretation of the findings from duplex ultrasonography requires experience, but basing management on objective data seems to be a logical advance.

PATIENTS WITH VENOUS ULCERATION

In patients presenting with venous leg ulcers, up to half of the cases will have only superficial venous incompetence.[18–20] In these patients, ligation and stripping of the superficial veins usually results in rapid ulcer healing. There is unlikely to be any advantage to varicose vein surgery in patients with deep-vein incompetence, especially if this involves the popliteal vein.[21–24] Removal of superficial veins where there is occlusion of the deep veins makes the problem worse. The aim of venous investigation in these circumstances is to identify the extent of the problem in the superficial veins, but confirm that the deep venous system is normal. Clinical examination and CW Doppler are unreliable at confirming that the deep venous system is patent and competent. Duplex ultrasonography reliably assesses patency of the deep veins. Investigation in this group of patients aims to define the location and nature of the venous problem (superficial veins or deep veins, incompetence or obstruction) and to assess the overall venous function of the limb using a plethysmographic method.

In summary, the following information will determine the treatment plan in a patient presenting with chronic venous insufficiency:

1. Is incompetence confined to the superficial venous system?
2. Are the deep veins competent?
3. Have the deep veins been damaged by a previous deep-vein thrombosis?
4. Is there residual obstruction of the deep veins?

PREOPERATIVE VEIN LOCALIZATION

The most common situation in which vein localization is helpful is the popliteal fossa. A wide range of anatomic patterns is seen in this region. The location of the junction of the SSV with the popliteal vein is very variable. Identification of this point using an imaging technique has been widely advocated, but never assessed to determine whether it actually improves the outcome of venous surgery (Fig. 41–5). Such localizations greatly assist the surgical procedure and hopefully reduce the likelihood of neurologic injury following popliteal fossa exploration. The marking of perforating veins[25] and residual segments of the LSV is also reported and greatly facilitates their ligation and removal at surgery.

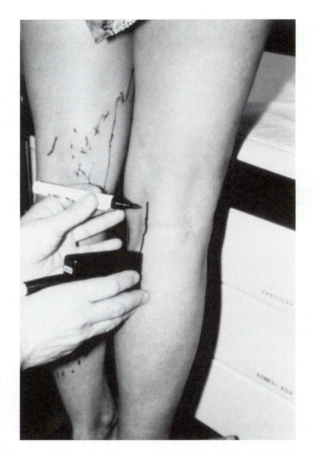

Figure 41–5. Preoperative duplex ultrasound localization of the SSV in the popliteal fossa.

CONCLUSION

Those who regularly use duplex ultrasonography in the management of venous disease are convinced of its value in improving the outcome of treatment, but no objective study has ever been carried out to prove this. Good surgery depends on full preoperative assessment of patients. At the SFJ, duplex is more accurate than clinical assessment and CW Doppler in patients with primary varicose veins. In recurrent varices, duplex ultrasonography is the most reliable investigation. In the popliteal fossa, clinical examination and CW Doppler are less sensitive to SPJ and popliteal vein incompetence than duplex ultrasonography. Duplex is helpful in resolving the complex anatomy of the popliteal fossa. In patients with recurrent varices it provides a precise indication of the surgery that was conducted previously, indicating where this has failed or if recurrence has occurred in some other part of the superficial venous system.

In patients presenting with venous ulceration, duplex ultrasonography is as reliable as phlebography in demonstrating the status of the deep veins, and identifies a substantial proportion of patients who may benefit from varicose vein surgery.

The exact role of duplex ultrasonography has not been objectively demonstrated in the management of patients with varicose veins—and it probably never will. This will not prevent its widespread application in the management of such patients!

REFERENCES

1. Thibault PK, Lewis WA. Recurrent varicose veins. Part 1: evaluation utilizing duplex venous imaging. *J Dermatol Surg Oncol.* 1992;18:618–624.
2. Katsamouris AN, Kardoulas DG, Gourtsoyiannis N. The nature of lower extremity venous insufficiency in patients with primary varicose veins. *Eur J Vasc Surg.* 1994;8:464–471.
3. Gaitini D, Torem S, Pery M, Kaftori JK. Image directed Doppler ultrasound in the diagnosis of lower limb venous insufficiency. *J Clin Ultrasound.* 1994;22:291–297.
4. Quigley FG, Raptis S, Cashman M, Faris IB. Duplex ultrasound mapping of sites of deep to superficial incompetence in primary varicose veins. *Aust NZ J Surg.* 1992;62:276–278.
5. Bradbury AW, Stonebridge PA, Callam MJ, et al. Recurrent varicose veins: assessment of the saphenofemoral junction. *Br J Surg.* 1994;81:373–375.
6. DePalma RG, Hart MT, Zanin L, Massarin EH. Physical examination, Doppler ultrasound and colour flow duplex scanning: guides to therapy for primary varicose veins. *Phlebology.* 1993;8:7–11.
7. McMullin GM, Coleridge Smith PD. An evaluation of Doppler ultrasound and photoplethysmography in the investigation of venous insufficiency. *Aust NZ J Surg.* 1992;62:270–275.
8. van der Heijden FH, Bruyninckx CM. Preoperative colour coded duplex scanning in varicose veins of the lower extremity. *Eur J Surg.* 1993;159:329–333.
9. Somjen GM, Royle JP, Fell G, et al. Venous reflux patterns in the popliteal fossa. *J Cardiovasc Surg Torino.* 1992;33:85–91.
10. Baker SR, Burnand KG, Sommerville KM, et al. Comparison of venous reflux assessed by duplex scanning and descending phlebography in chronic venous disease. *Lancet.* 1993;341:400–403.
11. Hanrahan LM, Kechejian GJ, Cordts PR, et al. Patterns of venous insufficiency in patients with varicose veins. *Arch Surg.* 1991;126:687–690.
12. Bradbury AW, Stonebridge PA, Ruckley CV, Beggs I. Recurrent varicose veins: correlation between preoperative clinical and hand-held Doppler ultrasonographic examination, and anatomical findings at surgery. *Br J Surg.* 1993;80:849–851.
13. Quigley FG, Raptis S, Cashman M. Duplex ultrasonography of recurrent varicose veins. *Cardiovasc Surg.* 1994;2:775–777.
14. Redwood NF, Lambert D. Patterns of reflux in recurrent varicose veins assessed by duplex. *Br J Surg.* 1994;81:1450–1451.
15. Abu-Own A, Scurr JH, Coleridge Smith PD. Saphenous vein reflux without incompetence at the saphenofemoral junction. *Br J Surg.* 1994;81:1452–1454.
16. De Maeseneer MG, De Hert SG, Van Schil PE, et al. Preoperative colour coded duplex examination of the saphenopopliteal junction in recurrent varicosis of the short saphenous vein. *Cardiovasc Surg.* 1993;1:686–689.
17. Sarin S, Shields DA, Farrah J, et al. Does venous function deteriorate in patients waiting for varicose vein surgery? *J R Soc Med.* 1993;86:21–23.
18. Shami SK, Sarin S, Cheatle TR, et al. Venous ulcers and the superficial venous system. *J Vasc Surg.* 1993;17:487–490.
19. Darke SG, Penfold C. Venous ulceration and saphenous ligation. *Eur J Vasc Surg.* 1992;6:4–9.
20. van Rij AM, Solomon C, Christie R. Anatomic and physiologic characteristics of venous ulceration. *J Vasc Surg.* 1994;20:759–764.
21. Burnand K, Thomas ML, O'Donnell T, Browse NL. Relation between postphlebitic changes in the deep veins and results of surgical treatment of venous ulcers. *Lancet.* 1976;i:936–938.
22. Stacey MC, Burnand KG, Layer GT, Pattison M. Calf pump function in patients with healed venous ulcers is not improved by surgery to the communicating veins or by elastic stockings. *Br J Surg.* 1988;75:436–439.
23. Bradbury AW, Stonebridge PA, Callam MJ, et al. Foot volumetry and duplex ultrasonography after saphenous and subfascial perforating vein ligation for recurrent venous ulceration. *Br J Surg.* 1993;80:845–848.
24. Payne SP, London NJ, Newland CJ, et al. Investigation and significance of short saphenous vein incompetence. *Ann R Coll Surg Engl.* 1993;75:354–357.
25. Hanrahan LM, Araki CT, Fisher JB, et al. Evaluation of the perforating veins of the lower extremity using high resolution duplex imaging. *J Cardiovasc Surg Torino.* 1991;32:87–97.

42

Modern Treatment of Lymphedema

Cindy L. Felty, MSN, RN, C-ANP, and
Thom W. Rooke, MD

Lymphedema is an abnormal accumulation of protein-rich fluid in the interstitial space that occurs secondary to anatomic or functional obstruction in the lymphatics or the lymph nodes.[1] This condition, which affects more than 1% of the U.S. population and more than 150 million people worldwide, is often misdiagnosed and/or mismanaged by health professionals. Unfortunately, without proper treatment, the condition may lead to repeated infections, enlargement of the limb, thickening of the skin, disfigurement, and disability.

LYMPHATIC ANATOMY AND PHYSIOLOGY

The lymph system helps maintain water and protein balance in the tissues and assists the immune system in protecting against harmful substances. The system includes lymphatic vessels and lymph nodes, along with other specialized structures such as the spleen, thymus, and tonsils. *Lymph* is a clear, colorless fluid formed by the transudation of plasma into the tissue spaces. The composition of lymph varies depending on its location, but it generally includes proteins and lymphocytes and may contain certain foreign substances such as bacteria. Lymph fluid is continually removed from the tissues in order to maintain the body's balance of fluid and protein. As edema develops, tissue pressure builds up and tends to push fluid from the interstitial spaces into the lymph vessels. Valves located in the lymphatics ensure that the lymph flows in only one direction.[2] Small lymphatics join to form larger ones, and the biggest lymph channels eventually combine into two separate lymph ducts through which lymph fluid ultimately returns to the blood. Lymph from the upper left side and lower part of the body flows primarily into the thoracic duct, while lymph from the right side of the head, neck, chest, and right arm empties into the right lymphatic duct located in the right side of the chest. The rate of lymph flow can be increased by skeletal muscle contraction, increased heart rate, and passive movements from other body parts. The velocity of lymph flow may increase by tenfold over resting values during exercise.

Lymphedema develops when the lymphatic load exceeds the transport capacity of the lymphatic system. When this occurs the tissue becomes inundated with protein-

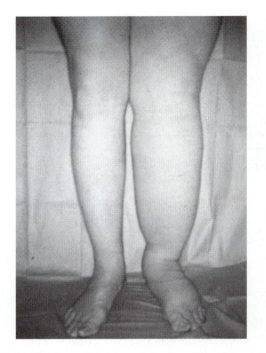

Figure 42–1. Primary lymphedema. Painless unilateral swelling of the leg and foot. The toes may appear squared. The edema does not resolve with overnight elevation of the extremity.

rich edema fluid. Without treatment, the protein-rich interstitial fluid is eventually replaced by fibrous tissue and collagen, which can lead to progressive fibrosis and, in later stages, irreversible tissue enlargement.

Lymphedema is often classified by stages. The first stage, also called the *reversible stage,* is manifested by edema of a pitting nature. The edema is soft and the swelling typically resolves overnight with simple elevation of the affected limb. If the lymphedema remains untreated, it produces a progressive hardening of the tissues in the affected areas, which occurs because of scarring and the proliferation of connective and/or adipose tissue. This stage of lymphedema, known as the *irreversible stage,* is manifested by edema that does not resolve with overnight elevation. At this point the lymphedema loses its pitting character and the skin begins to thicken. Stage 3 (or lymphostatic *elephantiasis*) is manifested by a tremendous increase in the volume of the affected limb. The hardening of the dermal tissues and papillomas that subsequently develop give the patient the appearance of having elephant skin (Fig. 42–1).

ETIOLOGY

There are two basic types of lymphedema: *primary* and *secondary.* Primary lymphedema occurs without any obvious cause. It is more common in females and occurs more often in the lower extremity. It is thought to arise from an inborn defect in the development of lymphatic vessels. Primary lymphedema can be present at birth or may occur before the age of 1, in which case it is classified as *congenital* lymphedema. Lymphedema arising between the age of 1 and 35 is referred to as *lymphedema praecox.*[3] *Lymphedema tarda* is generally the name given to primary lymphedema occurring after the age of 35.[4] Congenital lymphedema, which occurs in a familial pattern, is referred to as Milroy's disease.[3]

Secondary lymphedema is caused by injury, scarring, or excision of the lymph nodes. It may be the result of surgery in which lymph nodes are removed, or it can occur as a side effect of radiation therapy. Secondary lymphedema is occasionally caused by trauma or by chronic infections of the lymph system. Infections of the lymphatic system are generally bacterial in nature, with streptococci being the most common pathogen. In other parts of the world, especially in the tropics, secondary lymphedema is usually caused by parasitic infections.

EVALUATION

Before treatment is initiated the physician should attempt to define the cause of the edema. For patients older than 40 years of age, malignancy must be excluded.[5] Cancer (with or without surgery or radiation treatment) is responsible for 94% of upper extremity and 52% of lower extremity secondary lymphedema.[6]

The diagnosis of lymphedema can often be made by a history and physical examination alone. The patient may present with an insidious onset of painless, progressive swelling of the extremity, which starts at the ankle and progresses to involve the entire limb. Physical examination of the extremity sometimes reveals a square appearance to the toes, and the skin is frequently thick and/or the edema is hard and nonpitting.[5] The skin may have a red discoloration due to recurrent episodes of lymphangitis and cellulitis. Secondary skin changes such as verrucae and small vesicles (containing clear lymph fluid) may also be present.

Lymphedema should be distinguished from edema due to systemic causes.[5] Noninvasive venous evaluation is often needed to rule out occult venous disease. It has been noted, however, that secondary lymphedema may complicate long-standing venous insufficiency.[7] Other diagnoses such as lipedema, congestive heart failure, cellulitis, renal disease, myxedema, compartment syndrome, bursitis, arteriovenous anomalies, orthostatic edema, and muscle rupture may mimic lymphedema.

Lymphangiography is the "gold standard" test for diagnosing lymphedema. It is performed by cannulating a small lymph channel on the dorsum of the hand or foot and injecting a lipid-soluble contrast material. Unfortunately, it is possible for acute lymphangitis to result from this invasive procedure, and lymphangiography should therefore be avoided whenever possible.

Lymphoscintigraphy provides a safe and simple alternative to demonstrate whether edema is of lymphatic origin. Technetium-99m labeled colloid is injected into the web spaces of the foot or hand.[8] Images are obtained as the colloid progresses along the limb at 30-minute, 1-hour, 3-hour, and 6-hour intervals. Imaging of the lymph vessels is possible using this technique, and candidates for microvascular anastomosis can sometimes be identified.[9]

Magnetic resonance imaging (MRI) and computed tomography (CT) can be used to distinguish some of the features of lymphedema and to exclude an obstructing mass. It is possible with MRI or CT to evaluate the subcutaneous tissue; the presence of multiple branching, nonenhancing tubular structures in an enlarged subcutaneous tissue compartment is suggestive of lymphedema.[10] The presence of mild to moderate skin thickening may also be helpful in the diagnosis.[11]

MEDICAL TREATMENT

The goal of medical treatment for lymphedema is to prevent it from occurring, or if it occurs, to treat the disease in the early stages. Treatment is aimed at (1) removing excess fluid and dissolved substances (protein) from the lymphedematous area; (2) preventing fluid reaccumulation; (3) maintaining the smallest size possible for the lymphedematous limb using the simplest methods available; and (4) avoiding factors that can aggravate or worsen the edema. A final treatment goal is to provide information to the patient about lymphedema that will assist in the long-term management of the disease process.

The nonsurgical management of lymphedema usually involves one or more of the following approaches.

Limb Elevation

The patient is instructed to elevate the limb to 45 degrees, using either a foam wedge or a lymphedema sling (Fig. 42–2). Elevation is typically performed during the night, or during the day when possible.

Pumps

Vasopneumatic compression pumps are a part of many treatment programs (Fig. 42–3). The goal is to progressively move fluid along the limb in a distal-to-proximal direction. Vasopneumatic compression devices come with either single-chamber or multiple-chamber sleeves, and treatment sessions generally last 1 to 8 hours depending on the pump type. One advantage of this approach is that patients can usually use the vasopneumatic compression pumps at home. The cost of the pump and the sleeve generally ranges from $1,000 to $10,000, and most insurance companies reimburse vaso-pneumatic compression pumps for the treatment of lymphedema.

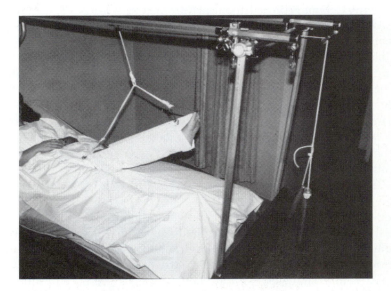

Figure 42–2. Elevating the affected limb at least 45 degrees using a lymphedema sling or a specifically designed table (or foam wedge) can help reduce edema.

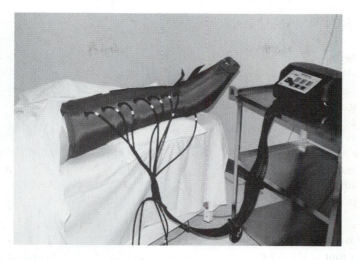

Figure 42–3. Lymphapress. Multiple-chamber devices such as this sequentially inflate in a distal-to-proximal direction, effectively moving fluid from the foot toward the body. Vasopneumatic pumping can be performed at home for convenience.

Massage

Manual massage is an old concept that is becoming more popular in the United States and worldwide (Fig. 42–4). Massage moves the edema fluid from the affected limb(s) toward the trunk of the body, and is usually performed one to two times per day. Manual lymphatic drainage has been shown to stimulate lymphatic flow and to reduce the swelling of the extremities.[12] When performed correctly and regularly, it is possible to keep the tissues soft and decompressed for an indefinite period of time.[13]

Bandaging

Compression bandaging can be performed after each vasopneumatic compression or massage session (Fig. 42–5). Bandaging of the extremity not only keeps fluid from reaccumulating in the limb, but also increases venous and lymphatic drainage. The bandages may be worn at night as well as during the day.

Exercise

An exercise program generally involves a light, remedial program designed to increase venous and lymphatic drainage. These exercises are typically performed while the patient is wearing compressive bandaging.

Complex Physical Therapy

Complex physical therapy combines several different treatment approaches, including manual lymphatic drainage, compressive bandaging of the extremity, lymphedema extremity exercises, education (especially about the importance of meticulous skin care), and ultimately the use of a compression garment.

The "modern" treatment of lymphedema usually emphasizes a multimodality approach, although this concept has been employed for decades. A retrospective study by Stillwell in 1977 evaluated 120 patients with lymphedema who were seen in the Mayo Clinic Department of Physical Medicine and Rehabilitation. The majority of these patients presented following unilateral radical mastectomy; the average age was 62 years. Treatment consisted of multiple modalities including pneumatic compression,

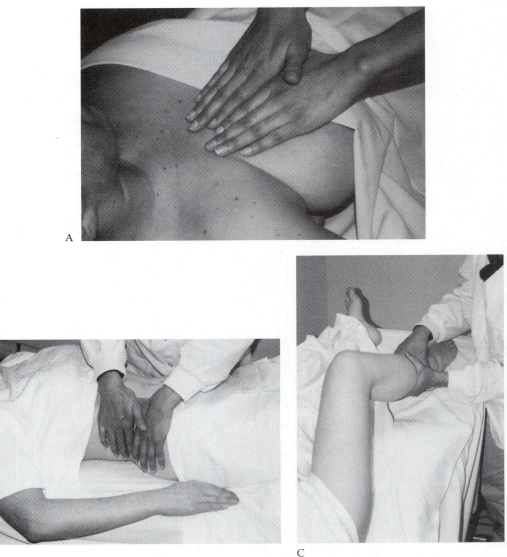

Figure 42–4. Manual lymphatic drainage (MLD) is performed by the physical therapist on a patient with leg lymphedema: (**A**) MLD is initiated in axillary regions to prepare and clear lymph nodes around the thorax. (**B**) Therapy is then used to stimulate and empty nodes in the trunk area. (**C**) The leg is massaged, pushing fluid proximally while the therapist progresses distally along the limb.

manual massage, elevation of the affected limb, exercise, and elastic support. An average reduction in limb volume of 33% was achieved using this approach.[14]

Boris et al.[13] reported in 1994 on CLT (complex lymphedema therapy), a technique of manual lymph drainage, compressive bandaging, and exercises that was utilized to treat 38 patients for a period of 1 month. Eighteen of these patients had unilateral lower extremity lymphedema, 16 were females with arm lymphedema secondary to

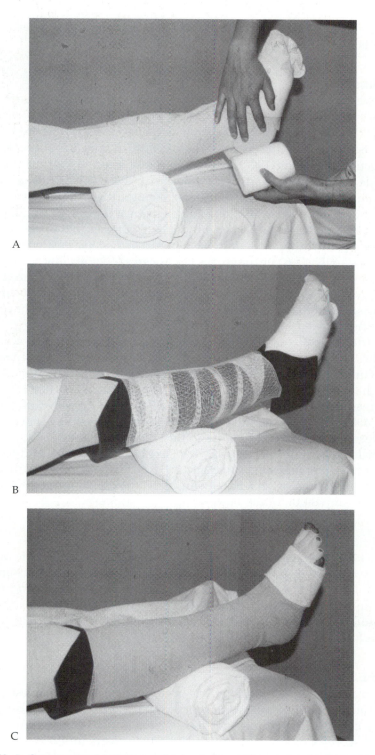

Figure 42–5. Compressive bandaging maintains limb reduction during the interval between MLD treatment, and at night for maintenance therapy. (**A**) Cotton stockinette, malleolar foam pads, and cotton padding are applied next to the skin. (**B**) Foam padding is applied over this to even the compressive forces. (**C**) Short stretch wraps such as Komprex are wrapped over the foam to provide limb compression.

breast surgery, and 4 had bilateral leg disease. Reduction of edema averaged 73% in those patients with arm disease and 88% in patients with leg edema.[13]

Drug Treatment

Some pharmacologic therapies are effective in the treatment of lymphedema. The prompt administration of antibiotics is important in the treatment of acute infection such as cellulitis and lymphangitis. Patients with lymphedema who are known to have recurrent episodes of cellulitis are often instructed to initiate oral antibiotics at the first sign of infection. Penicillin VK 250 to 500 mg four times a day for 7 to 10 days is generally adequate. For those patients who break through with recurrent infections (more than four to six times a year) despite following an appropriate treatment, Penicillin VK or another antibiotic can be taken by the patient for 1 week out of every month.

Another class of drugs, the 5,6 benzopyrones (Coumarin) have been used in Australia and Europe for many years to improve high-protein edemas by increasing extravascular proteolysis.[12] The 5,6 benzopyrones have been shown in clinical studies to stimulate the tissue macrophages that ultimately remove excess protein from the interstitial space. This promotes tissue softening and decreases chronic inflammation in the affected limb. The drugs are not currently FDA approved in the United States; however, clinical trials are being initiated to determine the efficacy of this medication.

In one trial, 50 patients with arm or leg lymphedema were randomized to either benzopyrones or placebo. In the group receiving the active agent there was a decrease in mean volume excess from 46% down to 26% in the arm and a decrease from 25% to 17% in the leg. Treated patients reported fewer attacks of cellulitis and noted a relative increase in mobility and softness of the limb.[15] The accepted dose of Coumarin is generally 400 to 800 mg/day. Although generally safe, these drugs have been reported to cause liver inflammation and failure in rare cases.[16,17]

Regular long-term diuretic therapy has generally not been found to be useful in the treatment of lymphedema. Although fluid is removed from the extremity, the interstitial concentration of protein remains high, potentially leading to an increase in fibrosis and inflammation of the tissues.[18]

Skin Care

Meticulous skin care is encouraged. Patients are instructed to moisturize dry skin using a lanolin-based lotion or similar agent. Antifungal creams or powders are prescribed as indicated. Instruction must be given on proper care of toenails and protection of the limb from injury or trauma. Patients are educated on the signs and symptoms of infection and are instructed to respond quickly to infections, often with an as-needed prescription for antibiotic therapy.

Graduated Elastic Compression

After the lymphedematous extremity has been reduced to the smallest possible size, the limb should be measured for an appropriate graduated elastic compression garment. The use of a compression garment remains the key to maintaining limb size for most patients (Fig. 42–6). Compression garments come in many different styles and colors. In our institution, we generally measure the patient for a custom-fit garment to ensure that the exact measurements of the limb are duplicated; most patients with significant swelling or an unusually shaped leg need a custom-made stocking in order to obtain an optimal fit. The garment should ideally be long enough to cover all swollen portions of the limb (Fig. 42–7).

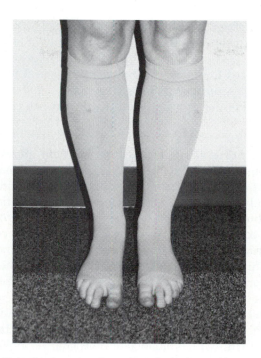

Figure 42–6. After limb size is reduced, graduated elastic stockings are worn to maintain limb size.

Before fitting a stocking, circumferential measurements are taken at predetermined locations before and after a pumping or massage session. The limb is considered ready for fitting when measurements stop decreasing on two consecutive assessments. It is important that the garment compression be appropriate. Lower extremities with lymphedema generally require 40 to 60 mm Hg pressure to control the swelling, while

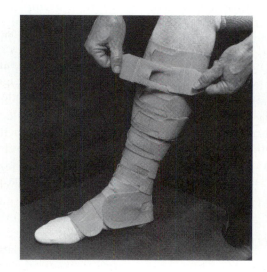

Figure 42–7. The CircAid device is applied to a limb to enhance graduated compression in patients with edema not responsive to elastic compression alone.

arm sleeves generally deliver 30 to 40 mm Hg pressure. The patient is encouraged to continue reduction treatment until the compression garment has arrived and a correct fit is confirmed.

Patients are instructed to replace their stockings every 3 to 6 months, depending on the type of stocking. After correct fit is ensured, the patient should purchase an additional garment so that one is available to wash and one is available to wear.

Maintenance Therapy

Once the patient is measured for a compression garment, plans and instructions are geared toward maintaining the limb in a reduced state. Maintenance therapy involves instructing the patient on how to elevate the limb while sleeping, continuing proper skin care, and promptly intervening when infection occurs. Patients are instructed to treat infections vigorously, and are often given a prescription for antibiotics to fill in the event that an infection develops and they are unable to reach their physician. Patients must be instructed about when to purchase a new garment and how to know when the garment is fulfilling its job. Correct fit is stressed in the educational process, since this largely determines how successful the patient will be in the lymphedema maintenance program.

Another important component of therapy is weight control. Patients should maintain their ideal weight in order to better control swelling in the affected limb. Salt restriction is advised along with avoidance of excessive alcohol consumption.

If patients will be using a vasopneumatic device or continued massage at home, they and/or their significant other need to be properly instructed. The patient should be given a name of a local distributor to contact to arrange for purchase or rental of a vasopneumatic device and the corresponding sleeve. If possible, patients should be encouraged to try more than one device; comfort, ease of operation, and cost are all important factors that need to be considered when purchasing a pump. When a patient treated with MLD returns home to continue massaging the extremity, a follow-up visit is usually arranged to ensure that the massage is being performed correctly.

Patients are encouraged to exercise at home on a regular basis while wearing their compression garment. Biking, swimming, and walking are excellent forms of exercise that enhance further massage of the extremity.

Once the patient returns home, he or she will need to implement the maintenance therapy program that has been outlined, taking into account normal routines for the day. Careful assessment of the patient's home situation allows the caregiver to assist in establishing a routine and enables the patient to perform the necessary treatments over the course of the day, hopefully with minimum alteration in usual lifestyle.

One of the most important things that caregivers can provide patients with is a source of support. Patients seen in our clinic are encouraged to return for regular follow-up care, and the nurses routinely call them within a week or two to assess how they are doing with any new treatment program. This is often the time when many questions arise regarding maintenance therapy in the home environment, and it provides a good opportunity for nurses to (1) emphasize the importance of continued maintenance therapy and (2) assist in devising creative alternatives for accomplishing this.

SURGICAL TREATMENT

A number of surgical procedures have been suggested as means to treat lymphedema, and they have all met with varying success. Fewer than 10% of patients with lymphedema are candidates for operative treatment.[19] The recommended operations are generally classified as either *reduction* operations (where the goal is to remove excess tissue and decrease the volume of the extremity) or *physiologic* operations (where the goal is to improve lymphatic drainage of the extremity). None of the operations should be considered "curative." The Homan and Charles operations are classic procedures that reduce the volume of the extremity. The Homan operation involves resection of a portion of the edematous and underlying tissues; with closure of the wound the size of the limb is in essence reduced. The Charles operation (described in 1912) involves complete excision of the skin, subcutaneous tissue, and fascia.[20] The muscle is subsequently covered with a split-thickness skin graft that is taken from healthy skin. More success with the surgical procedures has been reported in the upper extremity than in the lower extremity. Criteria for consideration of surgical intervention include extensive lymphedema that is not manageable by conservative means. Depending on the circumstances, repeated severe episodes of lymphangitis might also be considered an indication for surgical intervention.

Procedures to surgically restore lymphatic flow include lymphatic-to-venous anastomosis,[20-23] lympho-lympho anastomosis,[22] lymph vessel autotransplantation, and cross-femoral lymph vessel transposition.[24] *Lymphovenous anastomosis* is possible between lymphatic vessels (that are proximal to an obstruction) and nearby small veins; this allows lymph from the obstructed area to flow directly into the venous system. Lymphovenous operations performed at our institution show an initial 50% patency rate.[21] Lymphatic autotransplantation, in which lymphatic vessels are removed from one portion of the body and used to bypass the blockage in another part of the body[20,25] require the presence of large donor lymphatic vessels. Long-term patency following these microsurgical operations has been unpredictable. Another surgical procedure, the "enteromesenteric bridge," may be tried in selected cases of proximal lower extremity obstructive lymphedema.[26] A tunnel is constructed to allow a segment of ileum to be brought down beneath the inguinal ligament; this forms a "bridge" that is sutured down over the uppermost normal nodes of the lower extremity. Of eight reported patients where this procedure was performed, six showed sustained clinical improvement.[24]

Potential complications of surgical procedures include poor healing of the incision leading to infection and prolonged hospital stays, poor cosmetic results, a mandatory long period of bedrest following the surgical procedure, and failure to provide significant relief of swelling. In addition, the patient is usually required to wear a compression garment after the surgery.

PSYCHOLOGICAL CONCERNS

It is important to address the patient's psychological concerns regarding potential long-term disfigurement. Lymphedema is a chronic disease that has a significant impact on the patient's life. Without treatment, the limb may continue to swell and worsen over time. The swelling of the limb can cause heaviness and even limit the motion of the extremity. Repeated episodes of cellulitis and lymphangitis are common, and this may mean repeated hospitalizations with resultant continuous medical care and expenses. Because of the effect of heavy, strenuous work on swelling, patients with lymphedema may be limited in the jobs that they are able to perform and the lifestyle that they can lead. Often patients limit their participation in exercise because of uncomfortable sensations in the affected limb, which can lead to weight gain and a subsequent increase in the overall size of the affected limb.

All of these considerations regarding the effect of lymphedema on the patient suggest that close follow-up and continued reassessment of the patient's progress must be a part of any program. Many times the patient is told to just "live with the limb swelling." This is not necessary, because with daily care and maintenance treatments, it is usually possible for the patient to keep the limb down to a manageable size and lead a normal lifestyle.

REFERENCES

1. Browse NL, Stuart G. Lymphedema: pathophysiology and classification. *J Cardiovasc Surg.* 1985;26:91–106.
2. Edwards JM, Kinmonth JB. Lymphovenous shunts in man. *Br Med J.* 1969;4:579–581.
3. Allen EV. Lymphedema of the extremities. *Arch Intern Med.* 1934;54:606.
4. Kinmonth JB, Taylor GW, Tracy GD, Marsh JD. Primary lymphoedema: clinical and lymphangiographic studies of a series of 107 patients in which the lower limbs were affected. *Br J Surg.* 1957;45:1–10.
5. Spittell JA, Schirger A. Edema, peripheral. In: Taylor RB, ed. *Difficult Diagnosis.* Philadelphia: WB Saunders; 1985:130–137.
6. Gloviczki P, Calcagno D, Schirger A, et al. Non-invasive evaluation of the swollen extremity: experiences with 190 lymphscintographic examinations. *J Vasc Surg.* 1989;9:683–690.
7. Schirger A, Peterson LFA. Lymphedema. In: Allen EV, Barker NW, Hines EA, eds. *Peripheral Vascular Diseases.* Philadelphia: WB Saunders; 1980:823–851.
8. Stuart G, Gaunt JL, Croft D, Browse ML. The value of lymphoscintigraphy in the investigation lymphoedema. In: *Immunology and Hematology, Res Mon Ogr* 1982;2:209–213.
9. Cambria RA, Gloviczki P, Naessens JM, Wahner HW. Non-invasive evaluation of the lymphatic system with lymphoscintigraphy: a prospective, semi-quantitative analysis in 386 extremities. *J Vasc Surg.* 1993;18:773–782.
10. Huang A, Fruauff A, DiCarmine F, et al. Case report 861: primary lymphedema of the left lower extremity. *Skeletal Radiol.* 1994;23(6):483–485.
11. Hagjis NS, Carr DH, Banks L, Pflug JJ. The role of CT in the diagnosis of primary lymphedema of the lower limb. *AJR.* 1984;144:361–364.
12. Foldi M. Physiology and pathophysiology of lymph flow. In: Clodius L, ed. *Lymphedema.* Stuttgart: Georg Thieme; 1977:1–11.
13. Boris M, Weindorf S, Lasinski B, Boris G. Lymphedema reduction by noninvasive complex lymphedema therapy. *Oncology.* 1994;8(9):109–110.
14. Stillwell GK. Management of arm edema. In: Stoll BA, ed. *Breast Cancer Management—Early and Late.* Chicago: Heinemann Medical and Year–Book Medical; 1977:213–242.
15. Casley-Smith J, Piller N, Morgan RG. Behandlung chronischer Lymphödeme der Arme und Beine mit 5,6-Benzo-(alpha)-pyron: placebokontrollierte Doppelblind-cross-over-Studie Über die Dauer von êinem Jahr. *Therapiewoche.* 1986;12:1068–1076.
16. Cox D, O'Kennedy R, Thomas RD. The rarity of liver toxicity in patient treated with Coumarin (1,2-benzo-pyrones). *Human Toxicol.* 1989;8(6):501–506.
17. Casley-Smith JR. Frequency of Coumarin hepatotoxicity. *Med J Aust.* 1995;162(7):391. Letter; Comment.
18. Foldi E, Foldi M, Weissleider H. Conservative treatment of lymphedema of the limbs. *Angiology.* 1985;36:171.
19. Gloviczki P. Treatment of acquired lymphedema—medical and surgical. In: Ernst CB, Stanley JC, eds. *Current Therapy in Vascular Surgery—2.* Philadelphia: Decker; 1991:1030–1036.
20. Savage RC. The surgical management of lymphedema. *Surg Gynecol Obstet.* 1984;159:501.
21. Gloviczki P, Fisher J, Hollier LH, et al. Microsurgical lymphovenous anastomosis for treatment of lymphema: a critical review. *J Vasc Surg.* 1988;7:647–652.

22. Campisi C, Boccardo F, Tacchella M. Reconstructive microsurgery of lymph vessels: the personal method of lymphatic-venous-lymphatic (LVL) interpositioned grafted shunt. *Microsurgery.* 1995;16(3):161–166.
23. Campisi C, Boccardo F, Alitta P, Tacchella M. Derivative lymphatic microsurgery: indications, techniques, and results. *Microsurgery.* 1995;16(7):463–468.
24. Hurst PAE, Stuart G, Kinmonth JB, Browse LN. The long-term results of the enteromesenteric bridge operation in the treatment of primary lymphedema. *Br J Surg.* 1985;72:272–274.
25. Baumeister RG, Siuda S, Bhomert H, et al. A microsurgical method for reconstruction of interrupted pathways: autologous lymph-vessel transplantation for treatment of lymphedemas. *Scan J Plas Reconstruc Surg.* 1986;20:141–146.
26. Egorov YS, Abalmasov KG, Ivanov VV, et al. Autotransplantation of the greater omentum in the treatment of chronic lymphedema. *Lymphology.* 1994;27(3):137–143.

Index

Page numbers followed by *t* and *f* refer to tables and figures, respectively.

Page numbers followed by *t* and *f* refer to tables and figures, respectively.

Page numbers followed by *t* and *f* refer to tables
and figures, respectively.

Page numbers followed by *t* and *f* refer to tables
and figures, respectively.

Page numbers followed by *t* and *f* refer to tables
and figures, respectively.